Protocols in Neonatology

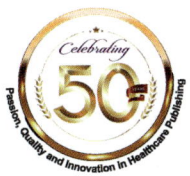

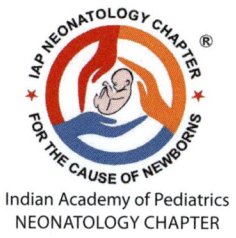

Indian Academy of Pediatrics
NEONATOLOGY CHAPTER

Protocols in Neonatology

Second Edition

Editors-in-Chief

Rhishikesh Thakre
DM (Neonatology) MD DNB DCH FCPS FIAP
Director
Neo Clinic and Hospital
Aurangabad, Maharashtra, India

Srinivas Murki
DM (Neonatology) MD
Chief Neonatologist
Department of Neonatology
Paramitha Children's Hospital
Hyderabad, Telangana, India

Chief Academic Editor

Ranjan Kumar Pejaver
FRCP FRCPCH (UK) FIAP FNNF
Chief Neonatologist
People Tree Hospitals
Professor
Department of Neonatology
Kempegowda Institute of Medical Sciences (KIMS)
Bengaluru, Karnataka, India

Associate Editors

Sandeep Kadam
DM (Neonatology) MD
Neonatal Fellow (Au)
Senior Neonatal Consultant
KEM and Ratna Memorial Hospital
Pune, Maharashtra, India

Naveen Bajaj
DM (Neonatology) MD
Neonatal Fellow (Canada)
Consultant Neonatologist
Deep Hospital
Ludhiana, Punjab, India

Sanjay Wazir
DM (Neonatology) MD
Director
Department of Neonatology
Cloudnine Hospital
Gurugram, Haryana, India

Ashish Jain
DM (Neonatology) AIIMS
Assistant Professor (Pediatrics)
Department of Neonatology
Maulana Azad Medical College
New Delhi, India

Forewords

Ashok Deorari
Pramod Jog

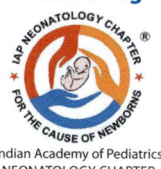

Indian Academy of Pediatrics
NEONATOLOGY CHAPTER

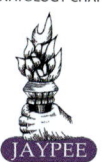

JAYPEE BROTHERS MEDICAL PUBLISHERS
The Health Sciences Publisher
New Delhi | London

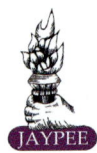
Jaypee Brothers Medical Publishers (P) Ltd

Headquarters
Jaypee Brothers Medical Publishers (P) Ltd
4838/24, Ansari Road, Daryaganj
New Delhi 110 002, India
Phone: +91-11-43574357
Fax: +91-11-43574314
Email: jaypee@jaypeebrothers.com

Overseas Office
J.P. Medical Ltd
83 Victoria Street, London
SW1H 0HW (UK)
Phone: +44 20 3170 8910
Fax: +44 (0)20 3008 6180
Email: info@jpmedpub.com

Website: www.jaypeebrothers.com
Website: www.jaypeedigital.com

© 2020, Jaypee Brothers Medical Publishers

The views and opinions expressed in this book are solely those of the original contributor(s)/author(s) and do not necessarily represent those of editor(s) of the book.

All rights reserved. No part of this publication may be reproduced, stored or transmitted in any form or by any means, electronic, mechanical, photocopying, recording or otherwise, without the prior permission in writing of the publishers.

All brand names and product names used in this book are trade names, service marks, trademarks or registered trademarks of their respective owners. The publisher is not associated with any product or vendor mentioned in this book.

Medical knowledge and practice change constantly. This book is designed to provide accurate, authoritative information about the subject matter in question. However, readers are advised to check the most current information available on procedures included and check information from the manufacturer of each product to be administered, to verify the recommended dose, formula, method and duration of administration, adverse effects and contraindications. It is the responsibility of the practitioner to take all appropriate safety precautions. Neither the publisher nor the author(s)/editor(s) assume any liability for any injury and/or damage to persons or property arising from or related to use of material in this book.

This book is sold on the understanding that the publisher is not engaged in providing professional medical services. If such advice or services are required, the services of a competent medical professional should be sought.

Every effort has been made where necessary to contact holders of copyright to obtain permission to reproduce copyright material. If any have been inadvertently overlooked, the publisher will be pleased to make the necessary arrangements at the first opportunity. The **CD/DVD-ROM** (if any) provided in the sealed envelope with this book is complimentary and free of cost. **Not meant for sale**.

Inquiries for bulk sales may be solicited at: jaypee@jaypeebrothers.com

Protocols in Neonatology

First Edition: 2016
Second Edition: **2020**

ISBN 978-93-89188-48-6

Printed at: Samrat Offset Pvt. Ltd.

Editorial Board

Editors-in-Chief

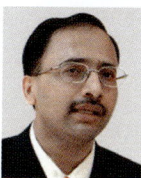

Rhishikesh Thakre
DM (Neonatology) MD DNB DCH FCPS FIAP
Director
Neo Clinic and Hospital
Aurangabad, Maharashtra, India

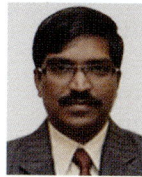

Srinivas Murki
DM (Neonatology) MD
Chief Neonatologist
Department of Neonatology
Paramitha Children's Hospital
Hyderabad, Telangana, India

Chief Academic Editor

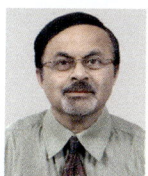

Ranjan Kumar Pejaver
FRCP FRCPCH (UK) FIAP FNNF
Chief Neonatologist
People Tree Hospitals
Professor
Department of Neonatology
Kempegowda Institute of Medical Sciences (KIMS)
Bengaluru, Karnataka, India

Associate Editors

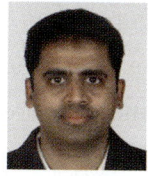

Sandeep Kadam
DM (Neonatology) MD Neonatal Fellow (Au)
Senior Neonatal Consultant
KEM and Ratna Memorial Hospital
Pune, Maharashtra, India

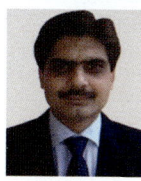

Naveen Bajaj
DM (Neonatology) MD
Neonatal Fellow (Canada)
Consultant Neonatologist
Deep Hospital
Ludhiana, Punjab, India

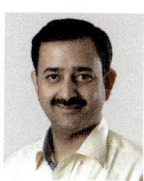

Sanjay Wazir
DM (Neonatology) MD
Director
Department of Neonatology
Cloudnine Hospital
Gurugram, Haryana, India

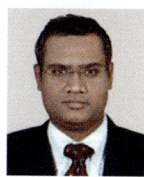

Ashish Jain
DM (Neonatology) AIIMS
Assistant Professor (Pediatrics)
Department of Neonatology
Maulana Azad Medical College
New Delhi, India

Members, Editorial Committee

Dinesh Chirla
MD DM (Neonatology) FRCPCH (UK)
Neonatal Fellow (Australia) Fellow in PICU (UK)
Director
Neonatology and Pediatric Intensive Care
Rainbow Children's Hospital Group
Hyderabad, Telangana, India

G Pramod Reddy MD DCH
Director and Head
Department of Neonatology
Fernandez Hospital
Hyderabad, Telangana, India

Nandkishor Kabra
DM (Neonatology) MD (Ped) DNB (Ped)
MSc (Clinical Epidemiology, Canada)
President, IAP Neonatology Chapter (2019–20)
Chief Neonatologist and Director
Neonatal Intensive Care Unit (NICU)
Surya Hospitals
Mumbai, Maharashtra, India

Rajesh Kumar
MD DM (Neonatology)
Director and Chief Neonatologist
Rani Children Hospital
Ranchi, Jharkhand, India

Deepak Chawla
DM (Neonatology) MD
Associate Professor
Department of Pediatrics
Postgraduate Institute of Medical
Education and Research (PGIMER)
Chandigarh, India

Binu Ninan
MD DNB DCH
Professor and Head
Department of Neonatology
Sri Ramachandra University
Chennai, Tamil Nadu, India

Bishwajit Mishra MD
Director, Intensive Care
Department of Pediatrics
Jagannath Hospital
Bhubaneshwar, Odisha, India

VC Manoj MD
Unit Head
Department of Neonatology
Jubilee Mission Medical College and
Research Institute
Thrissur, Kerala, India

Indian Academy of Pediatrics—Neonatology Chapter

OFFICE BEARERS 2019–20

Chairperson	:	Dr Nandkishor Kabra
Hon. Secretary	:	Dr Naveen Bajaj
Treasurer	:	Dr Rajesh Kumar
Joint Secretary	:	Dr Suman Rao
Imm. Past Chairperson	:	Dr Sanjay Wazir
Executive Members		
East Zone	:	Dr Arjit Mohapatra, Dr Vinod Kumar
West Zone	:	Dr Tushar Parikh, Dr Sanjay Ghorpade
North Zone	:	Dr Ashwani Singhal, Dr Bhawan Deep Garg
Central Zone	:	Dr Dinesh Kumar Chirla, Dr Tejopratap Oleti
South Zone	:	Dr VC Manoj, Dr AK Jaychandran

INDIAN ACADEMY OF PEDIATRICS OFFICE BEARERS 2019

President	:	Dr Digant D Shastri
President Elect, 2020	:	Dr Bakul J Parekh
Imm. Past President	:	Dr Santosh T Soans
Vice President	:	Dr Jaydeep Choudhury (East Zone)
		Dr Satish V Pandya (West Zone)
		Dr Rekha Harish (North Zone)
		Dr Shrinath B Mugali (South Zone)
		Dr M Surendranath (Central Zone)
Secretary General	:	Dr Remesh Kumar R
Treasurer	:	Dr Upendra Kinjawadekar
Editor in Chief, IP	:	Dr Dheeraj Shah
Editor in Chief, IJPP	:	Dr NC Gowrishankar
Secretary, Liason	:	Dr Sangeeta Yadav
Secretary Admin	:	Dr Sandeep Bapu Kadam

Contributors

Amita Kaul DNB (Ped)
Associate Chief
Neonatal and Pediatric Intensive Care Services
Surya Mother and Child Superspecialty Hospital
Pune, Maharashtra, India

Anjali Kulkarni
MD FRCPCH Fellowship in Neonatology (Au)
Head
Neonatal Intensive Care Unit
Bombay Hospital and Medical Research Center
Mumbai, Maharashtra, India

Anu Thukral DM (Neonatology) MD DNB MNAMS
Assistant Professor
Department of Pediatrics
All India Institute of Medical Sciences (AIIMS)
New Delhi, India

Anuradha Bansal MD
Neonatal Division
Department of Pediatrics
Government Medical College and Hospital
Chandigarh, India

Archana Kadam MD DNB (Ped)
Developmental Pediatrician
KEM Hospital and Jehangir Hospital
Pune, Maharashtra, India

Ashish Jain DM (Neonatology) AIIMS
Assistant Professor (Pediatrics)
Department of Neonatology
Maulana Azad Medical College
New Delhi, India

Ashish Mehta MD Fellowship in Neonatology (Au)
Director
Arpan Hospital
Ahmedabad, Gujarat, India

Ashwani Singal
DM (Neonatology) DNB (Neo) MD (Ped) DNB (Ped)
Senior Consultant (Neonatology and Pediatrics)
Sapling Hospital
Ludhiana, Punjab, India

Asim Kumar Mallick MD DCH
Professor and In-charge
Neonatal Unit
Department of Pediatrics
Nil Ratan Sircar (NRS) Medical College and Hospital
Kolkata, West Bengal, India

Balla Kalyan Chakravarthy MD DM
Consultant Neonatologist
Department of Neonatology
St. John's Medical College and Hospital
Bengaluru, Karnataka, India

Baswaraj Tandur DNB (Ped)
Senior Consultant
Vijay Marie Hospital
Neonatal Department
Hyderabad, Telangana, India

Binu Ninan MD DNB DCH
Professor and Head
Department of Neonatology
Sri Ramachandra University
Chennai, Tamil Nadu, India

C Aparna MD DM (Neonatology)
Consultant Neonatologist and Head
Department of Neonatology
Ankura Hospital for Women and Children
Hyderabad, Telangana, India

Chetana Naik MS (ENT) DORL
Consultant ENT Surgeon and Neurotologist
Hospicio Hospital, ENT and Vertigo Clinic
Margao, Goa, India

Deepak Chawla DM (Neonatology) MD
Associate Professor
Department of Pediatrics
Postgraduate Institute of Medical
Education and Research (PGIMER)
Chandigarh, India

Deepak Pande MD (Per) DCH
Consultant Pediatrician
Jamnagar, Gujrat, India

Deepak Sharma
MD (Pediatrics) DNB (Neonatology, Gold medalist) MNAMS
Consultant Neonatologist
Department of Neonatology
National Institute of Medical Science
Jaipur, Rajasthan, India

Dinesh Chirla
MD DM (Neonatology) FRCPCH (UK)
Neonatal Fellow (Australia) Fellow in PICU (UK)
Director
Neonatology and Pediatric Intensive Care
Rainbow Children's Hospital Group
Hyderabad, Telangana, India

Femitha P DM (Neonatology) MD
Consultant
Kerala Institute of Medical Sciences
Department of Neonatology
Thiruvananthapuram, Kerala, India

Giridhar Sethuraman MD DM (Neonatology)
Associate Professor
Department of Neonatology
Chettinad Hospital and Research Institute
Chennai, Tamil Nadu, India

Hemasree Kandraju MD DNB (Neo)
Consultant
Department of Neonatology
Fernandez Hospital
Hyderabad, Telangana, India

Jaikrishan Mittal MD DM (Neonatology)
Consultant Neonatologist
Neo Clinic
Jaipur, Rajasthan, India

K Sankarnarayanan
CCT (Neo) CCT (Ped) MRCPCH DM (Neo) MD (Ped)
DNB (Ped) DCH
Senior Consultant Neonatologist
Madras Mission Medical Hospital
Chennai, Tamil Nadu, India

Kiran Sathe
DNB (Ped) DCH Clinical Research Fellowship (Ped) Fellow
Pediatric Nephrology (IPNA ISPN)
Associate Consultant
Department of Pediatrics and Pediatric Nephrology
Sir HN Reliance Foundation Hospital
Mumbai, Maharashtra, India

Leslie Lewis MD DCH
Professor
Department of Pediatrics
Kasturba Medical College
Manipal, Karnataka, India

LS Deshmukh DM (Neonatology) MD
Professor and Head
Department of Neonatology
Government Medical College and Hospital
Aurangabad, Maharashtra, India

Manish Mittal MD
Consultant Neonatologist
Cocoon, Neoclinic
Jaipur, Rajasthan, India

Monika Kaushal
DM (Neonatology) MD Visiting Fellowship RCPCH
Head
Department of Pediatric and Neonatology
Zulekha Hospital
Dubai, UAE

N Chandra Kumar
MD (JIPMER) DNB MNAMS DM (Neonatology) DNB (Neo)
Neonatologist
Department of Neonatology
Cloudnine Hospitals
Chennai, Tamil Nadu, India

Nandkishor Kabra
DM (Neonatology) MD (Ped) DNB (Ped)
MSc (Clinical Epidemiology, Canada)
President, IAP Neonatology Chapter (2019–20)
Chief Neonatologist and Director
Neonatal Intensive Care Unit (NICU)
Surya Hospitals
Mumbai, Maharashtra, India

Contributors

Naveen Bajaj DM (Neonatology)
MD Neonatal Fellow (Canada)
Consultant Neonatologist
Deep Hospital
Ludhiana, Punjab, India

Naveen Jain DM (Neonatology) MD DNB
Department of Neonatology
Kerala Institute of Medical Sciences
Thiruvananthapuram, Kerala, India

Nishad Plakkal
MD Fellowship in Neonatal-Perinatal Medicine
Associate Professor
Department of Neonatology
Jawaharlal Institute of Postgraduate Medical Education and Research (JIPMER)
Puducherry, India

Pradeep Suryawanshi
MD DCH Fellowship in Neonatal Perinatal Medicine (Au)
Professor and Head
Department of Neonatology
BVU Medical College
Sahyadri Hospital
Pune, Maharashtra, India

Pramod Gaddam MD
Director
Department of Neonatology
Fernandez Hospital
Hyderabad, Telangana, India

Preetha Joshi
MD Fellowship in NICU and PICU Critical Care Transport and Cardiac ICU
Senior Consultant
Department of Pediatric and Neonatal Critical Care
Kokilaben Dhirubhai Ambani Hospital and Medical Research Institute
Mumbai, Maharashtra, India

Rajesh Kumar MD DM (Neonatology)
Director and Chief Neonatologist
Rani Children Hospital
Ranchi, Jharkhand, India

Rajiv Sharan DNB MNAMS
Consultant Pediatrics
Tata Motors Hospital
Jamshedpur, Jharkhand, India

Raktima Chakrabarti
MD Fellowship in Neonatology (Germany)
Consultant Pediatrician and Neonatologist
Apollo Cradle and Miracle Mediclinic
Gurugram, Haryana, India

Ranjan Kumar Pejaver FRCP FRCPCH (UK) FIAP FNNF
Chief Neonatologist
People Tree Hospitals
Professor
Department of Neonatology
Kempegowda Institute of Medical Sciences (KIMS)
Bengaluru, Karnataka, India

Rhishikesh Thakre
DM (Neonatology) MD DNB DCH FCPS FIAP
Director
Neo Clinic and Hospital
Aurangabad, Maharashtra, India

Rohit Arora MD
Clinical/Research Fellowship (UWO, Canada)
Head
Department of Neonatology
Apollo Cradle
Gurugram, Haryana, India

Sachin Shah
MD DM (Neonatology) Fellowship in Neonatology (Australia) Fellowship in Pediatric critical care (Canada)
Director
Neonatal and Pediatric Intensive Care Services
Surya Mother and Child Superspeciality Hospital
Pune, Maharashtra, India

Sandeep Kadam DM (Neonatology)
MD Neonatal Fellow (Au)
Senior Neonatal Consultant
KEM and Ratna Memorial Hospital
Pune, Maharashtra, India

Sanjay Aher DM (Neonatology) MD
Director
Neocare Hospital
Nashik, Maharashtra, India

Sanjay Wazir DM (Neonatology) MD
Director
Department of Neonatology
Cloudnine Hospital
Gurugram, Haryana, India

Shamsher Singh Dalal DM (Neonatology) MD (Ped)
Professor and Head
Department of Pediatrics
Command Hospital Air Force
Bengaluru, Karnataka, India

Snehal Thakre MS DNB (Opht)
Professor
Department of Ophthalmology
MGM Medical College and Hospital
Aurangabad, Maharashtra, India

Somashekhar Nimbalkar MD
Head
Neonatal Intensive Care Unit
Shree Krishna Hospital
Pramukhswami Medical College
Anand, Gujarat, India

Sreeram S MD (Ped) DM (Neonatology)
Consultant
Neo BBC Children's Hospital
Paramitha Children's Hospital
Hyderabad, Telangana, India

Srinivas Murki DM (Neonatology) MD
Chief Neonatologist
Department of Neonatology
Paramitha Children's Hospital
Hyderabad, Telangana, India

Suman Rao MD DM (Neonatology)
Professor and Head
Department of Neonatology
St. John's Medical College and Hospital
Bengaluru, Karnataka, India

Surg RAdm Sheila Samanta Mathai
VSM MD DNB DM (Neonatology)
Command Medical Officer
Consultant Neonatologist, Indian Navy
Eastern Naval Command
Visakhapatnam, Andhra Pradesh, India

Tanushri Mukherjee
Consultant Neonatologist
Department of Pediatric and Neonatal Critical Care
Cloudnine Hospital, Malad
Mumbai, Maharashtra, India

Tanveer Bashir DNB (Neonatology)
Consultant Neonatologist
Department of Neonatology
Fernandez Hospital
Hyderabad, Telangana, India

Tejopratap Oleti DM (Neonatology) MD
Consultant
Department of Neonatology
Fernandez Hospital
Hyderabad, Telangana, India

Tushar B Parikh
DNB DM (Neonatology) Fellowship in Neonatal Perinatal Medicine (Australia)
Consultant Neonatologist
KEM Hospital and Motherhood Hospital
Pune, Maharashtra, India

VC Manoj MD
Unit Head
Department of Neonatology
Jubilee Mission Medical College and Research Institute
Thrissur, Kerala, India

Venkat Kallem DNB
Neonatologist
Fernandez Hospital
Hyderabad, Telangana, India

Vinay Joshi MD (Peds) DM (Neonatology) Fellowship
PICU and PCICU, University of Toronto, Canada
Fellowship Neonatal and Perinatal Medicine
University of NSW, Australia
Senior Consultant
Department of Pediatrics and Neonatal Critical Care
KD Ambani Hospital
Mumbai, Maharashtra, India

Vinay Kumar Rai MD
Consultant Neonatologist
Department of Neonatology
Cloudnine Hospital
Gurugram, Haryana, India

Vinay Mishra MD
Consultant Neonatologist
Department of Pediatric and Neonatal Critical Care
KD Ambani Hospital
Mumbai, Maharashtra, India

From the Desk of IAP Neonatology Chapter

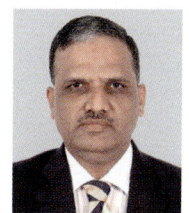

It gives me immense pleasure to write a foreword for revised edition of *Protocols in Neonatology*. This book has been conceived and edited by two of the very well-respected astute clinicians, teachers, and academicians par excellence in the field of Neonatal Perinatal Medicine—Dr Rhishikesh Thakre and Dr Srinivas Murki. A lot of effort of contributors, reviewers, and editors has gone in making this protocol book that is updated on the basis of currently available best evidence. It is one of the best protocol books for care of newborns that I have seen for a long time.

India's newborn healthcare is steadily improving; however, a lot more needs to be done. The *Protocols in Neonatology* is a concise, precise, and practical book that is useful for newborn healthcare providers, students pursuing pediatrics and fellowship in Neonatology, Neonatologists, and Pediatricians alike. It covers every part of management aspects of common neonatal problems encountered in day-to-day practice. This book is written in simplified scientific language and is extremely useful for providing bedside clinical care.

I am confident that this evidence-based protocol book will be of immense help in improving the quality of care and outcomes of newborns throughout India.

Nandkishor Kabra
DM (Neonatology) MD (Ped) DNB (Ped)
MSc (Clinical Epidemiology, Canada)
President, IAP Neonatology Chapter (2019–20)
Chief Neonatologist and Director
Neonatal Intensive Care Unit (NICU)
Surya Hospitals
Mumbai, Maharashtra, India

Foreword

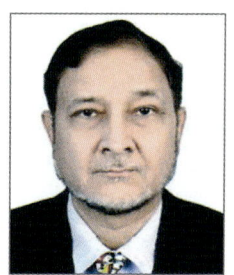

Ensuring healthy survival of all neonates is among the highest priorities of our times. The global community has committed itself to attain an under-five child mortality rate of less than 20 per 1000 live births in all countries by 2035. This would only be achieved if the neonatal mortality rate declines to less than 10 per 1000 live births. For India, this would be a two-thirds reduction from the prevailing level of 29 per 1000 live births.

India's success in reducing neonatal mortality, in particular, since the launch of the National Rural Health Mission has been modest. Nonetheless, the country mounted a spectacular effort in establishing newborn care corners and the special newborn care units, thus creating an impressive neonatal care infrastructure in the public sector. There has also been a concomitant expansion of neonatal care services in the private sector.

This massive expansion of neonatal care services has also brought to the fore an extraordinary need for skilled nurses and doctors. IAP Neonatology chapter envisioned the need of trained neonatal fellows to manage these facilities in the country. They have also recognized a felt need to have uniform standardized protocols for managing normal, at-risk and sick neonates. This compilation of protocols in neonatology is a timely step towards filling the gap for education translation for quality of care. These protocols are tailored to needs of neonatology fellow, resident doctors and practicing pediatricians.

I would like to congratulate the contributors, reviewers and the editorial team for an outstanding product. The credit goes to a very large team of neonatologists trained in India and abroad who have contributed in this endeavor. I am glad to see many young neonatologists contributing to this book. I know them for more than a decade. They are exceptional up-to-date educators with hands on experience in managing sick neonates. They have created simple protocols applicable in Indian context. It is heartening that these evidence-based protocols have been reviewed and critiqued by the most respected experts from all over the country. My special congratulations to Dr Rhishikesh Thakre and Dr Srinivas Murki for a job well done.

I am sure these protocols will help in providing safe care with focus on quality, so that healthcare is affordable and cost effective in the country.

Ashok Deorari MD FAMS FNNF
President, National Neonatology Forum (NNF), India, 2020
Professor and Head, Department of Pediatrics
Incharge, WHO Collaborating Center for Education and Research in Newborn Care
Chairman, Skills Center, Lead for QI in SEARO
All India Institute of Medical Sciences
New Delhi, India

Foreword

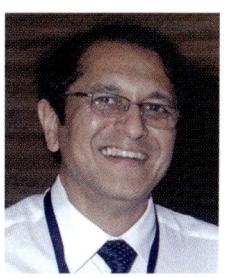

Publication of any book is a process as laborious as the process of delivering a baby. Maturity (contents and the quality), weight gain (number of pages) and intact survival (final copy) all have to be carefully looked after.

Protocols in Neonatology has gone through all these laborious processes and has come out as an exclusive book for newborn health-care providers giving instant guidelines for treatment, bringing uniformity in management and training minds for protocolized thinking. With each protocol the book provides concise, precise and up-to-date information which shall help standardize care in neonatal practice.

Textbooks published from the medically advanced countries do not focus enough attention on the prevailing problems and circumstances in the developing countries such as India. When a practitioner is confronted with a clinical problem, he can rarely turn to a textbook for help. What he needs at that time is not a recounting of a long list of differential diagnosis, but practical guidelines as to how to arrive at a particular diagnosis and how to proceed further.

With the help of history, focused examination and minimum investigations, one can reach a working diagnosis and lay down immediate priorities in management.

The goal behind publication of this book is to facilitate a logical and efficient stepwise approach to reasonable differential diagnoses for the common problems in a neonate. Moreover it would train the brain to approach a problem.

To put it in the words of Henry David Thoreau...*our lives are frittered away by detail; simplify, simplify*.

I am sure that the protocols will enhance the capabilities of students, house officers and clinicians guiding them towards optimal utilization of available investigative and therapeutic resources.

The explosion of knowledge in Neonatology is phenomenal and fast. If the medical advances and good clinical practice get coupled with effective advocacy, our increasing knowledge will benefit newborn care in our country.

Pramod Jog MD DNB FIAP
President, Indian Academy of Pediatrics (IAP) 2016
Standing Committee Member, International Pediatric Association (IPA) 2016–19
Steering Committee Member, GAVI (CSO) 2016–19
Senior Consultant, UNICEF, India
Associate Fellow, International Academy of Perinatal Medicine
Professor of Pediatrics, DY Patil Medical College, Pune, Maharashtra, India

Preface to the Second Edition

We are thankful and grateful to the learned readers for their overwhelming response to the 1st edition. We feel proud to announce the 2nd edition with inputs, feedbacks, suggestions and critical comments from the esteemed readers. The book *Protocols in Neonatology* continues to retain its original sections with a new added section on interpretation. The protocols have been thoroughly revised and updated. The contents have been made more

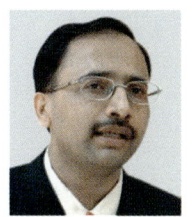 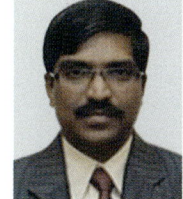

Rhishikesh Thakre **Srinivas Murki**

concise, precise, and evidence based. The entire emphasis has been to provide practical, reliable information to the residents, nurses, and clinicians for effective management and care of the well and sick newborns.

We sincerely feel and hope that this book will serve as an important bedside guide to diagnostic and therapeutic decision making in neonatal intensive care and stabilization units and serve as a valuable tool for all of us involved in delivering care to the newborns. We enjoyed the hard work in processing the book and hope the readers will find it enjoyable and benefit from it in delivering care of the newborns.

We express our gratitude to the Office bearers of Indian Academy of Pediatrics (IAP) Neonatology Chapter for having the faith in us and for their wholehearted support. We are grateful to Shri Jitendar P Vij (Group Chairman), Mr Ankit Vij (Managing Director), Ms Chetna Malhotra Vohra (Associate Director—Content Strategy) and Dr Savleen Kaur (Development Editor) of M/s Jaypee Brothers Medical Publishers (P) Ltd, New Delhi, India, for their zeal for perfection and professional attitude.

Rhishikesh Thakre
Srinivas Murki

Preface to the First Edition

We take great pleasure and pride in offering the *Protocols in Neonatology* to the learned reader. It is said that there are many ways to boil an egg. So also when it comes to managing newborn's, no two neonatal intensive care units (NICUs) are the same, so also the management by consultants within a NICU. It has been our endeavor to appraise and sensitize the reader to management of common disorders by providing precise, concise and relevant information, which should streamline the care of the sick newborn. Divided into theme-based sections, several topics of practical relevance are being covered under the headings—Clinical Approach to Sick Newborn; Care of Well Newborn; Care of Preterm/Low-birth Weight/High-risk Newborn; Neonatal Dilemmas; Specific Therapies, and Miscellaneous Topics. We hope this book serves as a ready-reference tool in a busy NICU.

A standardized approach and management enables the competent residents, fellows and pediatricians to quickly evaluate, identify and intervene before complications set it. We are confident that the protocols will be a step in this direction.

We are grateful to all our authors for their valuable contributions without which this book would not have seen the light of the day. We would appreciate and look forward to your feedback and comments.

We thank the office bearers of IAP Neonatology Chapter for having the faith in us. We appreciate all the support of Shri Jitendar P Vij (Group Chairman), Mr Ankit Vij (Group President) and Mr Tarun Duneja (Director–Publishing) of M/s Jaypee Brothers Medical Publishers (P) Ltd, New Delhi, India.

Rhishikesh Thakre
Srinivas Murki

Contents

SECTION 1: CLINICAL APPROACH TO SICK NEWBORN

1. IDENTIFICATION OF "AT RISK" NEWBORN AND ADMISSION TO SCNU/NICU   3
Rajiv Sharan
What is Triage? *3*
Emergency Signs *3*
Priority Signs *3*
Non Urgent Signs *4*
Criteria for Admission to SCNU/Level II NICU *6*

2. HYPOTHERMIA   7
Leslie Lewis
Indication for Temperature Screening *7*
Thermoneutral Environment *7*
Temperature Monitoring in Neonates *7*
Clinical Manifestations of Hypothermia *8*
Consequences of Hypothermia *9*
Management of Hypothermia *9*
Best Preventive Practices in Delivery Room *10*
Clinical Pearls *11*

3. RESPIRATORY DISTRESS   13
Rhishikesh Thakre
Definition *13*
Identify Severity *13*
Etiology *13*
Investigations (for All Newborns with Respiratory Distress) *17*
Management of Respiratory Distress *18*

4. NEONATAL SHOCK   23
Vinay Mishra, Preetha Joshi, Vinay Joshi
Definition *23*
Phases of Shock *23*
Role of Blood Pressure in Shock *23*
Types of Shock *24*
Evaluation of a Newborn with Shock *24*
Investigations and Monitoring *26*
Treatment Approach *26*
Therapeutic Targets in the Management of Neonatal Shock *28*
Outcomes *28*

5. SUSPECTED INFECTION — 32
Anuradha Bansal, Deepak Chawla

When to Suspect Neonatal Sepsis *32*
Classification of Neonatal Sepsis *33*
Investigations *34*
Management *36*
Adjunctive Therapies *39*

6. NEONATAL SEIZURES — 41
Ashish Jain

Definition *41*
Seizure Mimics *41*
Evaluation of Seizure *42*
Clinical Seizure Types *42*
Important Etiologies of Neonatal Seizures *42*
History and Examination *44*
Investigations *45*
Imaging *45*
Electroencephalography *45*
Prognosis *47*
Management and Drug Therapy of Neonatal Seizures *48*

7. JAUNDICE — 49
Srinivas Murki

Definition *49*
Assessing Severity of Jaundice *49*
Identifying Etiology *49*
Management *51*
Administration of Phototherapy *52*
Stopping the Phototherapy *52*
Practice Points *52*
Exchange Transfusion *53*
Guidelines for Management of Jaundice Neonates Born at <35 Weeks of Gestation *54*
Guidelines for Management Jaundice Neonates Born at ≥35 Weeks of Gestation *54*
Role of Intravenous Immunoglobulins *54*
IV Fluids/Fluid Supplement *54*
Prevention *54*

8. SUSPECTED CONGENITAL HEART DEFECT — 57
Monica Kaushal

Approach to Etiology *57*
Investigations *61*
Management *61*
Treatment *64*

9. FLUID AND ELECTROLYTE THERAPY — 67
Sandeep Kadam

How Much Fluids? *67*
Clinical Tips *68*
Electrolyte Supplementation *69*

  Which Fluids?   *69*
  Rate of Fluid Administration   *69*
  How much Dextrose?   *70*
  Monitoring of Fluid and Electrolyte Status   *70*
  Clinical Case Scenarios   *71*
  Common Electrolyte Problems   *73*

10. HYPOGLYCEMIA   77
Vinay Kumar Rai, Sanjay Wazir

  Definition   *77*
  Clinical Features   *77*
  Glucose Screening   *78*
  Management of Hypoglycemia   *79*
  Diagnostic Criteria to Define Hyperinsulinism   *80*
  Surgical Therapy   *81*
  Outcome   *81*

11. HYPOCALCEMIA   84
Surg RAdm Sheila Samanta Mathai

  Definition   *84*
  Clinical Suspicion of Hypocalcemia   *84*
  Etiological Approach   *85*
  First-Line Investigations   *85*
  Management   *85*
  Specific Treatment of Hypocalcemia   *86*

12. POLYCYTHEMIA   88
Raktima Chakrabarti

  Definition   *88*
  Assessing Severity of Polycythemia   *88*

13. FEED INTOLERANCE: GASTRIC RESIDUES   94
Rohit Arora

  Definition   *94*
  Clinical Symptoms of Feed Intolerance   *94*
  Management   *94*
  Family Counseling   *96*

14. BLEEDING NEWBORN   97
Rajesh Kumar

  Definition   *97*
  Types of Disorders   *97*
  Etiology   *97*
  Management   *99*
  Prevention of Bleeding   *100*

15. THROMBOCYTOPENIA   102
Binu Ninan

  Neonatal Thrombocytopenia   *102*
  Approach to Etiology   *102*
  Investigations   *102*
  Management   *105*

16. ANEMIA 107
Sanjay Aher

Identify the Severity *107*
Identify the Cause *107*
Physiologic Anemia of Infancy *108*

17. NEONATAL ENCEPHALOPATHY 116
Naveen Jain

Approach to a Baby with Neonatal Encephalopathy *116*
Causes of Neonatal Encephalopathy *116*
Assessment of Severity of Encephalopathy *117*
Imaging in Neonatal Encephalopathy *118*
Role of EEG and AEEG in Neonatal Seizures and NE *118*
Treatment of Neonatal Encephalopathy *118*
Early Detection of Neonatal Encephalopathy for Better Outcomes *118*
Prevention of Hypoxic Ischemic Encephalopathy *119*

18. FLOPPY INFANT 120
Preetha Joshi, Tanushri Mukherjee

Definition and Assessment *120*
Identify the Problem *120*
Etiology *121*
Investigations *124*
Principles of Management (Supportive) *125*

19. SUSPECTED INBORN ERRORS OF METABOLISM 127
Naveen Bajaj

Categories of Inborn Errors of Metabolism *127*
Clinical Clues to IEM during Neonatal Period *127*
Investigations for Suspected IEM *127*
Screening Metabolic Tests to Identify IEM *129*
IEM with Significant Encephalopathy *133*
Role of MRI *135*
Management *135*
Specific Treatment *136*
Prenatal Diagnosis *136*
Newborn Screening *136*

20. DISORDER OF SEX DEVELOPMENT 137
Tejopratap Oleti

Definition *137*
When should you Suspect that the Neonate have Disorder of Sex Development? *137*
Classification of Disorder of Sex Development *139*
History *139*
Physical Examination *139*
Investigations *141*
Approach for Diagnosis and Etiology *144*
Issues in Assignment of Gender *148*

21. NEONATAL TRANSPORT — 149
Sachin Shah, Amita Kaul

Indications for Transport   *149*
Contraindications for Transport   *149*
Transport Preparation   *150*
Type of Transport Teams   *151*
Caring during Transport   *151*
Modes of Transport   *152*
Transport in Specific Conditions   *152*
Deterioration of a Neonate during Transport   *152*
Practical Issues with Transport   *153*
Air Transport   *153*
Referring Center Responsibilities   *153*
Receiving Center Responsibilities   *153*
Transport Team Responsibilities   *153*
Neonatal Referral Documentation   *154*

22. ABDOMINAL DISTENSION — 158
Ashish Mehta

Evaluation and Examination   *158*
Medical Management of Bowel Obstruction   *161*

23. APNEA — 163
Rhishikesh Thakre

Definition   *163*
What is the Cause of Apnea?   *163*
First-Line Investigations   *163*
Management   *163*
Specific Therapy   *165*
Endpoint of Treatment   *166*
Failure of Medications   *166*

24. BLISTERING SKIN DISORDERS — 168
Rhishikesh Thakre

Mode of Delivery   *168*
Care in Delivery Room   *168*
Approach to Epidermolysis Bullosa   *168*
Principles of Management of Epidermolysis Bullosa   *169*
Importance of Nail Involvement   *170*
Investigations   *170*

25. SYSTEMIC FUNGAL INFECTIONS — 171
Rhishikesh Thakre, Srinivas Murki

Candida Species   *171*
Clinical Manifestations   *171*
Diagnosis   *172*
Treatment   *172*

SECTION 2: CARE OF WELL NEWBORN

26. EVALUATION IN DELIVERY ROOM — 177
Deepak Pande

Preparation before Birth *177*
Postnatal Care of Newborn *180*
Potential Harmful Practices in Delivery Room *183*

27. FIRST EVALUATION IN OUTPATIENT DEPARTMENT — 184
LS Deshmukh

Equipment Required *184*
Five Steps of Evaluation *184*
Important Considerations in History *185*
Sequence of Examination *185*
Communication and Documentation *190*
Neonatal Screening *190*

28. GROWTH MONITORING — 191
Shamsher Singh Dalal

Term Growth Charts *192*
Measuring Growth *193*
Target Growth Parameters *193*

29. NEWBORN METABOLIC SCREENING — 194
Asim Kumar Mallick

Components of Newborn Screening *194*
Basic Principles of Screening *195*
Types of Disorders to be Screened *195*
Ideal Age for Sample Collection *196*
Practical Tips *197*
Special Consideration *197*
Biochemical Technology Available to Detect Various Metabolic Inherited Disorders *198*

30. VITAMIN K — 200
C Aparna

Role of Prophylactic Vitamin K *200*
Role of Therapeutic Vitamin K *200*
Appendix: Vitamin K Forms *202*

31. NOT PASSED URINE IN THE FIRST 48 HOURS — 204
K Sankarnarayanan

Identification, Immediate Steps, and Potential Confounders *204*
Diagnosis of Oligoanuria *204*
Evaluation *204*
Physical Examination *205*
Urine Analysis *205*
Renal Ultrasound *205*
Micturating Cystourethrogram *206*
Radionuclide Scintigraphy *206*

Etiology of Acute Kidney Injury in Neonates *206*
Approach to a Baby with Oligoanuria *206*
Management *207*
Fluids *207*
Hyperkalemia *207*
Metabolic Acidosis *208*
Hyponatremia *208*
Nutrition *208*
Renal Replacement *208*

32. NOT PASSED STOOLS IN THE FIRST 48 HOURS — 209
Leslie Lewis

Timing for First Passage of Meconium *209*

33. DIRECT JAUNDICE — 212
Sreeram S

Clinical Features *212*
Investigations *212*
Management *214*
Prognosis *215*

34. CONGENITAL HYDRONEPHROSIS — 216
Jaikrishan Mittal, Manish Mittal

Physical Examination *216*
Radiologic Studies *217*
Approach *218*

35. COMMON PROBLEMS IN NEWBORN IN OUTPATIENT DEPARTMENT — 220
Nishad Plakkal

Diaper Rash *220*
Colic: the Crying Infant *221*
Not Enough Milk! *221*
Health Supplements *222*
Hemangiomas *222*
Jaundice *223*
Breast Discharge *223*
Natal/Neonatal Teeth *223*
Oral Thrush *224*
Phimosis *224*
Seborrheic Dermatitis/Cradle Cap *225*
Transitional Stools/Diarrhea *225*
Umbilical Discharge/Bleeding *225*
Umbilical Hernia *226*
Vaginal Bleeding *227*
Bathing/Skin Care of the Preterm Infant at Home *227*
Eye Discharge *227*
Regurgitation *228*
Constipation/Infrequent Stools *228*
Neonatal Sleep Myoclonus *228*

36. OPTIMIZING BREASTFEEDING IN A NORMAL NEWBORN   229
Anu Thukral

Breastfeeding Initiation and Maintenance   229
Assessing Breastfeeding Adequacy   230
Issues/Concerns for Breastfeeding in the first few days and their Management   230

37. GOLDEN HOUR CARE FOR PRETERM   234
Ashwani Singal

Preparation Prior to Birth   234
Care of Preterm at Birth   234
Stabilization in Nursery   236

38. COLIC   238
Rhishikesh Thakre

Definition   238
Etiology of Colic   238
Clinical Features   239
Diagnosis   239
Management of Colic   239
Role of Medications   240

SECTION 3: CARE OF PRETERM/LOW BIRTH WEIGHT/HIGH RISK NEWBORN

39. KANGAROO CARE   243
Suman Rao, Balla Kalyan Chakravarthy

Definition   243
Components of Kangaroo Mother Care   243
Advantages of Kangaroo Mother Care   243
Procedure   243
Preparations for the Kangaroo Mother Care Provider   244
Preparations for the Baby   244
The "Kangaroo Mother Care Position"   244
Duration of Kangaroo Mother Care   245
Monitoring a Baby in Kangaroo Mother Care   246
Discharge and Follow-up   246
Don'ts of Kangaroo Mother Care   246
Discontinuation of Kangaroo Mother Care   246
Overcoming Bottlenecks in Kangaroo Mother Care Implementation   247

40. LOW BIRTH WEIGHT FEEDING   248
Sandeep Kadam

Strategies to Optimize Breast Milk in Mothers with Low Birth Weight Baby   250
Developmental Origins of Health and Disease   254

41. NUTRITIONAL SUPPLEMENTATION   255
VC Manoj

Role of Human Breast Milk   255
Supplementation in Preterm Breastfed Infants   255
Supplementation in Formula/Animal Milk Fed Preterm Infants   257

42. DISCHARGE PLANNING — 260
VC Manoj

Timing of Discharge *260*
Planning *260*

43. RETINOPATHY OF PREMATURITY SCREENING — 263
Snehal Thakre

Indications *263*

44. HEARING SCREENING — 269
Chetana Naik

Importance of Hearing Screening *269*
Hearing Loss *270*
Hearing Tests to Identify Deafness in a Child *270*
Early Management *271*

45. FOLLOW-UP OF THE HIGH-RISK NEWBORN — 272
Archana Kadam

Components of the Developmental Follow-up *274*

46. IVH AND PVL SCREENING AND CLASSIFICATION — 280
Pradeep Suryawanshi

Intraventricular Hemorrhage *280*
Periventricular Leukomalacia *284*

47. DEVELOPMENTAL SUPPORTIVE CARE — 287
Rhishikesh Thakre

Steps for Developmental Supportive Care in Nursery *287*
Interventions for Developmental Supportive Care in NICU *288*
Documentation *290*

48. ANTENATAL CORTICOSTEROIDS — 291
Rhishikesh Thakre

Impact of Antenatal Steroids on Preterm Outcome *291*
Indications *291*
Onset and Duration of Action *292*
Adverse Effects *292*

49. BREAST MILK STORAGE AND HANDLING — 293
Rhishikesh Thakre, Srinivas Murki

Procedure *293*
Transporting Breast Milk *293*
Thawing Breast Milk *293*
Warming Breast Milk for Feeding *294*

50. IMMUNIZATION IN LOW BIRTH WEIGHT INFANTS — 295
Rhishikesh Thakre

Basic Principles *295*
Timing *295*
Dosing *295*

Vaccine Administration *295*
Schedule for Hepatitis B Vaccination for Preterm/Low Birth Weight Babies *295*
Thiomersal Issue *296*
Vaccination in Bleeding Disorder Infant *296*
Immunocompromised Infant *297*

SECTION 4: NEONATAL DILEMMAS

51. CRYPTORCHIDISM 301
Rhishikesh Thakre, Srinivas Murki

At Risk Groups *301*
Retractile Testis *301*
Ectopic Testis *301*
Cryptorchidism *301*
Physical Examination *302*
Manipulations *302*
Diagnostic Techniques *303*
Management *303*

52. BABY BORN TO HIV POSITIVE MOTHER 304
Hemasree Kandraju, Venkat Kallem

Risk of Transmission *304*
Interventions for Prevention of Mother-to-Child Transmission *304*
Principles of Infant Feeding for Human Immunodeficiency Virus Exposed Infants *306*
Care during Postpartum Period *306*
Care and Follow-up of the Infants Born to Human Immunodeficiency Virus Positive Mother *306*
Care of Human Immunodeficiency Virus Positive Infant *308*

53. BABY BORN TO HBsAG POSITIVE MOTHER 309
Giridhar Sethuraman

Factors Associated with High Rate of Mother-to-Child Transmission *309*
Clinical Manifestations and Treatment *309*
Practice Points *310*
Management *310*

54. BABY BORN TO MOTHER HAVING TUBERCULOSIS 311
Rajesh Kumar

Identify the Problem *311*
Identify Severity/Red Signs *311*
Identify Cause—History, Physical Examination *311*
Clinical Features *311*
Laboratory Investigations *312*
Newer Tests *312*
Management: General or Specific *312*
Indications for Separation of Infant Born to Mother with TB *312*
Algorithm *314*

55. BABY BORN TO MOTHER WITH CHICKENPOX — 315
Rhishikesh Thakre

- Timing of Chickenpox Infection *315*
- Risk of Transmission *315*
- Management of Newborns with Maternal Chickenpox during Delivery *315*
- Chickenpox Exposure during Postnatal Wards or at Home from Siblings *316*
- Chickenpox Exposure within the Neonatal Unit *316*
- Implications for Practice *317*

56. BABY BORN TO VDRL POSITIVE MOTHER — 318
Naveen Bajaj

- Physical Examination for Evidence of Congenital Syphilis *318*
- Major Findings in Early Congenital Syphilis *318*
- Clinical Manifestations of Late Congenital Syphilis *319*
- Serologic and Diagnostic Tests *319*
- Treatment Options *321*
- Follow-up *321*

57. BREASTFEEDING AND MEDICATIONS — 324
Anjali Kulkarni, Kiran Sathe

- Common Medications during Pregnancy *324*
- Breastfeeding and Medications *327*
- Ways to Minimize Infant Drug Exposure *327*

58. STEM CELL BANKING: SCOPE AND PRACTICE — 330
Femitha P

- Umbilical Cord Blood Banking *330*
- Types of Cord Blood Banking *331*
- Practice Pointers *331*

59. DECLARING NEWBORN DEATH — 333
Rhishikesh Thakre, Srinivas Murki

- When not to Initiate Newborn Resuscitation? *333*
- When to Consider Discontinuation of Resuscitation in a Newborn? *333*
- When to Declare Patient Dead after Initiating Resuscitation? *333*
- Documentation *334*
- Nursing Responsibility *334*

SECTION 5: SPECIFIC THERAPIES

60. ANTIBIOTIC POLICY IN NEONATAL INTENSIVE CARE UNIT — 339
Hemasree Kandraju

- Selection of Empiric Antibiotic Therapy *339*
- Re-Evaluating the Antibiotic Regime *340*
- Modification of Antibiotic after the Availability of Antibiogram *341*

61. SURFACTANT REPLACEMENT THERAPY — 346
Dinesh Chirla

Indications of Surfactant Therapy   *346*
Factors Influencing Surfactant Therapy   *346*
Choice of Surfactant   *346*
Timing of Surfactant Therapy   *347*
Early Administration of Surfactant Followed by Brief Ventilation and
Extubation to Continuous Positive Airway Pressure (Insure Strategy)   *347*

62. CONTINUOUS POSITIVE AIRWAY PRESSURE — 352
Nandkishor Kabra

Indications   *352*
Contraindications   *352*
Components of Continuous Positive Airway Pressure   *352*
Intubate, Surfactant and Extubate (Insure) Procedure   *354*
Assessment Checklist for Continuous Positive Airway Pressure   *355*

63. INTUBATE, SURFACTANT, EXTUBATE (INSURE) PROCEDURE — 356
Nandkishor Kabra

Indications   *356*
Eligibility Criterion   *356*
Poor Candidates   *356*
Procedure   *356*
Before Extubation Ensure   *356*
Clinical Pearls   *356*

64. BLOOD COMPONENT THERAPY — 357
Pramod Gaddam, Deepak Sharma, Tejopratap Oleti

Indications for Transfusion   *357*
Precautions Before Transfusion   *358*
Packed Red Blood Cells   *358*

65. TOTAL PARENTERAL NUTRITION — 364
Tushar B Parikh

Broad Outline of Total Parenteral Nutrition Therapy   *364*
Nutrients in Total Parenteral Nutrition   *365*
Energy Needs   *366*
Lipids in Total Parenteral Nutrition   *367*
Multivitamins in Total Parenteral Nutrition   *368*
Minerals   *368*
Calculation for Total Parenteral Nutrition   *369*
Compounding and Setting-up Total Parenteral Nutrition   *369*
Monitoring While on Total Parenteral Nutrition   *371*
Complications Related to Total Parenteral Nutrition   *371*
Concept of Aggressive Nutrition   *371*
Starter Packs in Total Parenteral Nutrition   *372*

66. OXYGEN THERAPY — 373
Rhishikesh Thakre, Srinivas Murki

Indications for Oxygen Therapy *373*
Source of Oxygen *373*
Selection of an Oxygen Delivery Device *374*
Practical Considerations in Oxygen Delivery *375*
Monitoring Oxygen Therapy *376*
Oxygen Toxicity *376*
Weaning Oxygen *377*
Oxygenation Status *377*

67. CHEST PHYSIOTHERAPY — 378
Tanveer Bashir, Rhishikesh Thakre

Indications *378*
Contraindications *378*

SECTION 6: INTERPRETING TESTS

68. NEONATAL SEPSIS SCREEN — 383
Rhishikesh Thakre, Srinivas Murki

White Blood Cells Count *383*
Neutrophil Count *383*
Peripheral Blood Smear *383*
C-Reactive Protein *384*
Erythrocyte Sedimentation Rate *384*
Gastric Aspirate *385*
Blood Culture *385*
Practical Utility *385*

69. C-REACTIVE PROTEIN — 387
Rhishikesh Thakre

Technical Issues *387*
Factors Affecting Results *387*
Clinical Implications *387*
Clinical Limitations *388*
Clinical Pearls *388*

70. BLOOD CULTURE — 389
Rhishikesh Thakre, Srinivas Murki

Indications *389*
Technique of Blood Culture *389*
Practice Pointers *389*
Rationale for a Blood Culture on Treatment or Once Treatment is Already Initiated *390*
Causes of Persistence of Positive Blood Culture *390*

71. THYROID FUNCTION TEST — 392
Rhishikesh Thakre

How Reliable are Clinical Features for Diagnosis of Congenital Hypothyroidism? *392*

72. INTERPRETING NEONATAL X-RAYS — 396
Rhishikesh Thakre, Tanveer Bashir, Srinivas Murki

Radiation Protection Measures *396*
Steps for Interpretation *397*
Indications for Lateral View *398*
Common Errors in X-Ray due to Technical Problem *398*
Clinical Pearls *399*

73. CONGENITAL RENAL DISORDERS — 401
Rhishikesh Thakre, Tanveer Bashir

Antenatal Hydronephrosis *401*
Vesicoureteric Reflux *401*
Multicystic Dysplastic Kidney *401*
Solitary Kidney *402*
Ureteropelvic Junction Obstruction *402*
Posterior Urethral Valves *403*
Prune Belly Syndrome *403*
Ureterovesical Obstruction *403*
Ureteroceles *403*

SECTION 7: MISCELLANEOUS TOPICS

74. PARENT COUNSELING — 407
Ranjan Kumar Pejaver

Qualities of a Good Counselor *407*
When do we need to Counsel during Perinatal Period? *407*
General Principles of Parent Counseling *408*
Some Technical Aspects of Perinatal Counseling *409*
Withdrawal of Care *409*

75. DISINFECTION AND STERILIZATION — 411
Srinivas Murki, Rhishikesh Thakre

Basic Concepts *411*
Disinfection *411*
Sterilization *414*

76. HANDWASHING — 416
Srinivas Murki, Rhishikesh Thakre

Indications (World Health Organizaton, Five Moments of Hand Hygiene) *416*
Purpose of Handwashing *416*
Steps of Handwashing *416*
Types of Hand Hygiene *417*
Microorganisms on Skin *417*
Pre-Requisites of Handwashing Agents *417*
Choice of Handwashing Agents: Soap Versus Antimicrobial *417*

Precautions in Soap Use *418*
Choice of Antimicrobial Solution *418*
Hand Drying *418*
Methods to Improve Handwashing *418*

77. PAIN MANAGEMENT 420
Somashekhar Nimbalkar

Nonpharmacologic Strategies *422*
Pharmacologic Agents *424*
Reduction of Painful Procedures *427*

78. COPING WITH DEATH 429
Rhishikesh Thakre

Implications for Practice *429*
Before Death *429*
During the Last Moments *430*
After Death *430*

79. BIRTH INJURY 431
Rhishikesh Thakre

Caput Succedaneum *431*
Cephalhematoma *431*
Subgaleal Hemorrhage *431*
Skull Fractures *431*
Epidural Hemorrhage *431*
Subdural Hemorrhage *432*
Subarachnoid Hemorrhage *432*
Erb's Palsy *432*
Klumpke's Palsy *432*
Facial Nerve Palsy *432*
Phrenic Nerve Injury *433*
Laryngeal Nerve Palsy *433*
Spinal Cord Injury *433*
Nasal Septal Dislocation *433*
Congenital Muscular Torticollis *433*
Clavicular Fractures *434*
Fracture Long Bones *434*

80. BEST PRACTICES IN NEONATAL INTENSIVE CARE UNIT 435
Srinivas Murki, Rhishikesh Thakre

Interventions to Prevent Preterm Brain Injury *435*
Infection Control Practices *436*
Respiratory Distress Syndrome Management *436*
Neonatal Jaundice Management *437*
Postasphyxia Management *437*
Ineffective Interventions in Neonatal Intensive Care Unit *437*

81. CHECKLISTS 439
N Chandra Kumar

Predischarge Checklist for VLBW Infant   *439*
Predischarge Checklist for Normal Newborn   *442*
Surgical Checklist for Newborn   *444*
Checklist for Preparation of Formula Feed   *446*
Central Line-Associated Bloodstream Infection (CLABSI) Bundle Checklist   *446*
Exchange Transfusion Checklist   *447*
Ventilator-Associated Pneumonia (VAP) Bundle Checklist   *450*

82. USE OF NEONATAL INTENSIVE CARE UNIT CHARTS, ALGORITHMS, CALCULATORS: MOBILE APPS AND WEBSITE LINKS 451
Baswaraj Tandur

Charts   *451*
Algorithms   *452*
Disease Diagnosis Tools   *452*
Mobile Apps   *453*
Calculators   *454*

INDEX 459

SECTION 1

Clinical Approach to Sick Newborn

SECTION OUTLINE

1. Identification of "At Risk" Newborn and Admission to SCNU/NICU
2. Hypothermia
3. Respiratory Distress
4. Neonatal Shock
5. Suspected Infection
6. Neonatal Seizures
7. Jaundice
8. Suspected Congenital Heart Defect
9. Fluid and Electrolyte Therapy
10. Hypoglycemia
11. Hypocalcemia
12. Polycythemia
13. Feed Intolerance: Gastric Residues
14. Bleeding Newborn
15. Thrombocytopenia
16. Anemia
17. Neonatal Encephalopathy
18. Floppy Infant
19. Suspected Inborn Errors of Metabolism
20. Disorder of Sex Development
21. Neonatal Transport
22. Abdominal Distension
23. Apnea
24. Blistering Skin Disorders
25. Systemic Fungal Infections

CHAPTER 1

Identification of "At Risk" Newborn and Admission to SCNU/NICU

Rajiv Sharan

WHAT IS TRIAGE?

Triage is a process of rapidly examining all sick newborn when they arrive in hospital in order to place them in one of the following categories with the help of TABC concept. The basic purpose of triage is to ensure that sickest newborn gets earliest treatment.

Concept of TABC

When sick newborn arrives in emergency department of a hospital the assessment is done based on TABC concept where:
- T stands for temperature
- A stands for airways
- B stands for breathing
- C stands for circulation, consciousness/coma and/or presence of convulsion.

EMERGENCY SIGNS

If any of the following are present (alone or in combination):
- *T:* Moderate or severe hypothermia (Temperature <35.9°C).
- *A:* No chest movement or no air entry in lungs/obstructed airways and/or central cyanosis.
- *B:* Not breathing/severe respiratory distress with increased work of breathing as evidenced by respiratory rate >60/minute with nasal flaring and/or chest retractions and/or grunting/gasping/head bobbing.
- *C:* Capillary refill time >3 seconds and/or poor pulse and/or decreased urine output.
    - Color of baby mottled or pale with or without cyanosis.
    - Presence of unconsciousness as evidenced by no response or minimal response.
    - Presence of convulsion.

PRIORITY SIGNS

If any of the following are present (alone or in combination):
- *T:* Mild-hypothermia (temperature ~ 36.0–37.4°C) or fever (temperature >37.5°C)
- *A:* Decreased air entry in either lungs ± chest signs by auscultation, e.g. crackles or wheezing.
- *B:* Fast breathing respiratory rate >60/minute ± retractions.
- *C:* Capillary refill time <3 seconds but decreased urine output.

Apart from above signs presence of the following features also classifies the newborn as having priority signs:
- Low-birth weight (weight <1,800 g)
- Irritability/restlessness/jitteriness
- Refusal to feed
- Abdominal distension
- Severe jaundice
- Severe pallor
- Bleeding from any site (apart from physiological vaginal bleed in female)
- Major congenital anomaly
- Large baby (weight >4 kg)
- Redness around umbilical area with or without pus discharge.

NON URGENT SIGNS

Newborns with nonurgent signs are mostly well and can wait for their turn to be addressed. TABC assessment in newborn with nonurgent sign is normal and usually newborns present with following features:
- Physiological jaundice
- Transitional stools
- Developmental peculiarity
- Minor malformations
- Rashes.

When and Where to Triage?

The process should begin as soon as the newborn arrives in the emergency department of the treatment facility or hospital or outpatient department of the hospital.

Time for Triaging

The process to triage newborns in having three above listed signs should take minimum time. The staff nurse on duty should complete the triage stratification at the earliest. It is important that they should know how to look for several signs at the same time for rapid assessment.

Who should Triage?

Triaging should be done by experienced clinical staff nurse with involvement of the junior nurses.

How to Triage?

Triaging of newborns shall be a rapid assessment with focus on TABC concept. After completing TABC assessment the various other features as mentioned above should be taken into account. The basic purpose of triage is to ensure that sickest newborn gets earliest treatment.

Keep in mind the concept of TABC. First assess temperature, then airway, breathing, circulation and lastly consciousness level/coma/convulsion.

Temperature assessment (Flowchart 1): To assess the temperature one should feel the newborn's soles and abdomen.
- If abdomen and soles both are warm, the newborn has normal temperature.
- If soles are cold and abdomen is warm, the newborn is suffering from mild hypothermia/cold stress.
- If the soles and abdomen are cold, the newborn has moderate/severe hypothermia.

Axillary thermometer should be used to record the newborn's temperature. Any other positive finding should be noted.

Flowchart 1: Assessment of temperature.

Temperature: Feel soles and abdomen and check temperature
↓
Decision: Classify degree of hypothermia if any positive sign
↓
Action: Manage hypothermia
↓
Management: Keep the baby under radiant warmer

Note: Normal newborn baby is usually warm.

CHAPTER 1
Identification of "At Risk" Newborn and Admission to SCNU/NICU

Newborn having hypothermia needs warming. The method of warming depends on the actual temperature.

Airway and breathing assessment (Flowchart 2): Airways and breathing pattern is assessed simultaneously for the sake of saving time. The following points should be looked for:
- Is the newborn breathing/gasping/grunting/having head bobbing or nasal flaring?
- Is the airway obstructed?
- Is the newborn blue?
- Does newborn have severe respiratory distress with or without retractions?

Any positive finding should be addressed on urgent basis and airways should be made patent. Oxygen is usually started before a definite diagnosis is made.

Circulation assessment (Flowchart 3): To assess if the newborn has circulatory problems one should:
- Look for cold and clammy skin.
- Look for capillary refill time (CRT) and note if it is more than or less than 3 seconds.
- Look for weak and fast pulse rate.

Prolonged CRT (>3 sec) is a surrogate marker of poor peripheral perfusion. Fast and weak pulse with decreased urine output in this setting may herald a shock like state. Such newborns need warmth and oxygen. An intravenous (IV) line should be inserted and bolus 20 mL/kg of normal saline/Ringer's lactate (NS/RL) initiated over 15–20 minutes. Color of skin of the newborn may be an early catch to an experienced eye. Pallor, mottling, and cyanosis are key visual indicators of reduced circulation to skin.

Pallor signifies white skin coloration from lack of peripheral blood flow. Mottling/patchy skin discoloration, with patches of cyanosis is due to vascular instability or cold. Cyanosis can be a sign of shock or respiratory failure.

Assessment of consciousness level in newborns (Flowchart 4): AVPU scale ("alert, pain, unresponsive") can be used to rapidly assess the newborn. AVPU in comparison with GCS scale is read as: A = 15, V = 12, P = 8, U = 3.
- *A:* Is the newborn alert?
- *V:* Is the newborn responding to voice?
- *P:* Is the newborn responding to pain?
- *U:* Is the newborn not responding? (Unresponsive).

Any unresponsive newborn or newborn with convulsion needs immediate attention.

After placing the newborn under radiant warmer airways/breathing should be assessed and addressed. Peripheral IV line should be established at the earliest, RBS infused

Flowchart 2: Assessment of circulation.

Airway and breathing: Look for not breathing/cyanosis/respiratory distress
↓
Decision: Consider oxygen therapy if any positive sign
↓
Management: Clear airways/give positive pressure if required

Note: Normal breathing appears regular without excessive respiratory muscle effort or audible respiratory sound. While in abnormal breathing there is increased or excessive nasal flaring or abnormal muscle use or decreased or absent respiratory effort or noisy breathing.

Flowchart 3: Assessment of airway and breathing.

Circulation: Look for CRT >3 sec/week and fast pulse
↓
Decision: Consider IV access and oxygen therapy if any positive sign
↓
Management: Bolus 20 mL/kg (normal saline or ringer lactate)

(CRT: capillary refill time)
Note: Normal warm child is usually suggestive of normal circulation whereas cyanosis, mottling, paleness/pallor or obvious bleeding suggests abnormal circulation.

Flowchart 4: Assessment of consciousness.

```
┌─────────────────────────────────────────┐
│ Coma or convulsion: Look for consciousness │
│              level/AVPU scale            │
└─────────────────────────────────────────┘
                    ↓
┌─────────────────────────────────────────┐
│ Decision: Warm/protect airway/consider oxygen │
│ therapy/insert IV line if any positive sign   │
└─────────────────────────────────────────┘
                    ↓
┌─────────────────────────────────────────┐
│ Management: Check RBS/take blood sample/ │
│ injection phenobarbitone 20 mg/kg slowly over │
│       20 minutes if RBS is normal        │
└─────────────────────────────────────────┘
```

(AVPU: Alert, voice, pain, unresponsive)

Note: A normal conscious child has normal cry and responds to parents or to environmental stimuli such as light, etc. and has good muscle tone and moves extremity well whereas abnormal or decreased cry and poor response to parents/environment suggests abnormal conscious level.

checked and injection phenobarbitone 20 mg/kg slowly over 20 minutes in a convulsing baby.

CRITERIA FOR ADMISSION TO SCNU/LEVEL II NICU

All newborns with emergency/priority signs and some babies with nonurgent signs will require admission in hospital for further management or for observational purpose. Other indications that may require admission into special care neonatal unit/neonatal intensive care unit (SCNU/NICU) may be enumerated as:
- Birth weight ≤1,800 g.
- *Low-birth weight*: Babies between 2,500 g and 1,800 g; if the clinical examination shows the baby needs supervised treatment should be shifted to SCNU and not postnatal ward.
- Prematurity <34 weeks of gestation and any baby >34 weeks if is not sucking well.
- Suspicion of infection
- Clinical concern of respiratory problems like: (1) Apnea or cyanotic episodes, (2) Any respiratory distress causing concern.
- Clinical concern of gastrointestinal problems, e.g. feeding problems severe enough to cause clinical concern and bile stained vomiting or signs suggestive of bowel obstruction.
- Clinical concern of metabolic disorder, e.g. low serum glucose level and acidotic breathing.
- Clinical concern of neurological disorder. (1) Convulsion (2) Perinatal asphyxia.
- Congenital anomalies including surgically correctable lesions.
- Any clinical condition which may require initial period of observation.

SUGGESTED READING

1. Children and Infant—Recognition of a sick baby or child in the emergency department—NSW Policy Guidelines; 2011.
2. Emergency Triage Assessment and Treatment—World Health Organization Publication.

CHAPTER 2

Hypothermia

Leslie Lewis

INTRODUCTION

Hypothermia is an under-recognized contributor to neonatal morbidity (e.g. respiratory distress, hypoglycemia, intraventricular hemorrhage, and late-onset sepsis) and mortality. The normal body temperature is 36.5–37.5°C. Axillary temperature below 36.5°C is considered hypothermia and is graded by severity as shown in Table 1.

Visual assessment is a rapid screening tool for thermal well-being (Table 2). Any abnormality detected warrants confirmation by thermometer.

INDICATION FOR TEMPERATURE SCREENING

- All sick infants
- *At risk infants*:
  - Low birth weight (LBW) (<2.5 kg)
  - Intrauterine growth restriction (IUGR)
  - Immediate post resuscitation
  - On admission
  - During transport
  - During re-warming
  - During procedures/surgery.

THERMONEUTRAL ENVIRONMENT

It is a range of temperature during which the basal metabolic rate is minimum, oxygen utilization is least in a baby thriving well. This range of temperature depends on weight, gestation, and postnatal age (Tables 3 and 4). All newborns must be kept in thermoneutral environment (TNE).

TEMPERATURE MONITORING IN NEONATES (TABLE 5)

The preferred method for neonatal temperature monitoring is using digital thermometer in the axilla.

Table 1: Severity of hypothermia (WHO).

Mild	36–36.5°C
Moderate	32–35.9°C
Severe	<32°C

Table 2: Visual assessment for thermal well-being.

Trunk	Extremity	Impression
Pink	Pink	Normal
Pink	Pale	Cold stress
Pale	Pale	Hypothermia
Core axillary mismatch >2°C		Sepsis

Table 3: Recommended TNE for neonates below 96 hours of age.

Age	1,000–1,200 g (+ or – 0.5°C)	1,200–1,500 g (+ or – 0.5°C)	1,500–2,500 g (+ or – 1.0°C)	>2,500 and >36 weeks (+ or – 1.5°C)
0–12 hours	35	34	33.3	32.8
12–24 hours	34.5	33.8	32.8	32.4
24–96 hours	34.5	33.5	32.3	32

Table 4: Recommended TNE for neonates beyond 96 hours of age.

Age	<1,500 g (+ or – 1.5°C)	1,500–2,500 g (+ or – 1.5°C)	>2500 and >36 weeks (+ or – 1.5°C)
5–14 days	33.5	32.1	32
2–3 weeks	33.1	31.7	30
3–4 weeks	32.6	31.4	
4–5 weeks	32	30.9	
5–6 weeks	31.4	30.4	

Table 5: Sites of temperature recordings in neonates.

Body site	Type of thermometer	Normal temperature range (°C)	Advantages	Disadvantages
Axilla	• Hg in glass, electronic • Roof of the axilla	35.6–37.3	Safe and easy	• Influenced by environment • Core temperature 0.5°C more
Rectal	• Hg in glass, 3 cm from the anal margin • Thermistor, 5 cm from the anus	36.5–37.5	• Continuous • Core temperature monitoring • Useful in asphyxiating neonates undergoing hypothermia	• Perforation of the rectum • Infection/NEC
Skin	Thermocouple or thermistor attached over the right side of abdomen	• Term 35.5–36.6 • Preterm 36.2–37.5	• Faster display • Trends	Overheating due to skin probe displacement
Esophageal	InnerSense temperature sensor/feeding tube	36.5–37.5	• Simultaneous feeding • Intraoperative monitoring	Expensive probes
Ear	Infrared emission	35.5–37.3	Rapid assessment	Not reliable for sick neonate

(NEC: necrotizing enterocolitis).

CLINICAL MANIFESTATIONS OF HYPOTHERMIA

- Body and extremities cool to touch
- Acrocyanosis
- Skin mottling
- Bradycardia
- Apnea, shallow or irregular respiration
- Lethargic and decreased activity
- Hypotonia

- Diminished or absent reflexes
- Central nervous system depression.

Tip: No single sign is diagnostic of hypothermia. A high index of suspicion is necessary to identify.

CONSEQUENCES OF HYPOTHERMIA

- Hypoglycemia
- Hypoxia
- Metabolic acidosis
- Pulmonary vasoconstriction
- Altered surfactant production
- Poor weight gain
- Thermal shock and disseminated intravascular coagulation, progressing to death.

MANAGEMENT OF HYPOTHERMIA (TABLE 6 AND FLOWCHART 1)

- Rewarm slowly under the radiant warmer/incubator:
  - Set incubator/radiant warmer temperature 1–1.5°C more than infant temperature and increase every 30 minutes.
  - Monitor for blood glucose, electrolytes, blood gases, hypotension, and bleeding manifestations.

Tip: Fast rewarming lead to apnoea, hypotension, and seizures.

- *Supportive care:*
  - Nil by mouth
  - Intravenous (IV) fluids by 10% dextrose infusion 80 mL/kg on day 1 and subsequently based on fluid and electrolytes requirements as per postnatal age.
  - Supplemental oxygen if necessary.
- Vitamin K administration to prevent bleeding in moderate/severe hypothermia.
- Work-up for sepsis is recommended for hypothermia infants.

Radiant Warmer Versus Incubators

Each has its own advantages/disadvantages. Primarily the use would be defined by the familiarity, ease, and experience. Following babies may be candidates for incubator care:

- Care of extremely LBW babies for humidification.
- For isolating an infected baby to achieve barrier nursing.
- For use at low ambient temperature or when there is lot of convective currents where a radiant warmer fails to work.
- For transporting babies.

Bottom line is not the equipment but the personnel's ease of using the equipment.

Table 6: Treatment strategies for hypothermia.

	Mild (36–36.5°C)	Moderate (32–35.9°C)	Severe (<32°C)
Site of care	Mother	Mother*/Warmer	Warmer
Skin-to-skin care	Yes	Yes*	No
Breast feeding	Yes	Once stabilized	No
Blood sugar check	No	Yes	Yes
IV fluids	No	If feeding not possible	Yes
IV antibiotics	No	Consider	Yes
Vitamin K	No	Yes, if not given earlier	Yes
Recheck temperature	–	Every 15 minutes till normal, 4–6 hourly thereafter	Every 15 minutes till normal, 4–6 hourly thereafter

If facilities do not exist.

Flowchart 1: Algorithm for thermal management.

```
                    Record temperature
                            │
                            │  After resuscitation
                            │  On admission
                            │  All sick and "at risk" newborns
                            ▼
              Identify temperature <36.5°C
        ┌───────────────────┼───────────────────┐
        ▼                   ▼                   ▼
   Temperature         Temperature         Temperature
   36–36.5°C           32–35.9°C           <32°C
```

- **Temperature 36–36.5°C:**
  - Mother/baby together
  - Skin-to-skin contact
  - Ensure breastfeeding
  - Additional clothes
  - Warm environment
  - Avoid draft of air

- **Temperature 32–35.9°C:**
  - Nurse naked under warmer
  - Cover head (skin-to-skin, if no facilities)
  - Keep temperature of skin probe to 36.5°C in servo control mode
  - Check temperature every 15 minutes till normal
  - Consider supervised feeding
  - Administer oxygen, check blood sugar
  - Administer vitamin K (if not given), antibiotics
  - Do a sepsis workup

- **Temperature <32°C:**
  - Nurse naked under warmer
  - Cover head
  - Rapid warming till 34°C temperature
  - Keep temperature of skin probe to 36.5°C in servo control mode
  - Check temperature every 15 minutes till normal, w/f apnea, hypoglycemia
  - Administer IV fluids, oxygen, vitamin K, antibiotics, check blood sugar
  - Do a sepsis workup

Humidification

- Humidity should be started in all infants <31 weeks gestation at 85% humidity
- *Infants of 28–30 weeks:* If temperature remains stable for 24 hours, start to decrease humidity by 5% daily
- *Infants of <28 weeks:* Maintain humidity of 85% for first 7 days and if stable for 7 days, decrease humidity by 5% daily.

Distilled water in the humidification chamber is a source of infection, water should be changed daily and precautions should be taken in regular cleaning the chamber.

BEST PREVENTIVE PRACTICES IN DELIVERY ROOM (BOX 1 AND TABLE 7)

The "warm chain" is a set of 10 interlinked procedures to be taken at birth and during the following few hours and days to prevent hypothermia by minimizing heat loss in all newborns. Failure to implement any one of these procedures will break the chain and put the newborn baby at risk of hypothermia.

Thermal Care Strategies in Preterm Babies

Combination of strategies may be required to maintain temperature (<32 weeks) delivery room (Box 2).

Low cost thermal care support systems include the following:
- Direct contact with skin of the mother—kangaroo mother care—provides biologically controlled heat source. Baby is nestled to lie between the breasts so that baby's

CHAPTER 2
Hypothermia

Box 1: Warm chain.

- Warm delivery room
- Immediate drying
- Skin-to-skin contact
- Breastfeeding
- Bathing and weighing postponed
- Appropriate clothing/bedding
- Mother and baby together
- Warm transportation
- Warm resuscitation and
- Training and awareness raising.

Note: Neonatal temperature may start falling by 0.5–1°C every minute if not supported after birth.

Box 2: Preterm specific delivery room interventions.

- Ensure room is draft free and warm (26°C)
- Early skin-to-skin contact, if breathing well (>30 weeks)
- Use of plastic wrap (<32 weeks)
- Maintain temperature between 36.5°C and 37.5°C
- Use thermal mattress, if available (<32 weeks)
- Record temperature at the end of resuscitation and on admission
- Do not apply hot water bottles or heat packs/stones directly to a baby
- Avoid hyperthermia

Table 7: Prevention of hypothermia.

Source of heat loss	Preventive measures
Conduction	• Warm surface • Warm baby sheets/blankets • Head covering • Warmed solutions
Convection	• Room temperature 26.6°C (80°F) • Incubator • Keep neonate covered
Radiation	• Radiant warmer • Wrap neonate • Warm room
Evaporation	• Heated, humidified inspired gases • Humidification inside the incubator • Plastic bags/wrap for preterm (<28 weeks)

naked ventral surface is in direct contact with mother's bosom.
- Application of oil and liquid paraffin reduces evaporative heat loss.
- Use of thermocol box serves as a good insulating agent.
- Using solar based apparatus avoiding electricity.
- Overhead lamps/electric bulbs (200 W at 50–60 cm away).

CLINICAL PEARLS

- Hypothermia is more commonly due to ignorance rather than lack of equipment.
- Admission temperature is a strong predictor of morbidity, mortality, and quality of care.
- There is dose-response relationship with morbidity and mortality of hypothermia in preterm. **For every 1°C drop in temperature below 36.5°C in preterms, the risk of mortality increases by 28%.**

SUGGESTED READING

1. El-Radhi AS, Barry W. Thermometry in paediatric practice. Arch Dis Child. 2006;91(4):351-6.
2. Knobel R, Holditch-Davis D. Thermoregulation and heat loss prevention after birth and during neonatal intensive-care unit stabilization of extremely low-birthweight infants. J Obstet Gynecol Neonatal Nurs. 2007;36(3):280-7.
3. Laptook AR, Salhab W, Bhaskar B; Neonatal Research Network. Admission temperature of low birth weight infants: predictors and associated morbidities. Pediatrics. 2007;119(3):e643-9.
4. Mullany LC, Katz J, Khatry SK, et al. Risk of mortality associated with neonatal hypothermia in southern Nepal. Arch Pediatr Adolesc Med. 2010;164(7):650-6.

5. World Health Organization, Maternal and Newborn Health/Safe Motherhood. Thermal Protection of the Newborn: A Practical Guide. Geneva: 1997. World Health Organization; pp. 1-65.
6. World Health Organization. Pregnancy, Childbirth, Postpartum, and Neonatal Care: A Guide for Essential Practice. Geneva: World Health Organization; 2007.
7. Merenstein GB, Gardner SL. Handbook of Neonatal Intensive Care. St Louis: Mosby Elsevier, 2011; pp. 117-23.

CHAPTER 3

Respiratory Distress

Rhishikesh Thakre

DEFINITION

Respiratory distress is diagnosed if two or more signs are present:
- *Tachypnea:* Respiratory rate >60/min
- Grunt
- Work of breathing (e.g. subcostal, intercostal, supraclavicular, sternal indrawing, and flaring of alae nasi)
- Central cyanosis.

Note: Undress the baby and closely observe respiration. Count respiratory rate for 1 minute ensuring that the baby is quiet and normothermic. You are likely to make a mistake if the baby is crying.

IDENTIFY SEVERITY

- *Respiratory distress* is characterized by increased work of breathing.
- *Respiratory failure* is characterized by ineffective ventilation or oxygenation or both. It is characterized by abnormal respiratory rate (slow or fast) and worsening sensorium. It is a stage which left unattended may lead to respiratory arrest in short period of time.
- *Respiratory arrest* is no spontaneous breathing, cyanosis and nonresponsiveness. Apnea is periodic pause in breathing.

Note:
- Gasping respiration is labored, irregular breathing. It is a sign of respiratory failure.
- Presence of respiratory failure and respiratory arrest is life-threatening and immediate life-saving measures should be initiated skipping further evaluation.

Silverman Anderson Score (SAS) and Downe's score (Appendix) are two important clinical tools to assess the severity of respiratory distress. SAS is ideal for use in preterm infants and Downes score in term infants.

Oxygenation index (OI): Oxygen index is a good method to assess severity of respiratory distress in infants on mechanical ventilation or other respiratory support [OI = (Mean Airway Pressure × FiO_2)/PaO_2].

$AaDO_2$: Alveolar to arterial oxygen difference is also used as criteria for assessing the severity of respiratory distress.

ETIOLOGY

Respiratory distress in newborns is often due to lung and airway pathologies. Cardiac, neurological, and metabolic causes also may cause respiratory distress in newborn. History (Tables 1 and 2), onset and course of respiratory distress, clinical assessment (Tables 3 and 4),

SECTION 1
Clinical Approach to Sick Newborn

Table 1: Approach to respiratory distress—history.

History	Rationale
Onset	Timing of RD (age in hours) helps identify etiology. Onset within 6 hours of birth suggests birth process related cause. Late onset (>3 days) may suggest CHD. Abrupt onset suggests air leak or mechanical problem (tube block, tube displacement)
Duration	Short lasting suggests functional problem (TTNB, metabolic). Duration more than 2 weeks suggests chronic problem
Progress	Helps identify whether disease is the same, worsening or improving

(RD: respiratory distress; CHD: congenital heart disease; TTNB: transient tachypnea of newborn)

Table 2: Approach to respiratory distress—risk factors.

Ask for risk factors	Suggestive of
Worsening on bag and mask resuscitation	CDH, air leak
Prolonged labor, difficult labor, assisted delivery, fetal distress, meconium stained liquor	Asphyxial lung disease, MAS, birth injury
Elective cesarean section	TTNB
Maternal fever, foul liquor, prolonged labor, multiple per vaginal examinations, PROM >12 hours, PPROM, assisted delivery	Pneumonia, sepsis
No antenatal steroids to mother, infant of diabetic mother (IDM), Rh-isoimmunization, perinatal asphyxia	RDS
Polyhydramnios	CDH, TEF
Oligohydramnios	MAS, pulmonary hypoplasia
Maternal hypertension, preeclampsia	Asphyxia, MAS
Placenta previa or abruption	Shock
Family history of unexplained neonatal deaths, stillbirths	RDS, IDM, CHD, IEM
Post-feed worsening	GERD, isolated cleft palate, TEF, IEM
Relation with crying	Crying worsens cyanosis (CHD), crying relieves cyanosis (choanal atresia)
Chronic course, oxygen dependency	BPD, CHD (TAPVC), atypical infection (CMV, fungus, *Pneumocystis carinii*, chlamydia), Wilson- Mikity syndrome, Recurrent aspiration (GER, pharyngeal incoordination, H-shaped TOF), osteopenia of prematurity

(CDH: congenital diaphragmatic hernia; MAS: meconium aspiration syndrome; TTNB: transient tachypnea of newborn; PPROM: preterm premature rupture of the membrane; RDS: respiratory distress syndrome; TEF: tracheoesophageal fistula; IEM: inborn errors of metabolism; IDM: infant of diabetic mother; GERD: gastroesophageal reflux disease; CHD: congenital heart disease; BPD: bronchopulmonary dysplasia; TAPVC: total anomalous pulmonary venous connection; CMV: cytomegalovirus infection; GER: gastroesophageal reflux; TOF: tracheoesophageal fistula).

chest X-ray and 2D echocardiogram are useful in identifying the causes of respiratory distress (Tables 5 to 7 and Box 1).

History/Risk Factors/Focused Examination

See Table 1 to 3.

CHAPTER 3
Respiratory Distress

Table 3: Physical assessment.

Look	Rationale
Sensorium	Increased work of breathing in alert baby is respiratory distress and with worsening sensorium is respiratory failure. Abnormal sensorium is persistent irritability, lethargy or drowsiness
Color	Stable baby has color pink. Altered color [pale (anemia, shock)], plethora (polycythemia), dusky (cold stress, hypothermia, CHD, shock), cyanosis (cold stress, CHD, respiratory failure) gives clue to underlying problem
Tone/posture	A stable baby is active with good tone and responds to pain. Abnormal tone is reflected by posture (frog legged posture, extended posture) and suggests neurologic compromise
Response to touch	Nonresponsive to touch (e.g. Heel prick, IV insertion) is ominous
Cry	A stable baby has lusty cry. Weak, absent or shrill cry is ominous
Vital parameters (Temperature, HR, RR, BP, SpO_2)	To define the baseline status, to monitor the trend, to anticipate problems and identify complications
Work of breathing (e.g. Downe's score or Silverman-Anderson score)	To objectively define respiratory distress, monitor the trend and anticipate deterioration
Perfusion (HR, color, core-axillary temperature, CRT, urine output, BP)	To identify early shock. Monitor the trends. More the parameters abnormal, more is the possibility of shock. Fall in BP (hypotension) is late sign of shock and is ominous sign
Gestation	Preterms (<34 weeks) are at risk for RDS and rarely develop MAS. Post-terms are at risk for MAS. Late preterms (34–37 weeks) are vulnerable population
Weight	SGA and LGA are at risk for difficult delivery and MSAF
Danger signs (Grunt, cyanosis, worsening sensorium, apnea)	To identify life-threatening events and consider urgent transfer/ interventions

(HR: heart rate; RR: respiratory rate; BP: blood pressure; SGA: small for gestational age; LGA: large for gestational age; MSAF: meconium-stained amniotic fluid; CRT: capillary refill time)

Table 4: Systematic evaluation.

Inspection	
SGA	MAS, asphyxia, polycythemia
LGA	Birth trauma, asphyxia, polycythemia, RDS, CHD, hypoglycemia
Potter facies	Hypoplastic lungs
Barrel chest	MAS
Large caput, bruises	Difficult labor, prolonged labor predisposes to asphyxia
Frothing at mouth	Tracheoesophageal fistula
Meconium staining	MAS
Pallor	Anemia, shock
Plethora	Polycythemia
Cyanosis	CHD, severe lung disease, shunt, abnormal hemoglobin, air leak

Contd...

Contd…

Inspection	
Murmur, hepatomegaly, cardiomegaly, abnormal pulses, differential cyanosis	CHD, shunt
Fever, hypothermia, cold stress, umbilical sepsis, foul smell, pustules, discharge, petechiae, bleeding tendency, sclerema	Sepsis, pneumonia
Twins	Twin-to-twin transfusion
Inability to pass orogastric tube	TEF
Isolated cleft palate	Aspiration syndrome
Scaphoid abdomen, distal heart sounds, shift of heart sounds, ipsilateral decreased air entry	CDH
Temperature instability, core periphery temperature difference >3°C	Pneumonia
Absent femorals	Coarctation of aorta
Cardiomegaly	CHD, cardiomyopathy
Palpation: Tracheal deviation, displaced apical beat, thrill	
Auscultation: Assess air entry, breath sounds, adventitious sounds	

(SGA: small for gestational age; LGA: large for gestational age; MAS: meconium aspiration syndrome; RDS: respiratory distress syndrome; CHD: congenital heart disease; TEF: tracheoesophageal fistula).

Table 5: Interpreting pulse oximetry.

Neonate	Pulse oximeter	Interpretation
Well	Low	Check probe placement
Dusky	Normal	Cold stress, abnormal hemoglobin
Tachypnea/RD	<90% in room air	Hypoxia
Tachypnea/RD	Labile (Desaturates on crying or activity)	Shunt, PPHN
Tachypnea/RD	UL > LL (>10)	PPHN, shunt
Tachypnea/RD	LL > UL	TGA
Tachypnea/RD	No improvement	Shunt, PPHN

(PPHN: persistent pulmonary hypertension of the newborn; RD: respiratory distress; UL: upper limb; LL: lower limb)

Table 6: Differentiating respiratory and cardiac cause of respiratory distress.

	RS	CVS
Breathing	Retractions	Tachypnea
Cardiac evaluation	Normal	Gallop, weak pulses, hepatomegaly, absent femorals
Second heart sound	Split	Single
X-ray chest	Parenchymal lesion	Shape, size of heart abnormal, abnormal pulmonary vasculature
pCO_2	High	Low
Pulse oximeter	Improvement with oxygen	Not much improvement with oxygen, differential cyanosis
Hyperoxia test	PaO_2 >300 mm Hg rules out cardiac disease	PaO_2 does not >150 mm Hg

(RS: respiratory system; CVS: cardiovascular system)

Table 7: Identifying the lung pathology.

Isolated tachypnea	CHD, metabolic acidosis, anemia, hypoglycemia, temperature instability, renal failure
Grunt	Alveolar lung disease (e.g. RDS, pneumonia, MAS)
Stridor	Upper airway obstruction, laryngotracheomalacia
Cyanosis	CHD, severe lung disease, polycythemia, abnormal hemoglobin, CNS dysfunction

(CHD: congenital heart disease; RDS: respiratory distress syndrome; MAS: meconium aspiration syndrome; CNS: central nervous system)

Box 1: Clues to congenital heart disease.

- Cyanosis disproportionate to clinical status
- Differential cyanosis (UL saturation >LL saturation)
- Second heart sound—single
- Murmur
- Isolated hepatomegaly
- Sudden deterioration
- Lack of response to oxygen

(UL: upper limb, LL: lower limb)

INVESTIGATIONS (FOR ALL NEWBORNS WITH RESPIRATORY DISTRESS)

Hemoglobin (Hb)
- Hemoglobin <12 mg% suggests anemia
- Hematocrit >65% suggests polycythemia
- Drop in hemoglobin, 6–12 hours apart suggests antepartum hemorrhage.

Blood Sugar
- Blood sugar <40 mg% is hypoglycemia
- Target sugar at 50–150 mg%
- Management is initiated by glucostix and confirmed by blood sample.

Sepsis Screen
- It includes TLC, ANC, IT ratio, CRP, and ESR
- Two or more parameters, if abnormal, suggest positive sepsis screen
- Negative sepsis screen 24–48 hours apart rules out infection
- It is not a substitute to blood culture
- It should be done only if on history and clinical course one is unable to identify etiology if the newborn is sick.

Blood Culture
- It is gold standard for bacterial infection
- It should be drawn first if antibiotics are initiated
- It helps to identify duration and choice of antibiotic.

X-ray Chest
- It is indicated in all cases with respiratory distress (RD), suspected congenital heart disease (CHD), suspected air leak, and acute deterioration
- Look for lung volume, unilateral or bilateral lung disease, symmetric or asymmetric lesion and focal or diffuse lung pathology (Table 8).

Arterial Blood Gas
- It is indicated for silent tachypnea, worsening RD, shock or sensorium
- It identifies oxygenation (O_2) or ventilation (CO_2) or metabolic problem
- Look at the trend rather than one value
- Interpret pO_2 with oxygen therapy
- Interpret arterial blood gas (ABG) in light of clinical status.

Role of Imaging
Role of US Chest
- Diagnosing pleural diseases

Table 8: Radiological signs and etiology.

Radiological signs	Etiology
Low lung volume	RDS, pulmonary hypoplasia
High lung volume	MAS, TTNB, cystic lung disease, hyperventilation
Air bronchograms	RDS, pneumonia
Diffuse parenchymal infiltrates	TTN, MAS, pneumonia
Lobar consolidation	Pneumonia, CLE, CCAM
Pleural effusion	Pneumonia, pulmonary lymphangiectasia
Reticular granular pattern	RDS, pneumonia
Hyperinflation	TTN, MAS, pulmonary lymphangiectasia
Fluid accumulations in interlobar spaces	TTN, pulmonary lymphangiectasia
Cystic mass	CCAM, CDH, pulmonary sequestration
Pneumothorax/pneumomediastinum	Spontaneous, MAS, RDS, pneumonia

(RDS: respiratory distress syndrome; MAS: meconium aspiration syndrome; TTNB or TTN: transient tachypnea of newborn; CLE: congenital lobar emphysema; CCAM: congenital cystic adenomatoid malformation).

- Distinction of solid from cystic intrathoracic masses
- Evaluation of diaphragmatic excursion.

Role of CT Thorax
- Determination of anatomical sites of areas of cystic change
- Evaluation of mediastinal masses and their relationship to normal vascular structures
- Suspected vascular ring or sling with airway obstruction.

Role of 2D Echo
- To identify structural or functional heart disease
- Bedside assessment of perfusion, contractility and end diastolic area for cardiac function.

Box 2: Common and uncommon causes of respiratory distress (RD).

Most common causes of RD (in order of incidence):
- Transient tachypnea of the newborn
- Respiratory distress syndrome
- Meconium aspiration syndrome

Less common but significant causes:
- Infection (e.g. pneumonia, sepsis)
- Nonpulmonary causes (e.g. anemia, congenital heart disease, congenital malformation, medications, neurologic or metabolic abnormalities, polycythemia, upper airway obstruction)
- Persistent pulmonary hypertension of the newborn
- Pneumothorax

Role of MRI Chest
- Pulmonary sequestration (to show the vascular supply from below diaphragm, as well as the relationship of the sequestration to the diaphragm)
- Evaluation of presence and size of the pulmonary arteries when they cannot be delineated by cardiac catheterization or echocardiography (Box 2).

MANAGEMENT OF RESPIRATORY DISTRESS

It involves the supportive care, which is common to all newborns with respiratory distress and specific care, which is etiology specific.

Supportive Care
Thermal Care
- Ensure normothermia (36.5–37.5°C)
- Avoid cold stress, hypo- and hyperthermia
- Ensure skin temperature at 36.5°C under warmer during first week of life
- Minimize evaporative losses in <32 weeks
- Set temperature alarms.

CHAPTER 3
Respiratory Distress

Oxygen
- Oxygen may be administered by nasal prongs, nasopharyngeal or oxygen hood
- With respiratory distress, initiate by nasal prongs and with impending respiratory failure start with 100% oxygen by hood at 10 L/min
- Use humidified oxygen
- Avoid hypo- and hyperoxia
- Monitor SPO_2. Target SPO_2 to 90–95%
- Set pulse oximeter alarms.

Nursing
- Minimal handling
- Allow baby to be in position of maximum comfort
- Ensure airway is clear. Suction if visible secretions
- Use pain-control measures like touch, swaddling, sucrose for IV insertion, pricks for blood collection, and gastric tube insertion
- Club nursing procedures together
- Document all interventions.

IV Fluids
- Ensure adequate hydration
- No routine restriction of fluids
- Avoid fluid overload
- Monitor perfusion, glucose, and urine output.

Nutrition
- Nil by mouth (NBM) during the unstable phase
- Trophic feeds as early as feasible
- Gastric feeds once stable with graded increments
- Consider parenteral nutrition if NBM >72 hours.

Antibiotics
- No prophylactic antibiotics
- Start if infection cannot be ruled out
- Cover gram positive/negative organisms with broad-spectrum antibiotics
- Have an exit policy based on clinical course, sepsis screen, and blood culture.

Pressors
- Consider if the shock is fluid resistant
- Dopamine is the drug of choice
- Dobutamine is preferred if there is myocardial involvement
- Consider increments of 4 g/kg/min based on clinical response.

Infection Control
- Use disposables where indicated
- Ensure strict asepsis
- Handwashing before and after every baby contact
- Human milk-feeding as preferred feeds
- Minimize pricks. Maintain skin integrity
- Minimize duration of antibiotics
- Minimize duration of central lines, parenteral nutrition, and ventilation
- Have an audit of infection-control measures periodically.

Monitoring
- Assess sensorium, vital parameters, respiratory status, and perfusion periodically
- Review investigations and clinical course to plan action.

Indication for Respiratory Support
- Continuous positive airway pressure:
  – Preterm <35 weeks within the first 6 hours of birth:
    ◆ Respiratory distress (tachypnea, retractions, grunt—any 2 of the 3) or

- Any preterm <35 weeks:
  - SAS >3
- Term and late preterm infant
  - SAS >5 or Downes score >5.
- Noninvasive mechanical ventilation (NIMV) or mechanical ventilation:
  - *Impending respiratory failure:* Gasping or poor respiratory efforts
  - Respiratory failure [severe distress on continuous positive airway pressure (CPAP) with FiO_2 >70% and CPAP pressure >7 cm of water, PaO_2 <50 and $PaCO_2$ >50 and pH <7.20]
  - Cardiopulmonary failure
  - Recurrent apnea.

Referral Criterion in Office Practices

- Inability to maintain SpO_2 >90% in room air
- Worsening sensorium
- RD with poor circulation
- Worsening SAS or Downes score
- SAS or Downes score >7.

Note: In utero transfer of "High-Risk" or Early ex utero is preferable. Only after stabilization of general status and under supervision.

Ineffective or Potentially Harmful Practices

- Prophylactic surfactant for respiratory distress syndrome (RDS)
- Prophylactic CPAP for RDS
- Routine sodabicarb
- Alkali drip for persistent pulmonary hypertension of the newborn (PPHN)
- Hyperventilation for PPHN.

APPENDIX

QUANTIFY RESPIRATORY DISTRESS (TABLES A1 and A2 and FLOWCHART A1)

Table A1: *Silverman Anderson score* for preterms.

	Upper chest retraction	Lower chest retraction	Xiphoid retraction	Nares dilatation	Expiratory grunt
Grade 0	Synchronized	None	None	None	None
Grade 1	Lags on inspiration	Just visible	Just visible	Minimal	On stethoscope
Grade 2	See saw	Marked	Marked	Marked	Audible

Table A2: *Downe's score* for term infants.

	RR	Retractions	Cyanosis	Grunt	Air entry
Score 0	<60	None	None	None	Equal
Score 1	60–80	Mild to moderate	Room air	On stethoscope	Decreased
Score 2	>80	Severe	On FiO_2 >40%	Audible	Absent

(RR: respiratory rate).
Note: Interpret scores with the sensorium. An improving score with alert newborn suggests improvement. An improving score with worsening sensorium suggests deterioration. One time assessment is not enough. Look at the trends every hour to grade the respiratory status.

CHAPTER 3
Respiratory Distress

Flowchart A1: Algorithm for respiratory distress.

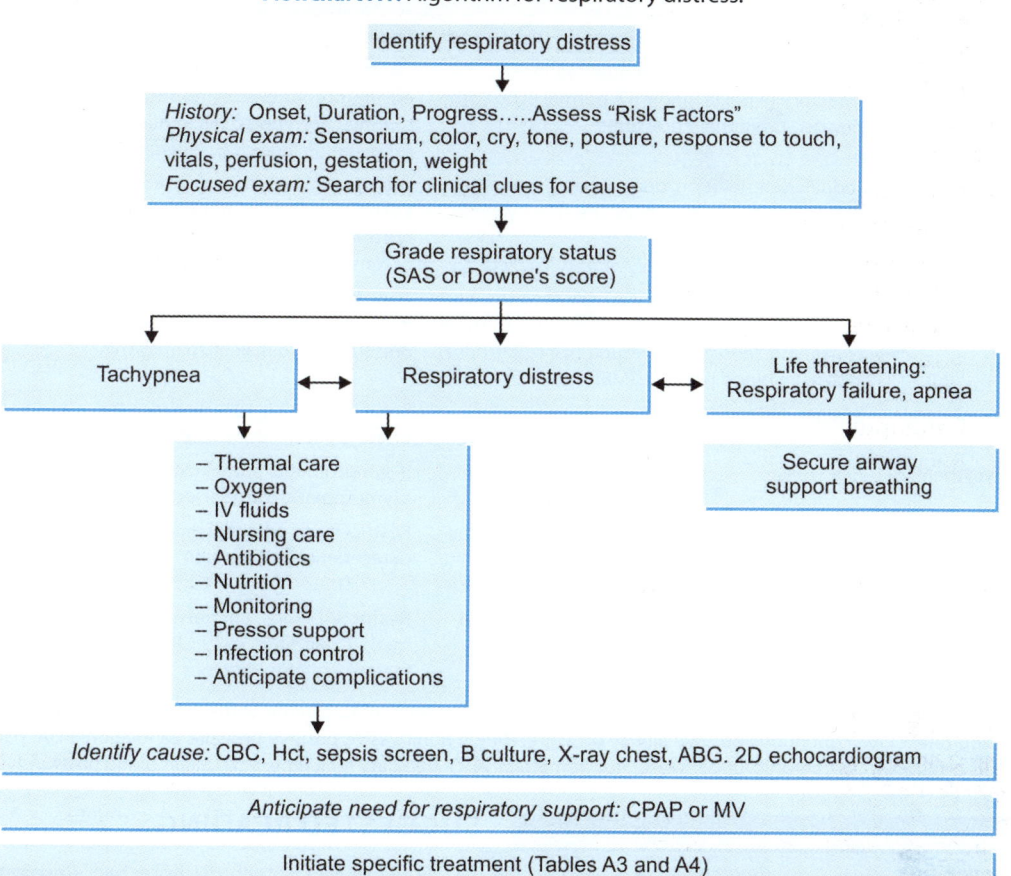

(SAS: Silverman-Anderson score).

Preterm with RD		
Initiate: Thermal care, oxygen, IV fluids, nursing care, antibiotics, nutrition, monitoring, infection control, anticipate complications		
Identify cause: CBC, Hct, sepsis screen, B culture, X-ray chest, ABG		
Silverman anderson score <3	**Silverman-Anderson score 4–6**	**Silverman-Anderson score >7**
Oxygen	Early CPAP	Exit from CPAP
	If FiO$_2$ >0.3, consider surfactant (INSURE)	If apnea, FiO$_2$ >0.7, CPAP pressure >7, respiratory failure = Consider intubation and ventilation

Table A3: Special issues and specific therapy.

Complications	Suspect	Treatment
PPHN	Labile oxygenation, differential cyanosis, refractory hypoxia, single S2, normal echo with elevated pulmonary pressures	Gentle ventilation, minimal handling, sedation, ensure normotension, normoglycemia, normothermia, normoelectrolytemia, antibiotics, track oxygenation index (OI), sildenafil
Air leak	Sudden deterioration, decreased air entry with shift of heart sounds to opposite side, cyanosis	Diagnostic tap in 2nd intercostals space on suspected side. Check for displaced tube, obstructed tube, if intubated. Air leak on ventilator or tension pneumothorax need ICD
Shock	Tachycardia, tachypnea, CRT >3 seconds, core axillary Temperature >2°C, cool extremities, Worsening sensorium, oliguria (<1 cc/kg/hour), low mean blood pressure (MBP)	10 cc/kg normal saline over 15–30 minutes, repeat if required, inotropes (titrate dopamine and or dobutamine to max of 20 g/kg/min)
Hypoglycemia	B Sugar <40 mg%	Bolus of 2 cc/kg 10% dextrose if symptomatic, titrate glucose infusion rate GIR), monitor sugar
Polycythemia	Hct >65%	If symptomatic, partial exchange transfusion, if asymptomatic consider extra fluids and reassess
PDA	Increasing oxygen requirement, unexplained metabolic acidosis, increasing ventilator requirement, murmur, bounding pulses	Restrict fluids, a dose of diuretic, indomethacin or paracetamol or ibuprofen
CLD	Oxygen dependency 28 days or more, clinical evidence of RD, radiology abnormality	Restricted fluids, enteral—parenteral nutrition, methyl xanthines, early CPAP/NIPPV + early surfactant, steroids, diuretics

(PPHN: persistent pulmonary hypertension of the newborn; ICD: implantable cardioverter-defibrillator; GIR: glucose infusion rate; CPAP: continuous positive airway pressure; NIPPV: noninvasive positive pressure ventilation; PDA: patent ductus arteriosus; CLD: chronic lung disease; Hct: hematocrit; CRT: Capillary refill time; MBP: Mean blood pressure)

Table A4: Specific treatment.

Condition	Treatment
Pneumonia	Antibiotics, MV
RDS	Surfactant, CPAP, MV
Air leak	Intercostal drain
Polycythemia	Partial exchange transfusion
Anemia	PCV transfusion
Shock	Fluid bolus, inotropes, steroids
CCF	Digoxin
Unexplained deterioration	Prostaglandin
TEF	Emergency surgery
CDH, CLE, CCAM, cleft palate	Elective surgery
Refractory hypoxia	HFV, iNO, ECMO

(RDS: respiratory distress syndrome; MV: mechanical ventilation; CPAP: continuous positive airway pressure; CCF: congestive cardiac failure; PCV: packed cell volume; CLE: congenital lobar emphysema; CCAM: congenital cystic adenomatoid malformation; HFV: high-frequency ventilation; iNO: inhaled nitric oxide; ECMO: extracorporeal membrane oxygenation; CHD: congenital heart disease; TEF: tracheoesophageal fistula).

SUGGESTED READING

1. Edwards MO, Kotecha SJ, Kotecha S. Respiratory distress of the term newborn infant. Paediatr Respir Rev. 2013;14:29-37.
2. Hany Aly. Respiratory disorders in the newborn: identification and diagnosis. Pediatr in Rev. 2004;25(6):201-8.
3. Hermansen CL, Lorah KN. Respiratory distress in the newborn. Am Fam Physician. 2007;76: 987-94.
4. Warren JB, Anderson JM. Newborn respiratory disorders. Pediatr in Rev. 2010;31:487-96.

CHAPTER 4

Neonatal Shock

Vinay Mishra, Preetha Joshi, Vinay Joshi

DEFINITION

Shock is a state of acute circulatory failure resulting in decreased tissue and organ perfusion which leads to depletion of oxygen and substrate in the cells. When this happens, anaerobic metabolism sets in, leading to accumulation of toxic waste products eventually causing cell death.

PHASES OF SHOCK

Shock is a progressive dynamic disorder which evolves over three phases—compensated, uncompensated, and irreversible.

Compensated Shock

In compensated shock, perfusion to vital organs, such as the brain, heart, and adrenal glands, is preserved. Clinical signs include pallor, tachycardia, cool extremities, and delayed capillary refill time (>3 sec) (Table 1).

Uncompensated Shock

During uncompensated shock, delivery of oxygen and nutrients to tissues becomes marginal or insufficient to meet demands. Clinical signs include hypotension, delayed capillary refill time, tachycardia, cold skin, tachypnea, and decreased or absent urine output (Table 1).

Table 1: Phases of shock.

	Compensated	Decompensated
Pulse	Tachycardia	Marked tachycardia; can arrest
Skin	White, cool, moist	White, "waxy", cold, marked diaphoresis
BP	Normal	Hypotension
Level of consciousness	Unaltered	Altered, ranging from drowsy to coma

Irreversible Shock

Irreversible shock is a retrospective diagnosis. Despite adequate resuscitation of circulation multiorgan damage sets in and ultimately leads to death.

> It may take hours for a compensated shock to become uncompensated shock but it takes few minutes for an uncompensated shock to become irreversible shock.

ROLE OF BLOOD PRESSURE IN SHOCK

There is currently no consensus on the best method to measure blood pressure in all cases. Invasive blood pressure measurement is widely accepted as the optimum method and its use is restricted to critically ill and those in refractory shock.

Oscillometric method is a noninvasive technique which serves as a surrogate marker. The measurements are taken with the infant in a comfortable position, using an appropriate size and position of cuff and in a restful state. The clinician should evaluate BP measurements within the context of the infant's history and current clinical assessment.

Full assessment of systemic blood flows and an individual baby's hemodynamic status is possible with fECHO for diagnosis and monitoring treatment.

- Hypotension is defined as mean arterial blood pressure less than the 10th centile for gestation/birth weight and postnatal age OR
- Mean arterial blood pressure in millimeters of mercury at or lesser than the mean gestational age in weeks. However, it is worth noting that this is only valid in the first 48 hours of life
- Hypotension is a late sign of shock

The variation in time (trend monitoring) might possibly be more informative than individual, static values. There is no research that has shown either technique for detection and management of BP leads to change in important clinical outcomes.

TYPES OF SHOCK

Many conditions and pathophysiologic disturbances are associated with shock and hypotension. Causes of neonatal shock are shown in Table 2.

EVALUATION OF A NEWBORN WITH SHOCK

Clinical manifestations of shock and hypotension are depicted in Table 3. But none of these alone can be used to diagnose shock. More the parameters affected, more is the likelihood of shock.

Diagnosis: Table 4 depicts certain clues which can help in diagnosing the type of shock and further management.

Table 2: Types of shock and causes of neonatal shock.

Sr. No.	Types	Causes
1.	Cardiogenic	Perinatal asphyxia, congenital heart disease, cardiomyopathy (IDM), heart failure, arrhythmias, or myocardial ischemia, bacterial toxins
2.	Hypovolemic	Acute blood loss—antepartum hemorrhage, umbilical cord accidents, traumatic birth, twin-to-twin transfusion, perioperative, IVH
3.	Distributive	Sepsis, vasodilators, myocardial depression, or endothelial injury
4.	Obstructive	Inflow obstructions: • TAPVR • Acquired inflow obstructions—air or thrombotic embolus • Increased intrathoracic pressure caused by high airway pressures or air-leak syndromes (e.g. pneumothorax) Outflow obstructions: • Pulmonary stenosis or atresia/aortic stenosis or atresia • Hypertrophic subaortic stenosis (IDM) • Coarctation of the aorta
5.	Dissociative	Profound anemia or methemoglobinemia

CHAPTER 4
Neonatal Shock

Table 3: Clinical manifestations of shock and hypotension.

Sr. No.	Parameter	Comments
1	Color	Subjective, influenced by light, skin temperature, race, hemoglobin status
2	Capillary refill time (CRT)	The normal range is <3 sec Subjective, may be delayed if there is hypothermia For most reliable assessment, base of the sternum is preferred
3	Central-peripheral temperature difference	Under normal conditions, core peripheral temperature difference is <2°C. If it is more than 3°C sepsis needs to be ruled out It is influence by body temperature, environmental temperature and the use of vasoactive drugs
4	Blood pressure	Hypotension suggests decompensated shock. It is a late sign BP is determined by cardiac output and systemic vascular resistance
5	Heart rate	Tachycardia may be seen with fever, anemia, pain, agitation, cry, bleeding, drugs, cardiac failure or arrhythmia. It influences the cardiac output and myocardial perfusion
6	Urine output	Denotes renal perfusion. It is a late marker. Oliguria is urine output <1 cc/kg/hr

Table 4: Clues which can help in diagnosing the type of shock and further management.

Hypovolemic shock: Insufficient circulatory blood volume

Causes	Clinical clues

• **Blood Loss:** Perinatal history
  – APH - Placental abruption/previa.
  – Uterine rupture
  – IVH
  – Pulmonary hemorrhage
  – DIC
	Pallor
	
	Bulging fontanelle
	ETT bleed

• **Plasma Loss**
  – Low oncotic pressure
  – Capillary leak
	Hydrops
	Sepsis

• **ECF Loss** – Insensible water loss	Extreme prematurity Gastroschisis Excessive weight loss Epidermolysis bullosa

Cardiogenic shock: Insufficient cardiac output, despite, sufficient blood volume in the ventricles d/t pump failure

– Myocardial dysfunction – IDM – Sepsis – Arrhythmia – Heart rate more than 220	Perinatal asphyxia ECG rhythm disturbances

• **Obstructive shock:** Obstruction to blood flow
  – Tension pneumothorax, pneumomediastinum CO_2 retention
  – Pulm atresia/stenosis
  – Obstruct TA, MA, TAPVC
	Hyper-expanded chest
	Reduced air entry
	Hyperoxia test

• **Distributive shock**
  – Peripheral vasodilatation
  – Sepsis
  – Supportive evidence
  – Drugs and neurogenic
	Wide pulse pressure

Contd...

SECTION 1
Clinical Approach to Sick Newborn

Contd...

Parameters	Cardiogenic	Hypovolemic	Early septic (warm)	Late septic (cold)
Blood pressure	Low	Low	Low	Low
CVP	High	Low	Normal	High
Pulse pressure	Decreased	Decreased	Normal	Decreased
Systemic vascular resistance	High	High	Low	High
Cardiac output	Low	Low	High/normal	Low
Core to peripheral skin temperature difference	Increased	Increased	Normal/decreased	Increased

INVESTIGATIONS AND MONITORING

- Continuous vitals monitoring should include heart rate to look for tachycardia and blood pressure for hypotension.
- Monitoring of perfusion and sensorium.
- Invasive intra-arterial blood pressure monitoring is preferred over noninvasive blood pressure, for the need of accuracy.
- Hourly urine output, preferably by placing a urinary catheter is an objective method to evaluate organ specific hypoperfusion.

Investigations:
- Complete blood count to look for anemia
- Total and differential white blood cell (WBC) counts
- C-reactive protein (CRP) and blood culture
- Blood sugar
- Blood grouping and cross matching
- Serum glutamic-pyruvic transaminase (SGPT)
- BUN and creatinine
- Creatine kinase-muscle/brain (CPK-MB)
- Coagulation profile assessment of organ perfusion
- Arterial blood gas (ABG)—assessment of acid-base status
- Serum lactate.
- Echocardiography and Doppler flow velocimetry—assessment of myocardial function and cardiac anatomy
- Inferior vena cava (IVC) collapsibility

Superior vena cava (SVC) flow in newborn infants has been reported to be a novel marker of systemic blood flow. Low SVC flow (<40 mL/kg/min) has been used to diagnose hypotension and to predict long-term outcome.

TREATMENT APPROACH

Appropriate supportive measures must be instituted as soon as possible including securing a patent airway, providing supplemental oxygen and positive-pressure ventilation, achieving intravascular or intraosseous access, and infusing 10 mL/kg of colloid or crystalloid (to repeat the same volume if needed).

Use of crystalloid or colloid solutions is appropriate unless the source of hypovolemia is hemorrhage, in which case whole or reconstituted blood is more appropriate.

First dose of broad spectrum antibiotic should be given as early as possible after collecting the blood culture if any infection is suspected.

Correction of negative inotropic factors such as hypoxia, acidosis, hypoglycemia, hypocalcemia, and other metabolic derangements will improve cardiac output.

There are three crucial steps in management of neonatal shock:
1. Optimize preload by volume expanders.
2. Improve cardiac contractility and vascular tone with the use of catecholamines.
3. Consider, case by case, use of steroids.

(Flowcharts 1 to 3).

Step 1: Volume Expanders—Practice Points

Fluid boluses are used only when there is evidence of hemorrhage or fluid loss. An

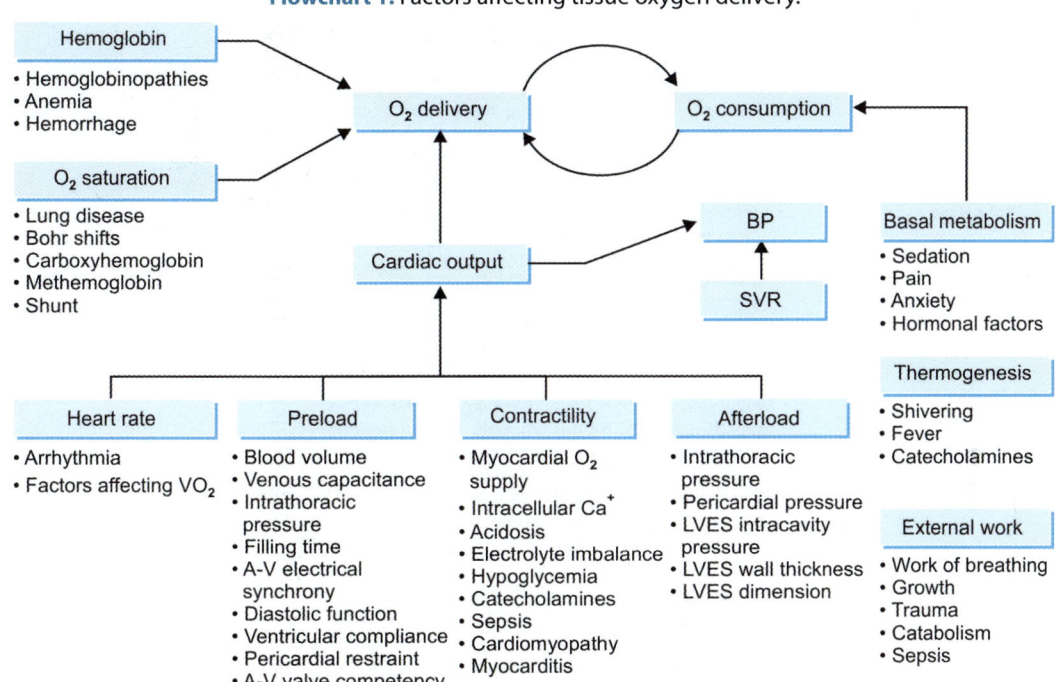

Flowchart 1: Factors affecting tissue oxygen delivery.

infusion of 10–20 mL/kg isotonic saline solution over 30 minutes is used to treat suspected hypovolemia if hematocrits more than 40% and cardiogenic process unlikely.

Routine use of volume expanders is not warranted as it may cause more harm than benefit.

Crystalloids are preferred over colloids in management of shock (compared in terms of cost, availability, safety, and effective therapeutic outcome).

Step 2: Use of Catecholamine

Despite adequate volume restoration, myocardial contractility and vascular tone may still be compromised due to the prior poor myocardial perfusion. In this scenario, inotropic agents and intensive monitoring may need to be continued. Knowledge about action and effects of inotropes helps in judicious use in appropriate situations (Table 5).

Dopamine, norepinephrine, and vasopressin are used to improve the systemic vascular resistance while dobutamine and milrinone are used to improve myocardial function.

In premature infants younger than 30 weeks' gestation, poor cardiac contractility is most common and they benefit from early institution of dobutamine.

Patients with septic shock benefit from dopamine as first-line management; it has been found to be more effective than dobutamine in correcting blood pressure for short-term treatment in these situations; however, the effect of these drugs on long-term outcome is unknown. Although adrenaline is used for cardiovascular compromise, its effect on mortality and morbidity has not yet been evaluated.

Evidence suggests that milrinone is not beneficial particularly in prevention of low systemic blood flow in ill, very-preterm

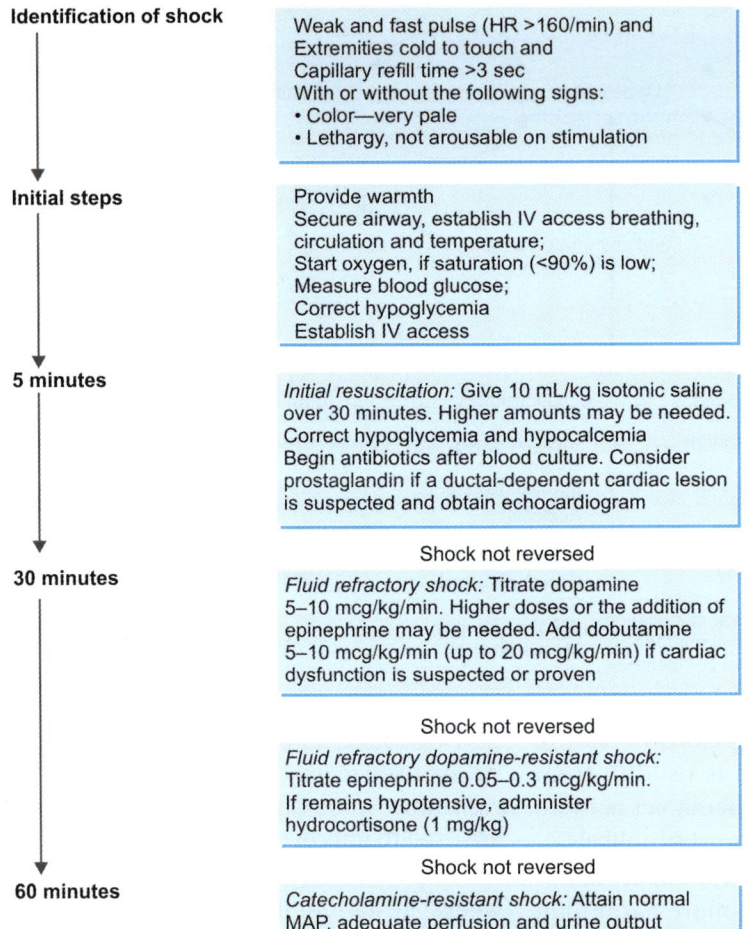

Flowchart 2: Suggested treatment algorithm for preterm.

Identification of shock
Weak and fast pulse (HR >160/min) and
Extremities cold to touch and
Capillary refill time >3 sec
With or without the following signs:
- Color—very pale
- Lethargy, not arousable on stimulation

Initial steps
Provide warmth
Secure airway, establish IV access breathing, circulation and temperature;
Start oxygen, if saturation (<90%) is low;
Measure blood glucose;
Correct hypoglycemia
Establish IV access

5 minutes
Initial resuscitation: Give 10 mL/kg isotonic saline over 30 minutes. Higher amounts may be needed.
Correct hypoglycemia and hypocalcemia
Begin antibiotics after blood culture. Consider prostaglandin if a ductal-dependent cardiac lesion is suspected and obtain echocardiogram

Shock not reversed

30 minutes
Fluid refractory shock: Titrate dopamine 5–10 mcg/kg/min. Higher doses or the addition of epinephrine may be needed. Add dobutamine 5–10 mcg/kg/min (up to 20 mcg/kg/min) if cardiac dysfunction is suspected or proven

Shock not reversed

Fluid refractory dopamine-resistant shock: Titrate epinephrine 0.05–0.3 mcg/kg/min.
If remains hypotensive, administer hydrocortisone (1 mg/kg)

Shock not reversed

60 minutes
Catecholamine-resistant shock: Attain normal MAP, adequate perfusion and urine output

Shock not reversed

Shock with normal BP and evidence of poor LV function: Consider milrinone (if normal renal function)

Cold shock with low BP and evidence of RV dysfunction: If PPHN, consider milrinone (if normal renal function)

Warm shock with low BP: Consider vasopressin or terlipressin in conjunction with inotropes

Refractory shock: Rule out and correct pericardial effusion, pneumothorax. Consider IVIG and closing PDA if hemodynamically significant

(HR: heart rate; BP: blood pressure; MAP: mean arterial pressure; LV: left ventricle; RV: right ventricle; PPHN: persistent pulmonary hypertension of the newborn; IVIg: intravenous immunoglobulin; PDA: patent ductus arteriosus; IV: intravenous; ECMO: extracorporeal membrane oxygenation).

CHAPTER 4
Neonatal Shock

Flowchart 3: Treatment algorithm for term newborns.

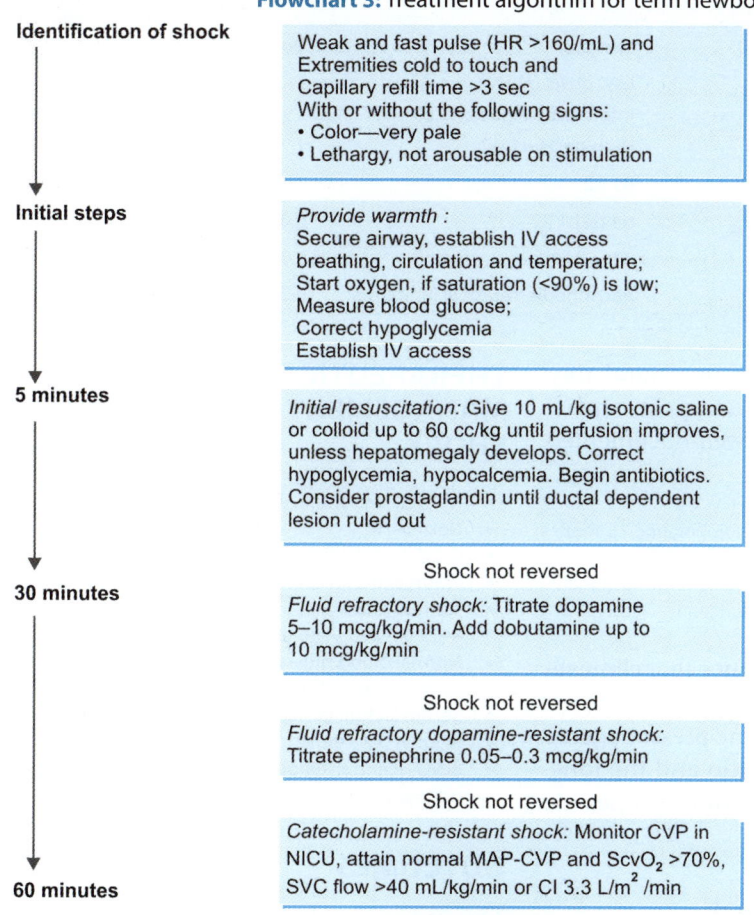

(CVP: central venous pressure; MAP: mean arterial pressure; $ScvO_2$: central venous oxygen saturation; SVC: superior vena cava; CI: cardiac index; VLBW: very low birth weight; PDA: patent ductus arteriosus; PPHN: persistent pulmonary hypertension of the newborn; ECMO: extracorporeal membrane oxygenation.

Table 5: Drugs in neonatal shock.

Sr. No.	Inotrope	Receptor	Dose
1.	Dopamine	Low dose: D1 D2 Intermediate dose: $\beta 1\ \beta 2$ High dose: $\alpha 1\ \alpha 2$	3–20 mcg/kg/min
2.	Dobutamine	$\beta 1\ \beta 2$	3–20 mcg/kg/min
3.	Epinephrine	$\alpha 1\ \alpha 2 \beta 1\ \beta 2$	0.05–0.1 mcg/kg/min
4.	Norepinephrine	$\alpha 1\ \alpha 2\ \beta 1\ \beta 2$	0.05–0.1 mcg/kg/min
5.	Milrinone	Phosphodiesterase III inhibitors	0.25–1 mcg/kg/min

neonates during the first postnatal day. However, use of milrinone in post-cardiac surgery as lusitropic agent is well-documented.

> **Tip:**
> - Dopamine should be the first choice inotrope if short-term improvement in blood pressure is the goal.
> - Dobutamine could be considered as a first line if there is documented myocardial dysfunction.

There is paucity of evidence that clinically important outcomes are improved by the use of any of these catecholamine pressor agents. The clinical risk/benefit ratio and the long-term consequences of use of inotropes are uncertain.

Step 3: Steroids in Shock

Use of steroids should be limited to catecholamine resistant shock states. The dose of hydrocortisone for refractory hypotension is 1–2 mg/kg/dose. If efficacy is noted, the dose can be repeated every 8–12 hours for 2–3 days, especially if low serum cortisol levels are documented before hydrocortisone treatment. There is no consensus on the choice, dose, and duration of steroid use.

THERAPEUTIC TARGETS IN THE MANAGEMENT OF NEONATAL SHOCK

- Normal sensorium, alertness
- Normal HR
- Capillary refill time <2 sec
- Warm extremities
- Normal CVP
  8–12 cm and ventilated 12–15 cm
- Normal blood pressure (age and sex)
- Urine output >1 mL/kg/hr
- Serum lactate (<1.2 mmol/L)
- Normal base deficit
- $ScvO_2$ (central venous O_2 saturation) >70 (usually not measured in neonates)

OUTCOMES

The outcome of shock in the newborns is guarded. The various factors associated with poor outcome are refractory shock, acute renal failure, neutropenia, deranged coagulation profile, and metabolic acidosis.

SUGGESTED READING

1. ACCCM consensus guidelines for treatment of shock in term infants and suggested modifications for preterm infants.

2. Carcillo JA, Fields AI; American College of Critical Care Medicine Task Force Committee Members. Clinical practice parameters for hemodynamic support of pediatric and neonatal patients in septic shock. Crit Care Med. 2002;30(6):1365-78.
3. Decembrino L, Ruffinazzi G, D'Angelo A, et al. Septic Shock in Neonates. In: Decembrino L, Angelo AD (Eds) Severe Sepsis and Septic Shock - Understanding a Serious Killer. Italy; 2012. pp. 285-308.
4. Fleer A, Krediet TG. Innate immunity: toll-like receptors and some more. A brief history, basic organization and relevance for the human newborn. Neonatology. 2007;92(3):145-57.
5. Goldstein B, Giroir B, Randolph A; International Consensus Conference on Pediatric Sepsis. International pediatric sepsis consensus conference: definitions for sepsis and organ dysfunction in pediatrics. Pediatr Crit Care Med. 2005;6(1):2-8.
6. Kluckow M, Evans N. Superior vena cava flow in newborn infants: a novel marker of systemic blood flow. Arch Dis Child Fetal Neonatal ED. 2000;82(3):F182-7.
7. Tibby SM, Murdoch IA. Monitoring cardiac function in intensive care. Arch Dis Child. 2003; 88(1):46-52.
8. Wynn JL, Wong HR. Pathophysiology and treatment of septic shock in neonates. Clin Perinatol. 2010;37(2):437-79.

CHAPTER

Suspected Infection

Anuradha Bansal, Deepak Chawla

INTRODUCTION

Evaluating a neonate presenting with suspected infection is one of the most difficult diagnostic challenges in neonatology. Clinical features of infection in a neonate are nonspecific and may be caused by noninfectious pathologies like metabolic derangements, electrolyte imbalance or hypothermia. Instituting treatment for sepsis without careful clinical and laboratory evaluation can result in overuse of antibiotics and emergence of multidrug resistant bacteria. On the other hand, due to high fatality rate associated with sepsis, missing diagnosis of sepsis and delaying the start of specific therapy can have grave consequences.

This protocol includes approach to diagnosis and management of neonatal sepsis which is defined as clinical syndrome characterized by systemic signs of infection and bacteremia in first month of life. It includes both systemic and deep seated localized infections, viz. septicemia, meningitis, urinary tract infection (UTI), pneumonia, septic arthritis, and osteomyelitis. This protocol does not include nonbacterial infections [e.g. malaria, TORCH (toxoplasmosis, rubella, cytomegalovirus and herpes simplex virus)] or superficial bacterial infections like conjunctivitis and oral thrush.

WHEN TO SUSPECT NEONATAL SEPSIS

Signs and symptoms of neonatal sepsis are usually subtle, hence a high degree of suspicion is required particularly in hospitalized very low-birth weight (VLBW) neonates. Various red flag signs include the following:
- *Temperature instability:* Hypothermia being more common in preterm low birth weight infants and fever in late onset sepsis (LOS) in term infants
- Lethargy, poor cry, and refusal to suck
- Poor perfusion, prolonged capillary refill time
- Feed intolerance (abdominal distension, vomiting, and increased prefeed residual)
- Direct hyperbilirubinemia
- Sclerema, bleed from any site/petechiae/purpura
- Hypotonia, absent neonatal reflexes, and seizures
- Brady/tachycardia
- Respiratory distress, apnea and gasping respiration
- Sudden increase in ventilatory requirement in a ventilated neonate
- Hypo-/hyperglycemia
- Metabolic acidosis.

However, all these signs and symptoms take some time to appear and the neonates who are in intensive care units especially VLBW and extremely low birth-weight (ELBW) may be very sick by the time these features appear. In such cases, monitoring of heart rate characteristics (HRC) in the form of reduced variability and transient deceleration in heart rate mediated by inflammatory mediators have been found to be highly suggestive of imminent sepsis.

Among infants who are discharged home, new onset of fever, cough, difficult or fast breathing, poor feeding, lethargy or convulsions are indicators of infection warranting admission and work up.

Fungal sepsis should be suspected in ELBW infants or preterm neonates (gestation <28 weeks) with persistent thrombocytopenia and unexplained hyperglycemia. Other risk factors include therapy with cephalosporins for >7 days, prolonged ICU stay, total parenteral nutrition, prolonged intubation, indwelling catheters, and administration of steroids.

CLASSIFICATION OF NEONATAL SEPSIS

- *Early onset sepsis (EOS)*: It refers to onset of symptoms within 72 hours of birth. Baby may be symptomatic at birth in severe cases. Infection is usually acquired from mother's genital tract in antenatal period or at the time of birth. It usually presents with pneumonia and respiratory distress, most common organisms being *Escherichia coli, Klebsiella,* and *Staphylococcus aureus*. Risk factors for EOS include the following:
  - *Prematurity/Low-birth weight*: It is one of the most strongly associated risk factors.
  - *Maternal chorioamnionitis*: It is defined as maternal fever (>38°C), leukocytosis (>15,000 WBCs/μL), uterine tenderness, foul smelling liquor, and maternal tachycardia and fetal tachycardia at delivery. Of these, measurement of maternal temperature during labor has been used as "EOS risk calculator" as fever is the essential criterion for diagnosis of maternal chorioamnionitis, other criteria are relatively insensitive. Also, incidence of chorioamnionitis varies inversely with gestational age.
  - *Prolonged rupture of membranes (>18 hours)*: In addition, perinatal asphyxia (5 min Apgar score ≤6), maternal UTI, unclean vaginal examinations (or >3 intrapartum vaginal examinations), prolonged labor (first and second stage >24 hours) and meconium-stained amniotic fluid have been associated with risk of EOS to variable extent.
- *Late onset sepsis*: LOS is defined as onset of symptoms beyond 72 hours of life. Infection is acquired postnatally either from the hospital or community. Common organisms are coagulase negative *Staphylococcus aureus* (CONS), *Staphylococcus aureus* and *Klebsiella* in former and *Staphylococcus aureus* in latter. LOS can present with septicemia, meningitis or deep-seated focal infection as mentioned above. Risk factors of LOS include the following:
  - In-hospital setting:
    ♦ Low-birth weight/prematurity
    ♦ Admission in intensive care unit
    ♦ Mechanical ventilation
    ♦ Invasive procedures including umbilical catheters
    ♦ Administration of parenteral fluids and total parenteral nutrition.

  In addition, hospitalized ELBW babies are also at risk of fungal sepsis.
  - The risk of community-acquired LOS is increased by:
    ♦ Poor hygiene
    ♦ Poor cord care
    ♦ Bottle-feeding
    ♦ Prelacteal feeds.

INVESTIGATIONS

Complete work-up in a septic neonate includes (Table 1):
- Blood culture sensitivity
- Complete blood count ±
- C-reactive protein (CRP)
- Cerebrospinal fluid (CSF) and urine culture when indicated.

Blood Culture Sensitivity

As suggested by the definition itself, blood culture should be and is the gold standard for the diagnosis of sepsis. A minimum of 1 mL blood should be inoculated in the culture bottle for a good yield. If two bottles have been provided, 2 mL blood should be drawn, 1 mL for each bottle. Sample should be inoculated for 72 hours minimum before declaring negative result. Sample should be drawn from peripheral vein only; cultures from indwelling catheters might yield false positive results due to colonizers.

With the help of BACTEC culture results may be obtained within 12–24 hours.

Septic Screen

Complete Blood Count

- *Total leukocyte count (TLC)*: Depression of TLC is more important than leukocytosis in diagnosis of EOS. However, this parameter

Table 1: Investigations for neonatal sepsis.

Test	Positive Result	Significance	Remarks
Blood culture	Any growth after 72 hours incubation	Gold standard	Minimum 1 mL sample in each bottle
CBC			
• ANC	Values less than normal for age as per Manroe's and Mouzinho's charts	Highly sensitive less specific	Should be performed at least 6–12 hours after birth
• I/T ratio	>0.27 in term and >0.22 in preterm	Most sensitive neutrophil index, less specific	
CRP	>10 mg/L	Highly sensitive less specific	Should be performed at least 6–12 hours after birth. Serial negative results may be helpful in deciding when to stop antibiotics in culture negative asymptomatic neonate
CSF analysis and culture cells Protein Sugar	>20/µL in term, >25/µL in preterm >100 mg/dL in term, >170 mg/dL in preterm <40 mg/dL in term, <20 mg/dL in preterm or CSF: blood sugar <0.5	Most sensitive parameter Most specific	CSF should be performed in all symptomatic neonates before starting antibiotics in suspected EOS and in all cases of suspected LOS

(CBS: complete blood count; ANC: absolute neutrophil count; CRP: C-reactive protein; CSF: cerebrospinal fluid; LOS: late onset sepsis).

has poor positive predictive accuracy in diagnosis of EOS and neutrophil count rather than leukocyte count is important.
- *Absolute neutrophil count (ANC)*: Just like TLC, neutropenia is more significant than neutrophilia. However, neutrophil count varies with age of newborn, lower limit being <1800/μL at birth, <7800/μL at 12–14 hours of age falling again to <1800/μL at 72 hours.
- *Immature neutrophils*: Immature neutrophil count has poor sensitivity and positive predictive accuracy in diagnosis of sepsis. However, immature-to-total-neutrophil ratio (I/T ratio) has best sensitivity of all neutrophil indices. It is calculated as:

$$\frac{\text{Immature polymorphs (band forms, metamyelocytes and myelocytes)}}{\text{Mature + immature neutrophils}}$$

Immature-to-total-neutrophil ratio also varies with age of the newborn declining from 0.16 at birth to 0.12 by 72 hours. Value beyond 0.27 in term and 0.22 in preterm neonates is significant. Although most sensitive, single elevated value of I/T ratio has low positive predictive accuracy in diagnosis of sepsis.

Note: In suspected EOS, neutrophil indices are more reliable if obtained 6–12 hours after birth as they require some inflammatory response to be there to be significantly abnormal.

Acute Phase Reactants

- *C-reactive protein (CRP)*: Just like other indices CRP has high sensitivity but poor specificity in diagnosis of sepsis. Values >10 mg/L are considered significant. For diagnosis of EOS, CRP is more valuable if test is performed after 6–8 hours of birth after the initiation of inflammatory response. Rather than a single value, serial CRP values <10 mg/L have high sensitivity in ruling out sepsis and may provide a basis for discontinuing antibiotics in an asymptomatic baby.
- *Procalcitonin*: Procalcitonin is another useful biomarker for sepsis. Its levels increase 2 hours after onset of infection and normalize after 2–3 days. It is more sensitive but less specific than CRP for diagnosis of sepsis. Values >0.5 ng/mL are suggestive of bacterial infection. However, procalcitonin levels show a physiological rise within 24 hours of birth and in some noninfectious conditions like respiratory distress syndrome, infant of diabetic mother and hemodynamic instability.

Hence, routine sepsis screen panels include neutrophil indices and CRP performed at least 6–12 hours after birth. Negative screen has high sensitivity in ruling out sepsis and is useful in deciding whether asymptomatic "at risk" neonates need antibiotics and whether antibiotics can be withdrawn in an asymptomatic culture negative "at risk" neonate.

Cerebrospinal Fluid Analysis

Signs and symptoms of meningitis may be subtle in newborn making it difficult to distinguish between septicemia and meningitis, hence, high index of suspicion is required for prompt diagnosis and management.

When to Perform CSF in EOS

- Blood culture positive sepsis
- Symptomatic neonates with positive laboratory evidence of sepsis
- Infants who worsen despite initial antibiotics.

All Cases of LOS

If the neonate is critically ill or likely to suffer cardiorespiratory compromise from lumbar puncture, antibiotics should be started and procedure deferred till the baby is stable.

CSF Parameters in Sepsis

- *Cytology*: Cell count of >20/µL (>25 in preterm) with >60% polymorphs is significant. Adjustment of neutrophils for RBCs is not required as it reduces sensitivity without much increase in specificity.
- *Glucose*: CSF hypoglycorrhachia (low CSF sugar <40 mg/dL in term and <20 mg/dL in preterm) is the most specific indicator of meningitis. Prior to lumbar puncture, a blood sugar level should be obtained to calculate CSF—blood glucose ratio, value <50% is indicative of sepsis.
- With a delay in sample processing >2 hours, CSF glucose and cells decline significantly, hence, prompt processing of sample is required.
- *Protein*: CSF protein of >100 mg/dL (>170 in preterm neonates) is highly suggestive of meningitis. CSF protein is the most sensitive indicator for ruling out meningitis.
- Culture.

Other Tests

- *Chest X-ray*: In case the baby has respiratory distress or apnea. Abdominal X-ray needs to be done in case of abdominal distension or feed intolerance.
- *Urine culture*: It is not routinely indicated in EOS. In suspected LOS, if the baby has fever, crying during micturition or direct hyperbilirubinemia, urine culture should be obtained by suprapubic aspiration or bladder catheterization. UTI is suggested by:
    - More than 10 WBCs/µL in 10 mL of centrifuged urine
    - Any organism identified in culture of suprapubic urine
    - More than 10^4 organisms/mL of catheterization sample.
- If fungal sepsis is suspected, suprapubic urine should be sent for fungal hyphae and blood culture sent in fungal culture medium. Sample should be incubated for 10 days before declaring the results to be negative. In case of indwelling catheters, sample should be obtained from both venepuncture site and catheter.

MANAGEMENT

Supportive Care

- Nursing in thermoneutral environment
- Maintain oxygen saturation in normal range, continuous positive airway pressure (CPAP) or mechanical ventilation if required
- Treatment of anemia, thrombocytopenia or disseminated intravascular coagulation (DIC) with appropriate transfusion
- Regular blood sugar monitoring for early detection and management of hypo- or hyperglycemia
- Monitoring hemodynamics, prompt detection, and management of shock with fluid boluses and inotropes
- Good nutritional support with breast milk or total parenteral nutrition, trophic feeds if full feeds are contraindicated.

Specific Treatment

- *Whom to treat*: A sepsis screen needs to be obtained and antibiotics started after obtaining blood culture in all of the following cases:
    - *Symptomatic neonates*: All babies who are symptomatic at birth should be worked up and managed for suspected EOS. They should undergo blood culture at birth, CBC ± CRP at 6–12 hours and CSF if baby is stable. However, if a critically-ill baby starts improving within 6 hours of life, noninfectious cause (respiratory distress syndrome, meconium aspiration syndrome, etc.) is more likely and in these cases, lumbar puncture may

be withheld and antibiotics may be discontinued if screen is negative and cultures are sterile.

All babies showing deterioration after 72 hours of life whether admitted or discharged home should have septic work-up (CBC ± CRP) done along with blood culture, lumbar puncture and urine culture (if febrile or direct jaundice) and started on empirical antibiotics, pending laboratory data, and culture reports.

- *Asymptomatic "at risk" neonates (Flowchart 1)*: These include all neonates with maternal chorioamnionitis, preterm neonates with prolonged rupture of membranes >18 hours or neonates with >2 risk factors for EOS. All these babies should have evaluation consisting of blood culture at birth and CBC ± CRP at 6–12 hours.
  - Antibiotics are started at birth and they can be stopped if laboratory data are normal, baby remains asymptomatic and cultures are sterile.
  - For term babies with rupture of membranes >18 hours or <2 risk factors only CBC ± CRP is done at 6–12 hours, if baby remains well and screen is negative, neonate is discharged home by 48 hours. If screen is positive, blood culture is drawn and antibiotics started pending culture sensitivity reports.

It is particularly important that antibiotics be started only when indicated (vide supra) because indiscriminate and prolonged use

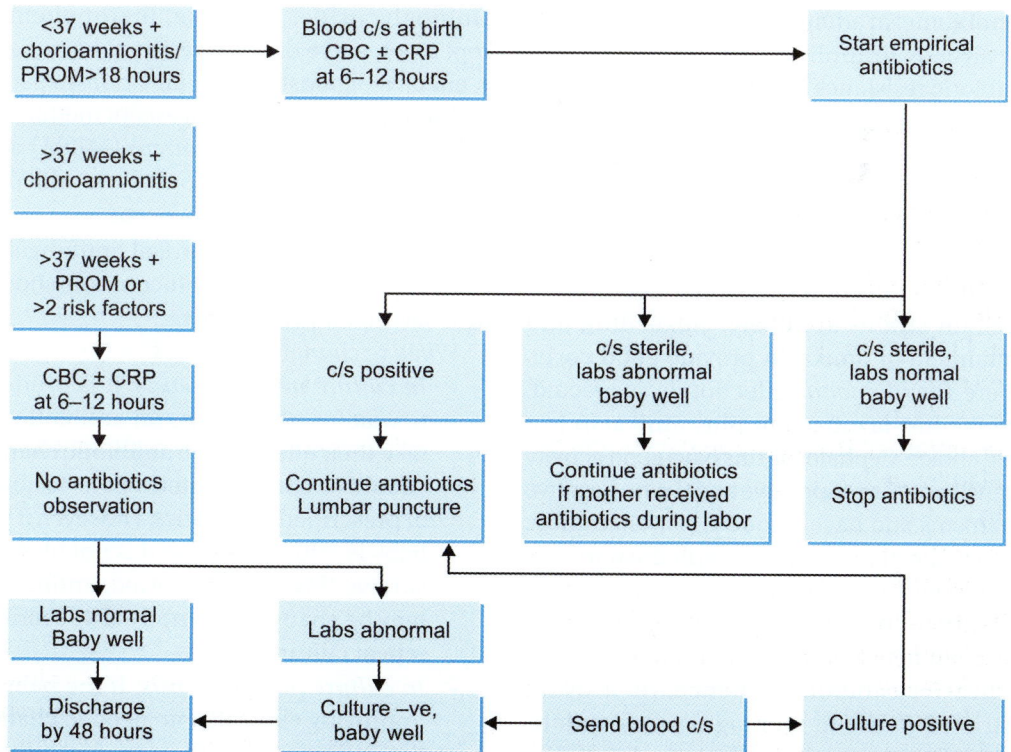

Flowchart 1: Approach to asymptomatic neonates with risk factors for EOS.

(EOS: early onset sepsis; CBC: complete blood count; CRP: C-reactive protein; PROM: premature rupture of membrane).

Table 2: Choice of antibiotics for neonatal sepsis.

Clinical situation	Septicemia or pneumonia	Meningitis	UTI
EOS—1st line 2nd line	Ampicillin + gentamicin Cefotaxime or piperacillin-tazobactam or ciprofloxacin + amikacin	Add cefotaxime	
LOS—1st line: • Community acquired • Hospital acquired 2nd line	Ampicillin + amikacin or gentamicin Cloxacillin + amikacin or gentamicin Same as EOS	Add cefotaxime	Cefotaxime + amikacin
3rd line	Meropenem + vancomycin	Meropenem + vancomycin	

(EOS: early onset sepsis; UTI: urinary tract infection).

of antibiotics particularly in preterm babies has been linked to increased mortality, risk of necrotizing enterocolitis, periventricular leukomalacia, and increased chances of wheezing in childhood due to alteration of microbiome. In addition, many neonatal units are already grappling with the menace of antibiotic resistance due to the same reason.

Choice of empirical antibiotics (Table 2): Choice of antibiotics depends on local antibiotic sensitivity patterns. Initial empirical therapy with ampicillin and gentamicin provides good coverage in EOS and community-acquired LOS. If the infection is hospital-acquired or resistant strains are likely, cloxacillin, and gentamicin or amikacin provide good cover. Where *Pseudomonas* infection is suspected, piperacillin-tazobactam plus amikacin is a good choice. Cephalosporins have good activity against most Gram-positive and Gram-negative organisms and have a good CSF penetration. However, extensive use of cephalosporins is associated with rapid development of drug resistance, particularly ESBL (extended-spectrum beta lactamase) and increased risk of invasive candidiasis, hence, their use is restricted to use in meningitis. Cefotaxime, used as ceftriaxone, is contraindicated in neonates because it displaces bilirubin from binding sites increasing the risk of kernicterus. Hence, use of cefotaxime is reserved only for cases of meningitis. In late onset of meningitis, antistaphylococcal agent like vancomycin should be added with or without aminoglycoside. Likewise, meropenem is kept as a reserve drug for resistant bacteria. It is effective against almost all Gram-negative and Gram-positive bacteria except methicillin resistant *Staphylococcus aureus* (MRSA) and *enterococcus*. Hence, vancomycin is added to cover for MRSA and enterococcus.

For fungal sepsis, empirical antifungal of choice is amphotericin B. Fluconazole should be reserved for prophylaxis.

- *When to change antibiotics*:
  - *In culture negative sepsis*: It is prudent to wait for 48–72 hours for antibiotics to take their effect. So no antibiotic change should be contemplated before 48 hours of prescribed antibiotics. However, if the baby is critically sick and is not likely to survive this window period, antibiotics may be changed promptly after sending repeat cultures.
  - *In culture positive sepsis*: If the baby is improving clinically, no need to change the antibiotics but therapy may be narrowed down to single sensitive drug after

sensitivity report except pseudomonas where two sensitive antibiotics must be used. If empirical antibiotics are sensitive but baby is worsening, antibiotics may be upgraded to second line drugs.

Duration of antibiotics: Duration of therapy depends on culture sensitivity report, sepsis screen, and clinical symptomatology as mentioned in Flowchart 2.

Hence, culture positive sepsis, whether EOS or LOS, should be treated for 10–14 days. *Staphylococcus* sepsis definitely requires 14-day therapy while for non-*Staphylococcus* cases, if baby becomes asymptomatic and CRP becomes negative, 10 days course may be sufficient. Meningitis is treated for 21 days. In Gram-negative meningitis, CSF should be repeated after baby becomes asymptomatic and antibiotics are continued for 21 days or for 14 days after sterilization of CSF whichever is longer. UTI is treated for 7–14 days depending on symptomatology. Deep seated bone and joint infections are treated for 6 weeks.

ADJUNCTIVE THERAPIES

- *Double volume exchange transfusion (DVET)*: DVET with cross-matched fresh whole blood has been used for management of severe sepsis with sclerema. However, its efficacy has not been proven in randomized controlled trials.
- *Immunoglobulins*: Currently available systematic reviews do not support the role of IVIG.
- *Granulocyte colony-stimulating factor*: There is no evidence that *granulocyte colony-stimulating factor* reduces mortality or morbidity in term or preterm septic neonates. However, it may be used to achieve rapid increase in neutrophil count in preterm neonates with severe neutropenia (ANC <500/μL).

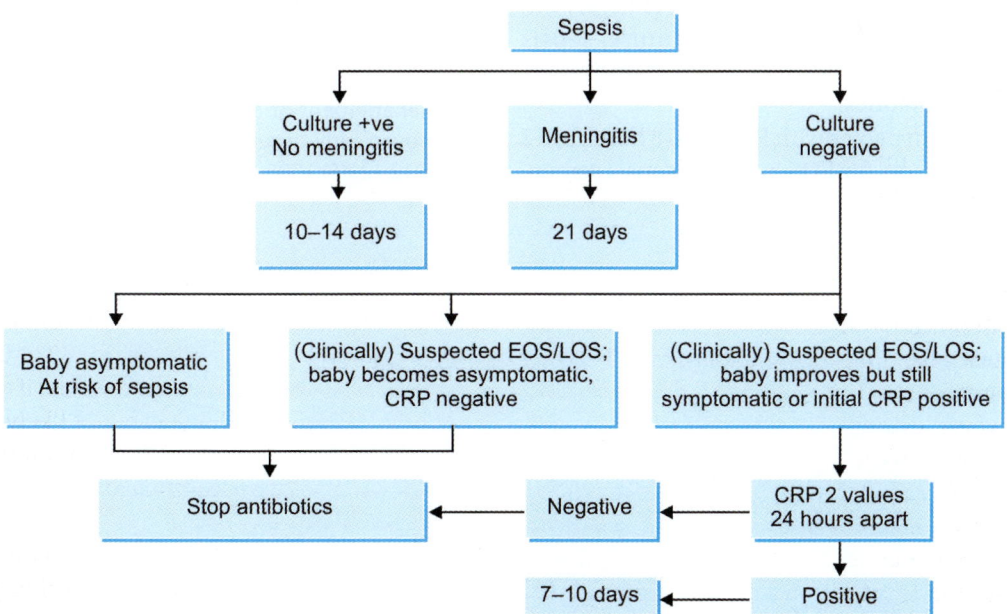

Flowchart 2: Duration of antibiotics in sepsis.

(EOS: early onset sepsis; LOS: late onset sepsis; CRP: C-reactive protein).

SUMMARY

- Signs and symptoms of sepsis are often subtle in neonates hence a high degree of suspicion is required.
- EOS is defined as onset before 72 hours of life and LOS as onset beyond 72 hours.
- Blood culture is gold standard for diagnosis. A minimum of 1 mL blood should be inoculated in each culture bottle to ensure a good yield.
- Sepsis screen (ANC, I/T ratio, CRP) is highly sensitive in ruling out sepsis but has a poor positive predictive value.
- All symptomatic neonates, unless an alternate diagnosis is proved, should have blood cultures and sepsis.
- Lumbar puncture should be performed in all neonates with culture positive sepsis, suspected LOS and symptomatic EOS before starting antibiotics. Asymptomatic "at risk" neonates do not require lumbar puncture at the start of antimicrobial therapy.
- All asymptomatic babies with maternal chorioamnionitis or preterms with premature rupture of membrane (PROM) >18 hours should have blood culture, sepsis screen at 6–12 hours and started on empirical antibiotics.
- For term babies with PROM >18 hours or >2 risk factors for EOS, perform sepsis screen, if positive send blood cultures and manage accordingly, otherwise discharge home by 48 hours. No need to start antibiotics empirically.
- First line therapy is ampicillin + gentamicin. If resistant strains are likely, cloxacillin + amikacin should be started. Cefotaxime should be added for meningitis. Combination of meropenem + vancomycin should be reserved for severe resistant cases.
- Duration of therapy is 10–14 days for culture proven sepsis, 21 days for meningitis and 7–10 days for probable sepsis. For asymptomatic babies "at risk" of sepsis, antibiotics should be stopped at 48–72 hours if the cultures are sterile.

SUGGESTED READING

1. Cotten CM. Antibiotic stewardship: reassessment of guidelines for management of neonatal sepsis. Clin Perinatol. 2015;42(1):195- 206, x.
2. Nizet V, Klein JO. Bacterial sepsis and meningitis. In: Nizet V, Klein JO (Eds). Infectious Diseases of the Fetus and Newborn Infant, 7th edition. Philadelphia, PA: Saunders; 2011. pp. 222-75.
3. Polin RA; Committee on Fetus and Newborn. Management of neonates with suspected or proven early-onset bacterial sepsis. Paediatrics. 2012;129(5):1006-15.

CHAPTER 6

Neonatal Seizures

Ashish Jain

DEFINITION

A neonatal seizure is a sudden paroxysmal depolarization of a group of neurons resulting in a transient alteration in sensory, motor, behavior, or autonomic activity, with or without an alteration of consciousness in the neonatal age group. Seizures in neonatal period are grouped in different ways; the most common grouping used is as:
- *Epileptic seizures*—phenomenon associated with corresponding electroencephalography (EEG) changes, e.g. clonic seizures.
- *Nonepileptic seizures*—clinical seizures without corresponding EEG correlate, e.g. subtle seizures.
- *EEG seizures*—abnormal EEG activity with no clinical correlation.

SEIZURE MIMICS

Jitteriness

Jitteriness is commonly associated with hypoxic-ischemic encephalopathy, hypoglycemia, polycythemia, hypocalcemia, and drug withdrawal. Features that differentiate jitteriness from seizures are as follows:
- Absence of abnormal gaze or eye movement seen during seizure activity.
- Provoked by stimulation of the infant, stretching a joint.
- Can be stopped with passive flexion or gentle restraint.
- Fast and slow component is absent during jitteriness.
- No EEG abnormality is seen in jitteriness.
- The frequency of jerks in jitteriness is faster (5–6/sec) as compared with 2–3/sec in seizures.
- Jitteriness is not associated with change in heart rate, respiratory rate, and blood pressure.

Benign Sleep Myoclonus

Bilateral symmetrical jerky myoclonic movements occur during sleep and the newborn is always neurologically normal. The myoclonic movements disappear on awakening of the newborn. These movements disappear by 2–3 months of age.

Hyperekplexia

This is associated with generalized stiffness while awake, exaggerated startle, and nocturnal myoclonus. Episodes of hypertonic and tonic spasms could occur due to tactile and auditory stimuli. If the episodes are severe it may present as acute life-threatening events (ALTEs). These ALTEs may be aborted by flexion of limbs and neck of the newborn.

Apnea

Nonepileptic apneas are more common in premature infants. Apnea is cessation of breathing for more than 15 seconds and often associated with bradycardia. As in seizure, apnea is not associated with tachycardia, changes in blood pressure, temperature instability, eye deviation, mouth deviation, or eye opening or closing.

EVALUATION OF SEIZURE

The evaluation of seizure in a newborn should include assessment of type of seizure, etiology, and prognostication.

CLINICAL SEIZURE TYPES

Neonatal seizures are categorized in four clinical types (Table 1): (1) subtle, (2) clonic, (3) tonic, and (4) myoclonic seizures. Each can be focal, multifocal, or generalized.

IMPORTANT ETIOLOGIES OF NEONATAL SEIZURES

Among neonates with seizures, the four most common etiologies are: (1) the hypoxic-ischemic encephalopathy (HIE) (38–48%), (2) neonatal hypoglycemia (3–7.5%), (3) hypocalcemia (2.3–9%), and (4) central nervous system (CNS) infection (5.5–10.3%). This pattern has not changed since 1990s. The complete list of the causes is very long. The following are some of the important causes.

Hypoxic Ischemia

- Moderate HIE present with subtle focal or multifocal fragmentary clonic seizures. Severe HIE present with myoclonic and tonic seizures and are difficult to control.
- The seizure present usually within first 24 hours.

Table 1: Clinical types of seizure.

Type	Frequency	Clinical/Presentation	EEG
Subtle	48%	Eyelid fluttering, eye deviation, fixed open stare, chewing, sucking, tongue thrusting, cycling, boxing, pedaling, limb movements, apnea (most often has either an accelerated or a normal heart rate when evaluated 20 seconds following its onset)	Usually normal
Clonic	32%	Rhythmic jerking (1–4 per second), consciousness usually preserved Focal limb or one side of face or body Multifocal irregular, fragmentary, non-Jacksonian migratory pattern	Usually abnormal
Myoclonic	13%	Synchronous single or multiple slow jerks of upper or lower limbs (or both) Usually associated with diffuse CNS pathology	Usually normal in focal or multifocal
Tonic	7%	Sustained period of muscle contraction without repetitive features Generalized tonic seizures mimic closely decerebrate or decorticate Posturing are most common in preterm babies with diffuse neurological dysfunction or major intraventricular hemorrhage Focal tonic seizures consist of sustained posturing of a limb or symmetric posturing of a limb or asymmetric posturing of the trunk or neck. EEG—usually abnormal	Usually normal

(CNS: central nervous system; EEG: electroencephalography)

- Metabolic disorders like hypoglycemia, hypocalcemia, syndrome of inappropriate antidiuretic (SIADH) secretion with hyponatremia and diabetes insipidus may coexist and trigger seizure.

Central Nervous System Infection
- Bacteria like group B *streptococci*, *Escherichia coli*, and *Listeria*.
- Viruses like *Coxsackievirus*, echovirus, rubella, *Cytomegalovirus*, and herpes (characteristic EEG).
- Others, toxoplasmosis and syphilis.

Intracranial hemorrhage and CNS trauma: Result from breech delivery or difficult forceps.
- Subarachnoid hemorrhage; usually asymptomatic or present with second day seizures.
- Periventricular hemorrhage; usually in preterm babies in first 3 days of birth.
- *Subdural hemorrhage:* Occurs in large babies after breech delivery and in first day of life.
- *Choroid plexus hemorrhage:* May at times occur in full-term infants.

Cerebral Artery Infarction
- These infants have normal Apgar score and investigations for infective or metabolic etiology.
- Early magnetic resonance imaging (MRI) imaging studies demonstrate the changes.
- May be provoked by deficiency of protein C and S, thrombocytosis, polycythemia, maternal lupus, maternal cocaine use, cardiac anomalies, and paradoxical emboli.

Metabolic Problems
- *Hypoglycemia* (blood glucose level <40 mg/dL): Most often occurs in infant of diabetic mother, small for gestational age (SGA), premature babies or may be associated with asphyxia or sepsis.
- *Hypocalcemia*: Calcium levels less than 7 mg/dL.

Early-onset hypocalcemia occurs in preterm babies, birth asphyxia, or trauma and infant of diabetic mother, and after exchange transfusion.

Late-onset hypocalcemia occurs following ingestion of cow's milk and high phosphate milk formula.
- *Hypomagnesemia* is defined as magnesium levels of less than 1.2 mg/dL and is often associated with hypocalcemia.
- *Hyponatremia*—results from SIADH secretion excessive renal salt loss, excessive administration of hyponatremic fluids.
- *Hypernatremia*: Seen with dehydration, renal diseases, and diabetes insipidus.
- *Pyridoxine dependency*: This is a rare autosomal recessive (AR) defect in inhibitory neurotransmitter GABA, which presents with early onset refractory seizures that are abolished within minutes by administrating pyridoxine 50–100 mg (normalization of EEG may be more gradual).
- *Inborn error of metabolism*: These groups should be considered when seizures are unresponsive to conventional treatment and there is positive family history, recent introduction of milk, acidosis, or distinctive odor is present.

Drug-associated Seizures
- Narcotic and sedative withdrawal leads to neurological signs like jitteriness, autonomic dysfunction, irritability, and occasionally seizures. Seizures occur within 2 days in case of heroin withdrawal or can be delayed for 1–2 weeks with methadone or barbiturates withdrawal.
- Inadvertent administration of local anesthetic into fetal circulation occurs through scalp injection or indirectly by

placental transmission during labor and delivery. Apart from seizures these babies have hypotonia, bradycardia, fixed and dilated pupils, and complete external ophthalmoplegia.
- Theophylline at toxic blood levels can also cause seizures.

Developmental Problems

- Both cerebral dysgenesis (heterotopias and neuronal disorganization) with normal cranial ultrasonography (USG) and MRI and phakomatoses (Sturge-Weber anomaly, neurofibromatosis, tuberous sclerosis) are associated with increased incidence of seizures.

Benign Neonatal Convulsions

- Benign familial neonatal convulsions (BFNC) are self-limiting (within 1–6 months). It is an autosomal dominant syndrome presenting with clonic seizures on the 2nd or 3rd day. The infant has no abnormal neurological signs in the interictal period and investigations reveal no apparent cause. Subsequent development is usually normal.
- Benign idiopathic neonatal convulsions (BINC or 5th day fits) refer to multifocal clonic seizures, the peak time of onset which is 5th day, generally ceasing within 15 days.

Syndromes

- Two rare syndromes, early myoclonic encephalopathy and early infantile epileptic encephalopathy are characteristically present in the 1st week with severe recurrent seizures and are associated with inborn error of metabolism and structural CNS abnormalities. Both lead to severe subsequent neurodevelopmental impairment.

HISTORY AND EXAMINATION

Detailed History

- Antenatal history, parental consanguinity, family history of convulsion or mental retardation.
- *Intrauterine infection*—fever, rash with lymphadenopathy.
- Maternal intake of alcohol, cocaine, heroin, or methadone.
- Increased perception of fetal movements due to fetal seizures.
- *Perinatal infection*—premature rupture of membranes (PROM), foul smelling liquor, mother on antibiotics
- Pudendal block.
- Difficult labor, forceps delivery or precipitate labor, requiring resuscitation at birth.
- Lethargy, poor feeding, drowsiness, and vomit after initiation of breast feed for inborn error of metabolism.
- Cow milk or top feeding for late-onset hypocalcemia.

Examination

- Record the time of onset, type of seizure associated eye movements and autonomic phenomenon, interictal period and level of consciousness.
- Record vital signs like heart rate respiration, blood pressure, capillary refill time, and temperature.
- Look for dysmorphic facies, obvious congenital anomalies.
- Look for forceps marks, skull fracture, subgaleal bleeds, bulging fontanel, and injection site mark on scalp. Look for neurocutaneous markers like hypopigmented patches. Hepatosplenomegaly
- Eye examination for chorioretinitis and abnormal eye movements.
- Record any unusual body or urine odor.

INVESTIGATIONS

Any investigation should be undertaken in a logical sequence and depending upon findings of detailed history and clinical examination. Attempt should be made to find common etiologies.

First-line Investigations

- Arterial blood gas, pulse oximeter, and vitals
- Hematocrit, blood sugar, serum sodium, calcium, and magnesium
- Septic screen including TLC (total leukocyte count), DLC (differential leukocyte count), ESR (erythrocyte sedimentation rate), CRP (C-reactive protein), IT ratio, blood culture, and CSF (cerebrospinal fluid) studies
- Cranial USG
- EEG (If available bedside).

Second-line Investigations

- CT scan/MRI
- TORCH (toxoplasmosis, rubella, cytomegalovirus and herpes simplex virus) screen, VDRL (venereal disease research laboratory test), blood ammonia
- CSF lactate, pyruvate, glycerine
- Urine for reducing substance, amino acids, and organic acid
- Urine and blood-drug level
- Specific enzyme level
- Gas chromatography Mass spectrophotometry/Tandem mass spectrophotometry (GCMS/TMS).

IMAGING

- Radiological investigations (ultrasound, CT, and MRI) of the cranium/head have a limited role in determining the presence or absence of clinical seizures or evaluating the efficacy of treatment with antiepileptic drugs (AEDs) in neonates.
- These investigations have role as part of the comprehensive evaluation of the etiology of neonatal seizures:
  - *Cranial USG*: Detects IVH, parenchymal hemorrhage, and gross CNS malformation. It does not detect cerebral arterial infarction, subdural, and subarachnoid hemorrhage.
  - *CT scan brain*: Can detect the developmental defects, subarachnoid hemorrhages and infections.
  - *MRI brain*: Best for the neuronal migration disorders or the smaller lesions.
- Even though the severe lesions detected on the neurosonography have generally a bad prognosis, in the absence of dysgenic brain, the prognostic value of these tests is limited.

ELECTROENCEPHALOGRAPHY

- Electroencephalography is the most accurate method for confirming that a clinical event is of epileptic origin, which is consistent with values and preferences of accurate diagnosis. Hence, should be performed whenever available. However, the standard method of diagnosis is the clinical recognition of neonatal seizures.
- The application of EEG to determine specific etiological factors is rather limited. Although, there are some EEG patterns that may be specific for certain neonatal brain disorders, these conditions are very little, represent a small proportion of risk factors and are no longer the critical diagnostic test for these disorders.
  - Hypsarrhythmia— nonketotic hyperglycinemia.
  - Comb-like rhythm of 5–7—Maple syrup urine disease (MSUD).

- 1-4 sharp and slow wave—pyridoxine dependency.
- Multifocal periodic pattern—herpes simplex.

- Studies titrating AED therapy to elimination of electrographic seizures have not been performed. Hence, in resource-challenged healthcare centers where EEG is not avail-

Flowchart 1: Algorithm of management of neonatal seizures.

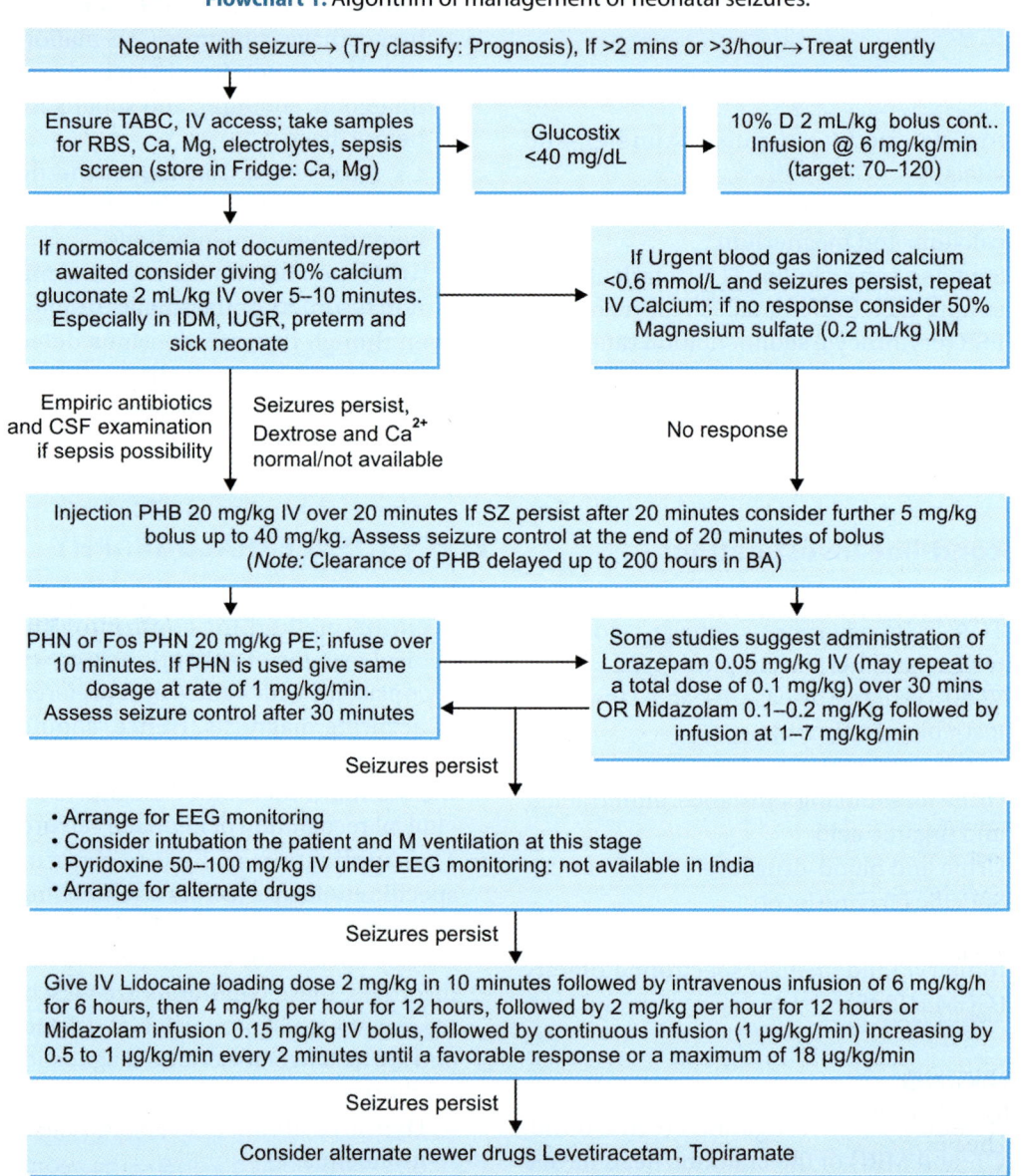

(RBS: random blood sugar; IDM: infant of diabetic mother; IUGR: intrauterine growth restriction; CSF: cerebrospinal fluid; EEG: electroencephalography; SZ: seizure).

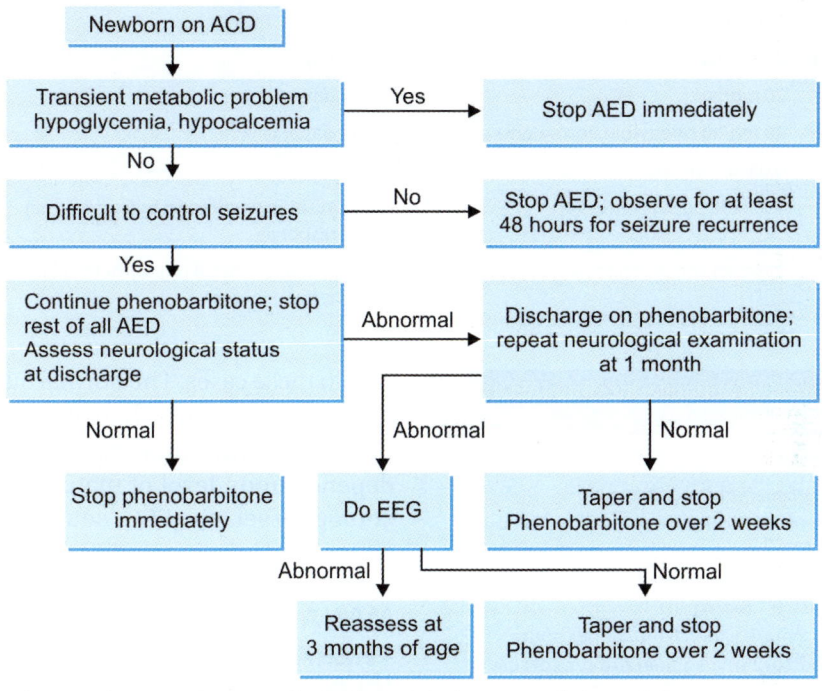

Flowchart 2: Algorithm on when to stop ACD.

(ACD: anticonvulsant medication; AED: antiepileptic drug; EEG: electroencephalography)

Table 2: Cause, incidence, and outcome of neonatal convulsions in term infants.		
Etiological factor	*Incidence (%)*	*Poor outcome*
Asphyxia	38–40	50
Cerebral arteriovenous infarction	20	0
Intracranial hemorrhage IVH (Grade II and above) sub acute hemorrhage (SAH)	12–20	90
		10
Congenital cerebral anomaly	5–10	100
Hypoglycemia	3–19	50
Hypocalcemia early		50
Hypocalcemia late		0
Infection	3–20	50
Inborn error of metabolism	1	Variable
Unknown cause	10–13	25

able, response to treatment is best assessed by clinical observation (Flowcharts 1 and 2).
- The EEG use in determining the prognosis of the neonatal seizures, include select patterns like burst suppression pattern, low voltage invariant pattern anteroelectrocerebral inactivity that indicates poor prognosis in both term- and preterm infants.

PROGNOSIS (TABLE 2)

The overall mortality in the neonatal seizures may be 10–15%. About 25–30% of the neonates having seizures in the neonatal period have some degree of the neurological sequelae. The chronic seizure disorder (epilepsy) in the later life is reported variably from 5% to

Table 3: Standard drugs used in neonatal seizures.

AED	Initial dose	Maintenance dose	Route
Phenobarbital	20 mg/kg	3–4 mg/kg per day	IV, IM, PO
Phenytoin	20 mg/kg	3–4 mg/kg per day	IV, PO
Fosphenytoin	20 mg/kg phenytoin equivalents	3–4 mg/kg per day	IV, IM
Lorazepam	0.05–0.1 mg/kg	Every 8–12 hours	IV
Midazolam	150–200 µg/kg IV infusion	1µg/kg/min IV infusion, increasing to 5 µg/kg/min until favorable response	IV
Lidocaine	2 mg/kg IV over 10 mins	6 mg/kg/hr for 6 hours IV, then 4 mg/kg/hr for 12 hours, then 2 mg/kg/hr for 12 hours	IV

Table 4: Alternative antiepileptic drug (AED) used in neonatal seizures.

Intravenous AEDs
- *High-dose phenobarbital:* >30 mg/kg
- *Pentobarbital:* 10 mg/kg, then 1 mg/kg per hour
- *Thiopental:* 10 mg/kg, then 2–4 mg/kg per hour
- *Midazolam:* 0.2 mg/kg, then 0.1–0.4 mg/kg per hour
- *Clonazepam:* 0.1 mg/kg
- *Lidocaine:* 2 mg/kg, then 6 mg/kg per hour
- *Valproic acid:* 10–25 mg/kg, then 20 mg/kg per day in 3 doses
- *Paraldehyde:* 200 mg/kg, then 16 mg/kg per hour
- *Chlormethiazole:* Initial infusion rate of 0.08 mg/kg per minute
- *Pyridoxine (B_6):* 50–100 mg, then 100 mg every 10 minutes (up to 500 mg)

Oral AEDs
- *Primidone:* 15–25 mg/kg per day in 3 doses
- *Clonazepam:* 0.1 mg/kg in 2–3 doses
- *Carbamazepine:* 10 mg/kg, then 15–20 mg/kg per day in 2 doses
- *Oxcarbamazepine:* No data on neonates, young infants
- *Valproic acid:* 10–25 mg/kg, then 20 mg/kg per day in 3 doses
- *Vigabatrin:* 50 mg/kg per day in 2 doses, up to 200 mg/kg per day
- *Lamotrigine:* 12.5 mg in 2 doses
- *Topiramate:* 3 mg/kg per day
- *Levetiracetam:* 10 mg/kg per day in 2 doses
- *Folinic acid:* 2.5 mg bid, up to 4 mg/kg per day

20% in these cases. The normal outcome may be expected in more than 50% of the cases.

In any individual case, the prognosis depends upon level of maturity, underlying etiology of seizure, EEG, neurological examination, and imaging studies of brain (Table 2).

MANAGEMENT AND DRUG THERAPY OF NEONATAL SEIZURES (FLOWCHARTS 1 AND 2)

Lidocaine should not be used if the infant has previously been treated with phenytoin and with underlying congenital heart disease (*see* Tables 3 and 4).

SUGGESTED READING

1. Handbook of Neonatology. The Neonatology Chapter of Indian Academy of Neonatology, 1st edition; 2013.
2. Martin RJ, Fanaroff AA, Walsh MC. Diseases of Fetus and Infant, Neonatal and Perinatal Medicine, 9th edition. Elsevier; 2011.
3. Volpe JJ. Neurology of the Newborn, 5th edition. Elsevier; 2008.
4. WHO/ILAE/IRCCS. Guidelines on Neonatal Seizures. World Health Organization Publication; 2011. pp. 1-100.

CHAPTER 7

Jaundice

Srinivas Murki

DEFINITION

- Icterus or jaundice is yellowish discoloration of skin, sclera, and mucus membrane.
- Jaundice should be observed in broad daylight.
- Jaundice should be differentiated from cholestasis by pigmented stools and no diaper staining.

ASSESSING SEVERITY OF JAUNDICE

Jaundice severity is assessed based on the onset, intensity of skin discoloration, associated clinical signs of hemolysis, laboratory reports and clinical features of bilirubin induced brain dysfunction. The features of severe or significant jaundice are as follows:
- Onset within the first 24 hours and/or rapid progression
- Jaundice affecting palms and soles
- Presence of risk factors for bilirubin encephalopathy such as:
  - Late preterm
  - Asphyxia
  - Sepsis
  - Intrauterine growth restriction
  - High bilirubin to albumin ratio
  - High free bilirubin
  - Metabolic acidosis.
- Clinical signs of hemolysis such as pallor, splenomegaly, onset within the first 24 hours and rapid progression.
- Clinical signs of bilirubin induced dysfunction with assessment from the bilirubin-induced neurologic dysfunction (BIND) score (Table 1)
- Total bilirubin levels >18 mg/dL after day 3 and age specific cut offs total bilirubin greater than the need for phototherapy (PT) on American Academy of Pediatrics (AAP) charts.

IDENTIFYING ETIOLOGY

Etiology of jaundice is evaluated from the history, course of jaundice, clinical

Table 1: BIND score.

	Mild (Score 1)	Moderate (Score 2)	Severe (Score 3)
Mental status	Sleepy and poor feeding	Lethargic and irritable	Semi coma and/or seizures
Muscle tone	Slight decrease	Hyper- or hypotonia depending on arousal state or mild nuchal/truncal arching	Markedly increased (opisthotonus) or decreased tone or bicycling movements
Character of cry	High pitched	Shrill	Inconsolable

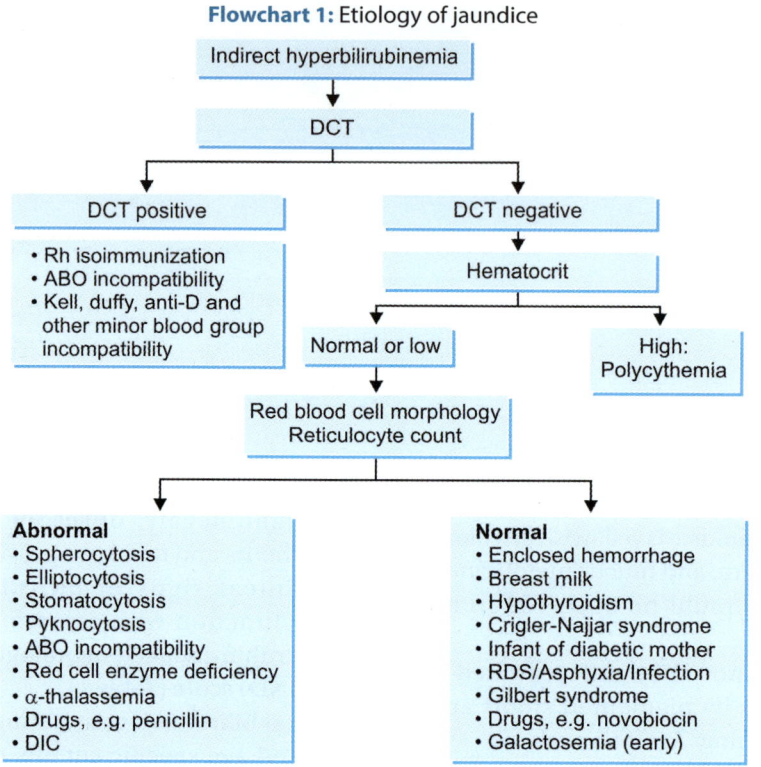

Flowchart 1: Etiology of jaundice

(DCT: direct Coombs' test; DIC: disseminated intravascular coagulation; RDS: respiratory distress syndrome)

examination, and laboratory reports. Any jaundiced infant should be first evaluated for hemolysis. In the presence of hemolysis it should be differentiated into immune and nonimmune hemolysis (Flowchart 1).

Signs of Hemolysis

- Onset of jaundice on day 1
- Rapid progression of jaundice
- Pallor
- Splenomegaly
- Packed cell volume (PCV) <40%
- Reticulocyte count >3%
- Peripheral smear showing marked anisopoikilocytosis, polychromasia, and nucleated RBCs.

Immune hemolysis should be suspected if:
- Mother blood group is O or Rh negative
- Baby blood group is AB or AB in presence of O blood group mother
- Baby is Rh positive and mother is RH negative
- Mother's ICT is positive and infant's direct Coombs' test (DCT) positive.

Practice point: False positive DCT can occur due to prozone phenomenon. Repeating DCT in dilution or with washed RBC will improve sensitivity.

Nonhemolytic jaundice can occur in the following situations:
- Cephalhematoma or subgaleal bleeds.
- Pallor in the absence of splenomegaly suggests internal or external bleeds.
- Family history of sibling with jaundice [glucose-6-phosphate dehydrogenase (G6PD) deficiency].
- Geographic origin of parents and rapidity of rise with mild or no clinical signs of hemolysis suggests G6PD deficiency
- Slow progression, absence of pallor, absence of bleed, weight loss and exclusive breast feeding suggest breast feeding jaundice (Table 2).

Evaluation of Jaundice (Table 2)

The evaluation of jaundice is described in Table 2.

Physical Examination

Physical examination has been shown in Table 3.

Investigations

Investigations have been shown in Table 4.

MANAGEMENT (FLOWCHART 2)

- Assess the severity of jaundice and risk factors for bilirubin encephalopathy

Table 2: Evaluation of jaundice.

History	Relevance
Fever and rash in mother during pregnancy	Intrauterine infection
Labor and delivery events	Asphyxia, trauma, use of oxytocin, delayed cord clamping
Maternal drugs (sulfonamide, nitrofurantoin, antimalarial)	Hemolysis in a glucose-6-phosphate dehydrogenase deficiency infant
Liver disease in family	Galactosemia, α-1 antitrypsin deficiency
Prolonged parenteral nutrition	Cholestatic jaundice

Table 3: Physical examination.

Physical examination	Relevance
SGA	Polycythemia, intrauterine infections (IUI)
Microcephaly	IUI
Pallor	Hemolytic anemia, extravasations of blood
Bruises, cephalhematoma	Increased bilirubin formation
Petechiae	IUI, sepsis, erythroblastosis
Hepatosplenomegaly	Hemolytic anemia, IUI, liver disease
Chorioretinitis	IUI
Urine staining diapers and clay color stool	Cholestasis

Table 4: Investigation.

Investigation	Relevance
PCV <40	Hemolysis or blood loss
Peripheral smear with anisopoikilocytosis, nucleated red blood cells, polychromasia	Hemolysis
Reticulocyte count >3%	Hemolysis or blood loss
Blood groups	Mother— O +ve, baby AB suggests isoimmunization. Mother Rh negative and baby Rh positive suggests isoimmunization
DCT	Positive suggests isoimmunization. Positive DCT with no blood group incompatibility suggests minor blood group incompatibility
G6PD levels	North west India and certain geographic locations
Conjugate bilirubin	>20% suggests conjugate hyperbilirubinemia
On follow-up	
BERA	• Done only if bilirubin is >18 or with signs of BIND • Better done at discharge or after 1 month. • Prolonged and increased latencies of wave III and V and decrease amplitude of wave III, V suggests bilirubin brain dysfunction
MRI	Basal ganglia hyperintensities in T1 and T2 weighted is suggestive bilirubin induced brain damage and possible risk of brain dysfunction

(PCV: packed cell volume; G6PD: glucose-6-phosphate dehydrogenase; MRI: magnetic resonance imaging; DCT: direct Coombs test)

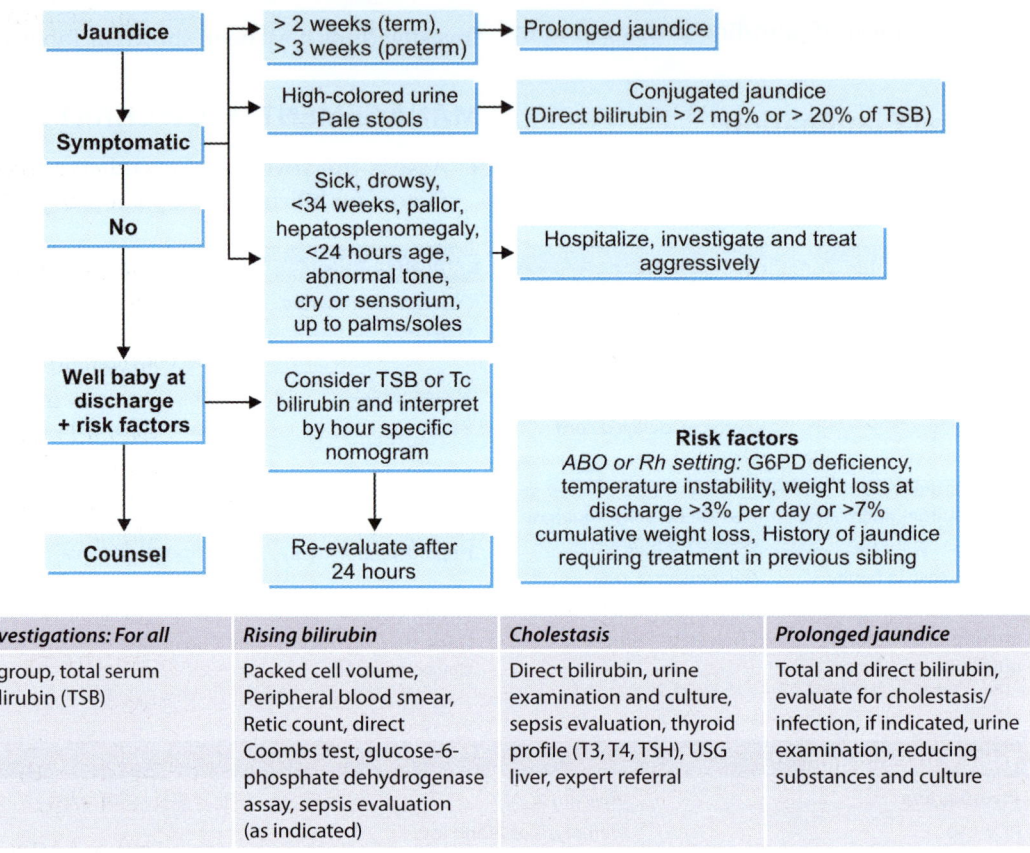

Flowchart 2: Management algorithm for a newborn with jaundice.

Investigations: For all	Rising bilirubin	Cholestasis	Prolonged jaundice
B group, total serum bilirubin (TSB)	Packed cell volume, Peripheral blood smear, Retic count, direct Coombs test, glucose-6-phosphate dehydrogenase assay, sepsis evaluation (as indicated)	Direct bilirubin, urine examination and culture, sepsis evaluation, thyroid profile (T3, T4, TSH), USG liver, expert referral	Total and direct bilirubin, evaluate for cholestasis/infection, if indicated, urine examination, reducing substances and culture

Note: Decision making is based on TSB. Do not subtract direct bilirubin fraction.

- Evaluate total serum bilirubin (TSB) levels
- Chart on AAP charts to decide on role of PT or exchange transfusion
- *Interpretation of AAP charts:*
  - Determine the need for PT
  - Infant age on X axis and TSB on Y axis (do not deduct direct from TSB)
  - Choose appropriate curve based on gestation and risk factors
  - The three curves on AAP charts indicate:
    1. *Top curve:* Infants at lower risk (≥38 weeks and well)
    2. *Middle curve:* Infants at medium risk (≥38 weeks + risk factors, or 35–37 6/7 weeks and well
    3. *Lower curve:* Infants at higher risk: (35–37 6/7 + risk factors)
- Risk factors include—isoimmune hemolytic disease, G6PD deficiency, asphyxia, significant lethargy, temperature instability, sepsis, acidosis or albumin <3.0 g/dL
  - For preterm and low birth weight babies NICE (National Institute for Health and Care Excellence) guidelines are used for PT.

ADMINISTRATION OF PHOTOTHERAPY

- Phototherapy is administered when the TSB levels are above the respective curves for

term (AAP charts) or preterms (Fanaroff/NNF guidelines).
- Special blue tube lights, special blue CFL lamps, and high intensity gallium nitride blue light emitting diodes are commonly used in dose if minimum of 15 µW/cm²/nm and ideally 30 µW/cm²/nm.
- Double surface and multiple PT is indicated if TSB rises rapidly (>0.5 mg/dL/hr), TSB is within 3 mg/dL of the threshold for exchange transfusion and/or TSB fails to respond to single surface PT within 6 hours
- While under PT, the baby's eyes and genitals (male infants) are to be covered without putting pressure on face and nose.
- Mother should be counseled for need to breastfeed on demand or every 2–3 hours
- The light should be as close to the baby as possible to increase the efficacy
- The efficacy depends on the type of light, surface area of exposure, intensity of light and baby condition:
  - *Type of light*: Blue light is the best as the spectrum of blue is best absorbed by bilirubin
  - *Intensity*: It can be improved by using LED or CFL light. The higher the intensity the better the efficacy. Intensity can also be increased by decreasing the distance between the lamps and baby
  - *Surface area*: It can be increased by double or triple surface light, by using fiber optic along with CFL/LED or by changing the position of the baby or by using reflectors
  - *Condition of baby*: Feeding the baby and ensuring euhydration status increases the efficacy.

STOPPING THE PHOTOTHERAPY

Stop PT once TSB values are at least 2 mg/dL below the PT cut-offs. Check for rebound rise in TSB after 8–12 hours in neonates with gestational age (GA) <35 weeks, birth weight <2000 g, G6PD deficiency or hemolytic diseases.

PRACTICE POINTS

- *Aggressive PT is the cornerstone for severe jaundice. Ensure adequate feeding while baby is under PT.*
- *Do not depend on transcutaneous bilirubin (TCB) or clinical estimation when baby is on PT.*
- *Monitor the progress of jaundice while under PT with frequent TSB measurements.*
- *Expose maximum body area and keep the baby under PT as much as possible.*
- *All management of jaundice is based on TSB and not on unconjugate bilirubin.*

EXCHANGE TRANSFUSION

Indications in Rh Incompatibility

- Hydrops fetalis and hemolysis
- Cord TSB >5 mg/dL
- Rise of bilirubin >0.5 mg/dL with Hb <9 g/dL or >1 mg/dL if Hb is >9 g/dL.

Indication in non-Rh cases: Based on AAP chart and risk factors.

Procedure for Exchange Transfusion

Blood exchange transfusion (BET) may be performed with:
- Umbilical vein cannulation which reaches inferior vena cava just below the right atrium junction
- Cannulation of umbilical vein and umbilical artery, or
- Cannulation of a peripheral artery (usually radial artery) and/or a large sized peripheral vein.

Single-catheter pull push technique: In this "central" technique, BET is usually performed by cannulating the umbilical vein (Fig. 1).

SECTION 1
Clinical Approach to Sick Newborn

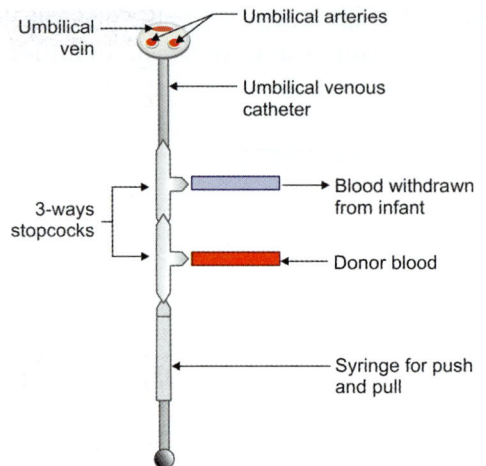

Fig. 1: Schematic diagram for performing a single-catheter pull push BET through the umbilical vein.

Table 5: Deciding about donor blood group.

Maternal group	Infant group	Donor blood group
O	O or A or B or AB	O
A or B or AB	O or A or B or AB	Baby blood group or O group
Rh negative	Rh positive or negative	Rh negative

- The procedure is performed ensuring normothermia and continuous monitoring of vital parameters.
- The area around the umbilical vein is cleaned using betadine. Sterile surgical eye cloth is placed over the umbilicus.
- A loose cord tie is placed around the base of the cord to prevent ooze.
- A French size 5 or 8 umbilical catheter prefilled with saline and attached to a 10 mL syringe is gently inserted into the umbilical vein.
- The venous catheter is advanced to the predetermined distance.
- Two three-way stopcocks or one four-way stopcock is attached to catheter.
- The four channels of connection to the umbilical catheter should, respectively (and in sequence), connect to the umbilical catheter, catheter draining the withdrawn blood, donor blood, and a saline prefilled syringe.
- All the connections should be saline filled to exclude air reaching the umbilical catheter. The catheter or the connections should never be kept open to the atmosphere to prevent any air embolism.
- The first aliquot of blood drawn from the neonate is used for laboratory tests.
- An aliquot of 5–8% of infants is estimated for removal of blood volume (more sick or smaller the baby smaller the size of aliquot). In a term infant the aliquot size is 15–20 mL to be withdrawn or infused at a rate of 5 mL/kg/min.

Double-catheter pull push technique: The umbilical artery and vein are cannulated. Blood from the umbilical artery is withdrawn and simultaneously equal volume blood is pushed through the umbilical vein. Two personnel are needed to operate each catheter and one person for monitoring the synchronization. An isovolumetric infusion and withdrawal is the advantage of this procedure.

Choice of blood group for donor blood (ABO and Rh typing) is shown in Table 5.

GUIDELINES FOR MANAGEMENT OF JAUNDICE NEONATES BORN AT <35 WEEKS OF GESTATION

These guidelines have been shown in Table 6.

GUIDELINES FOR MANAGEMENT JAUNDICE NEONATES BORN AT ≥35 WEEKS OF GESTATION (TABLE 7)

These guidelines have been shown in Table 7. (Beyond 24 hours)

Table 6: Guidelines for management of jaundice neonates born at < 35 weeks of gestation.

Birth weight (g)	Phototherapy (mg/dL)		ET (mg/dL)
	Healthy infant	Sick infant	
<1000	5–7	4–6	Variable
1,001–1,500	7–10	6–8	Variable
1,501–2,000	10–12	8–10	Variable
2,001–2,500	12–15	10–12	Variable

(ET: exchange transfusion)

Table 7: Total serum bilirubin levels (mg/dL).

Age (hr)	Low risk ≥38 weeks and well		Medium risk ≥38 weeks + risk factors* or 35–37 6/7 weeks and well		High risk 35–37 6/7 weeks + risk factors*	
	PT	ET	PT	ET	PT	ET
24	9	19	7	17	5	15
48	12	22	10	19	8	17
72	15	24	12	21	10	18.5
96	17	25	14	22.5	11	19
> 96	18	25	15	22.5	12	19

*Risk factors—isoimmune hemolytic disease; G6PD deficiency, asphyxia, significant lethargy, temperature instability, sepsis, acidosis or albumin <3.0 g/dL
(PT: phototherapy; ET: exchange transfusion)

ROLE OF INTRAVENOUS IMMUNOGLOBULINS

- Intravenous immunoglobulin (IvIg) is used in Rh/ABO incompatibility jaundice
- Use of IvIg prevents the need for exchange transfusion
- The treatment should be used in the early phase of jaundice
- Dose is 1 g/kg once daily for 2 days or 0.5 g/kg once daily for 5 days

IV FLUIDS/FLUID SUPPLEMENT

- It is indicated when baby is dehydrated or has significant weight loss
- No role of phenobarbitone in treatment of acute jaundice.

PREVENTION

- *Predischarge screening:* All babies should be screened before discharge for risk factors and/or TCB/TSB.
- Total serum bilirubin can be plotted in age specific Bhutani chart to decide on need for follow-up (Figs. 1 and 2).

Risk factors: Presence of one or more risk factors before discharge would need the baby for follow up 24 hours or on day 3 or day 4 of life (Box 1).

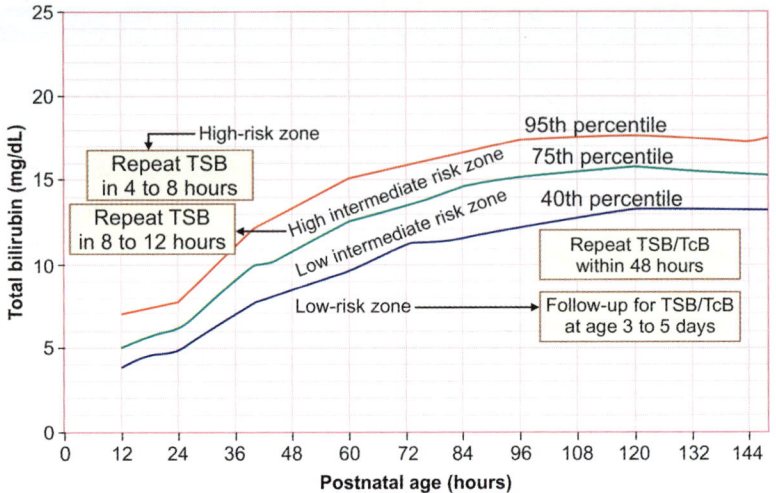

Fig. 2: An approach for a timed follow-up to repeat jaundice and bilirubin evaluation based on predischarge bilirubin testing by plotting TSB or TcB (<15 mg per 100 ml) on an hour-specific bilirubin nomogram A TcB >15 mg per 100 mL needs confirmation by laboratory TSB assay. Infants with early-onset extreme hyperbilirubinemia requiring intervention <48 hours were not included in the predictive nomogram because treatment with phototherapy and/or exchange transfusion had already been instituted.

(*Source*: Adapted from Kaplan et al.)

(TcB: transcutaneous bilirubin; TSB: total serum bilirubin).

Box 1

No role in jaundice management.

- Prophylactic phototherapy
- Sunlight
- Albumin infusion
- Routine IV calcium for exchange transfusion
- Supplementation of water, dextrose feeds
- Stopping breastfeeding in breast milk jaundice
- Routine phenobarbitone
- Herbal remedies
- Steroids

SUGGESTED READING

1. American Academy of Pediatrics Subcommittee on Hyperbilirubinemia. Management of hyperbilirubinemia in the newborn infant 35 or more weeks of gestation. Pediatrics. 2004;114(1):297-316.
2. Bell R, Bhutani VK, Bollman DL, et al. Severe Hyperbilirubinemia Prevention (SHP Toolkit), California Perinatal Quality Care Collaborative (CPQCC); 2005. Available from: http://www.cpqcc.org/quality_improvement/qi_toolkits/severe_hyperbilirubinemia_prevention_rev_october_2005.pdf. [Last accessed April, 2019].
3. Guruprasad G, Chawla D, Aggarwal S. *Management of Neonatal Hyperbilirubinemia*. In: Kumar P (Ed). NNF Clinical Practice Guidelines. 2010. Available from: http://nnfpublication.org/Uploads/Articles/0b79b423-4675-4420-98e6-5d14dd6fceaa.pdf. [Last accessed April, 2019].
4. Kaplan M, Wong RJ, Sibley E, et al. Neonatal Jaundice and Liver Disease. In: Martin R, Fanaroff A, Walsh M (Eds). Fanaroff and Martin's Neonatal-Perinatal Medicine: Diseases of the Fetus and Infant, 9th edition. Mosby Publications; 2010. pp. 1-2008.

CHAPTER 8

Suspected Congenital Heart Defect

Monica Kaushal

INTRODUCTION

Congenital heart diseases (CHDs) refer to structural or functional heart diseases, which manifest any time from birth, infancy or adulthood depending on the degree and severity of defect. Cardiac defect should be part of differential diagnosis in any unwell infant. High index of suspicion and systematic approach is vital for early diagnosis of CHD (Fig. 1).

APPROACH TO ETIOLOGY

Type of presentation, age at presentation, clinical evaluation, CXR, and ECG provide important clues in the diagnosis of most CHDs.

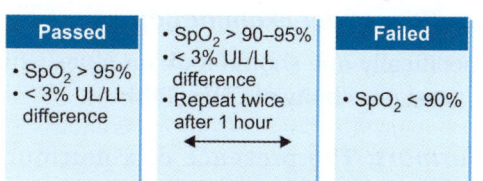

Fig. 1: Interpreting pulse oximeter screen for critical congenital heart defect.

(LL: lower limb; UL: upper limb)

Type of Presentation

Majority of symptomatic CHD infants present with one of the following as predominant problems—shock, cyanosis and/or respiratory distress.

Shock

Presence of signs of poor perfusion with associated murmur and cardiomegaly suggests cardiogenic shock. The manifestations are abrupt and life-threatening unless prompt measures are taken.
- In obstructive lesions affecting the left side of heart (e.g. hypoplastic left heart syndrome, critical aortic stenosis, and interrupted aortic arch), systemic perfusion is absent or markedly reduced.
- In obstructive lesions affecting the right side of heart (e.g. TAPVC, tricuspid atresia, and mitral atresia), the pulmonary blood flow is diminished resulting in decreased systemic blood flow, leading to shock.
- Defects with parallel pulmonary and systemic circulations [e.g. transposition of the great artery (TGA) with intact ventricular septum], mixing between the two circulations is decreased, leading to hypoxia, metabolic acidosis, cardiac failure, and shock.

Cyanosis

Closure of the ductus during the first few days of life precipitates clinical status causing profound cyanosis if:
- Ductus arteriosus is the only conduit of pulmonary blood flow, such as in patients with critically obstructive right heart lesions (critical pulmonary stenosis/atresia). Progressive cyanosis sets in as the ductus closes.
- Ductus arteriosus is the major supplier of systemic circulation as in critically obstructive left heart lesions (e.g. hypoplastic left heart and critical aortic valve stenosis). Poor perfusion leading to shock is the manifestation as the ductus closes.
- Ductus serves as a common channel mixing blood from pulmonary and systemic circulations (e.g. TGA). Such patients manifest with profound cyanosis and cardiogenic shock.

Cyanotic heart defects are clinically identified as those associated with increased pulmonary blood flow and those with decreased pulmonary blood flow.

Severe Respiratory Distress (Pulmonary Edema)

Signs include tachypnea, chest indrawing, hypoxia, leading to progressive increase in work of breathing. Sudden increase in pulmonary blood flow during transition due to fall in pulmonary pressure is the underlying cause. Examples include truncus arteriosus or patent ductus arteriosus or pulmonary venous circulation obstruction in total anomalous pulmonary venous connection (TAPVC) with obstruction.

Later Presentation

At times, critical CHDs are well at discharge only to deteriorate suddenly during 2–3 weeks of life. At every visit, the clinician should be alert for subtle signs.

Age at Presentation

Timing of presentation is influenced by type and severity of cardiac defect. Duct dependent lesions usually present after first 48 hours of birth.
- *Ductus dependent lesions*: This includes coarctation of the aorta (COA), interrupted aortic arch, aortic stenosis, hypoplastic left heart syndrome (HLHS), and TGAs. Sudden onset deterioration with poor perfusion is the hallmark.
- *Nonductal-dependent cyanotic lesions*: Nonductal-dependent cyanotic lesions have variable time period of manifestations. Tachypnea, mild cyanosis, and single second heart sound lead to suspicion of underlying defect. Truncus arteriosus, tetralogy of Fallot (TOF), and TAPVC are thus missed at the time of hospital discharge.

Newborn screening is a good screening tool for detecting critical congenital heart defects (CCHDs) (Table 1).

Clinical Evaluation

Clinical Manifestations

The manifestations depend on the type and severity of heart defect. Many are asymptomatic and detected on routine clinical examination. History and presence of certain symptoms and signs should raise suspicion of heart disease (Tables 2 to 4). Majority may deteriorate before a diagnosis is reached.

Cardiovascular Examination

Specifically one should look for clues which suggest possibility of CHD (Table 5).

Murmurs: The presence of a murmur is often associated with CHD. Murmur may be initially absent in HLHS, TGA, pulmonary atresia (PA) and cardiomyopathy, and aortic stenosis or ventricular septal defect (VSD). All murmurs are not pathological. Presence

CHAPTER 8
Suspected Congenital Heart Defect

Table 1: Newborn screen for CCHD (See Fig. 1).

For whom?	All well newborns
When?	At hospital discharge from birth
Why?	Identification of 7 disorders—hypoplastic left heart syndrome, pulmonary atresia (PA), TOF, TAPVC, TGA, tricuspid atresia (TA) and truncus arteriosus (TAC)
How?	Pulse oximeter
Where?	At hospital discharge, using oximeter probe placed over right hand (preductal) and either foot (pulse oximeter) and recording the SpO_2
Limitation?	Does not detect all left heart obstructive defects Does not detect acyanotic heart defects
Positive screen?	SpO_2 measurement <90% or SpO_2 measurement <95% in both upper and lower extremities on three measurements, each separated by 1 hour or SpO_2 difference >3% between the upper and lower extremities
Negative screen?	>95% in right hand or foot and <3% difference between right hand and foot
Counsel?	A negative screen does not rule out a heart defect

(CCHD: critical congenital heart defect; TAPVC: total anomalous pulmonary venous connection; TGA: transposition of great arteries; TOF: tetralogy of Fallot).

Table 2: Clinical clues to heart disease.

Symptoms	Signs
• Intermittent suckling • Sweating over forehead on feeds • Not gaining weight • Color changes on crying • Excessive crying • Repeated chest infections	• Murmur • Hyperdynamic precordium • Bounding pulses • Absent lower limb pulses • Unexplained hepatomegaly • Cyanosis on crying • Differential cyanosis • Single S2 • Hypertension • Anomalies • Progressive or refractory hypoxia

Table 3: Maternal/perinatal history.

ASK	Rationale
Preterm gestation	More common in preterm than term
Maternal illness	Diabetes, hypertension, epilepsy, 1st trimester fever, smoking, connective tissue disorders, TORCH infections increase risk of CHD in fetus
Maternal drugs	Phenytoin (PS, AS), lithium (e.g. Ebstein's anomaly) and alcohol (ASD, VSD)
Assisted reproductive technology (ART)	Risk for outflow tracts and ventriculoarterial connections
Family history	Increased risk if previous sibling affected

(AS: aortic stenosis; PS: pulmonary stenosis; ASD: atrial septal defect; CHD: congenital heart disease; VSD: ventricular septal defect).

SECTION 1
Clinical Approach to Sick Newborn

Table 4: Caveats in cardiac evaluation.

Murmur	• Murmur detection is subjective • Can be heard in about 1–2% of all newborns • Less than half of these murmurs indicate CHD
Cyanosis	• Clinical detection of cyanosis subjective and too late • Not all cyanosis is due to CHD • Anemia delays interpretation
Pulse	• Difficult to appreciate in newborn • Absent pulse is seen with LVOT obstruction • Presence of a pulse does not rule out LVOT obstruction
Cardiomegaly	• Strong predictor of heart disease (sensitivity: 85%, specificity: 95%, PPV: 95%) • Not a feature of all CHD • Can be due to noncardiac causes • An expiratory film of XRC may show pseudocardiomegaly
Cardiac failure	• Nonspecific signs • Not a feature of all CHD • Also seen due to noncardiac causes

(CHD: congenital heart disease; LVOT: left ventricular outflow tract; XRC: X-ray chest).

Table 5: Clinical cardiac examination.

Inspection	
Growth	Failure to thrive suggests complex/chronic heart disease
Cyanosis	Exaggerated on crying and relieves on rest
Ashen gray complexion	Suggests mixing of oxygenated/deoxygenated blood
Shock	Mottling, pale, delayed capillary refill time, weak pulses, cold extremities, drowsy, low BP
Work of breathing	Tachypnea, chest indrawing, grunt
Hyperdynamic precordium	Suggests right ventricular volume or pressure overload
Apical impulse	For cardiomegaly, dextrocardia,
Differential SpO_2	Upper limb SpO_2 >lower limb by 20%
Palpation	
Pulse	Bounding pulse (PDA), weak pulse (shock, obstructive left heart defects), fast or slow pulse (>200 or <100 bpm) suggests arrhythmia
Femoral pulses	Absent or weak with coarctation of aorta and interrupted aortic arch
Thrill	Suggests outflow tract obstruction
4 limb BP	A difference of >10 mm Hg is seen between upper and lower limb with left sided obstructive heart defects.
Hepatomegaly	Most reliable sign for CCF in newborns
Auscultation	
Second heart sound	Loud or single S2 suggests pulmonary hypertension, Single S2 beyond 48 hours suggests aortic atresia, pulmonary atresia or truncus arteriosus
Split of second heart sound	Widal or fixed split S2 (e.g. ASD, right ventricular volume overload),
Systolic clicks	Seen with semilunar valve stenosis, bicuspid aortic valve, and truncus arteriosus .
Mid-systolic clicks	Seen with mitral valve prolapse and with Ebstein's anomaly
S3 gallop	Cardiac failure
Pericardial rub	Suggests pericarditis or pericardial effusion

(ASD: atrial septal defect; CCF: congestive cardiac failure; PDA: patent ductus arteriosus).

Table 6: Characteristics of pathological murmur.

- Murmur intensity grade 3 or higher
- Harsh quality
- Pansystolic duration
- Loudest at upper left, upper right sternal border, or apex
- Abnormal S2
- Associated absent or diminished femoral pulses or noncardiac abnormalities

Table 7: Hyperoxia test results in neonates with cyanosis.

	PaO_2 (percent saturation) when $FiO_2 = 0.21$		PaO_2 (percent saturation) when $FiO_2 = 1$	CO_2
Normal	>70 (>95)		>300 (100)	35
Pulmonary disease	50 (85)		>150 (100)	50
Neurologic disease	50 (85)		>150 (100)	50
Methemoglobinemia	>70 (<85)		>200 (<85)	35
Cardiac disease				
Parallel circulation	<40 (<75)		<50 (<85)	35
Mixing with reduced PBF	<40 (<75)		<50 (<85)	35
Mixing without restricted PB	40–60 (75–93)		<150 (<100)	35
Differential cyanosis	Preductal 70 (95)	Postductal <40 (<75)	Variable	35–50
Reverse differential cyanosis	<40 (<75)	>50 (>90)		

of certain features suggests a pathological murmur (Table 6).

Hyperoxia test: The hyperoxia test is useful in distinguishing cardiac from noncardiac causes of cyanosis, especially pulmonary disease (Table 7).

Extracardiac abnormalities: Extracardiac abnormalities are frequently detected in children with CHD. Skeletal abnormalities, especially those of the hand and arm, are often associated with cardiac malformations. CHD may be a component of many specific syndromes and chromosomal disorders.

INVESTIGATIONS (TABLES 8 AND 9)

A normal neonatal electrocardiogram (ECG) has right axis deviation (QRS axis +90° to +180°) and a precordial pattern of right ventricular hypertrophy.

Lesions associated with a small right ventricle have the following:
- Left axis deviation for age (for pulmonary atresia intact ventricular septum typically +30° to +90°; for tricuspid atresia with normally related great arteries typically −30° to −90°)

Right atrial enlargement—Tall peaked P waves most easily identified in lead II.

MANAGEMENT

- *General supportive care*: Initial management begins with general care that includes cardiorespiratory support and monitoring to ensure sufficient organ/tissue perfusion and oxygenation:
  - Temperature maintenance.

Table 8: Role of investigations.

X-ray chest	• For lung fields, vascularity, pulmonary disease • Heart size, position • Massive cardiomegaly (Ebstein's anomaly) • Boot shaped heart (TOF), egg on string (d-TGA), snowman (TAPVC) • Situs aortic arch
ECG	• Rate and rhythm • P, QRS and T axes • Intracardiac conduction interval • Evidence for chamber enlargement or hypertrophy • Evidence for pericardial disease, ischemia, infarction, or electrolyte abnormalities
2D Echo	• For structure, function, flow, infective endocarditis
Catheterization	• For aortopulmonary collaterals in TOF, RV to coronary fistula in PA • For hemodynamics after initial palliative surgery

(PA: pulmonary artery; RV: right ventricle; TAPVC: total anomalous pulmonary venous connection; TGA: transposition of great arteries; TOF: tetralogy of Fallot).

Table 9: Findings on examination, X-ray and ECG of cyanotic heart disease.

	Physical examination		Chest X-ray			ECG	
Diagnosis	S2	Murmur	Heart size	PBF	Percent right aortic arch	QRS axis	Hypertrophy
TGA	Single	None	↑	↑	4	90–150	Nml
TOF	Single	Sys	Boot	↓	20	90–150	Nml
HLHS	Single	Sys	↑	VC		90–150	↓ LV forces
PA-IVS	Single	Sys	↑↑	↓		30–90	LVH, RAE
PS	Single	Sys	↑	↓		30–90	LVH, RAE
TAPVC	Split	Sys	↑/nil	↑VC		90–150	RAE
Tricuspid atresia	Single	Sys	↑	↓		–30 to –90	LVH, RAE
Truncus arteriosus	Single	Sys + dys	↑	↑	30	90–150	Nml
Ebstein's	Split	Sys	↑↑	↓		90–150	RAE

(ECG: electrocardiography; PBF: pulmonary blood flow; TAPVC: total anomalous pulmonary venous connection; TGA: transposition of great arteries; TOF: tetralogy of Fallot; RAE: right atrial enlargement; LVH: left ventricular hypertrophy; HLHS: hypoplastic left heart syndrome; PA-IVS: pulmonary atresia with intact ventricular septum; PS: pulmonary stenosis).

- Vital signs should be monitored.
- Four limb saturation and BP.
- Full lead ECG.
- If respiratory compromise, an adequate airway should be established immediately.
- Supplemental oxygen and/or mechanical ventilation instituted as needed.
- Patients with hypotension or poor perfusion require cardiopulmonary resuscitation.
- Placement of secure intravenous and intra-arterial catheters is most easily accomplished via the umbilical vessels.
- Correction and monitoring of acid-base balance.
- Metabolic derangements (hypoglycemia, hypocalcemia) corrected.
- Inotropic agents such as dopamine and dobutamine may be necessary to correct hypotension.

- In infants with severe polycythemia (>70%), an isovolumetric partial exchange transfusion should be performed with saline to reduce the hematocrit.
- If cyanosis is due to acquired methemoglobinemia, the offending agent is removed. In severe cases, methylene blue, 1% solution, in a dose of 1–2 mg/kg (0.1–0.2 mL/kg of a 1% solution) is infused intravenously over 5–10 min. The dose can be repeated in 1 hour if needed. Congenital methemoglobinemia does not respond to methylene blue.
- *Antibiotics*: Sepsis can lead to cyanosis and left ventricular dysfunction or pulmonary disease. As a result, unless another specific etiology is promptly identified, broad-spectrum antibiotics should be initiated after obtaining blood and urine cultures.
- *Specific CHD measures*: In most cases, cyanotic CHD is dependent upon a patent ductus arteriosus for pulmonary or systemic blood flow. Closure of the ductus arteriosus can precipitate rapid clinical deterioration.
- *Prostaglandin E1*: In infants who have a clinical suspicion for a ductal-dependent congenital heart defect, prostaglandin E1 should be administered until a definitive diagnosis or treatment is established (Table 10).

Prostaglandin E2 = Dinoprostone may also be used. Dose is—oral 20–25 mg/kg/hr and IV 0.003 mcg/kg/min initially and up to 0.02 mcg/kg/min.

- *Cardiac failure*: Babies with cardiac failure should be treated conventionally as follows:
  - Oxygen therapy
  - Restricted fluid intake to 120–150 mL/kg/day
  - Check urea and electrolytes for base line values
  - Frusemide 1–2 mg/kg once or twice daily
  - Spironolactone 1 mg/kg/day
  - Digoxin as follows, if necessary.

Digoxin:
- *Digitalization IV/IM*: 10 mcg/kg/dose total 3 doses at interval of 8 or 12 hours.
- *Maintenance*: 8 mcg/kg/dose every 24 hours.
- *Oral digitalization*: 15 mcg/kg/dose and total 3 doses at interval of 8–12 hours
- *Maintenance oral*: 10 mcg/kg/dose every 24 hours.

It is important to assess the effects on the individual and to adjust the dose according to clinical response. On those on long-term therapy we need to increase the dose according

Table 10: PGE1 use.	
When?	All suspected duct dependent heart defects or sudden deterioration without a cause
Strength?	500 mg/mL
Dilution?	5% D or Normal saline
Dose	0.05 mcg/kg per minute
	If duct dependent, 0.01 mcg/kg per min
	0.1 mcg/kg per min (maximum)
Complication?	Apnea, hypotension, tachycardia
Back up	Respiratory support
Deterioration?	Associated with pulmonary venous or left atrial obstruction (e.g. TAPVC, HLHS, cor triatriatum, severe mitral stenosis or atresia, or D-TGA associated with restrictive atrial shunting)

(HLHS: hypoplastic left heart syndrome; TAPVC: total anomalous pulmonary venous connection; TGA: transposition of great arteries).

to weight. Check electrolytes regularly and give potassium supplements, if needed. When digoxin toxicity is suspected check digoxin levels.

- *Arrhythmias*: Extrasystoles are common both supraventricular and ventricular. If there is no evidence of CHD, they should be monitored and urea and electrolytes and calcium and magnesium checked. May need ECG if persistent and referred for echo.
- *Paroxysmal supraventricular tachycardia*: It is the most common serious arrhythmia heart rate (HR) 180–300/min with normal QRS complexes on ECG. They often begin and end spontaneously but if persist for more than a few hours cardiac failure will develop. Look for abnormal P waves, short PR interval and delta waves suggestive of Wolff-Parkinson-White (WPW) syndrome.

TREATMENT

- Try vagal stimulation first ice bag on the face or immerse infant face in cold water for a few seconds. Try several times under ECG monitoring if no response.
- *Adenosine*: It is drug of choice. Give as fast as possible 50 mcg/kg/dose and increase by 50 mcg/kg/dose every 3–4 min to a maximum of 300 mcg/kg/dose. More recently larger doses have been suggested 0.2 mg/kg. Response is usually immediate with transient flushing and arrhythmia seen on ECG. Unfortunately recurrence is common but further dose can be given at 2–5 min intervals.
- *Cardioversion*: A hemodynamically unstable baby who does not respond to adenosine can be treated with direct current (DC) cardioversion with 0.5–2 Joules/kg.
- *Maintenance drugs*: Digoxin can be started at 5 mcg/kg twice daily or propranolol 0.5 mg–1 mg/kg/dose every 8 hours. Propranolol may cause apnea and hypoglycemia. Digoxin should not be given in WPW syndrome because of risk of enhancing antegrade conduction across the accessory pathway. Amiodarone may also be used. Do not give verapamil.
- *Atrial flutter and AV reciprocating tachycardia*: Rapid transesophageal atrial pacing.
- *Ventricular tachycardia*: It is associated with hypoxemia, shock, electrolyte disturbance, digoxin toxicity, and catecholamine toxicity, prolonged QTc syndrome and intramyocardial tumors.
  - Treatment:
    - Underlying cause rapidly sought and treated
    - Hemodynamic stable baby is given lidocaine bolus (1–2 mg/kg) followed by maintenance (20–50 µg/kg/min)
    - Hemodynamically compromised is given DC cardioversion 1–2 J/kg but will be ineffective in presence of acidosis. If severe acidosis must be treated.
- *Ventricular fibrillation*: It is a preterminal arrhythmia. There is coarse irregular pattern on ECG with no identifiable QRS complexes. There are no peripheral pulses or heart sounds on examination. Cardiopulmonary resuscitation should be instituted and defibrillation starting of 1–2 J/kg performed. A bolus of lidocaine 1 mg/kg followed by infusion should be started. Once the neonate is resuscitated the underlying problem is evaluated and treated.
- *Congenital heart block*: This may be—
  - Isolated
  - Associated with CHD—especially atrioventricular (AV) septal defects.
  - Associated with maternal lupus erythematosus and anti-ro antibodies.
  - May be noted in utero, or misinterpreted as fetal distress.

- Is often asymptomatic with HR about 50/min, narrow QRS, normal heart size requires no treatment unless there is associated heart disease or evidence of failure with HR 40/min.
- Treatment:
  - Firstly diuretics if heart failure.
  - Then isoprenaline infusion in 5% Dextrose, 0.2 mcg/kg/min.
  - Finally pacing.
- *Cardiac catheterization*: Cardiac catheter interventions can either be palliative by improving cyanosis or be corrective by relieving obstruction to flow.
  - Balloon atrial septostomy can relieve marked cyanosis in patients with transposition of great arteries (d-TGS) associated with restrictive atrial shunting, and in patients with a restrictive atrial septum associated with left-sided obstructive disease. In patients with D-TGA, this procedure can be performed at the bedside under echocardiographic guidance.
  - Balloon valvuloplasty can be effective in patients with critical pulmonary stenosis or aortic stenosis. Selected patients with pulmonary atresia are also candidates for balloon valvuloplasty.
  - Transcatheter occlusion of pulmonary arteriovenous malformations can also be performed.
- *Transport*: When it is necessary to transfer a neonate with cyanotic CHD from the birth hospital to another medical facility with pediatric cardiology expertise, the patient should be intubated and mechanically ventilated prior to and during transport if prostaglandin E1 is being administered. A successful transport involves two transition of care. Referring hospital staff, the transport team and accepting hospital staff. There should be detailed and complete communication of information between these teams under instructions of pediatric cardiologist.
  - Communication to referral hospital
  - Reliable vascular access and if possible umbilical vein catheter (UVC) to be inserted
  - Prostaglandin infusion with infusion pump
  - Inotropes if required
  - Parent airway so better to intubate and ventilate before transfer
  - Gastric decompression with orogastric tube
  - Acid base status and oxygen delivery should be checked with arterial blood gas sampling before transport. But better to avoid 100% oxygen for the risk of duct closure
  - Hemodynamic status including HR, BP, and distal perfusion should be reassessed (Flowchart 1).

Flowchart 1: Summary of approach to suspected congenital heart disease.

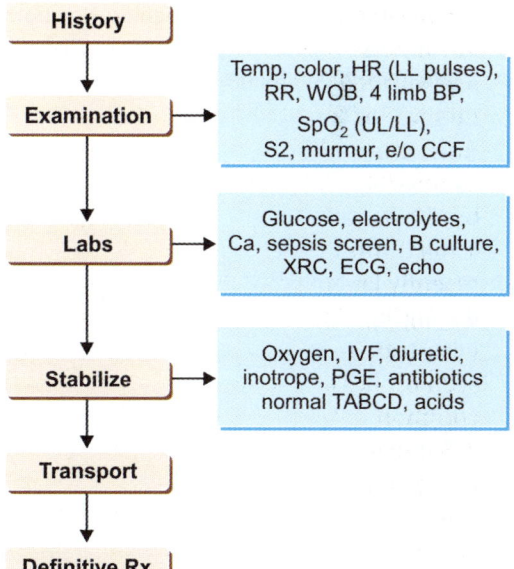

(HR: heart rate; LL: lower limb pulses; RR: respiratory rate; BP: blood pressure; UL: upper limb; Ca: calcium; WOB: work of breathing; CCF: congestive cardiac failure; PGE: prostaglandin; TABCDE: temperature airway breathing circulation dextrose).

SUGGESTED READING

1. Donofrio MT, Moon-Grady AJ, Hornberger LK, et al.; American Heart Association Adults with Congenital Heart Disease Joint Committee of the Council on Cardiovascular Disease in the Young and Council on Clinical Cardiology, Council on Cardiovascular Surgery and Anesthesia, and Council on Cardiovascular and Stroke Nursing. Diagnosis and treatment of fetal cardiac disease: a scientific statement from the American Heart Association. Circulation. 2014;129(21):2183-242.
2. Evans N. Echocardiography on neonatal intensive care units in Australia and New Zealand. J Paediatr Child Health. 2000;36(2):169-71.
3. Keane JF, Fyler DC, Lock JE. Nadas' Pediatric Cardiology, 2nd edition. WB Saunders, 2006. pp. 1-960.
4. Krishnan US. Approach to congenital heart disease in the Neonate. Indian J Pediatr. 2002;69(6): 501-5.
5. Liske MR, Greeley CS, Law DJ, et al. Tennessee Task Force on Screening Newborn Infants for Critical Congenital Heart Disease. Report of Tennesse Task Force on Screening Newborn Infants for Critical Congenital Heart Disease. Pediatrics. 2006;118(4):e1250-6.
6. Mahle WT, Martin GR, Beekman RH 3rd, et al.; Section on Cardiology and Cardiac Surgery Executive Committee. Endorsement of Health and Human Services recommendation for pulse oximetry screening for critical congenital heart disease. Pediatrics. 2012;129(1):190-2.
7. Moss S, Kitchener DJ, Yoxall CW, et al. Evaluation of echocardiography on the neonatal unit. Arch Dis Child Fetal Neonatal Ed. 2003;88(4):F287-9; discussion F290-1.
8. Rein AJ, Omokhodian SI, Nir A. Significance of a cardiac murmur as the sole clinical sign in the newborn. Clin Pediatr (Phila). 2000;39(9):511-20.
9. Riede FT, Wörner C, Dähnert I, et al. Effectiveness of neonatal pulse oximetry screening for detection of critical congenital heart disease in daily clinical routine--results from a prospective multicenter study. Eur J Pediatr. 2010;169(8): 975-81.
10. Strife JL, Sze RW. Radiographic evaluation of the neonate with congenital heart disease. Radiol Clin North Am. 1999;37(6):1093-107, vi.
11. Thangaratinam S, Brown K, Zamora J, et al. Pulse oximetry screening for critical congenital heart defects in asymptomatic newborn babies: a systematic review and meta-analysis. Lancet. 2012;379(9835):2459-64.

CHAPTER 9

Fluid and Electrolyte Therapy

Sandeep Kadam

INTRODUCTION

Fluid and electrolyte management is essentially a balancing act between intake and output. The process is dynamic and is affected by gestation, weight, postnatal age, disease, organ function, maternal drugs, and clinical status (Fig. 1). An understanding of body fluid compartment helps titrate fluid and electrolyte therapy (Table 1).

The goal is to ensure a delicate balance between fluids, electrolytes and dextrose to ensure optimum body composition and function. It is better to assess and individualize the approach, case by case, rather than rely on a cookbook formula.

HOW MUCH FLUIDS?

Fluids are administered taking into account the following:
- Maintenance or daily requirement (Tables 2 to 4)

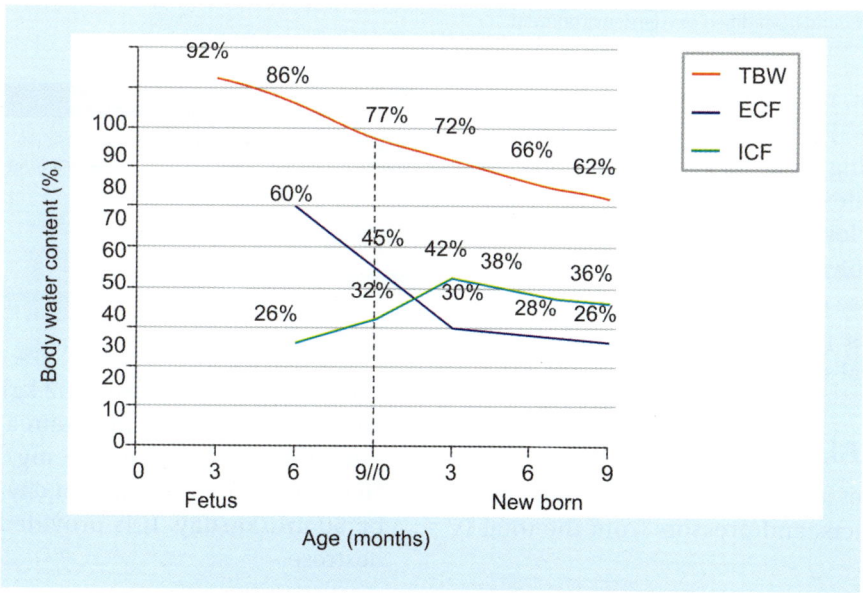

Fig. 1: Changes in body fluid compositions.
(TBW: total body weight; ECF: extracellular fluid; ICF: intracellular fluid).

Table 1: Total body water composition.

Intracellular compartment (40% body weight)	Extracellular compartment (20% body weight)	
	Interstitial tissues (15% body weight)	Plasma (5% body weight) Guide to therapy
Main electrolyte: K, PO_4 Regulates osmotic pressure	Main electrolyte: Na, Cl Regulates osmotic pressure	

Table 2: Maintenance fluid for term babies.

	Day of life						
	Day 1	Day 2	Day 3	Day 4	Day 5	Day 6	Day 7
Volume	60	75	90	105	120	135	150

Table 3: Maintenance fluid for preterm babies.

	Day of life						
	Day 1	Day 2	Day 3	Day 4	Day 5	Day 6	Day 7
1–1.5 kg	80	100	120	140	150	150	160
<1 kg*	100	120	140	150	160	160	180

*May need more fluid in extremely premature baby.

Table 4: Factors that influence water loss.

Factors that increase insensible water loss: Inversely related to gestational age and weight, respiratory distress, fever, radiant warmer, phototherapy, skin defects—omphalocele, gastroschisis, and nonhumidified oxygen/environment

Factors that decrease insensible water loss: Mature skin, heat shields, topical skin agents—paraffin, aquaphor, covering skin defects, and humidified oxygen/environment

- Deficit, reflected by acute weight change (Table 5)
- Ongoing losses (e.g. urine output, gastric aspirates, intercostal drain (ICD) drain, blood loss, etc.)
- Electrolyte imbalances
- Glucose status
- Disease process
- Clinical status.

Table 5: Identifying fluid deficit.

Degree of deficit	Weight loss (%)	Deficit fluid (cc/kg)
Mild	5	50
Moderate	10	100
Severe	15	150

- The initial fluids should be 10% dextrose (>1.2 kg) or 5% dextrose (<1.2 kg) with no additives in order to maintain a glucose infusion rate (GIR) of 4–6 mg/kg/min. Hence total fluid therapy on day 1 would be 60 mL/kg/day. It is provided as 10% dextrose.

CLINICAL TIPS

- Deduct amino acids, drug volume, blood products, and pressors from the total IV fluids.

- Sodium and potassium should be added after 48 hours of age and glucose infusion should be maintained at 4–6 mg/kg/min.
- Maintenance of fluid adjustment needs to take into consideration the insensible losses (Table 3).
- Strategies to reduce insensible loss include humidified incubators in extremely preterm babies, transparent plastic barriers over radiant warmers, emollients applications on skin, covering skin defects and using humidifiers in ventilators.

ELECTROLYTE SUPPLEMENTATION

- Sodium and potassium should be started in the IV fluids after 48 hours, each in a dose of 2–3 mEq/kg/day.
- Calcium may be used in a dose of 4 mL/kg/day (40 mg/kg/day) of calcium gluconate for the first 3 days in certain high-risk situations such as prematurity, infant of diabetic mothers.

WHICH FLUIDS?

The knowledge of body fluid composition guides the choice of fluids (Table 6).

- Gastric aspirates are replaced by half (1/2) normal saline (NS). Ileostomy losses are replaced by 0.9 NS.
- The composition of commonly used fluids and use are depicted in Table 7.

RATE OF FLUID ADMINISTRATION

- Calculate the 24 hour fluid requirement and use an infusion pump to administer mL/hr fluids.
- If infusion pump is not available, use a micro drip set. Adjust the rate (micro drops/min) = Volume of Fluid (mL)/24 hrs.

Table 6: Composition of body fluid compartment.

	ICF (mEq/L)	ECF (mEq/L)
Sodium	20	135–145
Potassium	150	3–5
Chloride	—	98–110
Bicarbonate	10	20–25
Phosphate	110–115	5
Protein	75	10

Table 7: Composition of commonly used fluids.

		Dextrose (g/L)	Na	K	Cl	Lactate	Ca	mOsm/L
Isotonic	NS		154		154			308
	RL		131	5	111	29	2	270
½ isotonic	½ NS		77		77			154
Electrolyte free solution	5%	50						278
	10%	100						556
Dextrose electrolyte solution	5% DNS	50	154		154			585
	D5½ NS	50	77		77			415
	D5 0.33% NaCl	50	57		57			381
	D5 0.2% NaCl	50	34		34			347
Pediatric maintenance	Isolyte P	50	25	20	22			368

HOW MUCH DEXTROSE?

The optimum requirement is decided by GIR which normally is 4–6 mg/kg/min to ensure blood glucose always above 45 mg%. The GIR needs to be increased or decreased either by altering the volume of fluid or concentration of dextrose.

The GIR can be delivered in variable ways depending on clinical requirement (Table 8).

MONITORING OF FLUID AND ELECTROLYTE STATUS

Body Weight

- Reflects total body water (TBW). Not very useful for intravascular volume.
- A serial weight measurement is a sensitive marker for over or under hydration in newborns.
- Loss of weight in term neonates of >2% per day or >10% of body weight is pathological and suggests fluid loss or inadequate fluids.
- Loss of weight in preterm neonates of >3% per day or >20% of body weight is pathological and suggests fluid loss or inadequate fluids.
- A weight loss of 1–2% daily and 10–15% of birth weight is physiological in term/preterm.
- Failure to lose weight in the first week of life suggests fluid retention and a need for evaluation of the underlying cause.

Clinical Examination (Table 9)

- Fluid status is assessed clinically for under or over hydration.
- Tachycardia suggests inadequate fluids or too much fluid.

Table 8: Glucose infusion rate calculator.

Dextrose % → mL/kg/day	5	6	7	7.5	8	9	10	11	12	12.5	14	15	20
10	0.3	0.4	0.5	0.5	0.6	0.6	0.7	0.8	0.8	0.9	1.0	1.0	1.4
20	0.7	0.8	1.0	1.0	1.1	1.3	1.4	1.5	1.7	1.7	1.9	2.1	2.8
30	1.0	1.3	1.5	1.6	1.7	1.9	2.1	2.3	2.5	2.6	2.9	3.1	4.2
40	1.4	1.7	1.9	2.1	2.2	2.5	2.8	3.1	3.3	3.5	3.9	4.2	5.6
50	1.7	2.1	2.4	2.6	2.8	3.1	3.5	3.8	4.2	4.3	4.9	5.2	6.9
60	2.1	2.5	2.9	3.1	3.3	3.8	4.2	4.6	5.0	5.2	5.8	6.3	8.3
70	2.4	2.9	3.4	3.6	3.9	4.4	4.9	5.3	5.8	6.1	6.8	7.3	9.7
80	2.8	3.3	3.9	4.2	4.4	5.0	5.6	6.1	6.7	6.9	7.8	8.3	11.1
90	3.1	3.8	4.4	4.7	5.0	5.6	6.3	6.9	7.5	7.8	8.8	9.4	12.5
100	3.5	4.2	4.9	5.2	5.6	6.3	6.9	7.6	8.3	8.7	9.7	10.4	13.9
110	3.8	4.6	5.3	5.7	6.1	6.9	7.6	8.4	9.2	9.5	10.7	11.5	15.3
120	4.2	5.0	5.8	6.3	6.7	7.5	8.3	9.2	10.0	10.4	11.7	12.5	16.7
130	4.5	5.4	6.3	6.8	7.2	8.1	9.0	9.9	10.8	11.3	12.6	13.5	18.1
140	4.9	5.8	6.8	7.3	7.8	8.8	9.7	10.7	11.7	12.2	13.6	14.6	19.4
150	5.2	6.3	7.3	7.8	8.3	9.4	10.4	11.5	12.5	13.0	14.6	15.6	20.8
160	5.6	6.7	7.8	8.3	8.9	10.0	11.1	12.2	13.3	13.9	15.6	16.7	22.2

Source: R Chowning, DH Adamkin. doi:10.1038/jp.2015.42.

CHAPTER 9
Fluid and Electrolyte Therapy

Table 9: Assessing hydration.

Fluid	Deficit	Excess
ECF (Interstitial)	Loss of skin turgor	Pitting edema, basal rales, wheeze
ECF (Intravascular)	Poor perfusion	High JVP, hepato-jugular reflex (HJR), BP
ECF (Transcellular)	Dry mouth, decreased tears,	Ascites, pleural effusion

(ECF: extracellular fluid; JVP: jugular venous pressure; BP: blood pressure).

- Hepatomegaly can occur with ECF excess.
- Fall in blood pressure is a late sign of shock.
- None of the markers of perfusion [e.g. heart rate (HR), respiratory rate (RR), blood pressure (BP), color, temperature, urine output, sensorium, etc.] in isolation are diagnostic of shock.
- The signs of dehydration are unreliable in neonates. With severe dehydration signs become apparent viz. sunken eyes and fontanel, cold and clammy skin, poor skin turgor and altered sensorium.

Serum Electrolytes

- Hyponatremia with weight loss suggests sodium depletion and would merit sodium replacement.
- Hyponatremia with weight gain suggests water excess and necessitates fluid restriction. Hypernatremia with weight loss suggests dehydration and would require fluid correction over 48 hours.
- Hypernatremia with weight gain suggests salt and water load and would be an indication of fluid and sodium restriction.

Urine Specific Gravity

The normal urine output is 1–3 mL/kg/hr, for specific gravity between 1.005 and 1.012 and for osmolarity between 100 mOsm/L and 400 mOsm/L.

Intravenous fluids should be *increased* in the presence of the following:
- Increased weight loss (>3%/day or a cumulative loss >20%)
- Increased serum sodium (Na >145 mEq/L)
- Increased urine specific gravity >1.020 or urine osmolality >400 mOsm/L
- Decreased urine output (<1 mL/kg/hr).

Similarly fluids should be *restricted* in the presence of the following:
- Decreased weight loss (<1%/day or a cumulative loss <5%)
- Decreased serum sodium in the presence of weight gain (Na <130)
- Decreased urine specific gravity <1.005 or urine osmolality <100 mOsm/L
- Increased urine output (>4 mL/kg/hr).

CLINICAL CASE SCENARIOS
Replacement of Fluid Deficit Therapy

- Moderate (10%) to severe (15%) dehydration fluid deficits are corrected gradually over 24 hours. For infants in shock, 10–20 mL/kg of normal saline is given immediately over 1–2 hours followed by half correction over 8 hours. The remaining deficit is administered over 16 hours.
- Assuming equal losses of fluid from the extracellular water (ECW) and intracellular water (ICW), the replacement fluid after correction of shock, should consist of N/2 (0.45 NS) composition.
- Concomitant hypokalemia worsens hyperglycemia in septic shock. Persistent hyperglycemia therefore warrants potassium estimation.
- High hematocrit with shock suggests severe intravascular depletion.
- Unexplained shock with hyperkalemia warrants ruling out adrenal pathology.

Extreme Prematurity (Gestation <28 Weeks, Birth Weight <1,000 g)

- Fluid requirement in the first week may be decreased substantially by reducing the insensible water loss (IWL) with the use of plastic transparent barriers or using double walled incubators.
- The initial fluids on day 1 should be electrolyte free and should be made using 5% dextrose solutions to prevent risks of hyperglycemia.
- Sodium and potassium should be added after 48 hours of life.

Respiratory Distress Syndrome (RDS), Bronchopulmonary Dysplasia

- Restrict fluids during the acute phase ensuring adequate hydration.
- Watch for diuresis during 2–3 days of life and adjust fluids accordingly.
- Avoid fluid overload during entire therapy.
- No weight loss or static weight in first 72 hours is a clinical marker of underlying pathology.
- Restricted water intake ensuring adequate hydration has a beneficial effect on the incidence of patent ductus arteriosus (PDA), bronchopulmonary dysplasia (BPD), necrotizing enterocolitis (NEC), and death.

Perinatal Asphyxia and Brain Injury

- Fluid restriction in this condition should be done only in the presence of hyponatremia. The intake should be restricted to two-thirds maintenance fluids till serum sodium values return to normal. Once urine production increases by the third postnatal day, fluids may be gradually restored to normal levels.
- Correction of acidosis precipitates hypokalemia.
- Do not routinely supplement calcium.
- Persistent hypocalcemia or hypokalemia warrants magnesium evaluation.
- Avoid hypo- or hyperglycemia.
- Persistent seizures or altered sensorium warrant Na/K estimation.
- High K suggests possibility of ongoing hemolysis, rhabdomyolysis or an adrenal pathology. Persistent low sodium may be associated with neurological sequelae.
- Persistent low Na is an ominous sign.

Oliguria/Renal Failure

- Urine output is not a reliable indicator for acute renal failure, especially in preterm.
- Ensure hydration by 40–60 cc/kg/day IVF (isotonic/dextrose) + urine output (24 hours) for calculating fluid requirements over next 24 hours.
- Presence of oliguria (<1 cc/kg/hr), unexplained weight gain warrants renal chemistry.
- Presence of low Na warrants fluid retention. Presence of high Na suggests possibility of renal tubular pathology.
- Hyperkalemia is a medical emergency.
- Increase fluids during the polyuric phase to maintain hydration.
- "Occult sodium" content of drugs need to be taken into consideration.

Patent Ductus Arteriosus

- In a symptomatic infant the first intervention needs to restrict fluids.
- Presence of isolated diastolic low blood pressure is an earliest marker of opening of ductus.
- Weight gain indicates development of cardiac failure. Ensure normokalemia before digitalizing. If no response to cardiac failure in 24 hours, check electrolytes.

CHAPTER 9
Fluid and Electrolyte Therapy

Flowchart 1: Approach to hyponatremia.

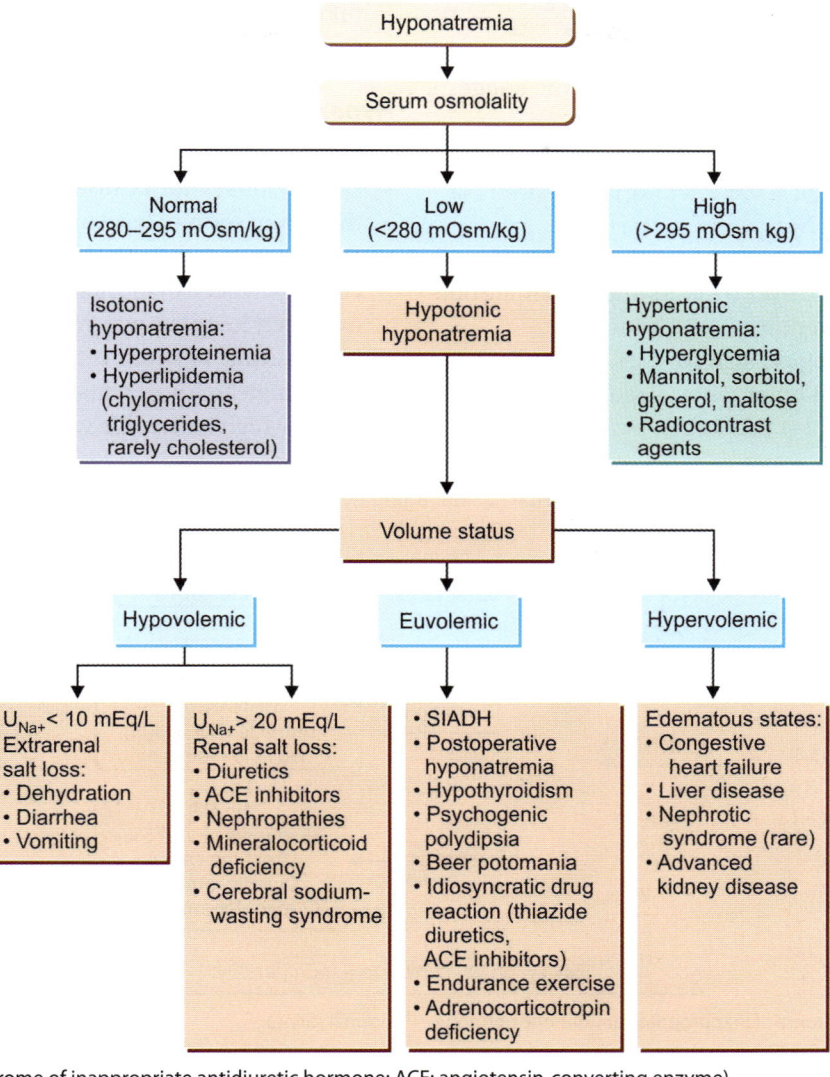

(SIADH: syndrome of inappropriate antidiuretic hormone; ACE: angiotensin-converting enzyme).

COMMON ELECTROLYTE PROBLEMS

Sodium (Na <130 mEq/L)

- Interpretation of sodium should always take into consideration the water content (Flowchart 1). Sugar content also influences the sodium concentration. For every rise of 100 mg% of sugar above 100 mg % sodium decreases by 1.6 mEq/L.
- If there is excessive free water intake relative to insensible and sensible water loss it leads to hyponatremia.
- With extremely premature infant or infants with increased sodium losses, inadequate sodium intake is the cause for hyponatremia.
- Deficits of chloride are 2/3 of sodium.

Correcting Hyponatremia (Flowchart 2)

- Check osmolality. Isotonic suggests pseudo-hyponatremia (e.g. hypertriglyceridemia/hyperproteinemia). Hypertonic suggests underlying hyperglycemia.
- Assess circulating volume.
- Na deficit = 0.6 × wt (kg) × (desired Na – current Na).
- Correct one-third of deficit in first 8 hours, one-third over 16 hours and remaining one-third over next 24–48 hours.
- Neurological signs or Na+ <120 mEq/L is a medical emergency. Treat promptly with 3% NS (2–4 mL/kg).
- Note that the $NaHCO_3$ 7.5% solution = 0.9 mEq Na^+/mL (if 3% NaCl not available).
- Correct underlying etiology.

Hypernatremia (Flowchart 3)

- Serum sodium level greater than 150 mEq/L.
- Usually, this is not a cause for concern until the serum sodium level has risen to greater than 150–155 mEq/L. Hypernatremia is commonly seen in the first few days of life in extremely low birth weight (ELBW) preterm infants and is most often the result of inadequate free water intake to compensate for very high insensible water loss.

Flowchart 2: Managing hyponatremia.

[Flowchart: Low Na → Yes: CNS symptoms → 3% NS; No → Volume overload → No NS, Fluid restriction (75%), Treat the cause; Volume depletion* → NS: wt × 1.5, D5½ NS + 20 mEq/L KCl, 3% NS:CSW+, Steroids (Adr. insuff), No fluid restriction; SIADH → No NS, Fluid restriction (75%), Treat the cause, Diuretic, oral salt, V2 receptor antagonist. Review drugs, correct to 6 mEq/per day]

(SIADH: syndrome of inappropriate antidiuretic hormone; NS: normal saline).

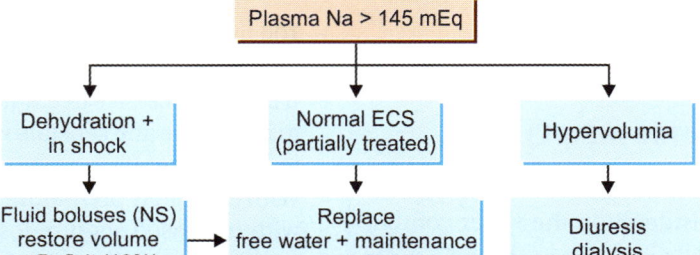

Flowchart 3: Managing hypernatremia.

(ECS: extracellular space).

- If there is water deficit suspect diabetes insipidus.
- If there is water and Na deficit most common cause is diarrhea.

Correction of Hypernatremia
- Estimate total body fluid deficit clinically or by change in weight.
- Rate of decrease should not exceed 0.5–1 mEq/L/hr.
- Rapid correction in hypernatremia may result in rebound cerebral edema.
- Free water deficit may be estimated as 4 cc/kg of free water needed for every mEq/l of Na above 145 mEq/L.
- Deficit will be replaced with free water (D5 or D10) remaining of deficit (total body fluid deficit—free water deficit) is replaced with NS.
- Adjust fluid on basis of clinical status and [Na].
  - If suggestive of volume depletion, repeat NS bolus.
  - If Na decreases too rapidly, either increase [Na] of fluid or decrease rate of IV fluid.
- If Na decreases too slowly, either decrease [Na] of fluid or increase rate of IV fluid.
- Replace ongoing losses as they occur.

Potassium

Acidosis leads to rise in potassium concentration in the blood or serum, whereas alkalosis leads to fall in potassium concentration. A handy rule is that 0.1 U of pH change results in a 0.3–0.6 mEq/L change in the serum potassium level.

Hypokalemia (K < 3.5 mEq/L)
Treatment is based on K^+ Level, clinical symptoms, renal function, transcellular shifts, and ongoing losses (Table 10).

Table 10: Management of hypokalemia.

Oral potassium	IV potassium
• Safer • Slower action • Liquid forms bitter, causes gastrointestinal upset • 2-4 mEq/kg/day • Maximum 120–240 mEq/day	• Cautious • IV fluids concentration 20 mEq/L • Increase to 40–60 mEq/L, ECG monitoring • *Dose:* 0.5–1 mEq/kg, over 1 hour. Maximum 40 mEq (Adults)
Continuous cardiac monitoring	

- Check history, acid base status, and if persistent magnesium levels.
- Replacement is done with KCl solution, per oral/IV, based on severity.
- Always search and treat the underlying cause.
- With digoxin ensure the serum potassium level is always more than 3.0 mEq/L.
- Electrocardiography manifestations include a flattened T wave, prolongation of the QT interval, or the appearance of U waves.
- Manifests as arrhythmias, ileus, and lethargy.
- Additional measures include K^+ sparing diuretics. If alkalosis with volume depletion, restore volume and treat hypomagnesemia.

Hyperkalemia (K >6 mEq/L)
- Check sampling error—avoid hemolyzed sample.
- Stop all potassium containing fluids.
- Electrocardiography manifestations of hyperkalemia are a progression from peaked T waves, as the earliest sign, to a widened QRS configuration, bradycardia, tachycardia, supraventricular tachycardia (SVT), ventricular tachycardia, and ventricular fibrillation.
- Measures to *stabilize* the heart—"work fast":
  - IV calcium over few minutes
  - IV bicarbonate—works best in acidosis
  - Insulin and glucose
  - Nebulized albuterol/salbutamol

- Measures to *remove* potassium—"work slow":
  - Loop diuretic
  - Exchange resin—rectally/orally
  - Dialysis—HD/PD

APPENDIX 1

	Fluid	Indication
1.	5% D	~IV maintenance for <1,000 g during first 24–48 hours ~Vehicle for ACT, aminophylline, calcium gluconate
2.	10% D	~IV Maintenance for >1,000 g for first 24–48 hours ~For hypoglycemia correction
3.	25% D	~For hypoglycemia correction ~For increasing glucose concentration
3.	NS	~Volume expander in shock ~Vehicle for phenytoin, sodium bicarbonate, Aminophylline ~Replacement of gastric aspirate ~Correction of hyponatremia
4.	RL	~Volume expander in shock
5.	½ NS	~Replacement of ileostomy losses
6.	3% NS	~Correction of symptomatic hyponatremia
7.	Isolyte P	~Maintenance IV fluid (>48 hours)

APPENDIX 2

Electrolyte content of common fluids.

Fluid solution	Concentration
100 cc of 0.9% NS	15.4 mEq of sodium
100 cc of 3% NS	51.3 mEq of sodium
100 cc Isolyte P	2.5 mEq Na, 2 mEq K
1 cc KCl (15%)	3.8 mEq potassium
1 cc KCl (10%)	2 mEq potassium
1 cc NaHCO$_3$ (7.5 %)	1 mEq of sodium
1 cc conc. RL	7 mEq of sodium

APPENDIX 3

Preparing desired percentage of dextrose using 5% D and 25% D, the most widely available glucose is 5% and 25% D. The formula for conversion of 5% dextrose to any other percentage is 5X – 25, where X is the required percentage of dextrose (*see* Table 7).

For example, to prepare 100 mL of 10% dextrose from 5% dextrose you need to add 5 × 10 – 25 = 25 mL of 25% dextrose; the rest, 100–25 would be 5% dextrose.

Example: To prepare 12.5% dextrose you require 5 × 12.5 – 25 = 37.5 mL 25% dextrose, the rest 100 – 37.5 = 62.5 mL would be 5% dextrose.

For 100 mL solution		
% Dextrose	25% D	5 % D
10%	25 mL	75 mL
12.5%	37.5 mL	62.5 mL
15%	50 mL	50 mL
17.5%	62.5 mL	37.5 mL
20%	75 mL	25 mL

SUGGESTED READING

1. Bhatia J. Fluid and electrolyte management in the very low birth weight neonate. J Perinatol. 2006;26(Suppl 1):S19-21.
2. Chawla D, Agarwal R, Deorari AK, et al. Fluid and electrolyte management in term and preterm neonates. Indian J Pediatr. 2008;75(3): 255-9.
3. Lorenz JM. Fluid and electrolyte therapy in the very low-birth weight neonate. NeoReviews. 2008;9(3):e102-8.
4. Modi N. Management of fluid balance in the very immature neonate. Arch Dis Child Fetal Neonatal Ed. 2004;89(2):F108-11.

CHAPTER 10

Hypoglycemia

Vinay Kumar Rai, Sanjay Wazir

INTRODUCTION

Hypoglycemia is a medical emergency. It is a potentially reversible cause of developmental delay/epilepsy.

DEFINITION

Neonatal hypoglycemia is defined as a proposed operational threshold of ensuring blood glucose above 45 mg/dL. The diagnosis is biochemical and not a clinical one.

CLINICAL FEATURES

Infants with hypoglycemia are usually *asymptomatic,* and in high-risk infants, hypoglycemia is often detected by routine monitoring of blood glucose. There is no single concentration or range of glucose concentrations that is associated with clinical symptoms. Presence of symptoms is a late sign. Symptoms are nonspecific and include one or more of the following—jitteriness and/or tremors, hypotonia, change in level of consciousness (irritability, lethargy, or stupor), apnea, bradycardia, and/or cyanosis, tachypnea, poor suck or poor feeding, weak or high-pitched cry and/or seizures. *There is no sign pathognomic for hypoglycemia.* Clinical examination must be focused to identify clues (Table 1).

Table 1: Clinical clues to hypoglycemia.	
Weight	<2 kg (LBW), >4 kg (LGA) are at risk for hypoglycemia
Gestation	All preterms (<34 weeks), late preterms (34–36 weeks) are at risk
SGA	All at risk for hypoglycemia
Well-being	Asymptomatic versus symptomatic has different treatments
Plethora	Polycythemia is a risk factor for hypoglycemia
Hypothermia	Thermal instability increases risk of hypoglycemia
Sepsis	Increases glucose requirements
Hepatomegaly, microcephaly, anterior midline defects, hemihypertrophy, macroglossia	Suggest central cause of hypoglycemia

(SGA: small for gestational age; LGA: large for gestational age)

- No single concentration or range of glucose concentrations that is associated with clinical symptoms.
- No glucose concentration or duration of hypoglycemia that can predict neurologic injury.

GLUCOSE SCREENING

Clinical detection of hypoglycemia is late and hence early detection in "at risk" newborns is mandatory. The glucose screening helps early detection and prevention of hypoglycemia (Tables 2 to 4 and Fig. 1).

Note:
- Collect blood for estimation of blood glucose in a fluoride vial. Do not estimate blood sugar in a hemolyzed sample.
- Glucose concentration measured in whole blood is 10–15% lower than that in plasma and may be further reduced if the hematocrit is high.
- Glucose oxidase (colorimetric method) or glucose electrode method are the two commonly used laboratory methods to assay blood glucose in the laboratory and are accurate and reliable.
- Monitor blood sugar every 12 hours in baby who is on total parenteral nutrition or intravenous (TPN/IV) fluid.

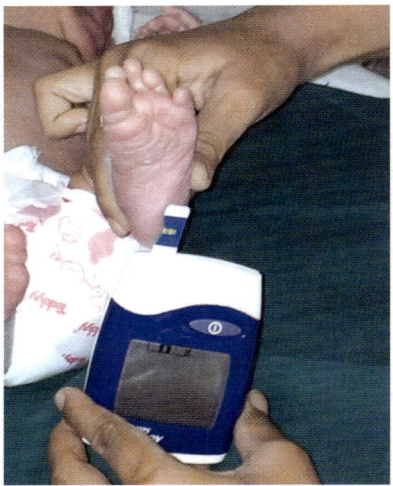

Fig. 1: Using glucometer.

Table 2: Blood glucose screening.

Whom?	Premature infants, Infants who are large or small for gestational age, Infants of diabetic mothers, Sick newborns (e.g. sepsis, hypothermia, asphyxia, etc.), Infants whose mothers were treated with beta adrenergic or oral hypoglycemic agents
When?	1–2 hours after birth
Relation to feed?	Prefeed
Maximum risk?	First 72 hours
Method?	Glucometer
Sample?	Capillary heel prick
Diagnosis?	<47 mg%
Confirmation?	Venous sample

Table 3: Schedule for blood glucose screening.

At-risk neonates	2, 6, 12, 24, 48 and 72 hours of life
Sick neonates	Every 6–8 hours (individualize as needed)
Neonates on parenteral nutrition	Initial 72 hours → every 6–8 hours After 72 hours → once a day

Table 4: Caveats for glucose sampling.

Blood or plasma glucose	Whole blood sugar value is about 15% less than that of plasma value
Stored glucose sample	Can give fallaciously low readings (Glucose can fall by 14–18 mg/dL per hour in samples that await analysis)
Arterial, venous or capillary glucose	Arterial samples have slightly higher value compared to venous or capillary samples

MANAGEMENT OF HYPOGLYCEMIA (FLOWCHART 1 AND 2)

Asymptomatic term or near term infants with blood sugar more than 25 mg% should be started on feeds and blood sugar checked after 30 minutes. If blood sugar is still low then one should start the parenteral therapy.

Identification and treatment of the cause of hypoglycemia is must (Table 5).

Parenteral glucose infusion is indicated in the following conditions:
- Symptomatic infants.
- Neonates with plasma glucose concentration less than 20–25 mg/dL.
- Neonates with persistent hypoglycemia after feeding defined as plasma glucose concentration below 40 mg/dL.
- Neonates who are unable to feed or intolerant of enteral feedings with plasma glucose concentrations below 40 mg/dL.

Management Algorithm for Hypoglycemic Neonate Requiring Intravenous Treatment (Table 6 and Fig. 1)

- Parenteral glucose therapy is administered as an initial bolus infusion 2 mL/kg of 10% dextrose in water over 1 minute.

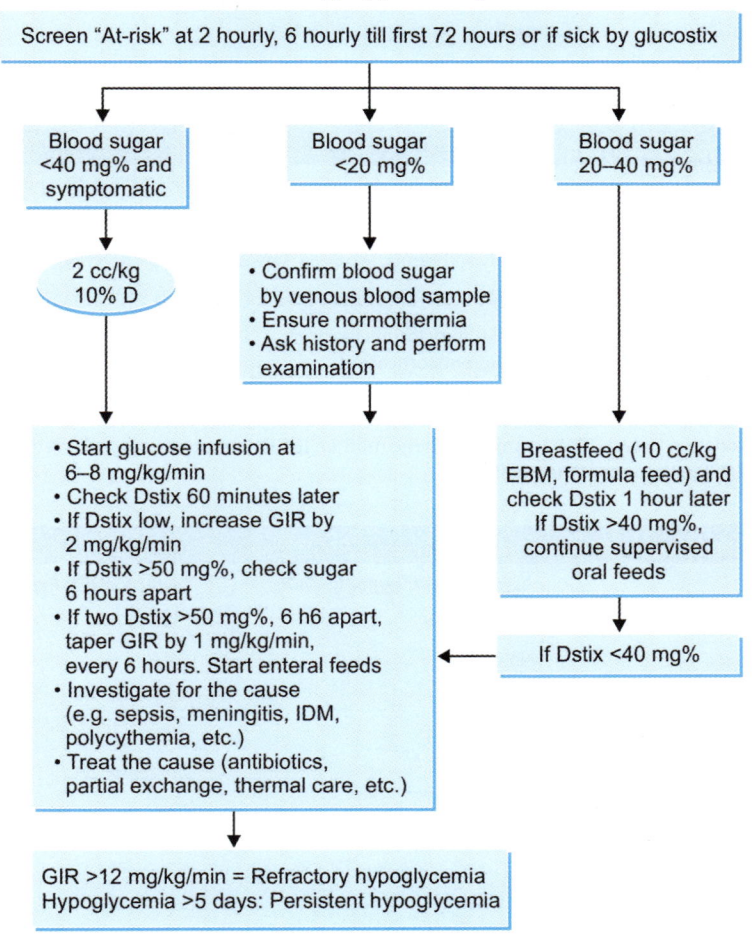

Flowchart 1: Hypoglycemia algorithm.

(GIR: glucose infusion rate).

SECTION 1
Clinical Approach to Sick Newborn

Flowchart 2: Approach to recurrent/persistent hypoglycemia.

```
                    Recurrent/Persistent hypoglycemia
                    Inv: Serum insulin, plasma FFA, plasma
                              lactate, urine ketones
                    ┌──────────────────┴──────────────────┐
                 Ketotic                               Nonketotic
                    │                                      │
              Serum lactate                              FFA
           ┌────────┴────────┐                  ┌─────────┴─────────┐
         Low:              High:              High:               Low:
    • Hypopituitarism  • Gluconeogenesis   • FAO defect      • Hyperinsulinism
    • GSD I            • Enzyme defect     • Carnitine defect
    • Ketotic hypoglycemia
                                                      │
                                          • Hydrocortisone
                                          • Diazoxide        If nonresponsive....
                                          • Octreotide, Glucoagon, Nifedepine
```

(FFA: free fatty acid; GSD I: glycogen storage disorder).

Table 5: Etiology for hypoglycemia.

Mechanism	Causes
Poor glucose production	Preterm, SGA, maternal drugs, IEM (e.g. galactosemia, FAO, etc.)
Increased glucose demand	Hypothermia, asphyxia, sepsis, severe Rh-incompatibility.
Hyperinsulinemia	IDM, IUGR, Islet cell adenoma, Beckwith-Wiedemann syndrome
Inadequate "anti-insulin" hormone	Pituitary insufficiency Adrenocortical def.
Iatrogenic	Fluid error, malposition UC

(FAO: fatty acid oxidation defect; IDM: infant of diabetic mother; IUGR: intrauterine growth restriction; SGA: small for gestational age; IEM: inborn error of metabolism).

Table 6: Management of hypoglycemia.

	Asymptomatic hypoglycemia	Symptomatic hypoglycemia
Feed trial	Yes	No
10% D bolus	No	Yes
IVF-GIR	No	Yes
Reassess	Yes	Yes
Low sugar persists	Start IVF	Increase GIR

(IVF: IV fluids; GIR: glucose infusion rate).

- After an initial bolus starts glucose infusion rate (GIR) at 6 mg/kg per minute.
- Check the blood glucose concentration 15 minutes after the bolus infusion.
- The clinician goal is to maintain the glucose value above 45 mg/dL in the first day, and more than 50 mg/dL thereafter.
- If the blood glucose remains <45 mg/dL, the GIR is increased in steps of 2 mg/kg/min (i.e. increase GIR infusion rate from 6 mg/kg/min to 8 mg/kg/min) to every 15 minutes with repeat checks on blood glucose after 15 minutes of starting new GIR infusion rate till the values are >45 mg/dL.
- If blood sugar remains well above 45 mg/dL, the frequency of checking can be every hour for the next 3 hours then every 6 hours.
- *Tapering of glucose infusion*: Once the blood glucose values stabilize above 45 mg/dL for about 24 hours or blood sugar is >100 mg/dL for 2 hrs, the infusion can be tapered off at 2 mg/kg/min every 6 hours. Once a GIR of 4 mg/kg/min is reached, the infusion can be stopped if the neonate is euglycemic.
- If baby is receiving TPN and he develops hypoglycemia, increase the daily fluid by 20 mL/kg/day.
- Symptomatic hypoglycemia in a baby who is on full enteral feeds is managed by reducing the feed by 50% of the requirement and give rest of the fluid through IV at 6 mg/kg/min.

Note:
Avoid using >12.5% dextrose infusion through a peripheral vein because of risk of thrombophlebitis.

Monitoring B glucose is done after 30–60 minutes and then every 6 hr until blood sugar is >50 mg/dL. After 24 hours of IV glucose therapy, once two or more consecutive blood glucose values are >50 mg/dL, the infusion can be tapered off at the rate of 2 mg/kg/min every 6 hours with sugar monitoring.

Table 7: Investigations for persistent hypoglycemia.

First line: Plasma insulin, serum cortisol, thyroid profile, serum ammonia, blood lactate, urine for ketones and reducing substances, serum free fatty acid level, serum level of beta hydroxybutyrate.

Second line: Serum 17-OHP, GALT assay, tandem mass spectroscopy, growth hormone, glucagon levels.

General Consideration during Hypoglycemic Episode

- Assess support and maintain airway, breathing, and circulation
- Maintain euthermia
- Correct acidosis
- Search and treat the underlying cause.

Persistent hypoglycemia should be suspected if GIR requirements are >12 mg/kg/min for more than 24 hours.

Prolonged hypoglycemia should be suspected when blood glucose levels remain unstable beyond 5 days.

- *Some important causes of persistent hypoglycemia*:
  - Hyperinsulinemia
  - Hypopituitarism
  - Adrenal insufficiency
  - Metabolic disorders like galactosemia, glycogen storage disease, etc.

Investigations for persistent hypoglycemia are depicted in Table 7.

DIAGNOSTIC CRITERIA TO DEFINE HYPERINSULINISM

- Glucose <40 mg/dL
- Insulin >2 microU/mL
- Glucose/insulin ratio <3:1
- Negative ketone bodies in plasma and urine (3-beta-hydroxybutyric acid <1 mmol/L)
- Glycemic reaction to glucagon administration >30 mg/dL (i.e. positive response) (Table 8).

Table 8: Treatment of hyperinsulinemic hypoglycemia.

Drugs	Dose
Hydrocortisone	5 mg/kg/day IV or PO in two divided doses for 24–48 hours
Diazoxide	10–25 mg/kg/day in three divided doses PO
Glucagon	100 mg/kg subcutaneous or intramuscular (max 300 mg), maximum of three doses
Octreotide	2–10 µg/kg/day subcutaneously two to three times a day

SURGICAL THERAPY

Surgical exploration is warranted in children older than several weeks of age in whom hyperinsulinism is proven and pharmacologic therapy fails to control hypoglycemia.

OUTCOME

Repeated or prolonged episodes of hypoglycemia may cause microcephaly, psychomotor retardation, cognitive deficits, epilepsy, and/or visual disturbances.

Magnetic resonance imaging before discharge is indicated in neonates with history of recurrent/persistent hypoglycemia. Selective posterior white matter and pulvinar edema were most predictive of clinical hypoglycemia, and watershed pattern of injury was seen more often in severe hypoglycemia. Pattern of cerebral injury depends on duration, degree of hypoglycemia, rate of cerebral blood flow, cerebral utilization of glucose, and also comorbidities. Regular follow up, developmental assessment at 20–24 months CGA (corrected gestational ages), and visual assessment should be done in all symptomatic hypoglycemic newborns. Even a single episode of hypoglycemia (<40 mg/dL) soon after birth was associated with a 50% reduction in the odds of achieving proficiency in literacy and numeracy at 10 years.

APPENDIX 1

How to calculate the GIR?

Glucose infusion rate is expressed in terms of mg/kg/min. It can be calculated using following formula:

GIR = Rate of IV fluids (in mL/kg/day) × % of dextrose infused divided by 144.

APPENDIX 2

How to prepare the desired concentration of glucose in intravenous fluid and how to mix various solutions for creating a desired concentration of glucose in IV infusate:

The formula for preparing 100 mL of fluid with a desired concentration of glucose using 5% dextrose and 25% dextrose solutions is given by the formula $5X - 25 = Y$, where X is the required percentage of dextrose and Y is the amount of 25% dextrose (in mL) to be made up with 5% dextrose to make a total of 100 mL.

For example, to prepare 100 mL of 12.5% dextrose, add $5 \times 12.5 - 25 = 37.5$ mL of 25% dextrose to 62.5 mL (100 – 37.5) of 5% dextrose.

How to increase GIR by 1 mg/kg/min: Add 2 mL/kg of 25% dextrose to the volume of fluid to be infused over 8 hours.

Drawback of this formula: For this formula to work, the GIR should be kept at or below a 10th of the total fluid intake in mL/kg/day.

For example, you cannot increase GIR beyond 10 mg/kg/min by using this formula if total fluid intake is 100 mL/kg/day; to increase GIR beyond this, fluid intake must be increased.

How to calculate GIR in an infant on oral feeds along with simultaneous intravenous infusion of glucose:

Glucose infusion rate while on feeding (mg/kg/min) = IV rate (mL/hr) × Dextrose conc. (g/dL) × 0.0167/wt (kg) + Feed rate (mL/hr) × Dextrose conc. (g/dL) × 0.0167/wt (kg).

Method of calculating GIR when 10% dextrose is used in IV fluid:

GIR (mg/kg/min) = IV fluid rate (mL/kg/day) × 0.07.

For example, if baby weight is 1.2 kg.

Steps:
1. fluid rate will be 80 mL/kg/day on day 1 of life.
2. dextrose conc. = 10%.
3. GIR will be 80 × 0.07 = 5.6 mg/kg/min.

Limitation of this formula—can be used only when concentration of dextrose is 10%.

Note:
- To convert mg/dL of glucose to mmol/L, divide by 18.
- To convert mmol/L of glucose to mg/dL, multiply by 18.
- 10% dextrose has 100 mg/mL of dextrose, 5% dextrose has 50 mg/mL, 7.5% dextrose has 75 mg/mL of dextrose.
- *Amount of dextrose in milk*: Breast milk = 7.1 g/dL, Term formula = 7.1 g/dL, Preterm formula = 8.5 g/dL.

SUGGESTED READING

1. Adamkin DH; Committee on Fetus and Newborn. Postnatal glucose homeostasis in late-preterm and term infants. Pediatrics. 2011;127(3):575-9.
2. Cornblath M, Hawdon JM, Williams AF, et al. Controversies regarding definition of neonatal hypoglycaemia: suggested operational thresholds. Pediatrics. 2000;105(5):1141-5.
3. Lilien LD, Pildes RS, Srinivasan G, et al. Treatment of neonatal hypoglycemia with minibolus and intravenous glucose infusion. J Pediatr. 1980;97(2):295-8.
4. Lorenzo F Jr, Pico MC, Bermúdez JM. Hipoglucemia neonatal. Protocolos Diagnóstico-terapéuticos de neonatología de la SEN-AEP, Ergon. Madrid, Spain.
5. Rosenthal M, Ugele B, Lipowsky G, et al. The Accutrend sensor glucose analyzer may not be adequate in bedside testing for neonatal hypoglycemia. Eur J Pediatr. 2006;165(2):99-103.
6. Wong DS, Poskitt KJ, Chau V, et al. Brain injury patterns in hypoglycemia in neonatal encephalopathy. AJNR Am J Neuroradiol. 2013;34(7):1456-61.

CHAPTER 11

Hypocalcemia

Surg RAdm Sheila Samanta Mathai

DEFINITION

Hypocalcemia in the term/preterm neonate is defined as a total serum calcium of <8/7 mg% (2/1.75 mmol/L) or serum ionized calcium of <4.4/4 mg% (1.1/1 mmol/L). It is a relatively common problem in neonates, though the exact incidence varies, ranging from 30 to 40% in preterms to 50% in infants of diabetic mothers (IDMs).

Babies at risk for early onset hypocalcemia include preterms, IDMs and those with birth asphyxia (Box 1). However, even normal newborns are prone to hypocalcemia soon after birth. In utero, calcium crosses the placenta against a concentration gradient mainly in the third trimester. After birth absorption of calcium from the newborn gut is dependent on the baby's calcium intake and vitamin D levels. Calcium concentration is relatively low in human breast milk and vitamin D levels in the neonate are entirely dependent on antenatal stores as intake from breast milk and exposure to sun in the first few days is limited. The physiological peak in calcitonin and the poor parathormone response to low calcium levels in the first few days after birth also add to the increased susceptibility to hypocalcemia in the first few days of life.

CLINICAL SUSPICION OF HYPOCALCEMIA

In a large number of cases, hypocalcemia is completely asymptomatic. The symptoms depend on the level of ionized calcium and usually appear if this falls to <0.9 mmol/L. Suspect hypocalcemia in a newborn who suddenly develops the following:
- Jitteriness
- Clonus
- Focal/multifocal seizures
- Tetany or tonic posturing
- Apnea or stridor particularly after crying.

Box 1 Etiology of neonatal hypocalcemia.

- Hypocalcemia occurring in the first 72–96 hours (early neonatal hypocalcemia) is usually mainly due to *prematurity, severe birth asphyxia,* and *maternal diabetes*. Premature infants have low stores, severely asphyxiated babies have hyperphosphatemia due to tissue damage and in infants of diabetic mothers mechanism is uncertain. Small for Gestational Age' babies are also prone to early hypocalcemia due to poor parathormone response.
- Hypocalcemia after 3–4 days of life (late neonatal hypocalcemia), can, in addition, be due to *maternal vitamin D deficiency* with low vitamin D stores in neonate, hypomagnesemia, hyperphosphatemia due to various causes and hypoparathyroidism.

CHAPTER 11
Hypocalcemia

Table 1: Clinical features suggesting etiology of hypocalcemia.

Finding	Interpretation	Remarks
Abnormal facies, skeletal shortness, congenital heart disease	Di George, CATCH22, other genetic causes of hypoparathyroidism	Do X-ray chest, echocardiography
Prematurity	Low stores and decreased intake	Recheck amount of calcium supplementation and Ca/P ratio
Potter's facies, edema	Renal insufficiency with possible hyperphosphatemia	Check antenatal ultrasonography finding of oligohydramnios
LGA, hypoglycemia	Suggestive of IDM	Recheck maternal glucose, glycosylated Hb

(LGA: large for gestational age; IDM: infant of diabetic mother)

ETIOLOGICAL APPROACH

- History, clinical examination, and investigations form the basis of finding the etiology (Table 1).
- If seizures are the initial manifestation other causes such as hypoglycemia, meningitis/sepsis, and intracranial bleeds should always be ruled out as soon as possible.
- History related to prematurity, maternal diabetes, need for resuscitation, and time of onset of symptoms give clues to the etiology.
- Cow's milk ingestion could suggest hyperphosphatemia.
- A physical examination should be done for neurological signs, dysmorphic features, congenital heart disease, and features of renal involvement to reach an etiological diagnosis.

FIRST-LINE INVESTIGATIONS

- Total serum calcium and ionized component
- *Serum albumin:* Serum calcium levels fall by 0.8 mg% for every 1 g% fall in serum albumin below 4 g%.
- ECG may show a prolonged QTc interval of >0.44 sec and should be done in all cases, if available.
- USG cranium may be done as part of seizure work-up.

- *Vitamin D:* Vitamin D_3 levels should be assessed in term babies with hypocalcemic seizures as this is not an uncommon cause due to the high level of low vitamin D levels in pregnant women in our country.

In a few cases, further investigations are required (Table 2). Parathormone levels and serum magnesium may be required in certain cases. EEG and MRI are rarely required. These should be considered only if there are seizures despite correction of hypocalcemia or there are abnormal neurological signs on follow-up.

MANAGEMENT

General monitoring of "at risk" neonates for serum calcium levels is recommended as follows:
- Asymptomatic preterm infant (>1,000 g) at 24 and 48 hours of life.
- Asymptomatic preterm infant (<1,000 g) at 12, 24, and 48 hours.
- Sick, stressed or symptomatic infant—as indicated, usually every 24–48 hours during the acute phase.

All babies at risk should get their daily requirement of calcium (60–120 mg/kg/day of elemental calcium), preferably orally. If this is not possible, continuous drip starting with 4–6 mL/kg/day of 10% calcium gluconate should be given. Pushes or boluses of calcium

SECTION 1
Clinical Approach to Sick Newborn

Table 2: Interpretation of investigations in hypocalcemia in the neonate.

Investigation	Interpretation	Causes	Remarks
Low vitamin D levels <30 mmol/L	Vitamin D deficiency	Maternal deficiency should be ruled out	Seen quite often in our country
Elevated serum phosphate >4.5 mg%	Renal insufficiency or hyperparathyroidism	Congenital renal problems	• Renal work-up essential • Rule out cow's milk ingestion
Magnesium level of <0.8 mmol/L	Hypomagnesemia	May be secondary to deficiency in mother	May also be seen in neonates on total parenteral nutrition not getting magnesium
Normal to moderately reduced $1,25(OH)_2D_3$, reduced alkaline phosphatase, reduced parathyroid levels	Hypoparathyroidism	May be secondary to maternal hyperparathyroidism or due to genetic causes	Look for skeletal defect (short 4th metacarpal) in mother
Absence of thymic shadows on chest X-ray and presence of conotruncal cardiac abnormalities	Suggests CATCH 22 or DiGeorge syndrome	Genetic defect in chromosome 22 leading to arch problems and hypoparathyroidism	Though uncommon, it is easy to suspect. Mutation studies required for confirmation
Urinary calcium excretion >4 mg/kg/day or 24-hour urinary calcium creatinine ratio more than 0.2	Hypercalciuria	May be primary or part of a renal tubular defect of parathyroid defect	May be seen occasionally

IV should be avoided. Meticulous care must be taken to ensure that the IV line is secure to prevent extravasation during the administration of calcium-containing fluids, as this can cause severe necrosis particularly in preterms.

SPECIFIC TREATMENT OF HYPOCALCEMIA

- *Asymptomatic hypocalcemia detected on screening of an "at risk" baby*: It is preferable to start IV maintenance doses of 4–6 mL/kg of calcium gluconate for at least 48 hours, after which oral supplementation can be given.
- *Symptomatic hypocalcemia (Flowchart 1)*: Patients with symptomatic hypocalcemia (seizures, tetany, severe jitteriness) should be given a bolus dose of 2 mL/kg/dose IV calcium gluconate 1:1 diluted with 5% dextrose over 10 minutes with heart rate (HR) monitoring to ensure that HR does not fall below 100/min or more than 20 beats/min from the baseline. A repeat bolus may be required if symptoms persist. A response to a bolus corroborates the diagnosis even before serum levels become available. Boluses should be followed by a continuous intravenous infusion of 6–8 mL/kg/day of calcium gluconate for the next 24–48 hours followed by normal maintenance doses orally thereafter. Daily requirement of vitamin D should always be ensured.
- *Symptomatic hypocalcemia unresponsive to calcium*: Send sample for calcium and magnesium estimation. Correct hypomagnesemia (<1.2 mg/dL) with 0.1–0.2 mL 50% $MgSO_4$ per kg deep intramuscular (IM). An empiric dose may be given if the test is not available. Dose may be repeated after 12 hours.
- Prolonged (>1 week) or resistant hypocalcemia not responding to addition of Mg

Flowchart 1: Algorithm for management of symptomatic neonatal hypocalcemia.

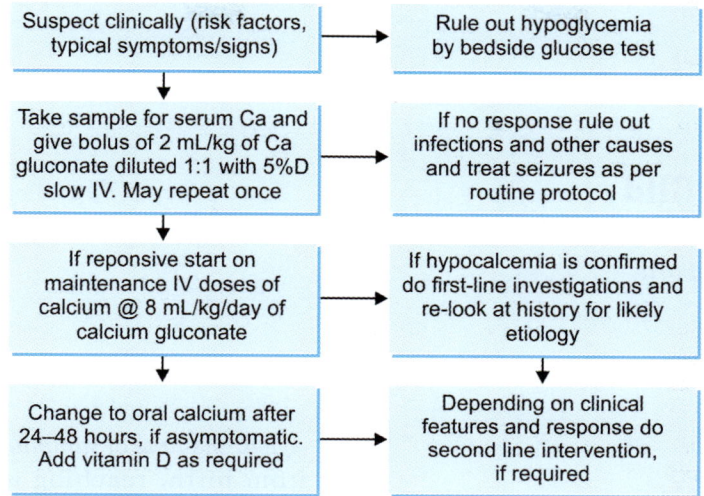

and vitamin D may be due to a syndromic cause, hypoparathyroidism or severe hyperphosphatemia. These may require phosphate binders and $1,25(OH)_2$ form of vitamin D in addition to higher doses of calcium. In most cases of hypocalcemia, which are controlled easily with calcium, the prognosis is excellent and the neonates do not manifest any long-term neurological deficits. Early onset hypocalcemia usually needs higher doses for the first 3–4 days after which it can be tapered though preterms must be given their normal daily requirements. Late onset hypocalcemia needs longer duration of treatment. Prolonged seizures leading to hypoxemia or syndromic causes of hypocalcemia have a guarded prognosis.

SUGGESTED READING

1. Fanaroff and Martin's Neonatal-Perinatal Medicine, Diseases of the Fetus and Infant, 10th edition, 2015.
2. Hansen AR, Eichenwald EC, Stark AR, et al. Cloherty and Stark's Manual of Neonatal Care. Wolters Kluwer; 2016.
3. Thomas TC, Smith JM, White PC, et al. Transient neonatal hypocalcemia: presentation and outcomes. Pediatrics. 2012;129(6):e1461-7.
4. WHO Guidelines. Hypocalcemia in the Newborn. [online] Available form: http://newbornwhocc.org/pdf/Hypocalcemia.pdf. [Last accessed April, 2019].

CHAPTER 12

Polycythemia

Raktima Chakrabarti

DEFINITION

Neonatal polycythemia is a pathological condition, which is characterized by increased venous hematocrit (Hct) for gestational and postnatal age. It is defined as:
- Hematocrit greater than two standard deviations (SD) above the normal value for gestational and postnatal age
- *Term infant*: Hct from a peripheral venous sample is greater than 65% or the hemoglobin is greater than 22 g/dL.

For practical purpose the Hct value is more important and considered, rather than the hemoglobin concentration.

Hct measurement depends on the following:
- *Site of blood sampling*: Hct are highest in capillary samples, intermediate in peripheral venous samples, and lowest in samples from the umbilical vein. Venous Hct are considered ideal, capillary samples may be used for screening, but all high values should be confirmed by a venous sample and result should be obtained from centrifuged sample. The venous Hct is generally 5–15% lower than the capillary Hct and diagnosis should be made if venous Hct is >65%.
- *Age at the time of sampling*: Hct increases from birth, reaching a maximum at approximately 2 hours of age, then decrease to levels in cord blood by 18 hours of age.
- *Method of Hct measurement*: Test results obtained from centrifuged samples are higher than those using automated cell counters and correlate better with blood viscosity.

ASSESSING SEVERITY OF POLYCYTHEMIA

Incidence and Risk Factors

Incidence of polycythemia is 1–5%. Chances of polycythemia increases in the following cases:
- Intrauterine hypoxia
- Intrauterine growth restriction
- Certain delivery procedures (e.g. delayed cord clamping, holding neonate below the level of the mother before cord clamping, stripping the cord toward the neonate at delivery)
- Placental transfusion (including twin-to-twin transfusion)
- Some congenital abnormalities (e.g. cyanotic congenital heart disease, renovascular malformations, congenital adrenal hyperplasia)

- Maternal insulin-dependent diabetes
- Perinatal asphyxia
- Down syndrome or other trisomies
- Beckwith Wiedemann syndrome
- Mother residing at a high altitude
- Multiple birth.

The terms polycythemia and hyperviscosity are often used interchangeably but they are not same. Polycythemia is significant only because it increases risk of hyperviscosity syndrome that is blood viscosity greater than 12 centipoise, measured at a shear rate of 11.5 per second. Whole blood viscosity can be affected by significant increases in any increase of red blood cells, white blood cells, platelets, plasma proteins, immunoglobulins or clotting factors. In neonates, the main culprit is excess of red blood cells. In case of hyperviscosity, slugging of blood occurs in blood vessels which results in decreased blood supply in different organs.

Blood viscosity and Hct have a linear relationship till the Hct is 65%. And it becomes exponential when the Hct exceeds 65%; it is such that a small increase in Hct is associated with a high increase in viscosity. So Hct exceeding 65% is a red flag sign because then suddenly a neonate can become symptomatic.

Identifying Cause

History

- Presence of risk factors should be obtained like:
  - Intrauterine or perinatal asphyxia
  - Maternal insulin dependent diabetes
  - Congenital anomalies or syndromes
  - Intrauterine growth restriction
  - Multiple birth (monochorionic twin and specifically the larger twin)
  - Large for gestational age.
- Previously delayed cord clamping and cord milking was considered to be risk factor but current multiple randomized studies have shown that risk of polycythemia and jaundice does not get increased by these processes.

So delayed cord clamping and milking should not be considered as risk factor.

- Any history of following symptoms:
  - Lethargy
  - Irritability/jitteriness
  - Tremors
  - Seizures
  - Cerebrovascular accidents
  - Respiratory distress
  - Cyanosis
  - Apnea.

Physical Examination

- Most of the cases are asymptomatic (74–90%)
- In case of symptomatic neonates, most of the signs/symptoms appear after 2 hours of life as Hct rises to the highest point at that point of time and gradually decreased by next 24–72 hours.
- The most common signs are gastrointestinal symptoms (poor feeding or vomiting) (17%), hypoglycemia (12%) and cyanosis/apnea (<10%).

Other signs are shown in Table 1.

Only in some cases symptoms may be delayed to second or third day of life. In these cases, the delayed increased Hct develops because of excessive extracellular fluid loss. And this volume depletion may exaggerate the expression of an already increased red cell mass or, in extreme cases; it can be the primary cause of the high Hct. Infants with no symptoms by 48–72 hours of age are likely to remain asymptomatic.

Symptoms of polycythemia are usually due to reduced tissue perfusion or associated metabolic abnormalities. However, these signs and symptoms may also occur with

Table 1: Signs and symptoms of polycythemia.	
General and metabolic	Lethargy, irritability, priapism, hypoglycemia, hyperbilirubinemia, and hypocalcemia
Cardiorespiratory	Cyanosis, tachycardia, and increased pulmonary vascular resistance
Respiratory	Respiratory distress
Gastrointestinal	Vomiting, poor feeding, necrotizing enterocolitis, and gallstone
Neurological	Hypotonia, abnormal cry, jitteriness, lethargy, seizure, tremor, and cerebrovascular accident
Hematological	Thrombocytopenia, disseminated intravascular coagulation but it is very rare
Renal	Decreased glomerular filtration rates, oliguria, hematuria, proteinuria, and renal vein thrombosis

many different neonatal disorders and may be associated with, but not caused by, the polycythemia.

Investigations

Laboratory screening: Screening is done only for high risk cases, which are mentioned before and for symptomatic cases. Screening is recommended in high risk cases at 2 hours of age, for a full term baby; if it is <65% then no further screening is required generally (in asymptomatic cases), if it is >65% then further screening at 6 hours, 12 hours, 24 hours, 48 hours, and 72 hours is required. Venous blood sample is the most reliable one; for practical purpose, capillary sample can be taken and abnormal values should be confirmed by venous sample.

Methods of Hct screening:
- *Automated analyzer:* Calculates from mean cell volume and hemoglobin
- *Microcentrifuge:* Blood is collected in microcapillary and centrifuged for 3–5 minutes at 10,000–15,000 rpm, plasma separates and packed cell volume is measured to calculate Hct
- More than 50% of infants with polycythemia have hyperviscosity. On the contrary, some infants with hyperviscosity are not polycythemia.
- As because other diseases can present with similar signs/symptom, other possible causes also should be sorted out like pneumonia, congenital heart disease, persistent pulmonary hypertension, intracranial hemorrhage, venous thrombosis, intracranial anomalies, or metabolic abnormalities, dehydration (loss of more than 7% of birthweight during the first 5 days of life may suggest dehydration).
  – Serum glucose and calcium levels
  – Bilirubin level (it is required because the increased RBC mass leads to an increased load of bilirubin precursors that can result in hyperbilirubinemia)
  – Arterial blood gases (ABG)—required to assess oxygenation in the symptomatic infant with respiratory distress and cyanosis
  – Platelet count.

Management

General

- All polycythemia infants should be closely monitored for neurologic and cardiovascular symptoms
- Serum bilirubin and serum glucose should be regularly monitored
- If hypoglycemia is detected (blood glucose <45 mg/dL) parenteral route for glucose supplementation is generally advisable with symptoms, and it is must for neonates with severe hypoglycemia (plasma glucose <25 mg/dL).

Flowchart 1: Algorithm for polycythemia.

```
Suspect polycythemia
(Screen high risk or symptomatic)
          ↓
Monitor 6-12 hourly serum glucose,
bilirubin and urine output and vital
          parameters
          ↓
Assess history and risk factors
   Confirm diagnosis (Hct)
          ↓
   ┌──────────────┴──────────────┐
Asymptomatic patients      Symptomatic patients
       ↓                          ↓
    Venous                Definitive treatment: PET
   hematocrit
   ┌───┬───┬───┐
65%-70% 70%-75% >75%
Monitoring Monitoring + Monitoring +
           increased     PET
           fluid intake
```

Note: Monitoring should be: 6–12 hourly vitals, symptomatology, urine output, serum glucose, serum bilirubin, and hematocrit by centrifuging venous blood in heparinized capillaries for 3–5 minutes @ 10,000–15,000 rpm.

(PET: partial exchange transfusion)

Specific

Management mainly depends on two factors:
- Absolute value of central venous Hct
- Presence or absence of symptoms (Flowchart 1).

Table 2: Management for asymptomatic newborn according to Hct.

Hematocrit	Action
65–70%	Monitoring
70–75%	Monitoring + Increased fluid intake
>75%	Monitoring + Partial exchange transfusion

For Asymptomatic Infants (Table 2)

Treatment depends on Hct value.
- *Hematocrit 65-70%*: They only need monitoring for symptoms and re-estimation of Hct (mainly 2, 12 and 24 hours). Further management depends upon the repeat values.
- *Hematocrit 70-75%*: Conservative management with hydration should be tried in these infants. An extra fluid (20 mL/kg) may be added to the daily fluid requirements. The additional fluid may be given by either enteral (supervised feeding) or parenteral route (IV fluids). The rationale for this therapy is hemodilution and the resultant decrease in viscosity. Along with this, cardiorespiratory monitoring, Hct monitoring, and serum glucose monitoring should be done every 6 hours. Serum bilirubin and urine output also should be monitored.
- *Hematocrit >75%*: Usually these infants are managed by partial exchange transfusion (PET); very rarely some clinicians follow conservative approach of observation with increased hydration.

In recent studies, including Cochrane review, it is shown that there is hardly any evidence of clinical benefit of intravenous fluid supplementation or PET in late preterm or term infants with asymptomatic polycythemia.

For Symptomatic Infants

The definitive treatment is PET. PET is removing some of the blood volume and replacing that volume with fluids so as to decrease the Hct to 55% (ideal). Isovolumetric PET reduces the Hct without causing hypovolemia.

> The required volume to be exchanged is:
> Volume to be exchanged = [Blood volume × (Observed hematocrit – Desired hematocrit)] ÷ Observed hematocrit

Blood volume is estimated to be 80–90 mL/kg in term babies and 90–100 mL/kg in preterm.

In general, the exchange volume is 15–20 mL/kg body weight.

Technique of Partial Exchange Transfusion (Two Approaches)

- *Peripheral route*: Blood is taken out from peripheral artery and replaced with normal saline via peripheral vein. This withdrawal and infusion can be done simultaneously (isovolumetric technique) or by serial aliquots of 10–15 mL/kg.
- *Central route*: Here blood is withdrawn through umbilical vein and normal saline is infused through peripheral venous route. Alternatively, the umbilical venous catheter may be used both withdrawal and infusion. But PET through central route is associated with increased risk of necrotizing enterocolitis.

Replacement fluid: Crystalloids like normal saline or ringer lactate are preferred than colloids as colloids are associated with more risk of infection.

Following PET, *feedings* should be withheld for 2–4 hours.

Effects of PET

- *Short term*: PET reverses the reduction in cerebral blood flow, oxygenation and microvascular flow velocity, cardiac index, and oxygen transport, polycythemia which are due to hyperviscosity but jitteriness may persist for 1–2 days. PET reduces the Hct quickly.
- *Long term*: This is a controversial issue. There is no evidence that it improves long-term outcome.

Complications of PET

- Necrotizing enterocolitis (NEC) may be increased especially PET done through central route
- Other gastrointestinal symptoms like abdominal distension, bloody stools, and vomiting. Again these are more common with central route.
- Infection
- Thromboembolic episodes
- Perforation of umbilical vein, portal vein, and ductus venosus

Outcome

- Effect of polycythemia or its treatment's long-term outcome is uncertain
- Long-term clinical outcome depends mainly on associated symptoms/conditions or underlying etiology/disorder.
- Generally, there is no adverse outcome in neurodevelopment.
- Only in some studies neurodevelopmental delay was found but it was independent of treatment and the brain dysfunction

is multifactorial; it is mostly due to the perinatal events caused by the risk factors which give rise to polycythemia.
- In one case, macular hemorrhage occurred due to polycythemia, but it is a rare complication.

SUGGESTED READING

1. Black VD, Lubchenco LO, Koops BL, et al. Neonatal hyperviscosity: randomized study of effect of partial plasma exchange transfusion on long-term outcome. Pediatrics. 1985;75(6): 1048-53.
2. Morag I, Strauss T, Lubin D, et al. Restrictive management of neonatal polycythemia. Am J Perinatol. 2011;28(9):677-82.
3. Ozek E, Soll R, Schimmel MS. Partial exchange transfusion to prevent neurodevelopmental disability in infants with polycythemia. Cochrane Database Syst Rev. 2010;(1):CD005089.
4. Sankar MJ, Agarwal R, Deorari A, et al. Management of polycythemia in neonates. Indian J Pediatr. 2010;77(10):1117-21.
5. Sundaram M, Dutta S, Narang A. Fluid supplementation versus no fluid supplementation in late preterm and term neonates with asymptomatic polycythemia: a randomized control trial. India Pediatr. 2016;53(11):983-6.

CHAPTER 13

Feed Intolerance: Gastric Residues

Rohit Arora

INTRODUCTION

The incidence of feed intolerance is estimated to be between 16% and 29%. Although the routine evaluation of gastric residues is a common neonatal intensive care unit (NICU) practice, studies indicate no benefit in terms of preventing sepsis, necrotizing enterocolitis (NEC), or feed intolerance.

DEFINITION

Gastric Residues

Gastric residuals (GRs) or gastric aspirates or pre-feed aspirates are the presence of food in the stomach from a previous feeding that is found at the start of the next feeding.

Feed Intolerance

The operational definition as given by the work of Moore and Wilson is the inability to digest enteral feedings presented as GRs more than 50%, abdominal distension or emesis or both, and the disruption of the patient's feeding plan.

CLINICAL SYMPTOMS OF FEED INTOLERANCE

- Gastric residuals
- Emesis
- Abdominal distension
- Visible bowel loops
- Altered stool character (diarrhea, guaiac positive or bloody)
- Temperature instability
- Apnea
- Bradycardia
- Pneumatosis intestinalis and necrotizing enterocolitis.

Table 1 describes the signs and symptoms related to feed intolerance, their assessment, and possible interventions.

MANAGEMENT

Following strategies may be adopted to prevent/minimize feed intolerance:
- *Antenatal steroids*: Significant reduction in incidence of NEC has been reported following antenatal steroid use. It enhances gastrointestinal maturation.
- *Breast milk*: Human milk has been reported to reduce the incidence of feed intolerance and NEC by up to sevenfolds compared to formula milk. It is better tolerated; causes faster gastric emptying. Presence of cytokines, growth factors, immunoglobulins, prebiotics, and probiotics contribute to the protective effects of breast milk.

CHAPTER 13
Feed Intolerance: Gastric Residues

Table 1: Signs and symptoms related to feed intolerance, their assessment, and possible interventions.

Symptoms of feed intolerance	Assessment	Intervention
Gastric residues	Is orogastric (OG) tube in correct placement?	Correct OG tube position by proper measurement. Place the baby in right lateral or prone position after feed.
	Are the residues nonbilious?	If baby is otherwise well and GRs >50% of the previous feed, refeed GR and subtract the volume of GR from next feed. Depending on the baby's condition decrease in volume or increasing the time between two feeds may be needed. Modified bolus or continuous feeding patterns are other interventions that might help. If baby is preterm and unwell with significant GRs then work on the lines of NEC as given below
	Are the residues bilious?	X-ray abdomen—supine/cross-table lateral CBC/blood gas/CRP/Electrolytes if baby is sick. Manage on the lines of NEC. Keep baby NPO, start antibiotics. Bilious GRs may also indicate intestinal obstruction. Extract any history of meconium passage and do X-ray abdomen.
Abdominal distension	Are the bowel sounds present or not? Has baby passed stool/meconium? Any significant increase in abdominal girth? Any tenderness / rigidity in the abdomen? Is the baby on CPAP?	Aspirate air/gastric residues if any. Glycerin tip suppository if no stool passed in last 24 hours. Check electrolytes if hypoactive bowel sounds. X-ray abdomen—supine/cross-table lateral. Put OG/NG tube if not already placed for baby on CPAP. R/O sepsis. Antibiotics if needed. Pediatric surgery consult if needed.
Emesis/vomiting	What's the color—clear / bloody / bile stained. What's the quantity? Is there GER as well?	If volume is large or bilious or blood stained then feeds need to be decreased or stopped. Modified bolus feeds over pump may be considered. X-ray/sepsis screen/paeds surgery consult etc. as per the case.
Apnea and bradycardia	OG/NG in correct place? Any evidence of GER? Are airway/breathing/circulation (ABC) intact?	Ensure ABC is protected. Correct the OG/NG position. Do X-ray if needed. Suction mouth/nose if necessary.

(CBC: complete blood count; CRP: C-reactive protein; GER: gastroesophageal reflux; GR: gastric residual; NEC: necrotizing enterocolitis; NPO: nil per oral; CPAP: continuous positive airway pressure; NG: nasogastric; R/O: rule out)

- *Introduction of early trophic feeds*: Trophic feeds are provided to facilitate gastrointestinal function and maturation to improve feed tolerance.
- *Oral medications and feed supplements*: Additives like human milk fortifier (HMF)/multivitamins/iron drops, etc. are regularly added to the human milk once babies are close to full feeds. Any additives to milk contribute to the osmolality and high osmolality delays gastric emptying. Breast milk has osmolality close to that of serum, i.e. approximately 300 mOsm/kg. If there is feed intolerance, such additives might need modification
- Management of patent ductus arteriosus (PDA) and sepsis and other coexisting conditions may contribute to feed intolerance. Management of such conditions like closure of PDA or treating sepsis with antibiotics may improve feed tolerance as well.
- *Prebiotics and Probiotics*: Prophylactic probiotic supplementation has been shown

to significantly reduce the incidence of NEC and death while facilitating feed tolerance and gut motility in preterm neonates. Most commonly studied probiotics are lactic acid bacteria and bifidobacteria. Unequivocal evidence exists regarding their benefits, however, few queries such as when to start and stop / what dose/duration interval, etc. need further clarification.
- Protocol for standard feeding regimens has been consistently shown to improve feeding patterns in very preterms.

FAMILY COUNSELING

Parents need to be counseled about immaturity of the gastrointestinal tract. Feed intolerance is expected with increasing prematurity. There is need for day-to-day counseling. Keeping the patient's family well informed on the neonate's condition helps to alleviate any surprise if changes arise. Information should be done in a clear and concise manner, making sure to answer any questions the family should have.

KEY POINTS

- Feed intolerance commonly manifests as gastric residues, abdominal distension with or without onset of apnea/bradycardia.
- In isolation, gastric residues should not be used for withholding of feeds. Presence of bilious vomiting, abdominal distension, abdominal wall erythema or ecchymosis, gross or occult blood in the stool, apnea, bradycardia, and temperature instability suggests possible pathology and need for detail evaluation of the underlying cause.
- Each unit must have a written protocol for enteral feeding practices which should be uniformly applied in clinical practice.

SUGGESTED READING

1. Cohen S, Mandel D, Mimouni FB, et al. Gastric residual in growing preterm infants: Effect of body position. Am J Perinatol. 2004;21(3):163-6.
2. Dasopoulou M, Briana DD, Boutsikou T, et al. Motilin and gastrin secretion and lipid profile in preterm neonates following prebiotics supplementation: a double-blind randomized controlled study JPEN J Parenter Enteral Nutr. 2015;39(3):359-68.
3. Dollberg S, Kuint J, Mazkereth R, et al. Feeding tolerance in preterm infants: Randomized trial of bolus and continuous feeding. J Am Coll Nutr. 2000;19(6):797-800.
4. Ewer AK, Durbin GM, Morgan ME, et al. Gastric emptying in preterm infants. Arch Dis Child. 1994;71(1):F24-7.
5. Gomella TL, Cunningham MD, Eyal FG. Neonatology: Management, Procedures, On-Call Problems, Diseases, and Drugs. New York: McGraw-Hill Medical; 2009.
6. Gonzales I, Duryea EJ, Vasquez E, et al. Effect of enteral feeding temperature on feeding tolerance in preterm infants. Neonatal Netw. 1995;14(3):39-43.
7. Hodges C, Vincent PA. Why do NICU nurses not refeed gastric residuals prior to feeding by gavage? Neonatal Netw. 1993;12(8):37-40.
8. Lucchini R, Bizzarri B, Giampietro S, et al. Feeding intolerance in preterm infants. How to understand the warning signs. J Matern Fetal Neonatal Med. 2011;24(Suppl 1):72-4.
9. Malhotra AK, Deorari AK, Paul VK, et al. Gastric residuals in preterm babies. J Trop Pediatr. 1992;38(5):262-4.
10. Srinivasjois R, Rao S, Patole S. Prebiotic supplementation in preterm neonates: updated systematic review and meta-analysis of randomized controlled trials. Clin Nutr. 2013;32(6):958-65.
11. Williams T, Choe Y, Price P, et al. Tolerance of formulas containing prebiotics in healthy, term infants. J Pediatr Gastroenterol Nutr. 2014;59(5):653-8.

CHAPTER 14

Bleeding Newborn

Rajesh Kumar

INTRODUCTION

The evaluation of bleeding disorders in neonates can be challenging because of subtle or nonspecific clinical presentations and difficulties in both obtaining adequate specimen for coagulation testing and interpreting the results of these tests in the context of developmental hemostasis. Neonates, especially preterms are at higher risk of bleeding due to decreased activity of certain coagulation factors and impaired platelet function. Bleeding disorders in neonates can be inherited, but are more often acquired. A systematic approach is required for proper management.

DEFINITION

Presentations suggestive of neonatal bleeding disorders include:
- Diffuse purpura/ecchymoses
- Oozing from the umbilical stump
- Excessive bleeding from peripheral puncture/heelstick sites
- Large cephalohematomas without significant birth trauma history or any subgaleal bleed
- Prolonged bleeding following circumcision
- Intracranial hemorrhage in a term or late-preterm infant without history of birth trauma
- Unexplained bleeding in a very low birth weight infant.

TYPES OF DISORDERS

Bleeding disorders are mainly classified into inherited and acquired causes. The other classification is bleeding related to platelet disorder or coagulation disorder. A simple physical examination is essential to identify the type of bleeding disorder.

ETIOLOGY

A good history and baseline investigations that include platelets, partial thromboplastin (PT), and activated partial thromboplastin time (APTT) are useful in further identifying the cause (Tables 1 to 3).

Laboratory investigation: Initial coagulation screen consists of complete blood count (CBC), PT and APTT. With the help of this screen, cause of bleeding can be suspected.

Normal PT and APTT values vary with gestational age and the postnatal age (Table 4). *Caution*: Abnormal laboratory report in neonate must be viewed with proper clinical finding because laboratory error in coagulation screen is common (Table 5).

SECTION 1
Clinical Approach to Sick Newborn

Table 1: Approach to bleeding newborn: Clinical examination.

Physical finding		Rationale
General appearance	Well neonate	Usually has inherited or immunological cause of bleeding
	Sick neonate	Usually has acquired cause of bleeding
	Dysmorphic features	Usually has inherited cause of bleeding
Type of bleeding	Petechial bleeding with small mucosal hemorrhage	Usually indicates thrombocytopenia
	Large bleeds	Usually indicates coagulopathy

Table 2: Approach to bleeding newborn: History.

History	Rationale
Was the baby sick or well at the onset of bleeding?	Well baby usually has inherited or immunological cause of bleeding. Sick baby usually has acquired cause of bleeding
H/o Vitamin K administration at birth	If baby has not received Vitamin K at birth, it is more likely to have hemorrhagic disease of newborn
H/o Maternal diseases such as ITP, pre-eclampsia	Baby tends to have thrombocytopenia due to these maternal illnesses
H/o Maternal exposure to drugs as aspirin	Aspirin can cause platelet dysfunction
H/o Maternal exposure to drugs as warfarin, anticonvulsants, rifampicin, and isoniazid	These drugs can cause coagulation disorder in neonates
Family history of bleeding disorders	More likely to have inherited bleeding disorder
Previous affected siblings	More likely to have inherited bleeding disorder. Alloimmune thrombocytopenia

(H/o: history of; ITP: immune thrombocytopenic purpura)

Table 3: Approach to bleeding newborn: Investigations.

Clinical condition	Platelet	Partial thromboplastin (PT)	Activated partial thromboplastin time (APTT)	Diagnosis
Sick neonate	↓	↑	↑	Disseminated intravascular coagulation
	↓	N	N	Sepsis, necrotizing enterocolitis, renal vein thrombosis
	N	↑	↑	Liver pathology
	N	N	N	Stress bleed
Well neonate	↓	N	N	Immune thrombocytopenia, bone marrow hypoplasia, Kasabach-Merritt syndrome
	N	↑	↑	Vitamin K deficiency bleed
	N	N	↑	Hereditary clotting factor deficiency
	N	N	N	Swallowed maternal blood, trauma, platelet function disorder, Factor XIII deficiency

Special Laboratory Tests

Peripheral smear examination: Always confirm low platelet count obtained by cell counters by peripheral smear examination. Size of platelet can also be examined and fragmented red blood cells (RBCs) can be seen in disseminated intravascular coagulation (DIC).

Apt test: It is used in ruling out swallowed maternal blood. Mix 1 part of gastric aspirate/vomitus/stool with 5 parts of distilled water. Centrifuge and separate the clear pink supernatant. Add 1 mL of 1% NaOH to 4 mL of supernatant. Maternal blood turns brown but fetal blood remains pink.

Table 4: Normal values PT and APT.

Test	Day 1	Day 5	Day 30
Term neonates			
PT (sec)	11.6–14.4	10.9–13.9	10.6–13.1
APTT (sec)	37.1–48.7	34.0–51.2	33.0–47.8
Preterm neonates (30–36 weeks GA)			
PT (sec)	10.6–16.2	10.0–15.0	10.0–13.6
APTT (sec)	27.5–79.4	26.9–74.1	26.9–62.5

(PT: partial thromboplastin; APTT: activated partial thromboplastin time)

d-Dimer test: It is required to confirm DIC.

PIVKA: For confirmation of Vitamin K deficiency. It can be done up to 72 hours after Vitamin K administration.

Antiplatelet antibodies: For confirmation of immune thrombocytopenia.

MANAGEMENT
General Measures

- Give Vitamin K: 1 mg IV if weight is ≥1.5 kg and 0.5 mg IV if weight is <1.5 kg
- If shock is present give whole blood as soon as possible
- Look for underlying cause and treat it.

Whole blood transfusion: If hematocrit (packed cell volume) is <40 whole blood should be transfused.

Platelet transfusion: Any bleeding neonate with platelet count <1,00,000/μL should be considered for platelet transfusion. For details regarding platelet transfusion, see the chapter on thrombocytopenia.

Fresh frozen plasma (FFP) transfusion: Indication of FFP transfusions are as follows:

Table 5: Laboratory errors in coagulation screen.

Variable	Source of error	Possible solution
Preanalytical	Insufficient sample volume and under-filling of collection tubes. Heparin contamination (sample collected from indwelling catheters or into a preheparinized syringe)	Establishment of standard protocols, techniques for specimen collection
	High hematocrit at birth (required citrate-to-blood ratio of 9:1 may not be achieved using standard collection tubes)	When the hematocrit exceeds 0.55 (55%), the reduced plasma volume requires a decrease in the volume of anticoagulant used to maintain the ratio of 9:1
Analytical	Elevated levels of bilirubin or lipids and hemolysis in neonates can interfere with optical density measurements used to determine end points of some coagulation tests	Additional centrifugation of the sample
Postanalytical	Defining appropriate reference ranges for neonates	Use of age-related reference ranges specific for analyzer-reagent combination used in the coagulation laboratory

- Coagulopathy with active bleeding
- Coagulopathy and invasive procedure planned
- Factor replacement when individual concentrates are not available (Factor II, V, VIII, IX, X, XI)
- At the initiation of heparin therapy, which group to be transfused is shown in Table 6.
- Transfuse FFP 15–25 mL/kg over 2–3 hours in term babies. Very low birth weight babies should be given 10–15 mL/kg over 2–3 hours
- Fresh frozen plasma can be stored in freezer compartment of freeze for 12 hours
- Once thawed, transfuse immediately and do not refreeze.

Specific measures: Disease specific measures in bleeding neonates are given in Table 7.

PREVENTION OF BLEEDING

It is important to anticipate bleeding disorder in neonates so that the serious bleeding can be prevented. In the conditions shown in Table 8, laboratory tests must be done even without overt bleeding (Flowchart 1).

Table 6: Selection of donor blood group for FFP transfusion.

Baby's blood group	FFP Group	
	1st preference	2nd preference
O	O	A, B, AB
A	A	AB
B	B	AB
AB	AB	—

(FFP: fresh frozen plasma)

Table 7: Specific therapy for a bleeding newborn.

Disease	Specific treatment
Vitamin K deficiency bleeding	Vitamin K by slow IV or by subcutaneously if venous access cannot be established. FFP for neonate with active bleeding. Vitamin K takes at least 6–8 hours to correct the coagulation deficiency
Immune thrombocytopenia	Do platelet count immediately after birth if born to mother with ITP. IVIG: Give if platelet count <100,000/µL. Dose: 1 g/kg/day for 2 days. Prednisolone: 2 mg/kg/day
Alloimmune thrombocytopenia	Transfuse platelet even if baby is asymptomatic if platelet count is <30,000/µL. Cranial USG to look for IC bleed
Hemophilia	In hemophilia A; Factor VIII concentrate: 50 IU/kg 8–12 hourly in severe bleed (intracranial bleed). In Hemophilia B; Factor IX concentrate: 100 IU/kg
DIC	Give Vitamin K 1 mg/kg. Keep platelet count >50,000/µL even if no active bleed. Consider DVET, if bleeding persists. In thrombotic DIC heparin should be given: 30 U/kg IV stat followed by 10 U/kg/hour to keep APTT 1.5–2 times of normal value. LMWH is preferred, the dose is 1.5 mg/kg/dose S/C 12 hourly.
Isolated altered gastric aspirate	If platelet count and coagulogram is normal or stress bleeding is suspected, give IV ranitidine. Dose: 0.5 mg/kg/dose twice daily in preterms and 1.5 mg/kg/dose in term babies

(DIC: disseminated intravascular coagulation; DVET: double volume exchange transfusion; ITP: immune thrombocytopenic purpura; IVIG: intravenous immunoglobulin; LMWH: low molecular weight heparin)

Table 8: Specific laboratory tests for different bleeding disorders.

Condition	Laboratory test
Necrotizing enterocolitis	Platelet count, PT
PDA treatment with Ibuprofen/ Indomethacin	Platelet count
Mother on warfarin, ATT, phenytoin	PT
Large hemangiomas	Platelet count
Cholestasis, liver pathology	PT

(PT: partial thromboplastin; PDA: patent ductus arteriosus; ATT: anti tuberculous therapy)

Flowchart 1: Approach to laboratory evaluation of coagulation in neonates to determine the etiology.

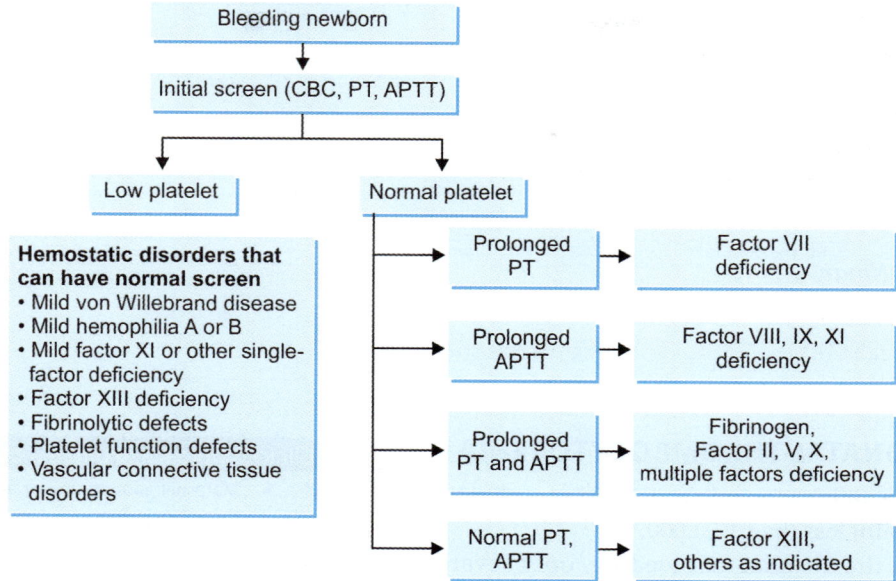

(APTT: activated partial thromboplastin time; CBC: complete blood count; PT: partial thromboplastin)

SUGGESTED READING

1. Andrew M, Paes B, Milner R, et al. Development of the human coagulation system in the healthy premature infant. Blood. 1988;72(5): 1651-7.
2. Gibson BE, Todd A, Roberts I, et al. British Committee for Standards in Haematology Transfusion Task Force: Writing group. Transfusion guidelines for neonates and older children. Br J Haematol. 2004;124(4):433-53.
3. Monagle P, Ignjatovic V, Savoia H. Hemostasis in neonates and children: pitfalls and dilemmas. Blood Rev. 2010;24(2):63-8.
4. Saxonhouse MA, Manco-Johnson MJ. The evaluation and management of neonatal co-agulation disorders. Semin Perinatol. 2009;33(1): 52-65.

CHAPTER 15

Thrombocytopenia

Binu Ninan

NEONATAL THROMBOCYTOPENIA

- Thrombocytopenia is defined as a platelet count less than 1,50,000.
- In the absence of bleeding, only severe thrombocytopenia (<50,000) needs to be evaluated.

APPROACH TO ETIOLOGY

- Thrombocytopenia in a well baby (Table 1)
- Thrombocytopenia in a baby with a syndrome or congenital anomalies
- Thrombocytopenia in a sick or unwell baby (Flowchart 1 and Table 2).

As a general rule, the cause in a well baby is immune-mediated consumption of platelets and in an unwell baby a combination of consumption and decreased production.

Infection continues to be a very common cause in preterm and term babies, and should be always looked for in all babies with severe thrombocytopenia.

Thrombocytopenia in a well baby is most often because of immune-mediated platelet destruction: alloimmune and autoimmune thrombocytopenia (Table 3). An initial step in the evaluation of thrombocytopenia in these infants is to determine the mother's platelet count.

Table 1: Clinical approach to thrombocytopenia.

Well baby	• Maternal alloimmune or autoimmune thrombocytopenia • Intrauterine growth restriction (IUGR) and babies born to mothers with pre-eclampsia • Hereditary disorder of platelets • Wiskott-Aldrich syndrome • Occult infection
Unwell or sick baby	• Birth asphyxia • Placental insufficiency with intrauterine chronic hypoxia • Bacterial infections, fungal infections • Congenital infections (TORCH) • Disseminated intravascular coagulation • Thrombosis like renal vein thrombosis • Exchange transfusions • Bone marrow infiltrations like in neuroblastoma or leukemia
Syndromic/ anomalies	• Thrombocytopenia with absent radius (TAR) syndrome • Fanconi's anemia • Chromosomal disorders due to trisomy 13,18, Turner syndrome • Kasabach-Merritt syndrome

INVESTIGATIONS

Complete Blood Count (CBC)

- Pancytopenia suggests a generalized systemic disorder or bone marrow affection. Platelet count is a sensitive marker of bleeding tendency.

Flowchart 1: Approach of neonatal thrombocytopenia.

```
                        Thrombocytopenia
    Exclude syndromic ──→
              ┌──────────────────┴──────────────────┐
              ▼                                     ▼
          Well baby                             Sick baby
              │                                     │
              ▼                                     ├──→ Sepsis (Complete workup
      Maternal platelet                             │     including blood culture)
         ┌────┴────┐                                │
         ▼         ▼                                ├──→ Perinatal asphyxia
      Normal      Low                               │
         │         │                                ├──→ Congenital infections
         │         └──→ Autoimmune                  │
         │              thrombocytopenia            ├──→ Other comorbid condition
         ├──→ Alloimmune                            │     RDS, NEC, PPHN
         │    Thrombocytopenia                      │
         │                                          ├──→ Thrombosis RVT
         ├──→ Maternal gestational                  │
         │    hypertension, IUGR                    └──→ Consumption
         │                                                DIC, ECMO, ET
         ├──→ Hereditary disorders
         │    of platelet
         │
         ├──→ Wiskott-Aldrich
         │    syndrome
         │
         └──→ Occult infection
```

(RVT: renal vein thrombosis; DIC: disseminated intravascular coagulation; ECMO: extracorporeal membrane oxygenation; ET: exchange transfusion; PPHN: persistent pulmonary hypertension of the newborn; RDS: respiratory distress syndrome; NEC: necrotizing enterocolitis; IUGR: intrauterine growth restriction)

Table 2: Evaluation of a newborn with thrombocytopenia.

Focused clinical evaluation	
Evaluation	**Look for**
Timing of onset	Gestational age
Localized or generalized	Well or sick baby
Bleed	Vital parameters
Family history	Site of bleed
Maternal illness	Pallor, petechiae, purpura
Intrapartum events	Jaundice
Medications	Ecchymosis, hepatosplenomegaly, congenital anomaly, dysmorphism, Bruit
Causes of refractory thrombocytopenia: • Drugs • Fungemia • Severe sepsis • Toxoplasmosis, rubella, cytomegalovirus and herpes simplex virus (TORCH) infections • Disseminated intravascular coagulation • Necrotizing enterocolitis • Hemangioma	

Table 3: Differentiating alloimmune from autoimmune thrombocytopenia.

Pathophysiology	Alloimmune thrombocytopenia Antifetal platelet membranes antibody	Autoimmune thrombocytopenia Maternal auto antibodies
History of maternal bleeding	No	Yes
Onset	Early	Early
Severity	Severe	Moderate
Risk of ICH	High	Low
Maternal platelet count	Normal	Low
Response to platelet transfusion	Good	Poor
Treatment	Platelet transfusion (antigen negative) in bleeding patient	Intravenous immunoglobulin or steroids in asymptomatic platelet transfusion in bleeding patient
Time to resolution	Days to weeks	Weeks to months
Risk of recurrence	Yes	No

(ICH: intracerebral hemorrhage)

- Low platelets may be due to increased destruction as in consumptive coagulopathy or due to decreased marrow production. Normal platelets with bleeding tendency is seen in hemorrhagic disease of newborn, drug intake, or localized bleeding like pulmonary or intraventricular.
- Platelet counts are 20–25% lower in infants who are small for gestational age.
- Presence of platelet clumps in low power field suggests adequacy of platelets.

Peripheral Smear

- The peripheral blood smear should be examined in any patient with a suspected platelet disorder. A low platelet count must be confirmed by review of the smear because clumping of platelets can cause a falsely low automated count, which may be easily detected on examination of the smear.
- Clumping of platelets can occur due to ethylenediaminetetraacetate (EDTA)-dependent antibodies and, if persistent, may require repeat collection of the blood sample in an alternative anticoagulant such as citrate.
- On a well-prepared slide, each platelet in a 100 field contributes approximately 15,000/mL to the total platelet count. A few fields should be counted and the results averaged to yield a platelet estimate. Examination of the smear also allows for examination of platelet morphology.

Coagulation Screening Tests (PT and PTT)

- Prothrombin time (PT) measures the extrinsic coagulation pathway (Factors II, V, VII, X) and partial thromboplastin time (PTT) assesses the intrinsic clotting system (Factors II, V, VIII, IX, X, XI, XII). Any PT greater than 17 seconds in a neonate of any gestational age and a PTT greater than 45–50 seconds in a term infant should be considered abnormal.

Subsequent tests: Based on clinical picture and results of initial screening tests other laboratory tests may be ordered to reach a conclusive diagnosis (sepsis screen, blood culture, cerebrospinal fluid study, arterial blood gas (ABG), D dimer assay, ultrasonography of skull, TORCH titers, genetic analysis and so on) (Table 4).

CHAPTER 15
Thrombocytopenia

Table 4: Laboratory errors in coagulation screening tests.

Error	Cause
Platelet count falsely low	• Platelets adhere to heel after stick • Errors in dilution (manual technique) • Adherence to tube • Dilution with EDTA
PT and PTT falsely high	• Decreased plasma/citrate ratio (due to either too small a sample or hematocrit >65%) • Contamination with heparin from indwelling lines
PT and PTT falsely low	• Sample contaminated with tissue thromboplastin from difficult venipuncture

(EDTA: ethylenediaminetetraacetate; PT: prothrombin time; PTT: partial thromboplastin time)

Table 5: Platelet transfusions.

Indications
- Platelets <100 × 10⁹/L and bleeding
- Platelets <50 × 10⁹/L and invasive procedure
- Platelets at any count, but with platelets dysfunction plus bleeding or invasive procedures

Without clinical bleeding
- Stable full-term: <20,000/cumm
- Sick full-term: <30,000/cumm
- Stable preterm: <30,000/cumm
- Sick preterm: <50,000/cumm

MANAGEMENT

General Principles

- Goal should be the *wellbeing of infant* rather than correcting the laboratory abnormalities.
- Therapy should be focused on treating the underlying disease such as septicemia, infection, shock, hypoxia, and acidosis in addition to the supportive therapy and replacing the appropriate blood components.
- Use blood components rather than whole blood wherever possible.
- Use blood products only when they are absolutely necessary (Table 5).

In a Sick Baby

- *Supportive care*: Nurse the infant in thermoneutral environment. Ensure oxygenation, perfusion, and euglycemia throughout. Correct hypoxia, acidosis, dyselectrolytemia, hypotension, and shock. Monitor the vital signs continuously in a sick infant.
- *Treatment of the cause*: The major focus should be on identifying and treating the underlying medical disorder.

Response to Platelet Transfusion

The neonate who presents with severe thrombocytopenia and responds well to platelet transfusions but requires them on a weekly basis is likely to have a disorder associated with decreased platelet production (i.e. congenital amegakaryocytic thrombocytopenia). In contrast, the need for frequent transfusions (every 1 or 2 days) strongly suggests increased platelet consumption. One unit of platelet transfusion increases platelet count by 50,000 unless there is ongoing destruction. Repeat platelet count should be done 12 hours of transfusion.

Specific Therapy

All infants born to mothers who have idiopathic thrombocytopenic purpura (ITP) should have a cord blood platelet count measured and be observed for any bleeding symptoms. For those with isoimmune thrombocytopenia and who have severe thrombocytopenia of less than 20,000 or clinical bleeding, intravenous immune globulin (IVIg) of 1 g/kg should be given. About 80–90% of babies respond to this.

Platelet transfusions are less effective and have a transient response. Platelet counts usually recover in 7–14 days.

The primary treatment for neonatal alloimmune thrombocytopenia (NAIT) is platelet transfusion and should be given to nonbleeding well neonates if platelet counts are less than 30,000. In neonates with intracranial hemorrhage or other major bleeding platelet transfusion are to be given if the platelet count is less than 50,000. But the platelets have to be either washed maternal platelets or human platelet antigens (HPA)-compatible platelets. If compatible platelets are not readily available, IVIG with or without random donor platelets can be used. IVIG is useful in this disorder just as with thrombocytopenia due to maternal ITP.

Cranial ultrasonography should be obtained in all cases of severe thrombocytopenia, especially with NAIT.

SUGGESTED READING

1. Bussel JB. Alloimmune thrombocytopenia in the fetus and newborn. Semin Thromb Hemost. 2001;27(3):245-52.
2. Christensen RD. Hematologic Problems of the Neonate. Philadelphia, PA: WB Saunders Company; 2000.
3. McFarland JG. Detection and identification of platelet antibodies in clinical disorders. Transfus Apher Sci. 2003;28(3):297-305.
4. Nuss R, Manco-Johnson M. Bleeding disorders in the neonate. Neo Reviews. 2000;1(10)e: 196-9.

CHAPTER 16

Anemia

Sanjay Aher

INTRODUCTION

Neonatal anemia is a common disorder, particularly in very preterm neonates. Giving red blood cell (RBC) transfusions to anemic infants is a very common practice in neonatal intensive care units (NICUs). Neonatal anemia can be due to blood loss (bone marrow hemorrhage), decreased RBC production (hypoplasia) or increased destruction of erythrocytes (hemolytic). Physiological anemia of the newborn and anemia of prematurity are the two most common causes of anemia in the neonates.

Definition: Neonatal anemia is defined as hemoglobin (Hb) or hematocrit (Hct) concentration greater than 2 standard deviation below the mean for postnatal age. For all practical purpose, a hematocrit <40% is considered anemia in the newborn.

IDENTIFY THE SEVERITY

The factors associated with severity are:
- Level of Hb or hematocrit. Lower the hematocrit, severe the anemia
- Acute onset is more severe than chronic
- Hemolytic anemia is more severe than nonhemolytic
- Presence of respiratory distress, tachypnea, feeding difficulty, murmur, and hepatomegaly suggest cardiac dysfunction.

IDENTIFY THE CAUSE (FLOWCHART 1)

- Differentiate true anemia from anemia of prematurity or anemia of infancy.
- The steps of identification of the cause include:
  - Rule out anemia due to decreased production from that due to hemolysis and increased loss (low reticulocyte count).
  - Rule out immune hemolytic anemia (Coomb positive).
  - Classify anemia with low versus normal or high mean corpuscular volume (MCV).
  - Differentiate anemia (normal or high MCV) from blood loss or infection from that due to nonimmune hemolysis (peripheral smear abnormal with nonimmune hemolysis).
- The features suggestive of hemolysis are:
  - Pallor with jaundice and splenomegaly.
  - Elevated reticulocyte count.
  - Peripheral smear showing marked anisopoikilocytes, spherocytes, nucleated RBCs, burr cells, and so on.

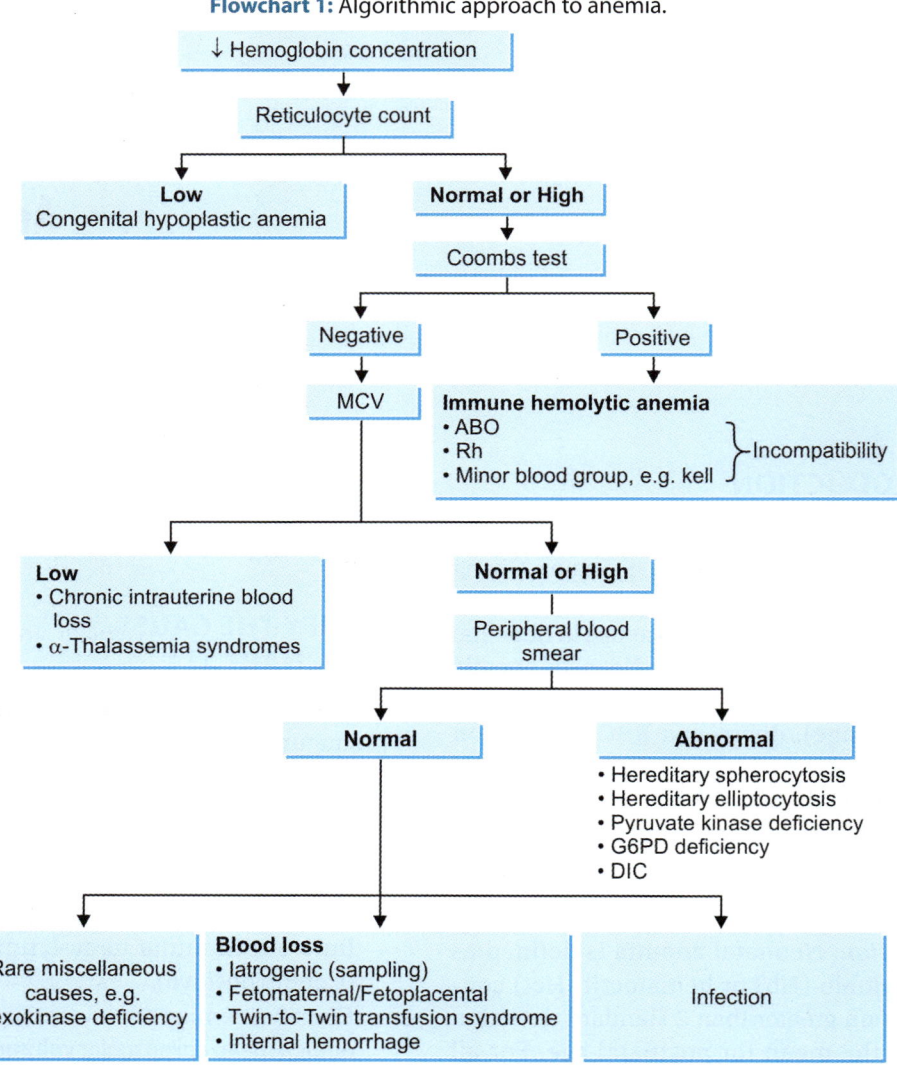

Flowchart 1: Algorithmic approach to anemia.

(DIC: disseminated intravascular coagulation; MCV: mean corpuscular volume; G6PD: glucose-6-phosphate dehydrogenase)

- Direct Coombs test differentiates immune from nonimmune hemolytic anemia.

PHYSIOLOGIC ANEMIA OF INFANCY

The normal developmental switch from fetal Hb to adult Hb replaces high-oxygenaffinity fetal Hb to low-oxygen-affinity adult Hb. This leads to delivery of a greater fraction of Hb-bound oxygen to the tissues. The Hb concentration continues to decrease until tissue oxygen needs are greater than oxygen delivery. Normally, this point is reached between 6 and 12 weeks of age, when the Hb concentration is 9–11 g/dL. As hypoxia is detected by renal or hepatic oxygen sensors, erythropoietin (EPO) production increases and erythropoiesis resumes. This condition is benign and does not require treatment.

Anemia of Prematurity

The physiologic anemia seen in preterm infants is more profound and occurs earlier than anemia of infancy. Various causes contribute to this condition. An important component in the first few weeks of life is blood loss due to sampling for many laboratory tests that these premature infants undergo. The erythropoietic response is also suboptimal, a significant problem because demands on erythropoiesis are heightened by the short survival of the RBCs from premature infants (approximately, 40–60 days instead of 120 days as in adults and children) and rapid expansion of the RBC mass that accompanies growth. The cause for this suboptimal erythropoiesis appears to be inadequate synthesis of EPO in response to hypoxia. The magnitude of deficiency is greatest in smallest and least mature infants. Deficiency of folic acid, vitamin B_{12} or vitamin E can aggravate anemia in these extremely premature infants. The anemia in preterm infants is largely caused by factors such as EPO deficiency. Combined treatment with EPO, iron, folate, and vitamin B_{12} during the first week reduces the need for transfusion in extremely low birth weight (ELBW) infants.

Causes and Approach of Neonatal Anemia (Table 1)

Anemia in the newborn infant results from three processes:
1. Underproduction of RBCs or hypoplastic anemia.
2. Increased destructions of RBCs or hemolytic anemia.
3. Loss of RBCs or hemorrhagic anemia.

Table 1: Approach to a newborn with anemia.

Symptoms and signs	
Hemorrhagic anemia	
Acute hemorrhagic anemia	• Presents at birth or with internal hemorrhage after 24 hours • Pallor not associated with jaundice and often without cyanosis and unrelieved by supplemental oxygen • Tachypnea is common, can have gasping respiration in severe bleedings • Vascular instability ranges from decreased peripheral perfusion to hypovolemic shock • Decreased central venous pressure (CVP) and poor capillary refill time (CRT) • Normocytic or normochromic red blood cells (RBCs) indices with reticulocytosis developing within 2–3 days
Chronic hemorrhagic anemia	• Unexplained pallor without cyanosis and unrelieved with supplemental oxygen • Minimal respiratory distress • CVP is normal or increased • Microcytic or hypochromic RBC indices with compensatory reticulocytosis
Asphyxia pallida (severe neonatal asphyxia)	• Pallor and cyanosis which improves with supplemental oxygen • Respiratory failure • Bradycardia • Normal CVP
Hemolytic anemia	
	• Jaundice is seen before diagnostic levels of Hb are obtained • Pallor after 48 hours of age • Hydrops fetalis in blood group incompatibilities and alpha thalassemia • Tachypnea • Hepatosplenomegaly

Contd...

Contd...

Hypoplastic anemia		
		• Presentation after 48 hours of age • Absence of jaundice • Reticulocytopenia
Other forms of anemia		
	Twin-twin transfusion syndrome	>20% difference in the birth weights of the 2 infants, with donor being the smaller twin
	Occult internal hemorrhage	• Intracranial—bulging anterior fontanel and neurologic signs (apnea, seizures and altered sensorium) • Visceral—abdominal mass or distension • Pulmonary hemorrhage—bloody tracheal secretions and partial or total radiographic opacification of a hemithorax
History		
Anemia at birth		
	Hemorrhagic anemia	• Third trimester vaginal bleeding or amniocentesis • Multiple gestation • Postpartum maternal fever • Nonelective cesarean delivery
	Hemolytic anemia	• Intrauterine growth restriction (IUGR) • Low Apgar score
Symptoms and signs		
	Anemia presenting after 24 hours of age	• Obstetric trauma • Unattended delivery • Perinatal fetal distress • Low Apgar scores
	Anemia presenting with jaundice	• Evidence of drug ingestion in late trimester that can lead to oxidative stress • IUGR • Family history of splenectomy, anemia, jaundice or cholelithiasis

Evaluation of Anemia

A good history, examination, and relevant laboratory investigations (Table 2) are useful in identifying the severity and etiology of anemia in the newborn.

Diagnosis

Management of Neonatal Anemia

Treatment of neonatal anemia may involve:
- Simple replacement transfusion
- Exchange transfusion
- Nutritional supplementation
- Treatment of underlying primary disorder.

Simple replacement transfusion:

Indications:
- Acute hemorrhagic anemia
- Ongoing deficit replacement
- Maintenance of effective oxygen-carrying capacity.

There are no universally accepted guidelines; however, those presented next are representative of most common practice.

Transfusion Guidelines

Guidelines for RBC transfusions differ worldwide and are based mainly on expert opinions. Use of these restrictive guidelines

Table 2: Approach to anemia: investigations.

Basic studies	
Hemoglobin	
RBC indices	• *Microcytic or hypochromic RBC indices*: Fetomaternal or twin-twin hemorrhage or alpha thalassemia (MCV < 90 fL) • *Normocytic or normochromic RBC indices*: Acute hemorrhage, systemic disease, intrinsic RBC defects or hypoplastic anemia
Corrected reticulocyte count (CRC)	• *Elevated CRC*: Antecedent hemorrhage or hemolytic anemia • *Low CRC*: Hypoplastic anemia
Blood smear	• *Spherocytes*: ABO incompatibility, hereditary spherocytosis • *Elliptocytes*: Hereditary elliptocytosis • *Pyknocytes*: G6PD deficiency • *Schistocytes or helmet cells*: Consumption coagulopathy
Direct Coombs test	Isoimmune or autoimmune hemolysis
Kleihauer-Betke test	Fetomaternal hemorrhage
Bone marrow aspiration	Congenital aplastic or hypoplastic anemia
TORCH titers	Congenital TORCH infections
Coagulation profile	Consumptive coagulopathy
Histopathology of placenta	Occult hemorrhage
Cranial or abdominal ultrasonography	Occult hemorrhage

(G6PD: glucose-6-phosphate dehydrogenase; MCV: mean corpuscular volume; RBC: red blood cell; TORCH: toxoplasmosis, rubella, cytomegalovirus and herpes simplex virus)

had reduced both the number of transfusions and donor exposures by 70–80% in last couple of decades, without an increase in length of stay or morbidity. In the premature infants in need of transfusion (PINT) study, it was demonstrated that transfusion threshold in ELBW infants can be moved downwards by at least 1 g/dL without incurring a clinically important increase in the risk of death or major neonatal morbidity (Table 3).

Product Specifications

Single donor: The use of single donor product for RBC transfusions for preterm infants is currently widespread in several units. An adult unit of RBC can be divided in up to 4 or 5 smaller units of 50 mL, so called Pedi-packs, which can be reserved for one specific neonate. The main advantage of Pedi-packs from single donor is the reduction in donor exposure in case multiple transfusions are required in a preterm infant.

Leukocyte filtration: The transfusion of latent intracellular viruses, such as cytomegaloviruses (CMV), can be greatly diminished by leukocyte depletion using filtration. CMV safe leukodepleted RBCs are often indicated in case of intrauterine blood transfusions.

Irradiation: To prevent graft-versus-host disease in immune compromised hosts, irradiation of cellular blood products, such as RBCs, is often advised for all intrauterine transfusions.

Preventative Measures/Alternatives for RBC Transfusions

Several measures have been proposed to reduce the number of RBC transfusions needed in preterm neonates, including:

Table 3: Indications for blood transfusion.

Hemoglobin (g/dL)	Mechanical ventilation or symptoms of anemia	PRBC volume
11 or less	Moderate or significant mechanical ventilation requirement (MAP > 8 cmH$_2$O and FiO$_2$ > 0.4)	15 mL/kg over 2–4 hours
10 or less	Minimal mechanical ventilation requirement (any mechanical ventilation or CPAP > 6 cmH$_2$O and FiO$_2$ > 0.4)	15 mL/kg over 2–4 hours
8 or less	No mechanical ventilation requirement and one or more of the following present: • 24 or more hours of tachycardia (HR >180) or tachypnea (RR > 80) • Increased oxygen requirement from the previous 48 hours • Elevated lactate concentration (2.5 mEq/L or more) • Weight gain <10 g/kg over previous 4 days while receiving 100 kcal/kg per day or more • Increase in episodes of apnea and bradycardia (10 or more in 24 hours period or 2 or more episodes in 24 hours requiring bag-mask ventilation) while receiving therapeutic doses of methylxanthines/caffeine • Undergoing any surgery	20 mL/kg over 2–4 hours (divide into two 10 mL/kg volumes if fluid sensitive)
Less than 7	No symptoms and absolute reticulocyte count < 100,000 cells/mL (RBC × reticulocyte count)	15 mL/kg over 2–4 hours

(CPAP: constant positive airway pressure; HR: heart rate; MAP: mean airway pressure; PRBC: packed red blood cell; RBC: red blood cell; RR: respiratory rate).

- Delayed cord clamping (DCC).
- Strict adherence to transfusion guidelines.
- Reduction of iatrogenic blood loss.
- Use of EPO.

Delayed Cord Clamping

Several randomized controlled studies have reported on the benefits of DCC in preterm infants. DCC implies waiting at least 60 seconds (up to maximum of 2–3 minutes after birth) before clamping the umbilical cord.

Latest newborn resuscitation program (NRP) 2015 guidelines also recommend DCC by 1 minute if baby is stable.

Laboratory Investigations using Cord Blood

The use of cord blood for the initial laboratory evaluation directly postnatally, significantly reduces the number of RBC transfusions in the first week of life.

Strict adherence to transfusion guidelines: Several studies have shown that adherence to a transfusion guideline reduces the number of RBC transfusions given.

Reduction of Iatrogenic Blood Loss

The use of microanalysis, smaller amounts of blood for diagnostic testing, indwelling lines with probes for intravenous or arterial lab measurements and transcutaneous instruments have largely reduced the amount of iatrogenic blood loss and thereby the need for RBC transfusions.

Erythropoietin

Several studies have investigated the role of EPO in reducing the transfusion volume or donor exposure in preterm infants. However, systematic reviews and meta-analyses of these studies have failed to show a clear benefit for early (n = 2,293 infants) or late (n = 1,361 infants) EPO administration. The major need for transfusion in preterm infants is in the first weeks of life, when there is no benefit yet of EPO administration. In addition, concerns have been raised about an increased risk for retinopathy of prematurity (ROP) after EPO use. In the Cochrane review for late EPO administration by Aher et al. no increased risk for ROP was found. The possible negative effects on ROP in early EPO administration are controversial. The Cochrane review on early EPO administration and effect on ROP is currently under revision and may soon be retracted.

Iron Supplementation

Iron is transported across the placenta from mother to child particularly during the last trimester of pregnancy. Therefore, infants delivered prematurely have a smaller supply of iron. In addition, preterm infants have an increased need for supplemental iron due to increased risk of iatrogenic blood loss related to frequent laboratory testing.

Supplemental iron seems to improve iron status after 2–3 months of age if started early in life. Effects of iron supplementation on the need for RBC transfusion are insufficiently studied. Although controversies on the benefits and optimal dosage of iron supplementation persist, most guidelines advise the use of extra iron (2–3 mg/kg) in preterm infants, starting early in life (when 100 mL/kg enteral feeding is tolerated).

The American Academy of Pediatrics recommends that preterm infants receive 2 mg elemental iron/kg per day; infants receiving EPO therapy should receive at least 6 mg/kg per day. After discharge, preterm infants continue to have increased iron needs because of rapid growth rate during the first postnatal year. There is a high rate of iron deficiency in preterm infants fed low-iron formula or breast milk. Recent data suggest that preterm infants with low serum ferritin concentrations might require additional iron supplementation.

Practice Points

- Limiting phlebotomy losses and starting iron therapy at 2 weeks of postnatal age might be effective preventive strategies against iron deficiency
- Delay cord clamping in stable babies after birth by 1 minute
- Try to restrict RBC transfusions to single donor as far as possible
- Think twice before transfusing a tiny neonate.

APPENDIX: ETIOLOGY OF ANEMIA

1. Anemia due to reduced production
   Hypoplastic anemia
   a. Congenital disease
      i. Diamond-Blackfan syndrome (congenital hypoplastic anemia)
      ii. Fanconi anemia
      iii. Transient erythroblastopenia of childhood
      iv. Atransferrinemia
      v. Congenital leukemia
      vi. Sideroblastic anemia
   b. Acquired disease
      i. *Infections*: Rubella, Syphilis, Parvovirus B_{19}, HIV and Cytomegalovirus
      ii. Aplastic crisis
      iii. Aplastic anemia
      iv. *Nutritional deficiencies*: Iron, folate, vitamin B_{12} and proteins

Contd…

Contd...

2. Immune hemolytic anemia (increased reticulocyte count and Coombs positive)
   Immune hemolysis
   a. Isoimmune hemolytic anemia
      i. ABO, Rh, minor blood group incompatibility
   b. Autoimmune hemolytic anemia
3. Anemia with low MCV
   a. Chronic inutero blood loss
   b. Alpha thalassemia
4. Anemia with normal or high MCV and abnormal peripheral smear
   a. Hereditary spherocytosis
   b. Hereditary elliptocytosis
   c. Hereditary pyropoikilocytosis
   d. G6PD deficiency
   e. DIC
5. Anemia with normal or high MCV and normal peripheral smear: Blood loss
   a. Antepartum period (1 in 1000 live births) blood loss
      i. *Loss of placental integrity*: Abruptio placentae, placenta previa, or traumatic amniocentesis (acute or chronic)
      ii. *Anomalies of the umbilical cord or placental vessels*: Velamentous insertion of the umbilical cord (10% in twins and almost all gestations with triplets), communicating vessels (vasa Previa), umbilical hematoma, or entanglement of the cord by the fetus
      iii. *Twin-twin transfusion*: Monozygotic multiple births
   b. Intrapartum period blood loss
      i. Fetomaternal hemorrhage
      ii. Cesarean delivery
      iii. Traumatic rupture of the umbilical cord
      iv. Failure of placental transfusion (umbilical cord occlusion, e.g. a nuchal cord or entangled or prolapsed cord
      v. Obstetric trauma (LGA infants, breech presentation or difficult extraction)
   c. Neonatal period blood loss
      i. Enclosed hemorrhage
         - Caput succedaneum
         - Cephalhematoma
         - Subgaleal (subaponeurotic)
         - Intracranial hemorrhage (subdural, subarachnoid or subependymal space)
         - Visceral parenchymal hemorrhage
      ii. Defects in hemostasis (consumption coagulopathy)
         - Congenital coagulation factor deficiency
         - Consumption coagulopathy
            – Disseminated congenital or viral infections
            – Bacterial sepsis
            – Intravascular embolism of thromboplastin
         - Deficiency of vitamin K-dependent coagulation factors (factors II, VII, IX, and X)
            – Failure to administer vitamin K at birth
            – Use of antibiotics
            – Maternal ingestion of anticonvulsants (carbamazepine, phenytoins), antituberculosis agents and vitamin K antagonists
      iii. Thrombocytopenia
         - Immune thrombocytopenia
         - Congenital thrombocytopenia with absent radii
         - Iatrogenic blood loss (symptoms may develop if a loss of >20% occurs within 48 hours period)

SUGGESTED READING

1. Aher S, Malwatkar K, Kadam S. Neonatal anemia. Semin Fetal Neonatal Med. 2008;13(4):239-47.
2. Aher SM, Ohlsson A. Late erythropoietin for preventing red blood cell transfusion in preterm and/or low birth weight infants. Cochrane Database Syst Rev. 2014;(4):CD004868.
3. Ohlsson A, Aher SM. Early erythropoietin for preventing red blood cell transfusion in preterm and/or low birth weight infants. Cochrane Database Syst Rev. 2012;(9):CD004863.
4. von Lindern JS, Lopriore E. Management and prevention of neonatal anemia: current evidence and guidelines. Expert Rev Hematol. 2014;7(2):195-202.

CHAPTER 17

Neonatal Encephalopathy

Naveen Jain

INTRODUCTION

Neonatal encephalopathy (NE) is a clinical syndrome of *disturbed neurological function* manifested as subnormal consciousness, poor cry, poor suck, swallow and feeding, decreased spontaneous movements, abnormal tone and reflexes, seizures and poor respiratory efforts or apnea.

APPROACH TO A BABY WITH NEONATAL ENCEPHALOPATHY

A baby with NE may be very sick with other organ dysfunction or have NE as the only/dominating manifestation.
- *Multiorgan dysfunction*: Most sick babies with abnormal TOPS (temperature, oxygenation, perfusion, and sugar) may have encephalopathy associated. Common causes of sick babies with multiorgan dysfunction and encephalopathy would be hypoxic ischemic encephalopathy (HIE) *and sepsis* (meningitis—encephalitis).
- *Encephalopathy as dominating manifestation*: Occasionally babies may have encephalopathy as the dominating picture like in metabolic disorders [hypoglycemia, inborn errors of metabolism (IEM)], bilirubin encephalopathy, cerebral malformations, intracranial hemorrhage, stroke, etc.

CAUSES OF NEONATAL ENCEPHALOPATHY

Hypoxic Ischemic Encephalopathy

If a neonate has NE manifesting at birth/very early in life, the term HIE or perinatal asphyxia *must be used only if a comprehensive evaluation* of maternal medical history, antecedent obstetric events, and neonatal evaluation including imaging, placental pathology *prove the cause* to be hypoxia/ischemia.

Presence of peripartum or intrapartum events, neonatal signs consistent with HIE, neuro-imaging and excluding all other causes of NE must be ensured before labeling HIE (to avoid false blame on obstetric care).
- Peripartum or intrapartum events—severe antepartum hemorrhage, cord prolapse, rupture uterus, severe maternal collapse (hypoxia–ischemia). Category III fetal heart rate patterns noted in a fetus with previous normal category I heart rate pattern points to an acute hypoxia ischemia [fetal bradycardia (<110) – tachycardia (>160), lack of beat to beat variability, prolonged late decelerations].
- Neonatal signs—need for extensive resuscitation at birth with need for positive pressure ventilation (PPV) at 10 minutes, chest compressions, APGAR <5 at 10 min-

utes, low pH <7.0 and high base excess (>–12) within 60 minutes of birth. Multiorgan dysfunction makes likelihood of HIE more.
- Neuroimaging—MRI (MRS) done at 7–21 days of life is most useful for prognosis. Deep cortical gray matter and watershed zone involvement are common patterns. Although ultrasound may be the only modality possible in sick babies, CT may be commonly available, both these lack sensitivity and specificity. Spastic quadriplegia and dyskinetic cerebral palsy (CP) are the most common manifestations of HIE. Although cognitive dysfunction, seizures, and neurosensory deficits also occur, isolated finding in the absence of above said pattern of CP are unlikely to be due to HIE.

Sepsis/Meningitis–Encephalitis

Sepsis/meningitis are important treatable causes of NE and must not be missed. Cerebrospinal fluid (CSF) examination must be a part of evaluation of all babies with NE/suspected sepsis. Newer investigations like polymerase chain reaction (PCR) test on CSF may help identify viruses that manifest as encephalopathy in early neonatal period.

Hypoglycemia

Blood sugar estimation must be done in all babies with encephalopathy; prompt treatment with dextrose can be lifesaving and can prevent major disability. Babies with symptomatic hypoglycemia have poor outcomes manifesting as cortical visual dysfunction (occipital lobe involvement), seizures, and CP.

Inborn Errors of Metabolism

Serum ammonia, serum lactate, urine ketones, and urine-reducing substances must be done in all babies with unexplained encephalopathy. If routine newborn screen has not been done, a blood, urine, and CSF examination must be done for metabolic diseases. Some of the IEMs are treatable with special diets.

Bilirubin Encephalopathy

Any baby with poor suck, lethargy in the first week of life must be evaluated for jaundice. Dyskinetic CP, hearing impairment are major manifestations of bilirubin encephalopathy.

Central Nervous System Malformations

Abnormal head size, craniofacial malformations, extra-neural anomalies may point to a central nervous system (CNS) malformation. Clue may be available from antenatal scans. All babies needing resuscitation at birth must have MRI to rule out birth defects before labeling as HIE.

Stroke

Stroke is being increasingly recognized as a cause of encephalopathy (seizures) in newborn.

Intracranial Hemorrhage

Birth trauma and other causes of intracranial hemorrhage (ICH) may be amenable to definitive surgical treatment and hence, a CT scan must be done if baby has acute presentation, pallor, bulging fontanel.

ASSESSMENT OF SEVERITY OF ENCEPHALOPATHY

The longer a baby remains encephalopathic the poorer the neurodevelopment outcomes are likely, irrespective of underlying cause. There are many scoring systems to evaluate

Table 1: Levene staging.

Features	Mild	Moderate	Severe
Consciousness	Irritability	Lethargy	Comatose
Tone	Hypotonia	Marked hypotonia	Severe hypotonia
Seizures	No	Yes	Prolonged
Sucking/Respiration	Poor suck	Unable to suck	Unable to sustain spontaneous respiration

severity of NE like Sarnat and Sarnat and Thomsons, but, the Levenes modification of Sarnat is the easiest to use. These scoring systems are designed for babies with HIE, but the physiological principles of NE progress in the same sequence and hence can be used for all NE situations (Table 1).

IMAGING IN NEONATAL ENCEPHALOPATHY

- Ultrasound
- CT scan
- MRI/MRS.

ROLE OF EEG AND aEEG IN NEONATAL SEIZURES AND NE

Babies with HIE/neonatal seizures will benefit by bedside video-EEG recording. This may help in differentiating abnormal movements or behaviors that mimic seizures. Amplitude-integrated EEG (aEEG) is easier to use by non-neurologists and is helpful in monitoring babies with HIE. A persistently abnormal aEEG at 48 hours or more is associated with an adverse neurodevelopmental outcome. A normal 6 hours aEEG has a good negative predictive value.

TREATMENT OF NEONATAL ENCEPHALOPATHY

Stabilization—ABC.

Specific Treatment

Treatment of Hypoxic Ischemic Encephalopathy

Optimizing post resuscitation care—ventilation, perfusion, blood sugars, fluid management, and optimal use of seizure medications anti-epileptic drugs.

Therapeutic hypothermia has evolved as a beneficial and safe therapy for HIE. Baby born at 35 weeks or more with peripartum events and neonatal signs is eligible for cooling. Best benefit is possible only if baby is enrolled early (by 6 hours age). Core temperature is maintained in a narrow range of 33.5–34.5°C for 72 hours and rewarmed slowly over 12 hours. The cooling may be best done by servo-controlled devices. In resource limited settings cool packs and bottles have been used. If monitoring of these sick babies with multiorgan dysfunction is done carefully in a neonatal unit, cooling is safe and effective. Cardiac rhythm abnormalities and thrombocytopenia are common adverse events.

EARLY DETECTION OF NEONATAL ENCEPHALOPATHY FOR BETTER OUTCOMES

Intact neurodevelopment is the most desired outcome of sick/at-risk neonates cared for by pediatricians. Good outcomes of baby's brain would depend on early detection of encephalopathy and timely correction of underlying pathology. Early signs of encephalopathy can be subtle and nonspecific and be confused with a normally sleeping baby.

It is important that units add "sensorium" (S)—the clinical measure of brain health to their primary evaluation/monitoring charts in addition to temperature (T), oxygenation (O), perfusion (P), and sugar (S) (STOPS). *Sensorium should be recorded* as active/sleepy by nurses in their monitoring charts of all sick babies *along with all other vital signs* hourly or as frequently as other vitals.

Healthy (active) babies are alert, look around, move frequently with range of movements, have a normal tone and arouse to touch, cry vigorously, show intent to suck, swallow easily, and have good respiratory efforts.

Healthy babies have a sleep wake pattern that cycles every 4–6 hours. They must not be sleepy for longer than this. A baby recorded as sleepy for longer than this duration in the neonatal unit must cause concern of encephalopathy.

PREVENTION OF HYPOXIC ISCHEMIC ENCEPHALOPATHY

- Moderate to severe HIE is associated with very high mortality and severe disability among survivors (up to 50%). Regular antenatal care, delivery in hospital with intra-partum monitoring, presence of personnel trained in neonatal resuscitation program, and preparedness of birthing facility are key determinant in decreasing incidence of HIE.
- *Monitoring of blood sugar*: Hypoglycemia as a cause of encephalopathy is mostly preventable. Monitoring of at-risk babies—preterm, intrauterine growth restricted (IUGR) babies, infant of diabetic mothers, all sick babies on intravenous fluids, and babies with lactation problems. Early detection by screening and prompt correction by feeding and IV dextrose will decrease risk of irreversible severe morbidity.
- To prevent severe hyperbilirubinemia and encephalopathy, highest priority should be given to universal bilirubin screening programs, education of parents and community and having a clear pathway for screening, tracking and treatment of hyperbilirubinemia.
- Prevention of sepsis.
- Newborn screening for metabolic diseases.
- Anomaly scans antenatal.

SUGGESTED READING

1. Bhardwaj K, Locke T, Biringer A, et al. Newborn bilirubin screening for preventing severe hyperbilirubinemia and bilirubin encephalopathy: a rapid review. Curr Pediatr Rev. 2017;13(1):67-90.
2. Chandrasekaran M, Chaban B, Montaldo P, et al. Predictive value of amplitude-integrated EEG (aEEG) after rescue hypothermic neuroprotection for hypoxic ischemic encephalopathy: a meta-analysis. J Perinatol. 2017;37(6):684-9.
3. Executive summary: Neonatal encephalopathy and neurologic outcome, 2nd edition. Report of the American College of Obstetricians and Gynecologists' Task Force on Neonatal Encephalopathy. Obstet Gynecol. 2014;123(4):896-901.
4. Rossouw G, Irlam J, Horn AR. Therapeutic hypothermia for hypoxic ischemic encephalopathy using low-technology methods: a systematic review and meta-analysis. Acta Paediatr. 2015;104(12):1217-28.
5. Thornton PS, Stanley CA, De Leon DD, et al. Recommendations from the Pediatric Endocrine Society for evaluation and management of persistent hypoglycemia in neonates, infants, and children. J Paediatr. 2015;167(2):238-45.

CHAPTER 18

Floppy Infant

Preetha Joshi, Tanushri Mukherjee

INTRODUCTION

Floppy infant or hypotonia is a well-recognized entity for a neonatologist and poses a challenge as hypotonia could be the presenting sign of both benign and serious disorder. Hypotonia is caused by disorders that affect any level of the nervous system—brain, brainstem, spinal cord, peripheral nerves, neuromuscular junction, and muscles. Early recognition, timely referral, and appropriate treatment are vital for good outcome.

DEFINITION AND ASSESSMENT

A hypotonic baby presents with:
- Abnormal posture
- Diminished resistance to passive movement
- Abnormal range of joint movement
- Delayed motor milestones.

Note: For assessing tone, the neonate should be alert but not crying. A key distinction is to determine whether the infant has low tone with or without muscle weakness. Hypotonia is decreased resistance of muscles to passive stretch. In contrast, weakness is diminished muscle power or strength. Weak infants are always hypotonic, but hypotonia is often present with normal strength.

IDENTIFY THE PROBLEM

Abnormal posture: The floppy infant assumes a frog-legged posture on supine position with hips abducted and knee flexed in supine position. On ventral suspension, baby cannot maintain limb posture against gravity and assumes the position of a rag-doll. There is decreased spontaneous movement.

There is diminished resistance to passive movement, as shown by pull to sit traction (when pulled-up from supine to sitting position, the head of the baby lags) and scarf sign (in supine position, hold one of infant's hands and try to put it around the neck as far as possible across the opposite shoulder. In the floppy infant, the elbow easily crosses the midline).

Traction response: Initiated by grasping hands and pulling the child to sitting position. After 33 weeks, there is considerable head lag, but neck flexors respond to traction by lifting head momentarily. At term, only minimal head lag is present. Presence of more head lag and failure to counter-traction by flexion of limb indicates postural hypotonia in newborn.

Vertical suspension: Place both hands in axillae; lift the baby straight up without grasping the thorax. In hypotonia, baby will slip off due to weakness of shoulders.

Ventral suspension/horizontal suspension: Suspend the infant in prone position horizontally. Normal infant maintains straight back and demonstrate flexion at elbow, hip, knee, and ankle. Hypotonic infant drapes over examiner's hand and limbs hang limply, like a rag-doll.

Identify the Severity/Red Flag Sign

- Severe respiratory distress needing assisted ventilation
- Encephalopathic baby with depressed sensorium
- Seizures
- Metabolic crisis.

Indications for hospitalization: All of the above and feeding difficulty with suspected aspiration.

ETIOLOGY (TABLES 1 AND 2)

Conditions where central and peripheral hypotonia may coexist:
- Familial dysautonomia
- Hypoxic ischemic encephalopathy
- Infantile neuroaxonal degeneration
- Lipid storage disease

Table 1: Examination of CNS.

Inspection	Decreased muscle bulk/Atrophy: SMA
	Fasciculation: SMA
Palpation	Confirm hypotonia examining for contractures
Primitive reflexes	Test for Moro's, suck, grasp, stepping, placing, and ATNR
Deep tendon reflex	Absent: SMA
	Decreased: Neuropathies, later myopathies
	Increased: Upper motor neuron lesion, congenital myasthenia
Visual/auditory	Normal: Neuromuscular disease
	Abnormal: HIE, metabolic/mitochondrial encephalopathy Muscle-eye-brain disease

(SMA: spinal muscular atrophy; ATNR: atonic neck reflex; HIE: hypoxic ischemic encephalopathy)

- Lysosomal disorder
- Mitochondrial disorder
- Perinatal hypoxia secondary to motor unit disease.

There are two approaches to diagnose. First identify the neuroanatomical site of the lesion (Table 3): UMNL (upper motor neuron lesion) or LMNL (lower motor neuron lesion). Second, whether hypotonia is associated with weakness or not. Hypotonia with progressive weakness suggests LMNL unless in acute stage of UMNL.

Table 2: Pattern of weakness and localization in floppy infant.

Anatomical site	Corresponding disorder
Central nervous system	*Perinatal:* Hypoxic ischemic encephalopathy, IVH, cerebral trauma, and spinal trauma
Anterior horn cell	*Anatomical:* Cerebral dysgenesis
	Chromosomal: Down syndrome, Prader-Willi syndrome, and Turner syndrome
	Infection: Meningitis, sepsis, and encephalitis
	Metabolic: Hypoglycemia, hypocalcemia, and hyponatremia
	Endocrine: Hypothyroidism
	Spinal muscular atrophy
	Hypoxic-ischemic myelopathy
	Traumatic myelopathy
Peripheral nerve	Congenital hypomyelinating neuropathy
	Familial dysautonomia
	Giant axonal neuropathy
	Metabolic and inflammatory neuropathy
Neuromuscular junction	Congenital myasthenic syndrome
	Transient neonatal myasthenia gravis
	Infantile botulism
	Hypermagnesemia
	Aminoglycoside toxicity
Muscles	Congenital myopathy
	Metabolic myopathy
	Congenital muscular dystrophy
	Congenital myotonic dystrophy

(IVH: intraventricular hemorrhage)

SECTION 1
Clinical Approach to Sick Newborn

Table 3: Identification of neuroanatomical site.

Clue	UMNL	LMNL
Deep tendon reflex	Brisk to normal	Depressed to absent
Postural reflex	Present	Absent
Muscle atrophy	Absent	Present
Fasciculation	Absent	Present
Abnormalities of other brain function	Present	Absent
Dysmorphic face	Present	Absent
Fisting, scissoring	Present	Absent
Seizure	Present	Absent
Other organ malformation	Present	Absent

(UMNL: upper motor neuron lesion; LMNL: lower motor neuron lesion)

Assessment of muscle power in infants is generally limited to inspection (Table 4).
- Frog-like posture and decreased spontaneous movement
- Poor swallowing ability, drooling, and oropharyngeal pooling of secretion
- Weak cry
- Paradoxical breathing pattern with intercostal and diaphragmatic palsy
- Inability to cough and clear airway secretion (cough test).

A detailed history, examination, and investigations are required to further diagnose the cause of hypotonia in a newborn (Tables 5 to 8).

Table 4: Distinguishing features of disorders of the parts of the motor system.

Site	Face	Arms	Legs	Proximal vs. distal	DTR
Central	0	+	+	> or =	N or Increased
Anterior horn cell	Late	++++	++++	> or =	0
Peripheral nerve	0	+++	+++	<<	Decreased
NM junction	+++	+++	+++	=	N
Muscles	Variable	++	+	>	Decreased

(DTR: deep tendon reflex; NM: neuromuscular)

Table 5: Detailed history, physical examination, and investigations.

History	
Antenatal	Decreased fetal movement in (congenital myopathy, myotonic dystrophy, SMA), polyhydramnios (due to decreased swallowing), breech presentation, TORCH infection, preterm delivery, drug or alcohol use
Perinatal	Birth trauma, asphyxia, need for resuscitation, delivery complication, fracture, APGAR score, low cord pH, seizure, and encephalopathic state
Family	Consanguinity, perinatal death or stillborn
Feeding	Feeding difficulty, drooling, pooling of saliva, and recurrent aspiration
Developmental	Delay in isolated motor development or affected cognition, vision, learning, auditory functioning or any neuroregression
Progress	Improving in HIE, deteriorating in spinal muscular atrophy, muscular dystrophy *Fluctuation:* Congenital myasthenia

(TORCH: toxoplasmosis other rubella cytomegalovirus and herpes infections; SMA: spinal muscular atrophy; HIE: hypoxic ischemic encephalopathy)

Chapter 18: Floppy Infant

Table 6: Clinical clues for etiology of a floppy infant.

	Physical examination
Dysmorphic facies	Down syndrome, Prader-Willi syndrome, lipidosis mucopolysaccharidoses, and congenital muscular dystrophy
Head size	*Microcephaly:* Cerebral palsy *Macrocephaly:* Congenital toxoplasmosis
Facial features	*Alert:* SMA *Expressionless:* Congenital myopathies, myotonic dystrophy, and myasthenia gravis Fish triangular mouth: Congenital myopathy and muscular dystrophy
Ptosis, ophthalmoplegia	Congenital myopathy, centronuclear myopathy, congenital myasthenia, and mitochondrial disease
Tongue fasciculation	SMA, denervation
Joint contracture, arthrogryposis, hip dislocation	Congenital myotonic dystrophy, intrauterine hypotonia due to varied causes
Stridor	Pontocerebellar hypoplasia, diaphragmatic SMA, congenital myasthenia, congenital myopathies, and hypotonic CP
Weak cry/cough	Hypotonic CP, SMA, congenital myopathies, and myasthenia
Pectus excavatum	Diaphragmatic SMA, congenital myopathies
Cardiomyopathy	Glycogen storage disease: Type 2 and 3
Hepatosplenomegaly	TORCH infection, MPS, glycogen and lipid storage disease, sepsis
Family members	Maternal grip myotonia, percussion myotonia, ptosis or distal weakness: Congenital myotonic dystrophy

(TORCH: toxoplasmosis other rubella cytomegalovirus and herpes infections; SMA: spinal muscular atrophy; CP: cerebral palsy; MPS: mucopolysaccharidosis)

Table 7: Clinical clues and supportive investigation of the floppy infant phenotype.

Condition	Clinical symptoms	Investigation
Central nervous system	Seizure, encephalopathy, cortical fist, scissoring, dysmorphology, increased DTR	MRI of brain, EEG, and IEM study
Spinal cord transection or disease	Hemangioma or tuft of hair in midline, scoliosis	MRI spinal cord
SMA	Tongue atrophy and fasciculation, paradoxical breathing, proximal muscle weakness with absent reflex. Alert sensorium	Molecular genetic study, EMG
Peripheral neuropathy	Distal weakness, absent DTR, and pes cavus	Nerve conduction study Molecular genetic study
Myasthenia gravis	Ocular and bulbar involvement Maternal similar history Fatigability	Tensilon test, EMG, antibody against acetylcholine receptors, and genetic study
Infantile botulism	Descending weakness, ptosis, unreactive pupil, constipation, dysphagia, and neuropathy	Isolation of clostridium difficile and its toxin from stool

Contd…

Contd...

Condition	Clinical symptoms	Investigation
Congenital muscular dystrophy	Associated brain and eye involvement. Decreased fetal movement, contracture, and arthrogryposis	Increased CPK Brain MRI
Congenital myotonic dystrophy	Polyhydramnios, decreased movement, V-shaped face, myotonia, premature cataract in mother	Muscle biopsy, molecular genetic test, and EMG of mother
Congenital myopathy	Slender features, nonprogressive weakness, feeding problem, malignant hyperthermia, and ptosis	Muscle biopsy. CPK and EMG not helpful genetic study
Glycogen storage disease: Pompe's disease	Cardiomegaly, large tongue, and hepatosplenomegaly	Peripheral smear: Vacuolated lymphocyte urine oligosaccharides, ECG, ECHO, acid maltase study, and muscle biopsy

(DTR: deep tendon reflex; EEG: electroencephalogram; IEM: inborn errors of metabolism; EMG: electromyography; CPK: creatinine phosphokinase; ECG: electrocardiography; SMA: spinal muscular atrophy)

Table 8: Suspected UMNL/central nervous system involvement.

	Investigation	Inference
General investigation	Electrolyte T3,T4, TSH	Low calcium, magnesium, sodium, and glucose. Hypothyroid
USG head	IVH, parenchymal bleed, porencephalic cyst, and ventriculomegaly	Hypotonic CP and HIE
MRI of brain	Hypoxic changes, bleeding, encephalocele, cerebral dysgenesis, and myelination abnormality	CP
Electroencephalogram	Seizure	CP, mitochondrial disease. Metabolic disease
Sepsis screen	CBC, CRP, blood culture, CSF, urine study, and X-ray of chest	Meningitis and sepsis
Karyotype	Chromosomal testing and FISH	Down, Turner, Prader-Willi syndromes,
Metabolic screen	Serum and urine amino acid, ABG, urine organic acid, serum ammonia, and LFT	Aminoacidopathy. Organic acidemia, FAOD, and GSD

(USG: ultrasonography; IVH: intraventricular hemorrhage; CP: cerebral palsy; HIE: hypoxic ischemic encephalopathy; CBC: complete blood count; CRP: C-reactive protein; CSF: cerebrospinal fluid; FISH: fluorescence in situ hybridization; ABG: arterial blood gas sampling; LFT: linear fractional transformation; FAOD: fatty acid oxidation disorders; GSD: glycogen storage disease)

INVESTIGATIONS

Investigation for Suspected Lower Motor Neuron Disease

- *Serum creatinine phosphokinase (CPK):* CPK level is increased in cord blood up to 5 times of adult value due to reflection of muscle damage during labor process. It reaches normal level by 5–10 days. CPK increased in congenital muscular dystrophy, mildly increased in spinal muscular atrophy (SMA). One should obtain CPK level before EMG study and muscle biopsy, as these investigations falsely elevate CPK level.

- *Electromyography*: The appearance of brief small-amplitude, polyphasic potential are suggestive of myopathy. The fibrillatory pattern, fasciculation, sharp wave, and motor unit potential that are large, prolonged, and polyphasic are characteristic of a denervation pattern. Repetitive nerve stimulation will detect disturbances in the neuromuscular junction.
- *Nerve conduction study*: As nerve conduction velocity (NCV) study measures only the fastest conducting fibers in a nerve, 80% of the total nerve fibers must be involved before slowing in conduction is detected. It differentiates axonal from demyelinating neuropathy. Demyelinating neuropathy causes greater slowing of conduction velocity. It also detects traumatic nerve injury.
- *Molecular genetic study*: SMN1 gene detection in SMA. 95% of patients of SMA are homozygous for absence of exon 7 and 8 of SMN1. Genetic tests also help in myotonic dystrophy and congenital myasthenic syndrome. With a genetic study, subsequent muscle biopsy is unnecessary in many patients.
- *Muscle biopsy*: The most important and specific diagnostic study of most neuromuscular disorders. Biopsy is taken from vastus lateralis muscle. An open biopsy is preferred as it gives sufficient tissue for subsequent biochemical, mitochondrial, and immunohistochemical study.
- *Nerve biopsy*: Sural nerve biopsy can detect neuropathy, but rarely used in the newborn period.
- *Tensilon test*: Edrophonium chloride temporarily reverses the weakness in myasthenic patients by blocking cholinesterase. Ptosis and oculomotor paresis are reliably tested. Subcutaneous (S/C) injection of 0.15 mg/kg produces a response within 10 minutes in newborn and IV 0.2 mg/kg in infant produces response within 1 minutes.
- *Electrocardiography (ECG) and 2D echo*: ECG detects cardiomyopathy and conduction defects in muscular dystrophy, inflammatory, and metabolic myopathy.
- *Pulmonary function test*: Muscular dystrophy and other progressive motor neuron disease.
- *Toxicology screen*.

PRINCIPLES OF MANAGEMENT (SUPPORTIVE) (FLOWCHART 1)

- Seizure treatment and monitoring
- *Physiotherapy*: Prevents contracture
- *Occupational therapy*: Appliances, improvement of posture, and facilitates activities of daily living
- Prevention and correction of scoliosis
- *Cardiac function*: Evaluation and treatment of heart failure and conduction abnormality
- *Respiratory support*: Assessment and requirement of invasive and noninvasive respiratory support. Influenza and pneumococcal vaccination
- *Feeding*: Nasogastric feeding, calorie-rich feed, gastrostomy tube. Management of gastroesophageal reflux disease (GERD).
- Prevention of obesity
- *Orthopedic*: Intervention to prevent and treat contractures
- Encouragement of overall learning and development process
- Social support group for family and counseling.

SECTION 1
Clinical Approach to Sick Newborn

Flowchart 1: Approach to a newborn with hypotonia.

```
History: Prenatal, neonatal, developmental, feeding, family history.
                              ↓
General physical examination: Dysmorphology, microcephaly, ptosis, facial expression
Systemic examination: Organomegaly, cardiac involvement, contracture, arthrogryposis
                              ↓
Neurological examination: Mental state, tone, reflex, strength, atrophy, fasciculation,
    seizure, cranial nerve, postural reflexes, primitive reflexes
              To differentiate between UMNL and LMNL
```

Hypotonic and strong
- Increased DTR
- Encephalopathic, seizure
- Global developmental delay
- Axial weakness
- Microcephaly
- Ankle clonus

Hypotonic and weak
- Decreased or absent DTR
- Preserved mental and social interaction
- Selective motor delay
- Weak antigravity muscles
- Atrophy, tongue fasciculation
- Paradoxical chest movement

Genetic studies: Karyotype, FISH, VLCFA → Trisomy, Prader-Willi, Zellweger

CT/MRI → HIE, Cerebral malformation

Creatine kinase, EMG, Nerve conduction study
- DNA-based mutation analysis → Spinal muscle atrophy, Congenital myotonic dystrophy, Congenital muscular dystrophy
- Muscle or nerve biopsy → Congenital myopathy

(FISH: fluorescence in situ hybridization; DTR: deep tendon reflex; VLCFA: very long chain fatty acid; MRI: magnetic resonance imaging; CT: computerized tomography; HIE: hypoxic ischemic encephalopathy; EMG: electromyography; UMNL: upper motor neuron lesion; LMNL: lower motor neuron lesion)

SUGGESTED READING

1. Crawford TO. Clinical evaluation of the floppy infant. Pediatr Ann. 1992;21(6):384-54.
2. Fenichel GM. The Hypotonic Infant. In: Fenichel GM (Ed). Clinical Pediatric Neurology: A Signs and Symptoms Approach, 5th edition. Philadelphia: WB Saunders Company; 2005. pp. 149-70.
3. Leyenaar J, Camfield P, Camfield C. A schematic approach to hypotonia in infancy. Paediatr Child Health. 2005;10(7):397-400.
4. Sarnat HB. Neuromuscular Disorders. In: Kliegman R, Behrman R, Jenson H, Stanton B (Eds). Nelson Textbook of pediatrics, 18th edition. WB Saunders Company; 2007. pp. 531-68.
5. Van Toorn R. Clinical approach to the floppy child. CME. 2004;22(8):449-55.

CHAPTER 19

Suspected Inborn Errors of Metabolism

Naveen Bajaj

INTRODUCTION

Inborn errors of metabolism (IEM) are a rare group of genetic disorders affecting the metabolic pathways leading to deficiency of end product, or accumulation of the substrate or intermediate metabolites leading to systemic derangements. IEM are under recognized and underdiagnosed and must be considered in the differential diagnosis of all sick infants with unexplained etiology.

CATEGORIES OF INBORN ERRORS OF METABOLISM

Broadly, IEM can be classified as follows:
- Disorders of carbohydrate metabolism.
- Disorders of amino acid metabolism.
- Disorders of organic acids metabolism.
- Disorders of fatty acid oxidation.
- Disorders of mitochondrial metabolism.
- Lysosomal and peroxisomal disorders.

CLINICAL CLUES TO IEM DURING NEONATAL PERIOD

Inborn errors of metabolism manifest with nonspecific presentations mimicking sepsis. A high index of suspicion is needed to diagnose IEM. The predominant sign needs to be identified and work-up is planned according to probable causes (Table 1).

All attempts must be made to examine the eye and fundus. Many of the IEM have classical findings in the eye (Table 2).

At times, suspicion of IEM is raised based on odor to body or urine (Table 3).

History is overlooked and many a times, a family history over 3–4 generations gives the clue. The absence of consanguineous marriage does not rule out an IEM (Table 4).

INVESTIGATIONS FOR SUSPECTED IEM (TABLE 5)

Collection of Blood Sample

- Collect while the baby is on feeds and before specific treatment is instituted. Test results may be falsely normal, if the child is kept nil by mouth.
- Free-flowing blood, preferably from arterial prick should be used to collect sample for ammonia and lactate. The samples should be transported in ice and immediately tested.
- Detailed history and including drug being given should be provided to the laboratory (e.g. sodium valproate therapy may increase ammonia levels).

Table 1: Clinical clues to inborn errors of metabolism

Feature	Conditions
Asymptomatic	Phenylketonuria (PKU), congenital hypothyroidism
Encephalopathy	Urea cycle disorders, organic acidemias, aminoacidurias
Dysmorphism	Peroxisomal disorders, Zellweger syndrome, lysosomal storage disorders, mucopolysaccharidosis (MPS), mucolipidosis, gangliosidosis, homocystinuria, Smith-Lemli-Opitz syndrome
Seizures	Pyridoxine dependent, folinic acid dependent, secondary to hypoglycemia, molybdenum cofactor deficiency, mitochondrial disorders, and lysosomal storage disorders
Hypotonia	Fatty acid oxidation (FAO) disorders, peroxisomal disorders, urea cycle disorders, mitochondrial disorders, Pompe's disease, and glycogen storage disorders (GSDs)
Lethargy	Aminoacidurias, organic acidemias, urea cycle disorders, fatty acid oxidation defects, and mitochondrial disorders
Jaundice or liver cell dysfunction	Galactosemia, hereditary fructose intolerance, tyrosinemia, citrullinemia, GSD type IV, α1-antitrypsin deficiency, hemochromatosis, Niemann-Pick disease, and fatty acid oxidation defects
Cardiac involvement	FAO disorders, carnitine deficiency, mitochondrial disorders, glycogen storage disease: type 2, Pompe's disease, and mucopolysaccharidosis
Hepato/splenomegaly	Lysosomal storage disorders, glycogen storage diseases
Abnormal posturing	Glutaric acidemia type 1

Table 2: Eye manifestations of inborn errors of metabolism.

Cherry red macular spots	Tay Sachs disease, galactosialidosis, Niemann-Pick disease, GM1 gangliosidosis
Lenticular cataracts	Galactosemia, fabry disease, mucopolysaccharidosis, cystinosis
Dislocated lens	Homocystinuria, Marfan syndrome, molybdenum cofactor deficiency, and sulfite oxidase deficiency
Retinitis pigmentosa	Abetalipoproteinemia, peroxisomal disorders, and mitochondrial disorders

Table 3: Inborn errors of metabolism with characteristic odor.

Odor	Condition
Fruity odor	Methylmalonic academia (MMA), propionic academia (PA)
Maple syrup like	Maple syrup urine disease (MSUD)
Musty	Phenylketonuria (PKU)
Sweaty socks like	Isovaleric academia
Malt like	Methionine malabsorption
Cat urine	3-methylcrotonic academia, 3-OH, 3-mehtylglutaric aciduria
Fish like	Trimethylaminuria, carnitine excess
Cabbage like	Tyrosinemia

Table 4: IEM and mode of inheritance.

Autosomal recessive	Autosomal dominant	X-linked recessive	Mitochondrial disorders
PKU	Marfan syndrome	Ornithine carbamylase deficiency	Kearns-Sayre syndrome
MSUD	Acute intermittent porphyria	Fabry disease	Leigh syndrome
GSD	Familial hypercholesterolemia	Pyruvate dehydrogenase deficiency	
Galactosemia			
Organic acidurias			
MCAD			
Zellweger syndrome			

Table 5: Investigations for suspected IEM.

1st line: Basic tests	2nd line: Metabolic screening tests	3rd line
• CBC • BUN, creatinine • Ca, PO$_4$, Mg • Liver enzymes • Uric acid • Creatine kinase • Cerebrospinal fluid (CSF) study • Cultures of blood, urine, CSF	• Blood sugar • S. Electrolytes • Urine for glucose-nonglucose reducing substances • Blood gas • Ammonia • Lactate, pyruvate • Quantitative plasma/urine amino acids • Urine organic acids • Acyl carnitine profile	• DNA studies and mutation analysis • Biopsy—liver, muscle and skin

SCREENING METABOLIC TESTS TO IDENTIFY IEM

- *ABG*: Metabolic acidosis with increased anion gap = *Organic academia*.
- *Hypoglycemia*:
  - *With ketosis*: Organic academia, glycogen storage disorders (GSDs)
  - *Without ketosis*: Maple syrup urine disease (MSUD), fatty acid oxidation (FAO) defects, and disorders of ketogenesis.
- *Hyperammonemia*: Urea cycle, organic acidemias.
- *Lactic acidosis*: Mitochondrial disorders, GSD, disorders of glyconeogenesis, FAO defects, aminoaciduria, and organic acidemia.
- *Lactate/Pyruvate (>20:1)*: Mitochondrial disorders, pyruvate carboxylase deficiency.
- *Quantitative amino acid profile*: Amino acid disorders.
- *Urine for organic acids*: Amino acid disorders.
- *Acyl carnitine profile*: FAO defects, organic acidemias.

Disorders Associated with a Positive Ferric Chloride Reaction

Disorder	Urine color
Phenylketonuria	Green
Hereditary tyrosinemia	Green, fading rapidly
Maple syrup urine disease	Grey-green
Histidinemia	Blue-green
Alkaptonuria	Dark brown
Diabetic ketoacidosis	Cherry red
Pheochromocytoma	Blue-green
Drug intoxications	Purple Purple Red-brown Green
Conjugated hyperbilirubinemia	Green

Serum Ammonia

- The venous ammonia sample must be collected, stored, and transported on ice to the laboratory.
- Specimen must be rapidly analyzed and not run as a routine test.
- It should be reported with an adjustment for the newborn age. An elevated ammonia level >100 umol/L indicates an abnormality in nitrogen balance.
- Samples collected without fasting or while the infant is receiving parenteral nutrition may have plasma ammonia concentrations two to three times higher than those found in fasted infants.
- With liver failure hyperammonemia occurs, but the plasma ammonia concentration is generally <500 umol/L.
- The key to differentiation of the cause of hyperammonemia is the presence or absence of acidosis, ketosis, or hypoglycemia (Flowchart 1).

Lactate/Pyruvate

- The samples must be obtained simultaneously.
- No tourniquet should be applied while collecting sample.
- The sample should be transported on ice and must be analyzed immediately in the laboratory.
- Pyruvate samples should be collected in perchlorate to prevent degradation (Flowchart 2).

Hypoglycemia

- Sampling has no relation with hypoglycemic episode as the yield is likely to be higher with IEM causing persistent hypoglycemia.
- Disorders associated with nonglucose reducing substances in urine include galactosemia, hereditary fructose intolerance, hereditary tyrosinemia, essential fructosuria, pentosuria, and severe liver disease with secondary galactose intolerance.
- Urine tests for ketones detect only acetoacetate, a positive urine dipstick test for ketones in an infant less than 1 month of age is indicative of severely altered metabolism, usually an organic acidemia or disorder of ketone body utilization (Flowchart 3).

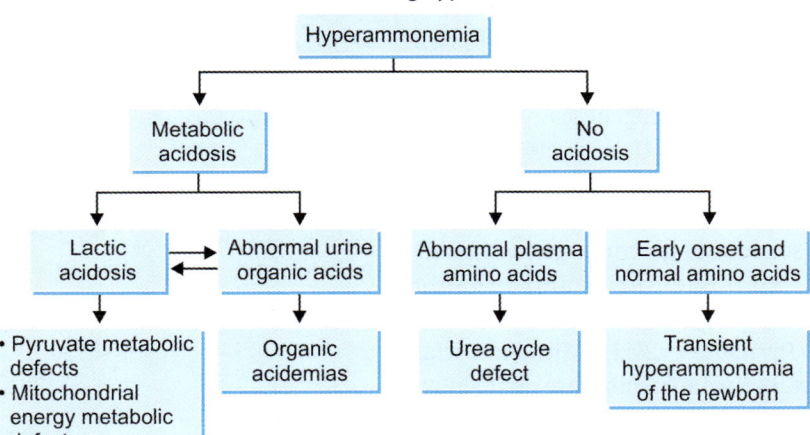

Flowchart 1: Evaluating hyperammonemia.

CHAPTER 19
Suspected Inborn Errors of Metabolism

Flowchart 2: Evaluating lactate/pyruvate.

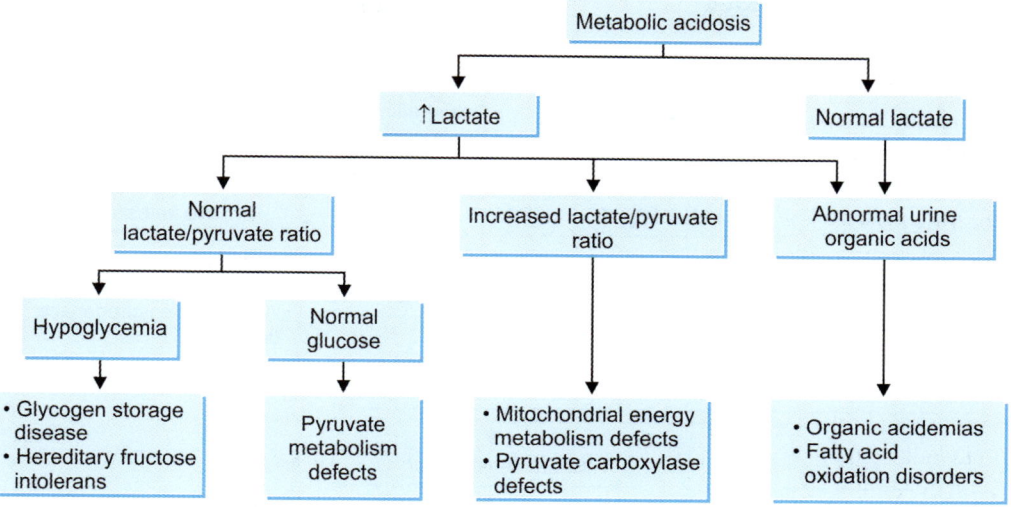

Flowchart 3: Evaluating persistent hypoglycemia.

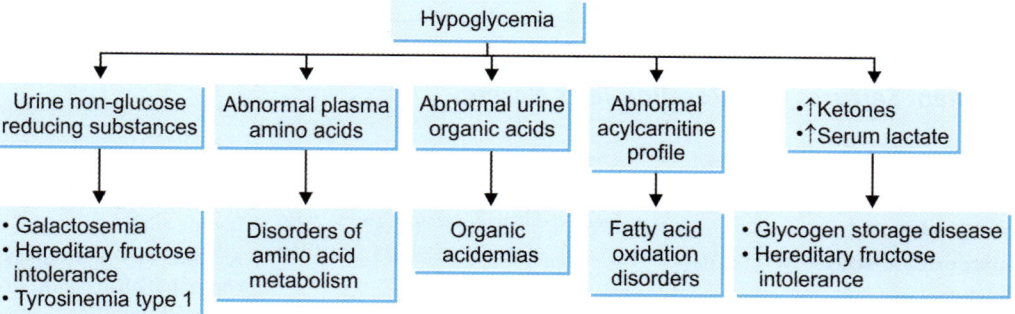

Flowchart 4: Approach to urea cycle defects.

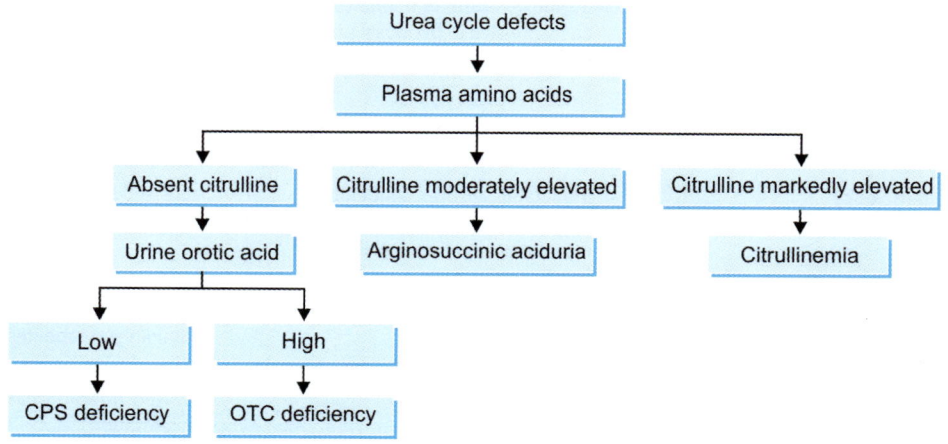

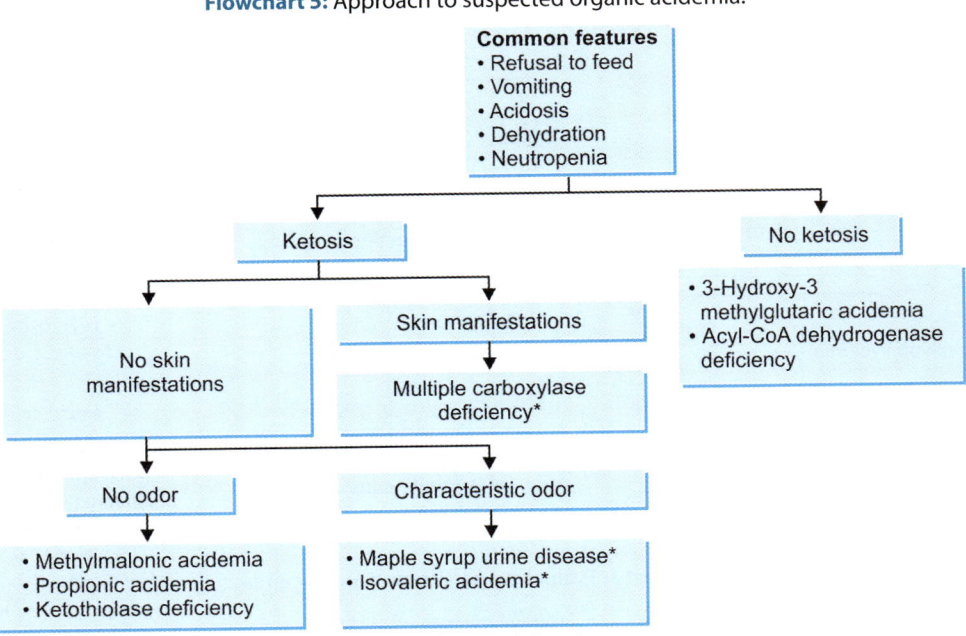

Flowchart 5: Approach to suspected organic acidemia.

* Indicates disorders in which patients have a characteristic odor.

Persistent Seizures with Baseline Tests Normal

Name	Onset	Characteristics	Diagnosis
Nonketotic hyperglycinemia	<48 hour	Lethargy, apnea, profound hypotonia, feeding difficulty, hiccups, and seizures	CSF: Plasma Glycine >0.08
Sulfite oxidase deficiency/ Molybdenum Cofactor deficiency	<5 days	• Drug resistant seizures, Lens dislocation • A low uric acid value may be noted in molybdenum cofactor deficiency	An elevated S. sulfocysteine concentration in plasma or urine is diagnostic
Pyridoxine-dependent seizures	Day 1>	Response of seizures to intravenous pyridoxine. A subset of neonates appears to be responsive to pyridoxal phosphate	
Folinic acid responsive seizures	Day 1>		Folinic acid (5–20 mg/day in divided doses)
GABA transaminase deficiency	Early	lethargy, hypotonia, hyper-reflexia, and a high-pitched cry	Detecting GABA in plasma or CSF
3-PGD deficiency	Early	Intractable seizures, congenital microcephaly, severe psychomotor retardation, hyperexcitability, and spastic tetraparesis	Decreased serine in fasting plasma and CSF
DPD deficiency	Early		A urine screen for purine and pyrimidine metabolites
GAMT deficiency	Early	Extrapyramidal signs	Low plasma creatine levels and elevated guanidinoacetate concentrations

Contd...

Contd...

Name	Onset	Characteristics	Diagnosis
GLUT-1 deficiency	3 weeks >	Reduced CSF glucose concentration	Respond to ketogenic diet
Disorders of pyruvate metabolism	Infantile	Lactic acidosis, ketosis, hyperammonemia, citrullinemia, and hyperlysinemia	On leukocytes or fibroblasts
Lactic acidosis and systemic manifestations	Infantile	Neuromuscular abnormalities, lactic acidosis, and other systemic manifestations cardiomyopathy, liver disease, and renal tubular defects	Metabolic studies detect tricarboxylic acid cycle disorders and fatty acid oxidation defects
Mitochondrial disorders	Variable		Mitochondrial respiratory chain analysis in muscle or mitochondrial or nuclear DNA analysis
Metabolic acidosis	Variable	Increased anion gap ketoacidosis	For organic acidemia
MSUD	By 1st week	Normal at birth. Neuroimaging findings are normal in the first few days after birth	Characteristic head MRI findings develop with time, including profound localized edema in the deep cerebellar white matter, dorsal brainstem, cerebral peduncles, posterior limb of the internal capsule, perirolandic white matter, and globus pallidus
Mevalonic academia Disorder of cholesterol Biosynthesis	Early	Dysmorphism, hepatosplenomegaly, anemia, and recurrent fevers	
Congenital disorders of glycosylation	Early	Multisystem involvement	MRI typically shows cerebellar hypoplasia
Neonatal myopathies Encephalomyopathies	Variable	Molecular testing for Rett syndrome should be considered in males who have unexplained encephalopathy and normal results on metabolic investigations	

IEM WITH SIGNIFICANT ENCEPHALOPATHY

Disorder	Characteristic findings
Organic acidemias (includes MMA, PA, IVA, MCD and many less common conditions)	Metabolic acidosis with increased anion gap; elevated plasma and urine ketones; variably elevated plasma ammonia and lactate; abnormal urine organic acids
Urea cycle defects (Flowchart 4)	Variable respiratory alkalosis; no metabolic acidosis; markedly elevated plasma ammonia; elevated orotic acid in OTCD; abnormal plasma amino acids

Contd...

Contd...

Disorder	Characteristic findings
Maple syrup urine disease	Metabolic acidosis with increased anion gap; elevated plasma and urine ketones; positive ferric chloride test; abnormal plasma amino acids
Nonketotic hyperglycinemia	No acid-base or electrolyte abnormalities; normal ammonia; abnormal plasma amino acids
Molybdenum cofactor deficiency	No acid-base or electrolyte abnormalities; normal ammonia; normal amino and organic acids; low serum uric acid; elevated sulfites in urine

(MMA: methylmalonic acidemia; PA: propionic acidemia; IVA: isovaleric acidemia; MCD: multiple carboxylase deficiency; OTCD: ornithine transcarbamylase deficiency)

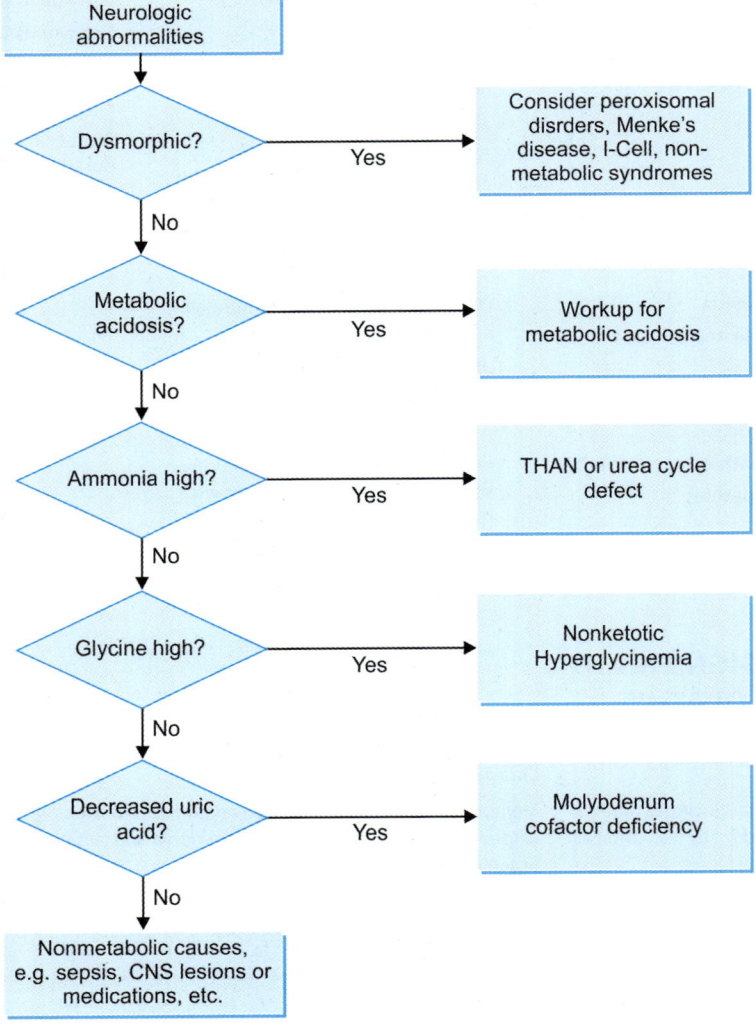

Flowchart 6: Approach to a newborn with neurological abnormalities.

ROLE OF MRI

- Abnormal hyperintense signal in the globus pallidus and periatrial white matter of the centrum semiovale is often present in mitochondrial disease.
- The globus pallidus is particularly vulnerable in metabolic disorders.
- Nonketotic hyperglycinemia and MSUD primarily affect the white matter.
- Different patterns of abnormality may suggest other underlying IEM. For example, basal ganglia "metabolic strokes" may occur in organic acidemias, and involvement of the caudate nucleus, in addition to the putamen, is seen in glutaric aciduria type I and juvenile Huntington disease.

MANAGEMENT

Management of Hyperammonemia

- Discontinue all feeds. Provide adequate calories by intravenous glucose and lipids. Maintain glucose infusion rate 8–10 mg/kg/min. Start intravenous lipid 0.5 g/kg/day (up to 3g/kg/day). After stabilization gradually add protein 0.25 g/kg till 1.5 g/kg/day.
- Dialysis is the only means for rapid removal of ammonia, and hemodialysis is more effective and faster than peritoneal dialysis, however, peritoneal dialysis may be more widely available and feasible. Exchange transfusion is not useful.
- *Alternative pathways for nitrogen excretion*: Sodium benzoate (IV or oral)—loading dose 250 mg/kg, then 250–400 mg/kg/day in four divided doses. Intravenous preparation is not available in India. Sodium phenylbutyrate (not available in India)—loading dose 250 mg/kg followed by 250–500 mg/kg/day.
- L-arginine (oral or IV)—300 mg/kg/day (intravenous preparation is not available in India) L-carnitine (oral or IV)—200 mg/kg/day.
- *Supportive care*: Treatment of sepsis, seizures, and ventilation. Avoid sodium valproate.

Acute Management of Newborn with Suspected Organic Academia

- The patient is kept nil per orally and intravenous glucose is provided.
- *Supportive care*: Hydration, treatment of sepsis, seizures, and ventilation.
- *Carnitine*: 100 mg/kg/day IV or oral.
- *Treat acidosis*: Sodium bicarbonate 0.35–0.5 mEq/kg/hr (max 1–2 mEq/kg/hr)
- Start Biotin 10 mg/day orally.
- Start vitamin B_{12} 1–2 mg/day I/M (useful in vitamin B_{12} responsive forms of methylmalonic acidemias)
- Start thiamine 300 mg/day (useful in thiamine-responsive variants of MSUD).
- If hyperammonemia is present, treat as explained earlier.

Management of Congenital Lactic Acidosis

- *Supportive care*: Hydration, treatment of sepsis, seizures, and ventilation. Avoid sodium valproate.
- *Treat acidosis*: Sodium bicarbonate 0.35–0.5 mEq/kg/hr (max 1–2 mEq/kg/hr).
- Thiamine up to 300 mg/day in 4 divided doses.
- Riboflavin 100 mg/day in 4 divided doses.
- Add co-enzyme Q: 5–15 mg/kg/day.
- L-carnitine: 50–100 mg/kg orally.

Treatment of Newborn with Refractory Seizures with No Obvious Etiology (Suspected Metabolic Etiology)

- If patient persists to have seizures despite 2 or 3 antiepileptic drugs in adequate doses, consider trial of pyridoxine 100 mg

intravenous. If intravenous preparation not available, oral pyridoxine can be given (15 mg/kg/day).
- If seizures persist despite pyridoxine, give trial of biotin 10 mg/day and folinic acid 15 mg/day (folinic acid responsive seizures).
- Rule out glucose transporter defect—measure CSF and blood glucose. In glucose transporter defect, CSF glucose level is equal to or less than one-third of the blood glucose level. This disorder responds to the ketogenic diet.

Management of Asymptomatic Newborn with a History of Sibling Death with Suspected IEM

- After baseline metabolic screen, start oral dextrose feeds (10% dextrose).
- After 24 hours, repeat screen. If normal, start breastfeeds. Monitor sugar, blood gases, urine ketones, and blood ammonia every 6 hours.
- Some authorities recommend starting medium chain triglycerides (MCT oil) before starting breastfeeds, however, palatabilty is a concern. (because of unpalatability of MCT oil).
- After 48 hours, repeat metabolic screen. Obtain samples for tandem mass spectrometry (TMS) and urine organic acid tests.
- The infant will need careful observation and follow-up for the first few months, as IEM may present in different age groups in members of the same family.

SPECIFIC TREATMENT

- Gene therapy.
- Enzyme replacement therapy.
- Transplantation—bone marrow, liver transplant fibroblast.

PRENATAL DIAGNOSIS

Most IEM are inherited as autosomal recessive trait having recurrence risk of 25% in each pregnancy. After confirmation of diagnosis in an index case, mutation analysis of affected baby and both parents are done. Prenatal diagnosis in subsequent pregnancies can be made by finding the same mutation from chorionic villous sampling or amniocentesis.

NEWBORN SCREENING

Many IEM can be diagnosed based on screening using tandem mass spectrometry. Screening should be done after 2 days and before 7 days of age. Sick and premature babies should also have metabolic screening performed by 7 days of life.

SUGGESTED READING

1. Burton BK. Inborn errors of metabolism in infancy: A guide to diagnosis. Pediatrics. 1998;102(6):E69.
2. Martin RJ, Fanaroff AA, Walsh MC. Fanaroff and Martin's Neonatal-Perinatal Medicine, 9th edn. Mosby; 2010. pp. 1-2008.
3. Scriver CR, Sly WS, Childs B, et al (Eds). The Metabolic and Molecular Basis of Inherited Diseases, volume 4. NewYork: McGraw Hill; 2001.

CHAPTER 20

Disorder of Sex Development

Tejopratap Oleti

DEFINITION

- The previously used nomenclature like "pseudohermaphrodite", "hermaphrodite" and "intersex" are replaced by the new term "disorder of sex development" (DSD) (Table 1).
- The neonates with discrepancy between phenotypic external genitalia, internal gonads and sex chromosomes at birth are considered to be having disorder of sex development.

WHEN SHOULD YOU SUSPECT THAT THE NEONATE HAVE DISORDER OF SEX DEVELOPMENT?

- Bilaterally nonpalpable testes (Fig. 1)
- Microphallus (stretched penile length <2.5 cm)
- Perineal hypospadiasis with bifid scrotum (Fig. 2)
- Clitoromegaly (clitoral width >6 mm or clitoral length >9 mm) (Fig. 3)
- Posterior labial fusion
- Gonads palpable in labioscrotal folds (Fig. 4)

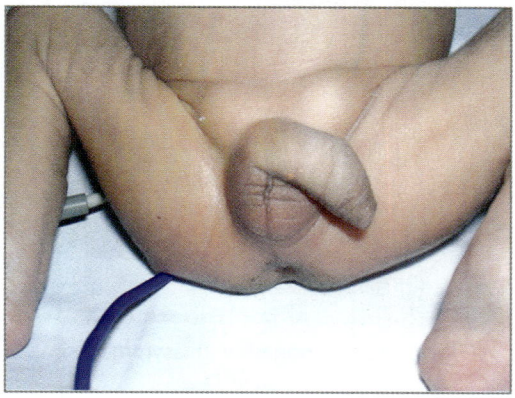

Fig. 1: Cryptorchidism with testes in inguinal region.

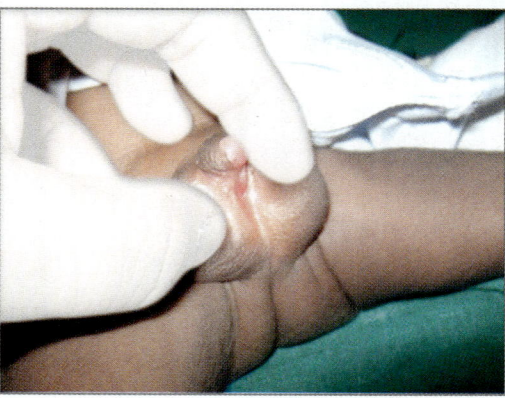

Fig. 2: Bifid scrotum, hypospadiasis and palpable gonads suggestive of 46 XY DSD with undervirilization.

SECTION 1
Clinical Approach to Sick Newborn

Table 1: Classification of disorders of sexual development (DSD).

46, XY DSD	46, XX DSD	Sex chromosome DSD

• Disorders of testicular development
  – Complete gonadal dysgenesis (Swyer syndrome)
  – Partial gonadal dysgenesis
  – Gonadal regression
  – Ovotesticular DSD
	• Disorders of ovarian development
	  – Ovotesticular DSD
	  – Testicular DSD (e.g. SRY+, dup SOX9)
	  – Gonadal dysgenesis
		• 45, x (Turner syndrome and variants)
		• 47, XXY (Klinefelter syndrome and variants)
		• 45, X/46, XY (mixed gonadal dysgenesis, ovotesticular DSD)
		• 46, XX/ 46, XY (chimeri, ovotesticular DSD)

• Disorders in androgen synthesis
  – Androgen biosynthetic defects (e.g. 17-hydroxysteroid dehydrogenase deficiency, 5α reductase deficiency, StAR mutations
  – Defect in androgen action (CAIS, PAIS)
  – LH receptor defects (e.g. Leydig cell hypo/aplasia)
  – Disorders of AMH and AMH receptor deficiency (persistent mullerian duct syndrome)
	• Androgen excess
	  – Fetal (21- and 11- hydroxylase deficiency)
	  – Fetoplacental (aromatase deficiency, POR)
	  – Maternal (luteoma, exogenous, etc.)	

• Others (e.g. severe hypospadiasis, cloacal exstrophy)	• Others (cloacal exstrophy, vaginal atresia, MURCS, other syndromes)	

(AMH: antimüllerian hormone; CAIS: complete androgen insensitivity syndrome; PAIS: partial androgen insensitivity syndrome; POR: P450-oxidoreductase)

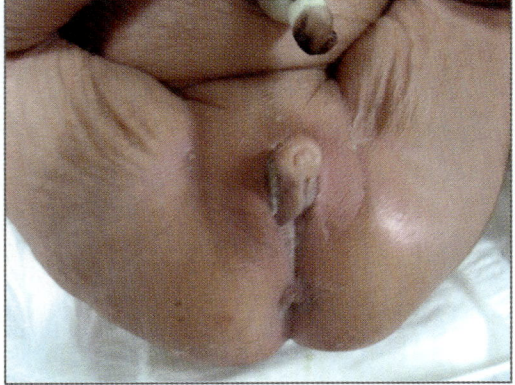

Fig. 3: Infant with 46 XX DSD with overvirilization having clitoromegaly and fusion of labia.

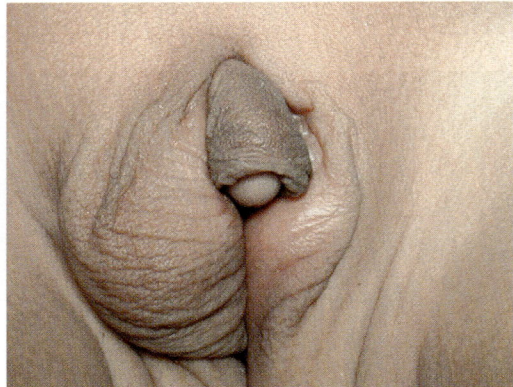

Fig. 4: Palpable gonads with asymmetry in mixed DSD.

- Hypospadiasis with unilateral nonpalpable gonad
- Discordant genitalia and sex chromosomes.

CLASSIFICATION OF DISORDER OF SEX DEVELOPMENT

The initial evaluation must include a detailed history which includes antenatal, postnatal aspects, physical examination, pelvic or abdominal ultrasonography, karyotype, and biochemical evaluation of gonadal and adrenal function. Further tests will be based on neonatal evaluation.

Based on the initial evaluation, the neonates can be categorized into following:
- Virilized XX
- Undervirilized XY
- Mixed sex chromosome pattern.

HISTORY

Apart from routine history taking, following aspects have to be more stressed while taking history:
- Intake of androgenic drugs like progesterones, danazol, testosterone or drugs which can modulate endocrine function like phenytoin, aminoglutethimide.
- Changes of virilization during pregnancy (placental aromatase deficiency, luteoma).
- Family history of early unexplained infant deaths [congenital adrenal hyperplasia (CAH)].
- Family history of primary amenorrhea or infertility.
- History of consanguinity (recessive disorders).

PHYSICAL EXAMINATION

The careful physical examination will give important clues regarding underlying diagnosis. The examination should include inspection and palpation of genitalia and

Table 2: External masculization score.

External masculization	Yes/No
Scrotal fusion	3/0
Micropenis	3/0
Urethral meatus	
Normal	3
Glandular (distal)	2
Penile (mid)	1
Perineal (proximal)	0
Right and left gonad (score for each)	
Scrotal 1.5	1.5
Inguinal 1	1
Abdominal 0.5	0.5

inguinal region and also number and location of urogenital openings need to be noted. The external genitalia examinations can also be scored with external masculinization score (Table 2). Healthy term neonates will have score of more than 12.

Penile Length

Penile length is measured on its dorsal surface from the pubic ramus to the tip of the penis (excluding any excess foreskin) after stretching the penis to the point of increased resistance. The ruler should be pressed down against the ramus to completely depress the suprapubic fat pad. Penile width (diameter) is measured at the level of midshaft. In a term infant, at birth, the normal penile length is ≥2.5 cm and normal penile diameter is ≥0.9 cm. These measurements should be adjusted for gestational age (Fig. 5).

Gonads

The scrotum, labia majora and inguinal area should be carefully palpated to look at the number and position of the gonads. The neonate should be examined in a warm room with warm hands in frog-leg position. Gonads palpable below the inguinal ligament are usually testes. The undescended testis

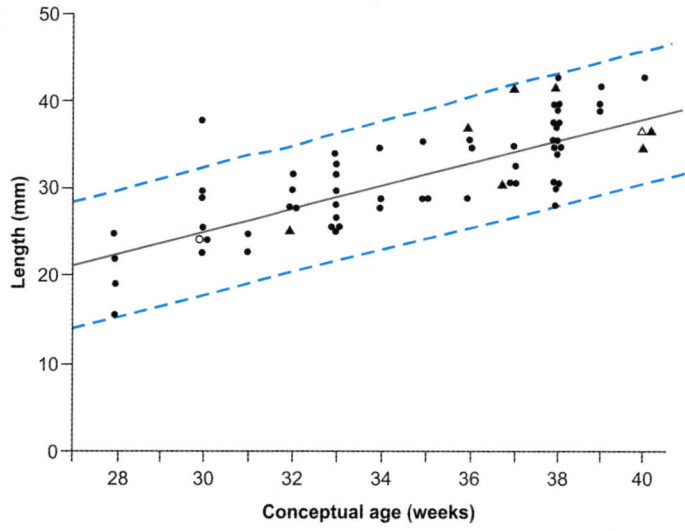

Fig. 5: Phallic length nomogram in neonates according to gestation (Feldman et al. 1975).

may be located in inguinal canal, superficial inguinal pouch, and root of scrotum or rarely in perineal, femoral or contralateral scrotal region.

Urethral Opening

The location of urethral opening in relation to other external genitalia will give us the clues for diagnosis. A single opening at the base of the phallus may be either an incompletely fused penile urethra (penoscrotal hypospadias) or a virilized urogenital sinus (e.g. internal connection between the vagina and urethra).

Clitoral Size

Clitoral width is measured by gently pressing the shaft of the clitoris between the thumb and forefinger to exclude excess skin and subcutaneous tissue. Normal clitoral width in a neonate ranges from 2 mm to 6 mm. The mean length of the clitoris depends on population characteristics. However, lengths of more than 9 mm are unusual in normal neonates. The clitoris may appear disproportionately more prominent in preterm infants because clitoral size is fully developed by 27 weeks gestation as there is less fat in the labia majora.

Virilization: Prader and Quigley (Fig. 6) had the description for assessing the development of external genitalia in female and male neonates, respectively. These standards are useful for documenting the characteristic phenotype of genital phenotype.

Anogenital Ratio

The anogenital ratio, which is independent of gestational age and body size, is the distance between the anus and posterior fourchette divided by the distance between the anus and the base of the clitoris. A ratio of >0.5 suggests virilization with some posterior labial fusion.

The hyperpigmentation around external genitalia can also give a clue for suspecting underlying CAH.

The examination should also focus on associated nongenital anomalies and dysmorphic features. The presence of nongenital anomalies usually excludes common forms of adrenal disorders. The genital anomalies might have been part of syndrome due to chromosomal anomalies or due to dyshormonogenesis [inadequate follicle stimulating hormone (FSH)/luteinizing hormone (LH) production]

CHAPTER 20
Disorder of Sex Development

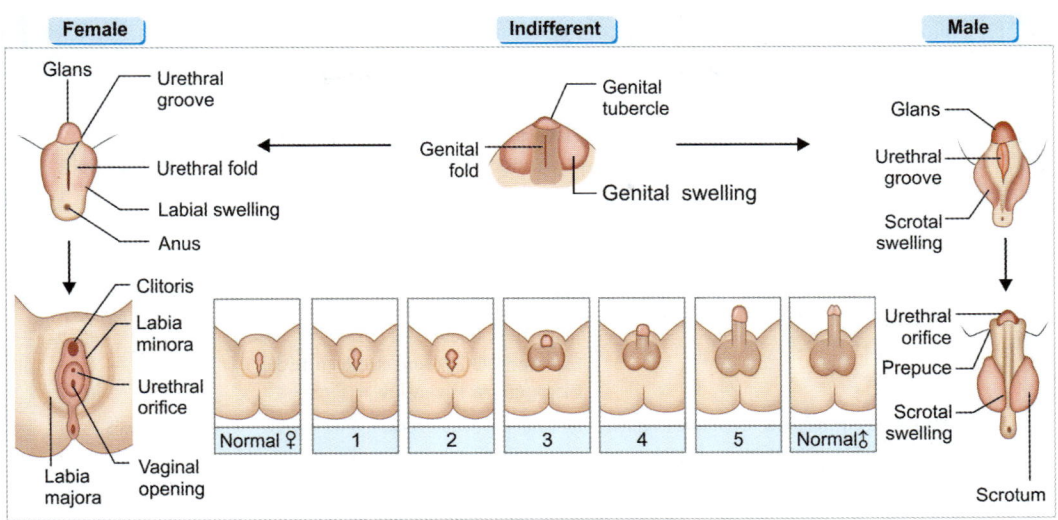

Fig. 6: Virilization of external genitalia (Prader grading).

Prader staging: 0: Normal female; 1: Female external genitalia with clitoromegaly; 2: Clitoromegaly with partial labial fusion forming a funnel-shaped urogenital sinus; 3: Increased phallic size with complete labioscrotal fusion forming a urogenital sinus with a single opening; 4: Complete scrotal fusion with the opening of the urogenital sinus at the base of the phallus; 5: Normal male.

Table 3: Abnormalities in genitalia and associated syndromes.

Abnormality	Syndrome
Hypospadiasis/Bifid scrotum	WAGR syndrome, Fryns syndrome, Fraser Syndrome, Smith–Lemili–Opitz syndrome, bladder exstrophy sequence
Micropenis	Prader–Willi syndrome, Noonan syndrome, CHARGE association, Anencephaly sequence, Carpenter syndrome
Cryptorchidism	Cloacal exstrophy sequence, Trisomy 13 and 18, Smith–Lemli–Opitz syndrome, Noonan syndrome, Fraser syndrome, Miller–Dieker syndrome, Rubinstein Taybi syndrome
Hypoplasia of labia majora	Prader–Willi syndrome, Trisomy 18, Robinow syndrome

or inadequate production of steroid precursor due to other metabolic disorders. The presence of gastrointestinal anomalies should make clinician to suspect altered cloacal development. For further details of associated anomalies, go through Table 3.

INVESTIGATIONS

- Karyotype and fluorescence in-situ hybridization (FISH) technique for sex chromosomes by using peripheral leukocytes. To rule out mosaics, at least 200 cells should be examined before giving final report.
- 17-hydroxyprogesterone to rule out common forms of CAH. If there is strong suspicion of CAH, then serial serum electrolytes should be done before final diagnosis.
- Evaluation for sex-determining region on the Y chromosome (SRY) gene using FISH and SRY specific probes to be considered to narrow the diagnosis.
- *For other forms of CAH:* 17-hydroxypregnenolone, dehydroepiandrosterone (DHEA), and 11-deoxycortisol (Table 4).
- *To rule out suspected central hypoadrenalism*: Cortisol and adrenocorticotropic hormone (ACTH) needs to be done.

Table 4: Clinical and biochemical characteristics—common forms of congenital adrenal deficiency.

Enzyme deficiency	Clinical features	Hormones	Electrolytes
21-hydroxylase	Ambiguous genitalia in female Addisonian crisis	Low cortisol and aldosterone Elevated 17 OHP, 21-deoxycortisol High androstenedione, testosterone, ± plasma rennin activity Estrogens relatively low in females	Acidosis Low sodium High potassium
11β-hydroxylase	Ambiguous genitalia in female Hypertension	Low cortisol, corticosterone, aldosterone, ± plasma rennin activity Increased androstenedione, testosterone levels Elevated DOC 11 and deoxycortisol Estrogens relatively low in females	± Alkalosis High sodium Low potassium
17α-hydroxylase	Ambiguous genitalia in male Hypertension	Normal corticosterone Increased mineralocorticoids Decreased androgens and estrogens Elevated DOC	± Alkalosis High sodium Low potassium
Aldosterone synthetase	No ambiguous genitalia Addisonian crisis in salt-wasting type only	Low mineralocorticoids All other hormones normal Elevated corticosterone, ± 18 hydroxy corticosterone	Acidosis Low sodium High potassium
3β-HSD	Ambiguous genitalia in male Addisonian crisis	Elevated DHEA and suppressible by dexamethasone Increased 17-hydroxypregnenolone, Δ^5 C21- and C19 steroids Low cortisol, aldosterone—androgens low in male, high in female	Acidosis Low sodium High potassium
P-450 oxidoreductase deficiency	Ambiguous or normal female Variable androgenization Maternal androgenization during pregnancy	Normal or low cortisol with low response to ACTH stimulation Elevated 17 OHP, testosterone, progesterone, corticosterone Low estradiol Combined P450c17 and P450c21 insufficiency	Normal to low sodium

(ACTH: adrenocorticotropic hormone; DHEA: dehydroepiandrosterone; DOC: deoxycorticosterone; HSD: hydroxysteroid dehydrogenase)

- Undervirilized male infants should undergo Luteinizing hormone, FSH, testosterone, dihydrotestosterone, antiMüllerian hormone (AMH), and human chorionic gonadotropin (hCG) stimulation test (Table 5).

Imaging

Ultrasound of abdomen and pelvis should be integral part of initial evaluation to study internal genitalia. Some cases may need retrograde urethrogram, cystoscopy/vaginoscopy, and MRI for detailed evaluation.

Molecular genetic studies also play an important role in identifying these complex disorders. Common genes which cause DSD and their inheritance pattern is mentioned in Table 6.

Chapter 20: Disorder of Sex Development

Table 5: Interpretation of hCG stimulation test.

Disorder	Testosterone	Testosterone: DHT	Testosterone: Androstenedione
17β HSD type 3 deficiency	Low	Normal	<0.8
5α reductase deficiency	Normal	>20:1	Normal
LH receptor defects	Low	Unresponsive	Normal
AIS	No increase from basal testosterone level	Normal	Normal

(AIS: androgen insensitivity syndrome; DHT: dihydrotestosterone; HSD: hydroxysteroid dehydrogenase; hCG: human chorionic gonadotropin; LH: luteinizing hormone)

Table 6: Showing genes known to cause disorders of sex development (DSD).

46 XY DSD	
Single gene disorders involving testicular development derangements	
Genitalia	*Genes/Chromosomes*
Dysgenetic testes	WT1, SF1, DHH, ATRX, ARX DMRT1(9p24.3), WNT4 (1p35)*, WWOX (16q23)
Dysgenetic testes or ovotestis	SRY, SOX9 NR0B1(Xp21.3)
Hormone synthesis	
LHGCR (G-protein receptor)	2p21
DHCR7 (Enzyme)	11q12-13
StAR (Mitochondrial membrane protein)	8p11.2
CYP11A1 (Enzyme)	15q23-24
HSD3B2 (Enzyme)	1p13.1
CYP17 (Enzyme)	10q24.3
POR (P450 oxidoreductase-electron donor)	7q11.2
HSD17B3 (Enzyme)	9q22
SRD5A2 (Enzyme)	2p23
Anti-müllerian hormone (Signaling molecule)	19p13.3-13.2
Anti-müllerian hormone receptor	12q13
Androgen receptor	Xq11-12**
46 XX DSD	
Disorders of ovarian development	
Ovotestis	SRY
Undetermined	SOX9
Androgen excess	
HB2HSD (Enzyme)	1p13
CYP21A2 (Enzyme)	6p21-23
CYP11B1 (Enzyme)	8Q21-22
POR (P450-electron donor)	7Q11.3
CYP19 (Enzyme)	15q21
Glucocorticoid receptor	5q13

*Associated with persistent müllerian structures
**Only hormonal derangement disorder with X-linked recessive inheritance. All other have autosomal recessive inheritance.

APPROACH FOR DIAGNOSIS AND ETIOLOGY (FLOWCHARTS 1 TO 3)

Management

Management of neonate with DSD should include multidisciplinary team.
- Neonatologist
- Pediatric endocrinologist
- Pediatric urologist
- Psychologist
- Clinical geneticist
- Clinical biochemist.

The goal evaluation and management includes:
- Looking for emergency conditions like Addisonian crisis
- Gender assignment with multidisciplinary approach
- Formulation of long-term management

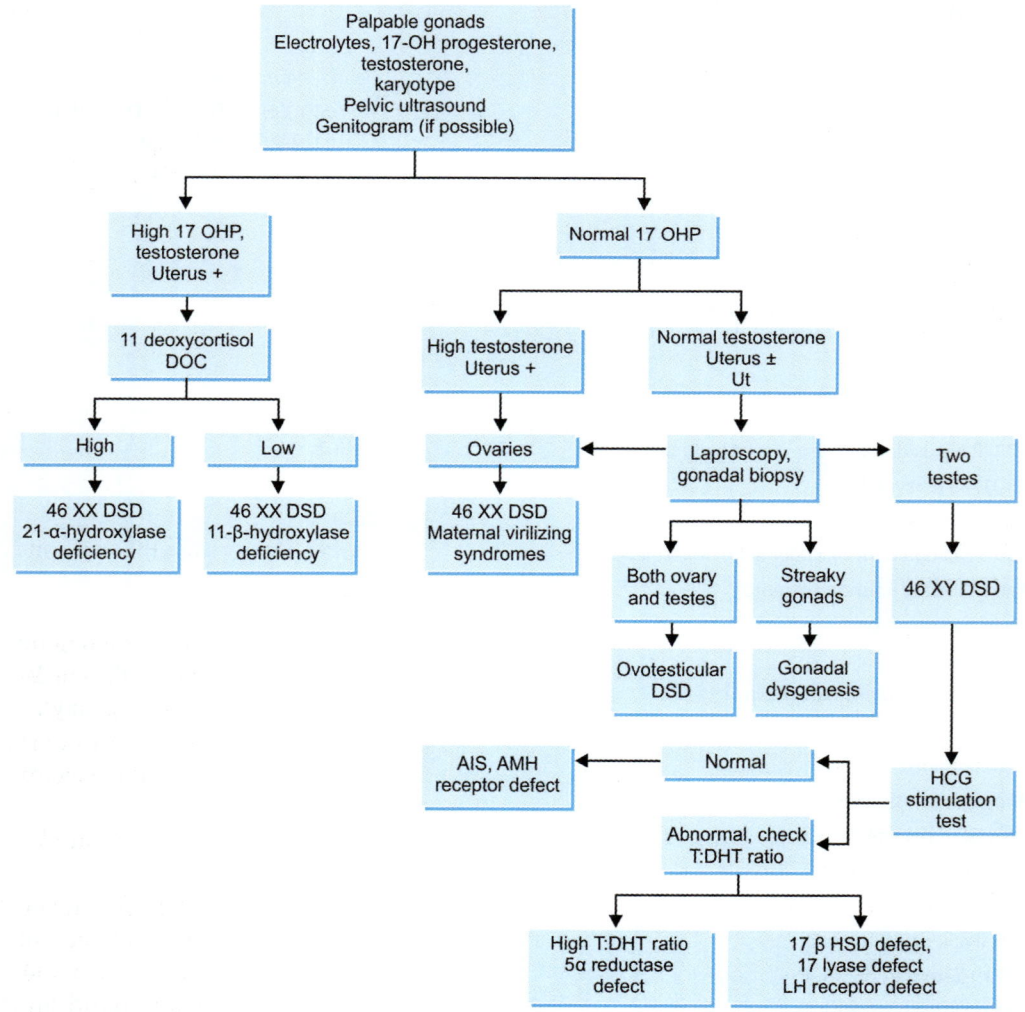

Flowchart 1: Practical approach to disorders of sexual differentiation.

(DHT: dihydrotestosterone; DOC: deoxycorticosterone; DSD: disorder of sex development; hCG: human chorionic gonadotropin; HSD: hydroxysteroid dehydrogenase; OHP: hydroxyprogesterone)

CHAPTER 20
Disorder of Sex Development

Flowchart 2: Approach to neonate with 46 XY disorder of sex development.

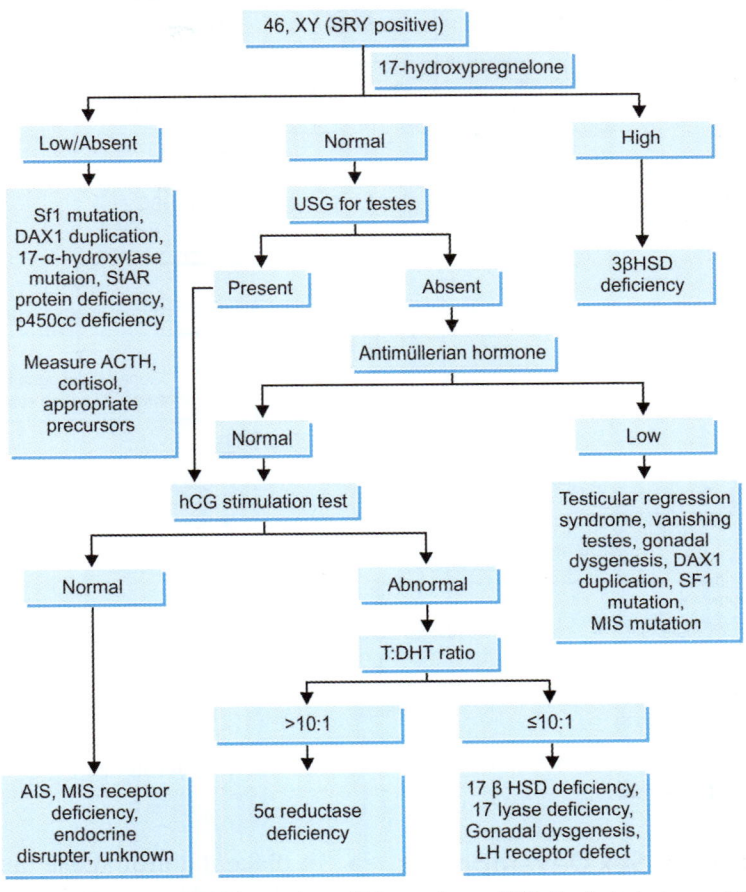

(ACTH: adrenocorticotropic hormone; AIS: androgen insensitivity syndrome; DHT: dihydrotestosterone; HSD: hydroxysteroid dehydrogenase; hCG: human chorionic gonadotropin; MIS: Müllerian inhibiting substance)

- Open communication with parents and other family members.

Immediate Management

- Addisonian crisis:
  - All the neonates need to be observed in the hospital for 2 weeks.
  - Till the results of hormone metabolites are available, electrolytes and blood pressure should be monitored.
  - Once the diagnosis is confirmed or if the neonate presents with signs and symptoms of Addisonian crisis, then neonate needs to be treated with hydrocortisone (50–100 mg/m^2 or 1–2 mg/kg/day).
  - Emphasis should be given to correct fluid, hypoglycemia and other electrolyte abnormalities.
  - Monitor vitals for signs of shock and respiratory failure.
- Look for associated genital and nongenital anomalies which need urgent intervention like anorectal and cardiac malformation.
- Gender assignment will depend on the underlying disease.

Flowchart 3: Approach to neonate with 46 XX disorder of sexual development.

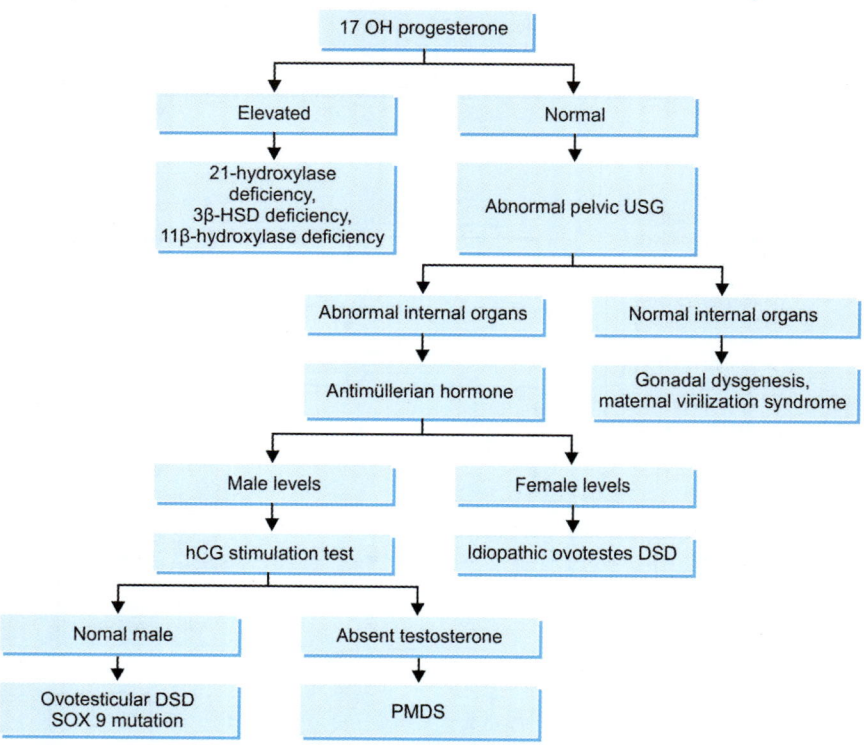

(DSD: disorder of sex development; HSD: hydroxysteroid dehydrogenase; hCG: human chorionic gonadotropin; PMDS: persistent müllerian duct syndrome)

46 XX Disorder of Sex Development

- *Congenital adrenal hyperplasia:* Most common are 21-α- and 11-β-hydroxylase enzyme deficiencies.
  Once the neonate is stabilized and recovered from Addisonian crisis, the longterm glucocorticoid (10–20 mg/m²/day in 3 divided doses) or/and mineralocorticoid replacement (fludrocortisone 0.05–3 mg/day) to be advised
  - During the stress periods like infection, the hydrocortisone dose needs to be increased to 3–5 times the normal
  - The female infants might require antiandrogens during puberty
- *Gestational hyperandrogenism:*
  - It occurs due to maternal CAH, virilizing tumors of adrenal or ovary, or exposure to androgenic drugs.
- In placental aromatase deficiency both mother and infant will be virilized.

46 XY Disorder of Sex Development

- *Congenital adrenal hyperplasia:*
  - Undervirilization can be due to 17α hydroxylase, 3β hydroxysteroid dehydrogenase deficiency (3β HSD), P450 side chain cleavage deficiency and lipoid hyperplasia (StAR protein deficiency)
  - The differential diagnosis and characteristic features are shown in Table 4.
- *Abnormal testicular activity:*
  - Presence of normal serum concentrations of antimüllerian hormone or inhibin-B shows normal Sertoli cell function.
  - Low AMH indicates abnormal testicular Sertoli cell function.

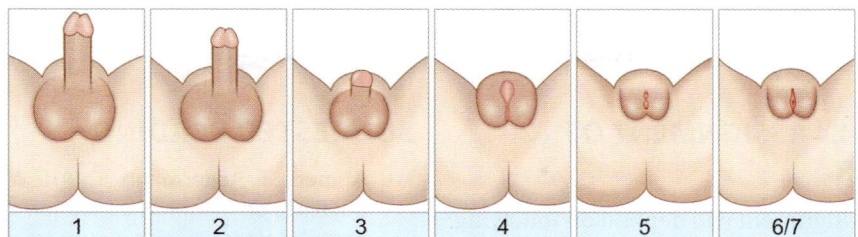

Fig. 7: Grading scheme for clinical classification of androgen insensitivity syndromes.

Grades are numbered 1–7 in order of increasing severity (more defective masculinization).
- Grade 1—normal masculinization in utero.
- Grade 2—male phenotype with mild defect in masculinization.
- Grade 3—male phenotype with severe defect in masculinization like small penis, perineoscrotal hypospadiasis, bifid scrotum and/or cryptorchidism.
- Grade 4—severe genital ambiguity of clitoral like phallus, labioscrotal folds, single perineal orifice.
- Grade 5—female phenotype with posterior labial fusion and clitoromegaly.
- Grade 6/7—female phenotype (grade 6 if pubic hair present in adulthood, grade 7 if no pubic hair in adulthood).

- These cases need surgery and hormone replacement therapy in later life.
- *Abnormal androgen synthesis and insensitivity*
  - Clinical grading of androgen insensitivity has been shown in Figure 7.
  - hCG stimulation test will differentiate different conditions (Table 5). It consists of:
    - Estimation of basal LH, FSH, testosterone, androstenedione, and DHT.
  - hCG: 500 units intramuscularly on alternate days for a total of 3 doses.
  - β hCG (confirms the adequate administration), testosterone, androstenedione and DHT have to be estimated on days 3 and 6.
  - A doubling of testosterone level by day 3 and 4 times increase by day 6 indicate normal response.
  - The normal ratio of testosterone to DHT and testosterone to androstenedione is normally less than 10:1 and more than 0.8, respectively.
- Increase in phallic length to 50 mg depot monthly injections of testosterone will suggest partial androgen insensitivity syndrome. In complete androgen insensitivity, there will not be any response.
- Testing for associated adrenal insufficiency can be done by ACTH stimulation test.

Sex Chromosome Disorder of Sex Development

- Mixed gonadal dysgenesis:
  - If there is measurable AMH or positive hCG stimulation test, the position of testes should be evaluated with imaging and surgical techniques
  - Majority of these neonates are assigned female sex, so the testes should be removed
  - The dysgenetic and streaky gonads need to be removed due to the risk of germ cell tumors in later life.
- Ovotesticular DSD:
  - Dysgenetic gonads should be removed
  - Sex assignment will depend on internal and external genitalia
  - Further surgeries will depend upon the gender assignment and child's behavior.
- Sex chromosomal abnormalities:
  - Turner syndrome and Klinefelter syndrome will have characteristic spectrum of abnormalities

- Will require hormone replacement therapy and surgery in later life.

ISSUES IN ASSIGNMENT OF GENDER

The sex assignment will depend on following:
- The penile length in 46 XY DSD infants and virilization in 46 XX DSD in terms of fusion of labioscrotal folds
- Exposure to intrauterine androgens or estrogens will influence gender identity and behavior formation in utero
- Parents need to be explained about options of medical and surgical therapy and their effect on future gender-related behavioral problems in the neonate.

SUGGESTED READING

1. Ahmed SF, Achermann JC, Arlt W, et al. UK guidance on the initial evaluation of an infant or an adolescent with a suspected disorder of sex development. Clin Endocrinol (Oxf). 2011;75(1):1226.
2. Houk CP, et al. Evaluation of the Infant with Ambiguous Genitalia In: Post TW (Ed). Up To Date. Waltham, MA: 2015.
3. Lambert SM, Vilain EJ, Kolon TF. A practical approach to ambiguous genitalia in the newborn period. Urol Clin North Am. 2010;37(2):195205.

CHAPTER 21

Neonatal Transport

Sachin Shah, Amita Kaul

INTRODUCTION

Neonatal transport is shifting a neonate from one setting or facility to another for further provision of expert care or evaluation. This may be inter- or intrahospital transfer. Transfer in itself does not constitute therapy and represents a time of increased risk.

Goal: The *right* newborn has to be taken at the *right* time, by the *right* people, to the *right* place by the *right* form of transport, and receive the *right* care throughout.

The neonatal transfers may involve stable or unstable newborns and can be categorized as:
- Emergency
- Urgent
- Nonurgent.

As a rule of thumb the team should be mobilized within 30 minutes for emergency transfers and within 2 hours for urgent transfer.

INDICATIONS FOR TRANSPORT

In general, transport is indicated if skills, resources or care of the woman and her unborn baby or infant in the local setting are inadequate to manage the possible complications.

Conditions that require transfer to a tertiary care center include the following:
- Gestational age <32 weeks
- Birth weight <1,500 g
- Respiratory distress requiring ventilatory support
- Hypoxic respiratory failure
- Congenital heart disease or cardiac arrhythmias
- Major congenital anomalies and/or inborn errors of metabolism
- Severe hypoxic ischemic injury
- Seizures
- Severe hyperbilirubinemia that may require exchange transfusion
- Sepsis with multiorgan dysfunction
- Need for surgical intervention unavailable at referring hospital.

The safest and best way to transport is in-utero.

CONTRAINDICATIONS FOR TRANSPORT

- Newborn with a condition incompatible with survival.
- The newborn's condition is unstable and threatening to deteriorate rapidly.
- Weather conditions are hazardous for travel.
- No experienced attendant/transport team available to accompany patient.

SECTION 1
Clinical Approach to Sick Newborn

TRANSPORT PREPARATION

Phase 1: Stabilize the Patient

Key Components
- Airway
- Breathing
- Circulation
- Dextrose
- Environment—temperature.

Focus of Evaluation
- What is the problem?
- What is being done?
- What effect is it having?
- What is needed now?

Assess the baby and depending on facilities available check for temperature, airway, breathing, circulation, and sugar (Table 1).

Available models for pretransport stabilization and care during transport are:
- *STABLE*: **S**ugar, **T**emperature, **A**rtificial breathing, **B**lood pressure, **L**aboratory work, **E**motional support.
- *SAFER*: **S**ugar, **A**rterial circulatory support, **F**amily support, **E**nvironment, **R**espiratory support.
- *TOPS*: **T**emperature, **O**xygenation (Airway and Breathing), **P**erfusion, **S**ugar stabilization of sick neonates before and care during transport to maintain euglycemia, normothermia, adequate oxygenation, and perfusion should be the utmost priority.

Phase II: Equipment Check

All the equipment required during transportation should be functional, available in various sizes and anticipated.

Power Backup

Ensure the equipment has battery backup and is fully charged prior to transport. A power

Table 1: Stabilization of newborn.

Temperature	• Record temperature before starting and on arrival • Use transport incubator, if possible. Thermocol box is an alternative • Ensure the palms and soles are pink • Cover the head, keep baby skin to skin contact with mother • Avoid drafts of air • Ensure temperature of 36.5–37.5°C.
Airway	• Keep the baby in sniffing position on a firm, flat surface • Avoid flexion or extension of neck • Suction, if required • Ensure suction apparatus is available—suction bulb, foot operated • If unstable, intubate prior to transport.
Breathing	• Note the work of breathing • Use objective parameters like SA score or Downes score • Note the trend of breathing • Have a backup of intubation, self-inflating bag • T-piece resuscitator is an alternative, if facilities exist • Monitor using pulse oximeter • Anticipate need for intubation and plan accordingly • Ensure oxygen supply if SpO_2 <90%.
Circulation	• Assess for HR, RR, color, sensorium, CRT, temperature, pulse volume, BP, and urine output • Consider need for fluid bolus, prior to starting • If fluids/inotropes are required, use syringe pump • Avoid fluid overload.
Dextrose	• Monitor glucostix • Target b glucose > 45 mg% • Ensure use of syringe pump if hypoglycemia.
Feeds/Fluids	• If unstable, ensure patent IV line • If stable, ensure breast feeds or expressed breast milk • Monitor for sugar • *Check all the medications received.*

source of current 240 V should be made available via a generator or an inverter.

Gas Supplies

Ensure enough gas supply for transport. Anticipate need for additional gas and have extra spares. Most of the cylinders with the transport incubator last for not more than 2 hours. Adaptors and supplies for change of cylinders should be readily available and the personnel should be familiar with changing of cylinders.

Specific Equipment Items

- *Ventilators*: Dedicated transport ventilators should be used. A T piece resuscitator is an option for noninvasive respiratory support. Backup of self-inflating bag and intubation set is mandatory.
- *Transport incubators*: Dedicated incubators should be used. Appropriate power source, battery backup should be available.
- *Restraints*: Ensure the infant is well strapped and does not change position during transport. Use of series of foam wedges and straps, adjustable as per requirement help restrain the infant within the transport incubator.
- *Syringe infusion pumps*: Ensure the syringe pump is adequately powered prior to start. A power source of 240 V should be available. Most of the pumps have a battery backup. Anticipate use based on duration of transport.
- *Monitors*: A pulse oximeter with battery backup should be used. A multichannel monitor is desirable. Note that the motion of the ambulance may cause artifacts. A signal extraction technology-based pulse oximeter is most suited.

Phase III: Personnel Preparation

- The composition of the transport team should be decided based on the clinical condition of the neonate.
- The minimum number of transport team members should be three, of which one is the driver. The other two team members should be a newborn trained doctor and nurse proficient in assessing, supporting and maintaining airway, breathing and support. Resuscitation skills are must.

Supervision

A person should be in-charge and available for consultation if any problem happens en route.

TYPE OF TRANSPORT TEAMS

Unit-based Transport Team

This team consists of trained doctors and nurses from within the nursery who are allotted the duty to get a sick infant from a nearby facility. Such a system works if the numbers of transports are less in volume.

Dedicated Transport Team

This team consists of dedicated and skilled team of doctors and nurses, who are specifically assigned the duty of transportation. They are not involved in NICU care. Such a system is best if there is a large volume of transport.

CARING DURING TRANSPORT

- Ensure warmth
- Easy access to the patient, always
- All lines and drains must be secured
- Neonate must be restrained and covered
- The incubator must be secured to the transport vehicle
- Anticipation is the key.

Table 2: Modes of transport.

	Ground ambulance	Rotor-wing aircraft	Fixed-wing aircraft
Departure times	Excellent	Excellent	Poor to fair
Arrival times	Fair to poor	Excellent	Good
Out-of-hospital time	Poor	Excellent	Fair to excellent
Patient accessibility	Good	Poor	Fair
Weather issues	Excellent	Poor	Fair to good
Cost	Low	High	High
	Up to 200 km	Up to 300 km	>200 km

MODES OF TRANSPORT (TABLE 2)

Factors influencing mode of transport include nature of illness, urgency of transfer, mobilization time, geographical factors, weather, traffic conditions, and cost.

TRANSPORT IN SPECIFIC CONDITIONS

Babies with Respiratory Distress

- Oxygen supply with nasal prongs/catheters should be used for mild hypoxia. If there is moderate distress, continuous positive airway pressure (CPAP) by T piece resuscitator is an option. If unstable, the infant should be intubated and stabilized prior to transport.
- Need for intubation should be planned and anticipated.
- Elective ventilation before transport may be considered if (A) Respiratory distress worsening with increasing oxygen requirement (FiO_2 of more than 60%); (B) Recurrent apnea; (C) Recurrent seizures; (D) Congenital heart disease on prostaglandin E1 infusion of more than 0.05 µg/kg/min (risk of apnea); (E) Congenital diaphragmatic hernia; (F) Limited space and skills to perform any resuscitation; and (G) Long distance travel of unstable patient.
- Surfactant replacement is indicated for intubated infants with respiratory distress syndrome before transport.

Air Leak Syndromes

- It is advisable to drain the pneumothorax adequately and preferably keep a chest tube in place before departure. During transport, underwater seal systems are bulky and difficult to manage in ambulance. The chest tube and its connections may move and get dislodged with the movement or vibrations of the ambulance hence should be well secured.

Esophageal Atresia

- The baby should be nursed prone.
- Airway should be clear.

Meningomyelocele

- The exposed swelling on the back should be covered with gauze piece soaked in normal saline and baby should lie on the side and not back during transport.

DETERIORATION OF A NEONATE DURING TRANSPORT

The strategies that can be used in case of acute deterioration are:

- Stop the vehicle and resuscitate.
- Avoid performing any procedures in a moving vehicle. Get to the nearest facility, stabilize, and then proceed.

PRACTICAL ISSUES WITH TRANSPORT

Thermal Issues

Hypo- and hyperthermia is common during transport. Periodic assessment of temperature is must.

Noise and Vibration

Vibration can derange lines and tubes, and affect monitoring equipment. A Masimo or Oxismart technology-based pulse oximeter is preferred as it is not affected by motion. Visual rather than audio alarms should be used where possible.

AIR TRANSPORT

- Ensure efforts to maximize oxygen delivery in hypoxic infants as the barometric pressure gets lowered in space. Ensure adequacy of hemoglobin and cardiac output. The tendency of air to expand at high altitude and exacerbate air leaks should be noted. Draining equipment should be readily available.
- Ensure the infant is well-strapped.

REFERRING CENTER RESPONSIBILITIES

- Ensure communication with the receiving unit. Based on clinical condition develop a treatment plan for stabilizing the patient, the optimal time, mode of transfer and transport personnel.
- Ensure that a bed is kept ready on arrival.
- Preparation and stabilization for transfer is the referring unit's responsibility.
- If the neonate is transported by the referring center, the referring health care provider is responsible for the patient until arrival at the receiving center.
- The referring center is responsible if the patient is being transported by its own team.
- If the transport team is from the receiving unit, the responsibility of the patient is with the team once it takes over the transport process.
- Consent forms must be obtained with parents counseled about the need for transfer.
- Parents should be encouraged to see and touch the infant and travel with the infant, if possible.
- Appropriate maternal/neonatal identification should be in place before transport.

RECEIVING CENTER RESPONSIBILITIES

- On arrival, assessment and stabilization of the neonate should be done and recorded.
- Verify the identification of the neonate before transport.
- Inform the parents on arrival the infant's condition, likely course, and possible intervention done or anticipated.
- Ensure the neonate's history, clinical interventions, and reports and investigations are received.
- Talk during ongoing transport with the team to anticipate problems on admission.
- The referral unit must be apprised of the progress and clinical outcome.

TRANSPORT TEAM RESPONSIBILITIES

- Note the summary of the patient regarding clinical condition, intervention, and investigations prior to transport.
- Anticipate, plan, and prepare for complications based on the clinical status.
- Ensure ongoing communication with the parents and receiving unit.

- Maintain records of the clinical status during transport.
- Hand over patient's records with forms filled appropriately.
- All untoward events should be recorded.
- Ensure all transport equipments are checked, drugs stocked and for next transport.

NEONATAL REFERRAL DOCUMENTATION

- Transfer sheets pre- and post-transport should be filled.
- The following documents should accompany the transported neonate:
    - Complete maternal prenatal record
    - Current maternal medical record
    - Current neonatal medical record
    - Any images in a format that can be reviewed by the receiving care team
    - Record of care during transport.

The referring center should maintain a record regarding disposition of transferred neonates.

Receiving Center Responsibilities

- Maintain a record of the transported neonate.
- Send a summary of care to the referring unit.

Legal Issues

- Ensure the parents are involved in decision making. Consent, documentation pre-, post- and during transport is must.
- If baby deteriorates during transport:
    - Stop the ambulance and initiate lifesaving measures including cardiopulmonary resuscitation (CPR).
    - Inform the parents and keep them updated on ongoing efforts.
- Professional indemnity insurance coverage is must for all team members.
- The ambulance should confirm to the regional transport authority norms.

APPENDIX: NEONATAL TRANSPORT EQUIPMENT

A. Organization and maintenance of neonatal transport equipment is the responsibility of the transporting facility.
B. Equipment to maintain a neutral thermal environment for the neonate should include:
   - Transport incubator
   - Thermometer
   - Blanket, insulating blanket, chemically-activated heat pack (appropriate for neonatal use), or plastic wraps.
C. The transport incubator should meet the following requirements:
   - Approved by the manufacturer for use during transport and installed in the transport vehicle with crashworthy restraints.
   - The equipment should comply with national safety standards. The transport incubator and monitoring equipment should not interfere with navigational instruments.
   - Have a heat source that requires minimal time for preheating and should maintain ambient temperature within the desired range of 29–36°C. The control for temperature setting should be readily accessible and easy to operate, and there should be provision for easy determination of ambient temperature. It is essential to have an alarm system that will recognize overheating or underheating.
   - Provide an environment in which the oxygen supply is constant and controllable.
   - Provide unrestricted visibility of the neonate with a functional independent

6. Leslie A, Stephenson T. Neonatal transfers by advanced neonatal nurse practitioners and paediatric registrars. Arch Dis Child Fetal Neonatal Ed. 2003;88(6):F509-12.
7. Shlossman PA, Manley JS, Sciscione AC, et al. An analysis of neonatal morbidity and mortality in maternal (in utero) and neonatal transports at 24–34 weeks' gestation. Am J Perinatol. 1997;14(8):449-56.
8. Stroud MH, Trautman MS, Meyer K, et al. Pediatric and neonatal interfacility transport: Results from a national consensus conference. Pediatrics. 2013;132(2):359-66.

CHAPTER 22

Abdominal Distension

Ashish Mehta

INTRODUCTION

Abdominal distension in neonates is associated with the spectrum of diseases, which extend from complete benign condition related to excessive crying to major surgical problem requiring emergency exploration. A timely referral to surgeon is important.

EVALUATION AND EXAMINATION

- History and clinical examination are important (Table 1).
- Abdominal examination should be done at least 1 hour after feed when baby is calm and relaxed. Normally, liver is palpable at least 2 cm below costal margin and lower poles of both kidneys are palpable in newborn.
- Abdominal distension in babies is mainly manifested by a protruding abdomen. There may be fullness or significant distension, unilateral or bilateral, localized or generalized. Note the mode of onset—acute, subacute, or chronic.

Common causes that will not require major investigation are:
- Aerophagia
- Excessive crying
- Continuous positive airway pressure (CPAP) belly while on ventilator.

Overall *approach to etiological diagnosis* is shown in Flowchart 1.

Causes of abdominal mass are summarized in Figure 1 and Table 2.

Abdomen distension related to gas (free gas/air-fluid levels): It can be due to pneumoperitoneum and intestinal obstruction.

Pneumoperitoneum

Perforation of any part of gastrointestinal (GI) tract can be due to poor bowel integrity [necrotizing enterocolitis (NEC) or localized perforation of any bowel segment due to ischemia], and excessive pressure (e.g. obstruction, tracheoesophageal fistula, instrumental) lead to pneumoperitoneum.

Intestinal Obstruction

It is divided into three parts.

1. Congenital Mechanical Obstruction

Intrinsic type includes atresia, stenosis, hypertrophic pyloric stenosis, cysts within bowel, imperforate anus.

Pyloric stenosis: Pyloric stenosis presents with nonbilious vomiting after age of 2–3 weeks. Sometimes, it is associated with jaundice

CHAPTER 22
Abdominal Distension

Table 1: Clinical approach to abdominal distension.

History	Significance
Gestation	Preterm infants are at risk for necrotizing enterocolitis. More the prematurity more the risk
Timing	Early onset (<24 hours of birth) indicates a surgical cause
Duration	• Acute onset suggests surgical cause. • Chronic duration suggests a local pathology, functional or metabolic cause
Associated complaints	• Vomiting, which is projectile, bilious, recurrent or bloody, is pathological. • Not passed stools in first 24 hours, inconsolable crying, not well between episodes, bleeding per rectum warrants search for underlying cause
Examination	**Significance**
Well or sick	• Well baby with abdominal distension has aerophagia or organomegaly. • Sick baby is likely to have a dynamic or adynamic obstruction
Position of umbilicus	• A mid-size position with distension suggests a generalized cause. • A downward shift of umbilicus suggests upper abdominal and an upward shift of umbilicus suggests a lower abdominal pathology. A transversely stretched umbilicus suggests free fluid
Per abdomen	Gastric residues (>50%), absent bowel sounds, is pathological
Perforation	Absent bowel sounds with unstable vital parameters and shock, tense shiny abdomen, transillumination positive

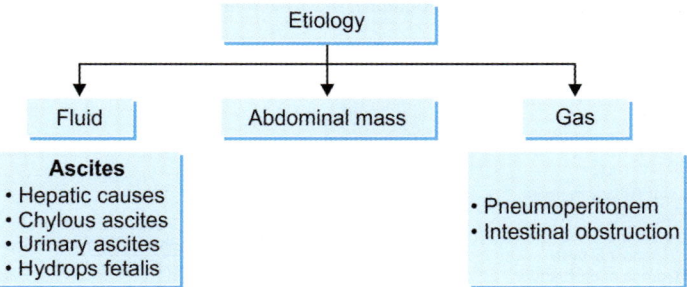

Flowchart 1: Approach to abdominal distention.

and hematemesis. X-ray abdomen shows large stomach with little or no gas below the duodenum. It is confirmed by USG.

Duodenal atresia: About 70% of duodenal atresia are associated with malformatione such as Down syndrome, GI and cardiac anomalies. It can be diagnosed prenatally by USG. History of polyhydramnios may be present. Baby presents with bilious vomiting after birth with upper abdomen distension. X-ray shows double-bubble appearance with no gas in large and small intestine.

Imperforated anus: About 50% of imperforated anus is associated with VACTERL anomalies. Baby may pass meconium if a rectovaginal or rectourinary fistula exists. A fistula is present in 80–90% of males and 95% of females.

Extrinsic type like peritoneal bands, aberrant vessels, hydrometrocolpos, duplication of the intestine also gives picture of obstruction with air-fluid levels and same symptomatology such as intrinsic obstruction.

Table 2: Abdomen distension related to abdominal mass.

Condition	Clinical features	Investigation	Management
Hydronephrosis	Palpable kidney and bladder, ascites may be present in severe cases	USG, IVP with MCU, blood urea and serum creatinine	Decompression of bladder and pelvis of kidney, corrective surgery after condition stabilizes
Wilms tumor	Usually unilateral may be associated with hemihypertrophy and aniridia	Urinalysis for hematuria, USG abdomen, IVP-distorted pelvicalyceal system	Avoid radiation therapy in the newborn period
Hemangioma of liver	Often a cause of unexplained hepatomegaly, it may be associated with a cutaneous hemangioma, bruit may be head over the liver.	• Thrombocytopenia may be present, USG, CT scan of abdomen, • Biopsy is contraindicated.	Large doses of steroids of, subtotal hepatectomy or ligation of hepatic artery
Neuroblastoma	Origin occurs in the adrenals and the tumor displaces the kidney downward and literally, the tumor might undergo spontaneous regression or may be malignant	Elevated VMA levels in urine, skeletal survey, bone marrow aspiration, IVP shows displacement of the kidney, calcification on plain X-ray abdomen, CT scan of abdomen to delineate tumor mass	Chemotherapy

(CT: computed tomography; IVP: intravenous pyelography; MCU: micturating cystourethrogram; USG: ultrasonography; VMA: vanillylmandelic acid)

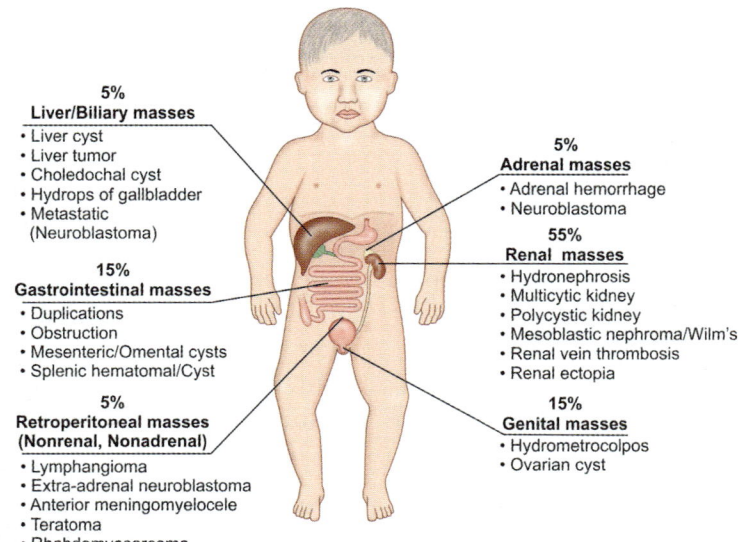

Fig. 1: Causes of abdominal mass.

2. Acquired Intestinal Obstruction

- *Malrotation with obstruction*: It may be associated with other congenital GI abnormalities such as annular pancreas, diaphragmatic hernia, and bowel atresia. Baby presents with bilious vomiting and may have passed normal stool. X-ray shows dilated bowel loops. Sign of shock and sepsis are often present, which at times misguides clinician for conservative or nonsurgical approach. Bilious emesis equals malrotation until proved otherwise.
- *Intussusceptions*: It is unusual in neonatal periods.
- *Peritoneal adhesions*: Due to meconium peritonitis, after abdominal surgery, idiopathic.
- Mesenteric thrombosis
- Strictures secondary to NEC
- Incarcerated inguinal hernia.

3. Functional Intestinal Obstruction

Immature bowel motility: It is mainly seen in extreme preterm babies, intrauterine growth restriction babies with compromised antenatal intestinal perfusion and in postsurgical babies.

Hirschsprung disease: It should be suspected in neonates who fail to pass meconium spontaneously by 24–48 hours after birth. Abdominal distension which develops is relieved by rectal stimulation. X-ray shows dilated bowel. Per rectal examination reveals giving in effect. Contrast enema may show transition zone. Rectal biopsy is the diagnostic investigation which shows absent of ganglion cells and hypertrophic nonmyelinated axons. Surgical intervention is required in form of colostomy (if enterocolitis or adequate decompression cannot be achieved) or primary pull-through procedure.

Paralytic ileus due to sepsis or by medication (narcotics or hypermagnesemia).

Meconium ileus: It is the most common cause of meconium peritonitis. X-ray shows air-fluid levels. About 99% of babies with meconium ileus have cystic fibrosis.

Decompression with continuous nasogastric (NG) suction will minimize further distension. Contrast enema can serve both diagnostic and therapeutic purpose. Surgical treatment is required, if the contrast enema fails to relive the obstruction.

Meconium plug syndrome: It develops in case of prematurity, sick and those with functional immaturity of the bowel with small left colon, seen in infant of diabetic mothers, Hirschsprung disease (rule out cystic fibrosis). Treatment is in the form of glycerine suppository, warm saline enema, and rectal stimulation.

MEDICAL MANAGEMENT OF BOWEL OBSTRUCTION

To manage bowel obstruction you should:
- Place the infant in an incubator for close observation and for temperature control
- Nurse supine with the head elevated
- Place an orogastric tube (8–10 FG). The amount and type (e.g. bile-stained, feculent) of fluid aspirated should be recorded
- Place nil by mouth
- Commence IV fluids. If signs of shock, may need fluid resuscitation with normal saline in 10–20 mL/kg aliquots. Give maintenance fluids plus mL for mL replacement of nasogastric aspirate with normal saline and 10 mmol KCl/500 mL
- Obtain abdominal X-rays (include supine and lateral decubitus view)

- Note that a relatively gasless abdomen is compatible with mid-gut volvulus
- It may be appropriate to commence antibiotics preferably after blood culture taken.
- Obtain blood for CBC, electrolytes, blood gas, and lactate (and blood cultures, if commencing antibiotics)
- Obtain a surgical consult.

Be aware that these infants frequently have associated problems of acidosis and shock.

SUGGESTED READING

1. Hutson JM, O'Brien M, Woodward AA, et al. Jones Clinical Paediatric Surgery: Diagnosis and Management, 6th edition. Blackwell Publishing; 2008.

CHAPTER 23

Apnea

Rhishikesh Thakre

DEFINITION

Apnea is clinically identified as:
- Pause in breathing of >20 seconds
- Pause in breathing associated with bradycardia or cyanosis.

Apnea Mimic

- Periodic breathing is a normal phenomenon in preterm. It is characterized by respiratory pauses >3 seconds duration with less than 20 seconds of breathing between pauses.
- Seizures presenting with apnea are associated with tachycardia.

WHAT IS THE CAUSE OF APNEA?

A thorough physical examination, the day of onset of symptoms, and basic laboratory investigations are essential in identifying the etiology of apnea (Table 1).

FIRST-LINE INVESTIGATIONS

Test	Rationale
Hb	Anemia or polycythemia
Sepsis screen	Suspected sepsis
Blood culture	Suspected bacterial infection

Contd...

Contd...

Test	Rationale
Cerebrospinal fluid study	Suspected meningitis or intracranial hemorrhage
Blood sugar	Hypoglycemia detection
Serum electrolytes	Electrolyte imbalance
Serum calcium	Detect hypocalcemia
USG skull	Intracranial hemorrhage or malformation

MANAGEMENT (FLOWCHART 1)

General

The Acute Apneic Episode

- Respond to the baby first and not to the alarm.

Table 1: Common causes of apnea.

Day 1–2	Day 3–6	Late
Hypothermia and hyperthermia		
Impending respiratory failure	Hypoglycemia, Hypocalcemia	Sepsis
Asphyxia	Sepsis	Fungemia
Sepsis	Impending respiratory failure	Anemia
Hypoglycemia	PDA	GER
Polycythemia	Massive IVH	NEC
	Apnea of prematurity	IEM

(GER: gastroesophageal reflux; IEM: inborn errors of metabolism; NEC: necrotizing enterocolitis; PDA: Patent ducuts arteriosus; IVH: intraventricular hemorrhage)

SECTION 1
Clinical Approach to Sick Newborn

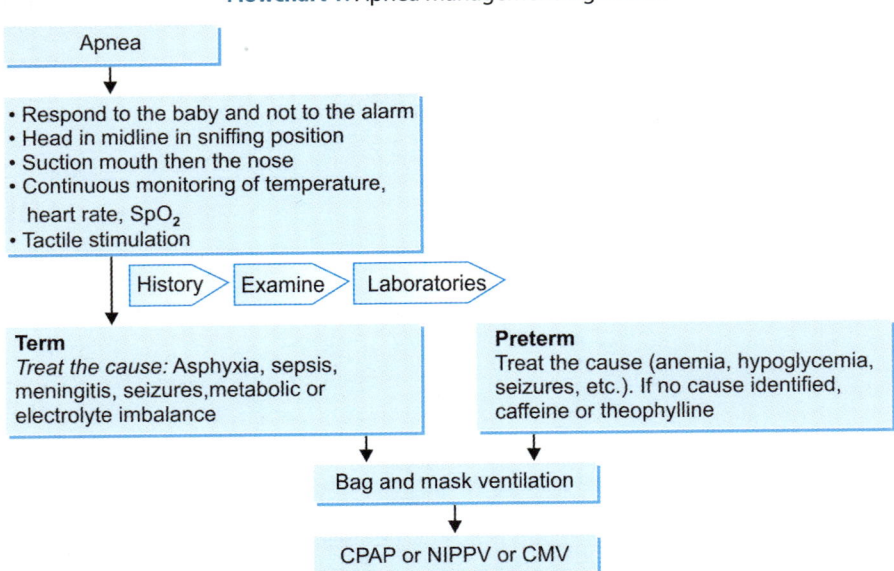

Flowchart 1: Apnea management algorithm.

(CPAP: continuous positive airway pressure; NIPPV: nasal intermittent positive pressure ventilation; CMV: cytomegalovirus).

- Ensure sniffing position. Avoid flexion or extension of neck.
- Stimulate the baby—tap the feet or cheek or rub the back.
- Suction first the mouth then nose. Avoid vigorous suction.
- Support ventilation with self-inflating bag, if still no response.
- Provide oxygen, 10% more than predeterioration stage.
- If still no response, initiate positive pressure ventilation.
- Look for clues on physical examination for the cause of apnea.

Stabilization of Apneic Infant
- Ensure normothermia. Avoid hypo- or hyperthermia. Nurse the infant in thermoneutral environment.
- Ensure ongoing monitoring with pulse oximeter.
- Ensure resuscitative equipment at the bedside.
- Ensure the infant on continuous cardio-respiratory monitor with alarm limits set.
- *Positioning*: Ensure the infant is kept in "sniffing" position. Prone or lateral position is preferred. Elevate the head end by 15–30°. If required place a roll below the shoulders to keep the airway patent.
- *Note*:
  - Blast of cold air during oxygen delivery is avoided. Ensure warm humidified gases.
  - Distension of stomach may come in the way of breathing. Ensure the stomach is aspirated.
  - Shift to orogastric tube. Nasogastric tube will further decrease the airway opening.
- Observe the infant during and after an apneic episode:
  - Assess temperature, color, cry, and activity.
  - Note the tone for limpness or flaccidity.
  - Neck position for "neutral" posture.
  - Note for change in HR or SpO_2 or both.

- Determine if there are any abnormal movements, change in color, eye movements or frothing.
- Note if there was any preceding intervention—insertion of feeding tube, suction, posture change, noise, etc.

SPECIFIC THERAPY

Apnea in Term Infant

Treatment of thermal instability, asphyxia, sepsis, meningitis, respiratory distress, seizures, hypoglycemia, metabolic or electrolyte imbalance or underlying cause relieves the symptoms.

Caffeine and methylxanthines are not of much use in term infants.

Apnea of Prematurity

- It is a diagnosis of exclusion. The incidence decreases with decreasing gestational age (Table 2).
- Pharmacologic interventions are indicated if the infant has 3 episodes of apnea within a 24 hour window that needs either stimulation or bag-mask ventilation.

Methylxanthines

Theophylline and caffeine are the drugs of choice for treatment of apnea in preterm infants. Caffeine has a longer half-life and is less toxic. Caffeine is preferred for the routine management of apnea of prematurity.

Table 2: Apnea and gestation.

Gestation	Incidence
<30 weeks	80%
30–31 weeks	54%
32–33 weeks	14%
>34 weeks	7%
Term	<2%

Table 3: Drugs for apnea of prematurity.

IV, PO	Aminophylline	Caffeine citrate
Loading dose	8 mg/kg	20–40 mg/kg
Maintenance dose	1.5–3 mg/kg/dose	5–8 mg/kg/dose
Dosing interval	q 8–12 hours	OD

Start: <10 days of life for <32 weeks or <1,250 g.
Stop: By 35 weeks of postmenstrual age.

Theophylline is a bronchodilator and in neonates with bronchopulmonary dysplasia (BPD) it offers the advantage of treating both apnea and bronchospasm (Table 3).

Caffeine Citrate

20 mg/mL containing the equivalent of 10 mg/mL of caffeine is available for either intravenous or oral use:
- *When:* <10 days of life.
- *Whom:* <32 weeks or <1250 g.
- *How long:* Till 35 weeks of postmenstrual age.
- *Plasma half-life:* 37–231 hours.
- *Therapeutic level:* 8–20 µg/mL.
- *Toxic level:* >30 µg/mL.

Theophylline

- *Plasma half-life*: 12–64 hours.
- *Therapeutic level:* 6–12 µg/mL.
- *Toxic level*: >20 µg/mL.
- *Administration*: Always infuse slowly over a minimum of 20 minutes. Rapid IV pushes have been associated with Sudden Death from Cardiac Arrhythmias (Table 4).

Doxapram

Doxapram is no longer preferred in apnea management due to concerns of: (A) Absence of evidence, (B) Need for IV infusion, and (C) Benzyl alcohol content with the drug which is known to displace bilirubin.

Table 4: Comparison of aminophylline and caffeine.

IV, PO	Aminophylline	Caffeine citrate
Loading dose	8 mg/kg	20–40 mg/kg
Maintenance dose	1.5–3 mg/kg/dose	5–8 mg/kg
Dosing interval	q 8–12 hours	OD
Side effects	Agitation, sleeplessness, irritability, seizures, feed intolerance, and hyperglycemia	Irritability

ENDPOINT OF TREATMENT

- Apnea free interval of at least 4–7 days
- 34 weeks+.

FAILURE OF MEDICATIONS

Continuous Positive Airway Pressure

Continuous positive airway pressure (CPAP) is initiated if the infant has spontaneous respiratory efforts. A CPAP pressure of 5 at FiO_2 of 0.5 is the usual starting support. CPAP merits continuous monitoring and good nursing support.

Nasal intermittent positive pressure ventilation (NIPPV) is another option to CPAP for noninvasive respiratory support.

Intermittent Mandatory Ventilation

Nonresponsiveness to medications or failure of CPAP may warrant intubation and positive pressure ventilation.

Criterion for Discharge

Apnea free for at least a week.

Areas of Uncertainty in Clinical Practice

- Kinesthetic stimulation for treating apnea in preterm infants.
- Prophylactic methylxanthine for prevention of apnea in preterm infants.
- The place of blood transfusion in treatment of apnea.
- Use of high flow oxygen by nasal cannulae.

Prognosis

Isolated apnea is not associated with a poor neurological outcome. Presence of comorbid conditions determines the outcome.

Implications for Practice

- Apnea is a sign and not a "diagnosis".
- Always search and treat the underlying cause.
- Apnea in term infants is rarely idiopathic.
- Apnea of prematurity is diagnosis of exclusion.
- All newborns less than 34 weeks gestational age are at risk for apnea and bradycardia.
- Respond to the baby and not to the alarm first.
- Unexplained apnea or recurrence suggests evaluation for pathology.
- Supportive care and evaluation of cause of apnea is must.
- Majority of apnea respond to medications. Ventilator support may be required for nonresponders.
- Continued follow-up is must.

SUGGESTED READING

1. Henderson-Smart DJ, Osborn DA. Kinesthetic stimulation for preventing apnea in preterm infants. Cochrane Database Syst Rev. 2002;(2):CD000373.
2. Henderson-Smart DJ, Steer P. Doxapram versus methylxanthine for apnea in preterm infants. Cochrane Database Syst Rev. 2000;(2):CD000075.
3. Henderson-Smart DJ, Steer PA. Doxapram treatment for apnea in preterm infants. Cochrane Database Syst Rev. 2004;(4):CD000074.
4. Henderson-Smart DJ, Steer PA. Prophylactic methylxanthine for preventing of apnea in preterm infants. Cochrane Database Syst Rev. 2000;(2):CD000432.
5. Henderson-Smart DJ, Subramaniam P, Davis PG. Continuous positive airway pressure versus theophylline for apnea in preterm infants. Cochrane Database Syst Rev. 2001;(4):CD001072.
6. Lemyre B, Davis PG, de Paoli AG. Nasal intermittent positive pressure ventilation (NIPPV) versus nasal continuous positive airway pressure (NCPAP) for apnea of prematurity. Cochrane Database Syst Rev. 2002;(1):CD002272.
7. Marchal F, Bairam A, Vert P. Neonatal apnea and apneic syndromes. Clin Perinatol. 1987;14(3):509-29.
8. Osborn DA, Henderson-Smart DJ. Kinesthetic stimulation for treating apnea in preterm infants. Cochrane Database Syst Rev. 2000;(2):CD000499.
9. Osborn DA, Henderson-Smart DJ. Kinesthetic stimulation versus theophylline for apnea in preterm infants. Cochrane Database Syst Rev. 2000;(2):CD000502.
10. Steer PA, Henderson-Smart DJ. Caffeine versus theophylline for apnea in preterm infants. Cochrane Database Syst Rev. 2000;(2):CD000273.

CHAPTER 24

Blistering Skin Disorders

Rhishikesh Thakre

INTRODUCTION

Epidermolysis bullosa (EB) is genetically inherited skin condition characterized by blister formation (0.5–1 cm) at site of skin friction due to fragile skin and mucous membrane.

MODE OF DELIVERY

Infants delivered via caesarean section have a lesser chance of skin injury. Assisted delivery leads to more skin injury compared to normal delivery. EB many a times has intrautero onset due to kicking activity. Presence of lesions in varying stages at birth suggests intrauterine origin.

CARE IN DELIVERY ROOM

Table 1 shows care in delivery room.

APPROACH TO EPIDERMOLYSIS BULLOSA (TABLE 2)

- Is skin or mucus membrane or nails involved?
- Is it localized or generalized?
- Are there severe lesions—scarring, pigmentation changes, cicatricial alopecia, absent or dystrophic nails, and mitten deformity of the hand or foot?
- Is there systemic involvement—eyes, teeth, gut, bones, muscles, urinary, or respiratory tract?

Two classical signs noted are:
1. *Koebner phenomenon*: Bleb formation on minimal trauma.
2. *Nikolsky's sign*: Skin breakdown on rubbing of the skin.

Table 1: Shows care in delivery room.

Care	Method	Rationale
Suction catheters	Soft. Minimal suction pressure	Vigorous suction erodes the mucosa. Scarring causes microstomia
Cord clamp	Use ligatures and not plastic clamps	Cord clamps irritate surrounding skin causing skin injury
Temperature	Avoid hyperthermia	Heat aggravates blistering. Aim for cool environment

Table 2: Identify the type of epidermolysis bullosa.

Type	Skin	Mucous membrane	Nail	Healing	Mode of inheritance
EB simplex	+	–	–	Bullae resolve without scarring and heal rapidly	AD
EB dystrophic	++	+	+	Leaving atrophic scars, Keloids and contractures	AR
EB junctional	+++	++	+	Denudation, scarring, and contractures Signs of GI/urinary obstruction and prenatal polyhydramnios	–

(AD: autosomal dominant; AR: autosomal recessive; EB: epidermolysis bullosa).

PRINCIPLES OF MANAGEMENT OF EPIDERMOLYSIS BULLOSA

- Skin care
- Avoidance of trauma
- Maintenance of fluids/electrolytes/nutrition
- Analgesia
- Help prevent contractures.

Skin Care

Open wounds are covered with nonadherent materials and extra padding is provided at sharp edges to prevent skin injury. Blisters are stuck with a sterile needle to avoid fluid accumulation and preventing the blister from spreading further. The affected area is covered with gauze of white petrolatum and fluid allowed to drain by gravity.

Bacitracin or silver sulfadiazine is applied daily for care of open or partially healed wounds. These are covered with gauze impregnated with white petrolatum.

Soft clothing for the infant is preferred as it reduces self-inflicted damage. White petrolatum is used liberally as it is a softening agent. Hands and feet are covered with socks and gloves.

Any erosion near the perineal area is treated with local application of a 50% white soft paraffin and 50% liquid paraffin mixture.

Handling Babies

Gentle handling and minimal handling is the key. Place the infant on a soft cloth such as a folded towel. Cover the intravenous (IV) line with gauze piece. Instead of rubbing the skin prior to blood collection or injections, prefer swabbing. Avoid pressure and traction during vein puncture to prevent skin injury or de-gloving. Use padded splints and ensure the edges are short and soft.

Suspecting Skin Infection

Features to suggest skin infection are:
- Features of cellulites (redness, discharger, or tenderness)
- Lymphangitis
- Presence of yellowish crusts or pus
- Fever.

Cultures should always be taken with suspected skin infection, followed by oral antibiotics.

Feeding

Oral feeding are preferred and promoted. Avoid frequent change of feeding tubes. Failure to thrive, feeding difficulty, constipation, anemia, and/or vitamin deficiencies are common nutritional problems experienced by EB patients.

Table 3: Multidisciplinary care.		
Ophthalmology	**Gastroenterologist**	**Plastic**
For conjunctivitis, blepharitis, corneal erosions or ulcerations, and ectropion	For esophageal strictures	For contractures or deformities
A speech therapist for communication delay	Dentist to prevent destruction or loss of teeth	Physical and occupational therapists

IMPORTANCE OF NAIL INVOLVEMENT

- Dystrophy and loss of the nails is a feature of autosomal recessive form of EB dystrophic form. Post healing, scars, keloids, and contractures are common.
- Mucous membranes and nails are usually not affected in EB simplex, an autosomal dominant form. Bullae resolve without scarring and heal rapidly.

INVESTIGATIONS

Immunofluorescence mapping, using EB-specific antibodies, and mutational analysis are required for subtyping of EB. Light microscopy helps to exclude other blistering diseases.

Initial severity of skin problem does not indicate later outcome.

Long-term consequences are related to scar formation, contractures, and deformity causing disability and loss of function. Multidisciplinary care is required (Table 3).

SUGGESTED READING

1. Cohn HI, Teng JM. Advancement in management of epidermolysis bullosa. Curr Opin Pediatr. 2016;28(4):507-16.
2. Watkins J. Diagnosis, treatment and management of epidermolysis bullosa. Br J Nurs. 2016;25(8):428-31.

CHAPTER 25

Systemic Fungal Infections

Rhishikesh Thakre, Srinivas Murki

INTRODUCTION

Fungal infection in general and *Candida* species in particular is one of the most common causes of late onset sepsis in newborns. Preterm infants and sick term infants in neonatal intensive care units (NICUs) are at increased risk for invasive fungal infection.

CANDIDA SPECIES

Candida organisms are saprophytic yeasts and normal constituents of microbial flora. Pseudohyphae formation is characteristic of candida and responsible for invasive nature. *Candida albicans* is the most common species. *Candida parapsilosis* is responsible for nosocomially acquired infection (central line infection), and other species such as *Candida stellatoidea, Candida lusitaniae, Candida krusei,* and *Candida glabrata* are rarely reported. Any *Candida* species may cause disease in neonates but certain risk factors predispose to fungemia (Table 1).

CLINICAL MANIFESTATIONS

Clinical manifestations vary depending on the site and severity of infection (Box 1). The clinical picture of systemic fungemia mimics bacterial

Table 1: Risk factors for candidiasis.

Gestational age <32 weeks	Umbilical catheters
Birth weight ≤1,500 g	Peripheral or central venous catheters
Apgar score <5 at 5 minutes	Abdominal surgery
Intubation/mechanical ventilation	Use of intralipid/TPN
Prolonged administration of antibiotics	Corticosteroid use
Use of broad-spectrum antibiotic (cephalosporin's)	

(TPN: total parenteral nutrition)

Box 1: Clues to fungal infection.
- Ashen gray skin complexion
- Indolent clinical course
- Persistently elevated C-reactive protein
- New-onset or persistent thrombocytopenia
- Sepsis with negative blood culture

sepsis. Symptoms are often more subtle and indolent. Among these, respiratory distress and apnea are the most common presenting signs. A significant proportion of neonates will present simultaneously with localized signs viz. pneumonia, meningitis, renal tract infection, ophthalmitis, osteomyelitis, endocarditis, liver abscesses, and skin abscesses. In majority of neonatal candidiasis two or more organs are affected at the time of presentation.

DIAGNOSIS

The gold standard for candidemia is positive culture for candida from normally sterile body fluid. Candida grows by 48–72 hours of incubation in routine blood culture bottle requiring no special media. Presence of Candida in wounds, skin, urine, or stool specimens is not diagnostic of disease. Culture negative fungemia is known. Overgrowth of bacteria on nonselective media can easily inhibit or hide the growth of fungi. Selective culture media can be made inhibitory to bacteria by maintaining a low pH (e.g. Sabouraud dextrose agar) or by including antibacterial agents in the media (e.g. gentamicin and chloramphenicol). Polymerase chain reaction testing is increasingly used in the diagnosis of fungal meningitis.

Screening for Disseminated Disease

Persistent symptoms, isolation of candidemia beyond 5 days of initiation of therapy, should prompt screening for disseminated disease (Box 2). Presence of dissemination alters the duration of treatment, risk of complication, and prognosis.

Box 2
Screening tests for systemic candidiasis.
- Culture of blood, urine, and cerebrospinal fluid
- Indirect ophthalmoscopy evaluation of the retina
- Echocardiographic evaluation of the heart
- Renal ultrasound
- Abdominal ultrasound focusing on liver for target lesions

Consequences of Missed or Delayed Diagnosis

Inappropriate treatment results in increased rates of intraventricular hemorrhage, chronic lung disease, retinopathy of prematurity requiring surgery, and increased risk of neurodevelopmental delay. The risk of mortality with invasive candidiasis is three times higher than that of uninfected infants of similar gestational age and birth weight. Untreated, the mortality exceeds 80%.

TREATMENT

Empiric Treatment

There is lack of evidence for routine empiric treatment. In some situations, empiric antifungal therapy for 48–72 hours may be considered in infants with thrombocytopenia (<100,000/cmm) or necrotizing enterocolitis or focal bowel perforation or weight of less than 750 g or <26 weeks gestation.

Definitive Treatment (Table 2)

Isolation of candida from sterile site warrants definitive therapy.

Amphotericin B is the drug of choice for invasive fungal infections. It is effective against most Candida species except for *C. lusitaniae*. Lipid formulations of amphotericin B offer no advantage over conventional form and its use should be restricted to patients who are refractory or intolerant to regular amphotericin B preparation. Amphotericin B should always be given in an infusion diluted with dextrose over few hours.

Flucytosine as a monotherapy is not used because of its innate ability to develop resistance. There is no parental preparation available.

Table 2: Antifungal agents.

Drug	Dose	Toxicity	Comments
Amphotericin B	1 mg/kg/day q 24 h IV	Anemia, hypokalemia, nephrotoxicity	Monitor blood urea nitrogen, creatinine, and K^+ daily initially and twice weekly if stable after 1 week; hold dose until K^+ <3 mEq/dL is corrected. Dilute in dextrose only and give infusion over 2–4 hr.
Lipid formulations of amphotericin B	3–7 mg/kg/day q 24 h IV	Less nephrotoxic than amphotericin B	Monitor renal function and K^+ as above
Flucytosine	50–150 mg/kg/day q 6 h PO	Bone marrow suppression, hepatotoxicity, and gastrointestinal symptoms	Good penetration into cerebrospinal fluid (CSF); must reduce dosage in patients with renal failure
Fluconazole	Loading 25 mg/kg f/b 12 mg/kg/day q 24 h PO, IV	Good penetration into CSF	Drug interaction with cytochrome P-450 system
Itraconazole	5 mg/kg/day q 24 h PO		Limited experience

Fluconazole is both safe and effective for invasive fungal infections. Up to half of *C. glabrata* and almost all of *C. krusei* isolates have been reported to be resistant to fluconazole.

Newer agents like caspofungin, voriconazole and posaconazole are not approved for newborn use.

Duration of Treatment

Treatment usually is continued for at least 14 days after the last positive blood-culture result in the absence of disseminated disease. Prolonged antifungal therapy (6 weeks) is recommended for disseminated candidiasis, endocarditis, endophthalmitis, and osteomyelitis.

Monitoring Laboratory Parameters during Treatment

- Liver and renal function at the time of diagnosis.
- Serum electrolytes and the hematologic, hepatic, and renal systems should be monitored weekly during treatment.
- In patients with persistent fungemia of more than 5 days, possibility of abscess formation should be ruled out.
- Persistent thrombocytopenia may indicate therapeutic failure.

Antifungal Prophylaxis

There is insufficient evidence for routine use of prophylactic oral antifungal agents in very low birth weight babies. NICUs with high rate of infection and those with large populations of <1000 g infants, prophylaxis may be considered. The major concern with fluconazole prophylaxis is the risk of emergence of resistance over time, and this issue is being evaluated. Best preventive practices are depicted in Box 3.

Malassezia furfur

This frequently affects babies receiving intralipid through a central venous catheter. Predominant lung involvement is characteristic and involvement of other organ systems is uncommon. Removal of indwelling central

Box 3: Good practices to reduce fungal infections.
- Increased compliance with hand hygiene standards
- Improved accuracy of the diagnosis of bacteremia
- Reduced line and line connection (hub) bacterial contamination
- Maximal barrier precautions for central line placement
- Improve nursing practices to maintain skin integrity. Avoid skin abrasions
- Decreased number of skin punctures
- Decreased duration of IV lipid infusion
- Decreased duration of central venous line use
- Early enteral nutrition preferably by breast milk
- Remove a central venous catheter on suspicion of severe fungal infection or within 24 hours of a positive culture for fungus
- Avoid use of antacids as increased gastric pH favors fungal colonization
- Use narrowest spectrum antibiotics possible
- Reduce duration of antibiotics. Stop antibiotics if cultures negative
- Use HEPA filtration ventilation systems and take measures for containment of dust, especially during hospital renovation and construction

(HEPA: high efficiency particulate air; IV: intravenous)

catheters and omitting intralipid along with amphotericin B resolves the infection.

Aspergillosis

Ventilation system contamination is a predisposing factor. It manifests as rapid necrotic eschar formation at injured skin areas. Demonstrating septate hyphae with 45° angles is characteristic of *Aspergillus* species.

SUGGESTED READING

1. Greenberg RG, Benjamin DK Jr. Neonatal candidiasis: diagnosis, prevention, and treatment. J Infect. 2014;69(Suppl 1):S19-22.
2. Kelly MS, Benjamin DK Jr, Smith PB. The epidemiology and diagnosis of invasive candidiasis among premature infants. Clin Perinatol. 2015;42(1):105-17, viii-ix.
3. Rios JF, Camargos PA, Corrêa LP, et al. Fluconazole prophylaxis in preterm infants: a systematic review. Braz J Infect Dis. 2017;21(3):333-8.

SECTION 2

Care of Well Newborn

SECTION OUTLINE

26. Evaluation in Delivery Room
27. First Evaluation in Outpatient Department
28. Growth Monitoring
29. Newborn Metabolic Screening
30. Vitamin K
31. Not Passed Urine in the First 48 Hours
32. Not Passed Stools in the First 48 Hours
33. Direct Jaundice
34. Congenital Hydronephrosis
35. Common Problems in Newborn in Outpatient Department
36. Optimizing Breastfeeding in a Normal Newborn
37. Golden Hour Care for Preterm
38. Colic

CHAPTER 26

Evaluation in Delivery Room

Deepak Pande

INTRODUCTION

The evaluation of newborn in the delivery room begins prior to birth. This involves the following:
- Formation of the team, team-briefing, delegation of responsibilities
- A focused history of the mother
- Assessment of risk factors
- Estimation of gestation (single or multiple, term or preterm) and the expected birth weight
- Antenatal counseling
- Preparation for resuscitation (environment, equipment, and personnel).

Postnatal evaluation of the newborn includes:
- Assessing the need for resuscitation (and provide resuscitation as per standard guidelines)
- Provision of preventive care: 6 cleans, cord clamping, thermal care, cord care, eye care, administration of vitamin K, and early initiation of exclusive breastfeeding
- Early skin to skin contact and exclusive breastfeeding
- Assessing gestation, birth weight, and stratifying level of care for the newborn
- Complete physical evaluation for malformation
- Ongoing assessment for danger signs
- Parental counseling.

Special interventions are needed for preterm care and are discussed elsewhere.

PREPARATION BEFORE BIRTH

Maternal History

Age
- Maternal age less than 18 years and advanced maternal age (>35 years) are risk factors for fetal growth restriction and for preterm birth.
- In younger age mothers, the newborn is at risk of neglect and abuse. With advanced maternal age, the risk of chromosomal abnormalities increases.

Medical Conditions
See Table 1.

Socioeconomic History
- Neonate born in a poor family is at increased risk of morbidity and mortality due to lack of access to affordable healthcare in addition to other risks.
- History of smoking, alcohol, or drug abuse in the mother can lead to specific problems

Table 1: Maternal medical conditions affecting the fetus.

Medical condition	Risk to the fetus-newborn	What to look for
Pregestational diabetes	Congenital malformations, macrosomia, birth injury, respiratory distress, hypoglycemia, polycythemia	Pregestation control of diabetes Diabetes control in the last trimester Drugs the mother was taking
Hypertension	IUGR, prematurity, asphyxia	Control of hypertension and the drugs (some drugs like ACE inhibitors and beta-blockers have effect on the fetus/newborn)
Thyroid disease	Hypothyroidism, hyperthyroidism, goiter	Maternal antibody status and drugs
Congenital/acquired heart disease	Congenital heart disease, IUGR	Fetal echocardiography, newborn screen for critical CHD
Connective tissue disease (SLE)	Congenital heart block, IUGR, prematurity	Fetal heart rate, maternal antibodies

(ACE: angiotensin-converting-enzyme; CHD: congenital heart disease; SLE: systemic lupus erythematosus; IUGR: intrauterine growth restriction)

in the newborn like fetal alcohol syndrome or drug withdrawal.

Past Obstetric History

The relevant history should be elicited with specific emphasis on congenital malformations or genetic disorders, breastfeeding, neonatal illness including hyperbilirubinemia, immunization, and developmental history of the siblings.

Antenatal History

Any deviations from the normal in the current pregnancy need to be noted including assisted reproductive techniques (especially donor gametes or surrogacy). Definite information which should be sought for includes:
- Fever with or without rash
- Multiple pregnancy
- Bleeding in early pregnancy
- Immunizations during pregnancy and preconception
- Urinary tract infection
- Medications used during pregnancy
- Blood group and indirect Coombs test status (if mother Rh negative)
- Screening tests done—ultrasound/Doppler, fetal echocardiography, biochemical screen for aneuploidy, amniocentesis, and chorionic villous sampling
- Fetal interventions—if any (like intrauterine transfusions).

Intrapartum Risk Factors

The major emphasis is on eliciting risk factors for asphyxia (need for resuscitation) and the risk of early-onset sepsis (Boxes 1 and 2).

In addition to the abovementioned risk factors, risks associated with the mode of delivery and type of anesthesia/analgesia also need to be considered. Elective cesarean without labor may increase the risk of transient tachypnea; use of general anesthesia may increase the need for resuscitation.

Preparing for Resuscitation

It is important to prepare, in advance, for resuscitation, in every delivery, as half the times asphyxia may occur without presence of any risk factor. The following general principles should be adopted for the preparation:

- All resuscitations should be conducted under strict asepsis.
- All resuscitation apparatus should be clean and sterile and where indicated, disposable.

> **Box 1: Maternal risk factors for early-onset neonatal sepsis.**
>
> - Confirmed or suspected invasive bacterial infection in mother (such as septicemia) at any time during labor, or in the 24-hour period before or after birth
> - Prelabor rupture of membranes
> - Spontaneous preterm labor (before 37 weeks of gestation)
> - Suspected or confirmed rupture of membranes for more than 18 hours
> - Intrapartum fever higher than 38°C
> - Confirmed or suspected chorioamnionitis
> - Multiple/unsterile per vaginal examination

> **Box 2: Intrapartum risk factors for asphyxia/need for resuscitation.**
>
> - Nonreassuring fetal heart rate pattern
> - Meconium stained amniotic fluid
> - Antepartum hemorrhage
> - Eclampsia/severe pre-eclampsia
> - Prolonged labor
> - Instrumental vaginal delivery
> - Maternal narcotic administration

- Delivery room temperature needs to be maintained between 25°C and 28°C; such temperature should be reached before the delivery, and maintained throughout the time the newborn is in the delivery room.
- Every delivery needs to be attended by a person skilled in neonatal resuscitation but if one or more risk factors are present, at least two skilled persons, out of whom at least one should be skilled in all the steps (including endotracheal intubation, umbilical vein cannulation, and administration of medications), should be present. For more difficult situations like extreme prematurity or diaphragmatic hernia, more number of skilled persons may be required, and so need to be informed in advance. In multiple gestations, number of persons required should be at least two per fetus.
- A list of equipment required for resuscitation should be available in the resuscitation corner and checked before delivery, not only to confirm their availability, but also to ascertain their proper functioning (Table 2).

Table 2: Neonatal resuscitation equipment checklist.

To be checked before each delivery		
Radiant warmer	Switched on, heating checked	
Baby receiving set—opened	3 sheets/towels, 1 baby cap—prewarm by placing them under radiant warmer	
	2 pads, 5 gauze pieces, scissors, bowl	
Suction	Tubing, Y-piece and 10 or 12 F catheter attached	
	Pressure checked (80–100 mm Hg)	
Suction catheters	6 F, 10 F, 14 F	2 each
Meconium aspirator		1
de Lee suction trap		1
Oxygen tubing attached to flow meter	Flow meter set at 10 L/min	1
Pulse oximeter with probe	Functioning checked, probe detached	1
Self-inflating bag/ T-piece resuscitator	Mask attached (depending on baby size)	1
	Functioning checked	

Contd...

SECTION 2
Care of Well Newborn

Contd...

To be checked before each delivery		
Face mask (term and preterm)		1 each
Oxygen reservoir	Checked and detached	
Feeding tube	8 F	1
Laryngoscope (blade 0 and 1)	Cleaned and checked	
Extra bulb, dry cells for laryngoscope		
Endotracheal tubes	2.5 mm, 3.0 mm, and 3.5 mm	2 each
Waterproof tape for fixing endotracheal tubes	Cut to size	2
Stethoscope (with neonatal head)	Check functioning	1
Inj. Adrenaline (1:1,000)	Prefilled, labeled 1:10,000 solution	2
Normal saline: 100 mL		1
Surgical blade		1
Umbilical catheter 4 F and 5 F		1 each
3-way stopcock		2
Syringes	1, 2, 5, 10, 20 mL	2 each
Gloves	6.5, 7.0 and 7.5	2 each
Neoflon 24 G		2
Tegaderm		2
Inj. Vitamin K1	Prefilled	1
Cord clamp		2
EDTA vial (small)	Labeled	1
Inj. Heparin (10 units/mL)		1
3-lead ECG monitor and leads		1 set
Clean plastic bag or plastic wrap	(for <32 weeks gestation)	1
Chest tube bag		1
Cheat drainage needle with trocar		1
Incision and drainage tray		1

POSTNATAL CARE OF NEWBORN

- *Assessing the need for resuscitation*: Once the baby is born, immediately evaluate the baby for the need of resuscitation, and proceed as per the resuscitation algorithm.
- For babies requiring resuscitation, some salient points to be remembered at all times.
    - Ensure that the baby's temperature is maintained in the euthermic range during and after resuscitation. Prevent hypothermia as well as hyperthermia.
    - Vigorous babies born through meconium stained amniotic fluid do not need tracheal suction.
    - Positive pressure ventilation (PPV) (with bag and mask, or T-piece resuscitator) is the most important step in neonatal resuscitation.

CHAPTER 26
Evaluation in Delivery Room

- Immediately after initiating PPV, check for rising heart rate (else chest rise with each positive pressure breath). If heart rate is not rising, immediately initiate Ventilation Corrective Steps (MR SOPA).
- Initiate PPV whenever required with room air in term babies and approximately 40% oxygen for preterm babies. Gradually increase oxygen if baby is not improving by looking at oxygen in the pulse oximeter which is an important adjunct in babies undergoing resuscitation.
- Target preductal SpO_2 values are as follows:
    - 60–65% at 1 minute
    - 65–70% at 2 minutes
    - 70–75% at 3 minutes
    - 75–80% at 4 minutes
    - 80–85% at 5 minutes
    - 85–95% at 10 minutes of birth.
- The most sensitive indicator, of a successful response to each step, is an increase in heart rate.
- During resuscitation, assess the improvement using the parameters of respiratory rate and heart rate. Such assessment should be made every 30 seconds during PPV, and every 60 seconds during coordinated chest compressions with PPV.
- Epinephrine needs to be repeated every 3–5 minutes, if heart rate remains below 60 beats/min despite adequate ventilation. Repeat doses of epinephrine should be given by IV route only, and not by endotracheal route.
- 10 mL/kg (intravenous or intraosseous, over 5–10 minutes) of normal saline or O negative blood can be used as volume expanders, when indicated.
- Failure of the baby to improve despite appropriate resuscitation should prompt the search for refractory cases like pneumothorax, congenital airway or lung malformation, congenital heart disease, severe metabolic acidosis or even hypoglycemia and sepsis.

Best Preventive Care Practices

- *The six cleans*: Clean hands of the birth attendant, clean surface, clean blade, clean cord tie, clean towels to dry the baby and then wrap the baby, clean cloth to wrap the mother.
- *Temperature of the neonate*: It should be recorded, and maintained between 36.5°C and 37.5°C.
- *Cord clamping:* It should be delayed for at least 1 minute (clamp between 1 and 3 minutes) in both, term and preterm babies not requiring resuscitation.
- *Cord care:* The cord should be kept dry. There is no need for routine application of antiseptic.
- *Eye care*: Both eyes should be cleaned, with separate, sterile gauze or cotton pieces, soaked in saline, from medial to lateral side, without application of any pressure.
- *Sterile linen*: All linen used to place, to dry, and to cover the baby, should be sterile.
- *Sterile equipment, consumables*: All equipment used for the baby should be sterile, and the consumables used should be single-use disposables, and sterile.
- *Administration of vitamin K*: It may be done immediately after birth or after the first feed. The dose is 0.5 mg for preterm, and 1 mg for term infants, given intramuscular in the anterolateral thigh.

Complete Head-to-toe Physical Evaluation

A quick survey should also be made to look for birth injuries, especially Erb's palsy in difficult deliveries, and any cuts or major bleeding. A head-to-toe evaluation is done to assess for presence of gross congenital malformations that may mandate admission to neonatal intensive care unit (NICU). Such malformations include, but are not limited to, neural tube defects, abdominal wall defects, ambiguous genitalia, anorectal malformations, trachea-esophageal fistula, and diaphragmatic hernia.

Minor congenital abnormalities like ear tags, cleft lip or palate, syndactyly or polydactyly may be noted, and parents counseled, for caring for the same.

> **Box 3** Indications for admission to NICU/SNCU.
>
> - Birth weight < 1,800 g
> - Gestational age < 34 completed weeks
> - Need for resuscitation after delivery—positive-pressure ventilation for >1 minute, use of chest compression or drugs, respiratory distress of tachypnea (rate > 60/min) persisting for >30 minutes, persistent cyanosis (saturation inappropriate for age)
> - Major congenital malformation—diagnosed or suspected
> - LGA, infant of diabetic mother
>
> (NICU: neonatal intensive care unit; SNCU: Special newborn care unit; LGA: Large for gestational age)

Early Skin-to-skin Contact and Exclusive Breastfeeding

All efforts should be made to establish early skin-to-skin contact between the mother and the baby in the delivery room, as soon as feasible, following the delivery. Early initiation of breastfeeding in the delivery room itself, and exclusive breastfeeding, should be promoted and advocated.

Assessing Gestation, Birth Weight, and Stratify Level of Care for the Newborn

A clinical estimate of the gestation should be made based on physical evaluation (Parkins score) to assign approximate gestation. The baby should be weighed (in the first hour after birth) and intrauterine growth status [small for gestational age (SGA), appropriate for gestational age (AGA), and large for gestational age (LGA)] determined.
- *Routine care*: Routine care is recommended for all newborns who established spontaneous respiration and/or cry at birth, have stable vital parameters and have no abnormality on physical examination.
- *Observational care*: Observational care is recommended for "at risk" newborns who need supervision and monitoring (SGA, LGA, infant of diabetic mother, brief PPV <1 minute) for babies requiring blood glucose monitoring, a specific order should be written in the case sheet regarding the timings and need for intervention.
- *Indications for admission to NICU*: Immediately after birth, the indications may be as shown in Box 3 (These may vary from unit to unit, and all units must make a uniform policy for admissions).

Ongoing Assessment for Danger Signs

Presence of hypothermia, hypoglycemia, decreased feeding, decreased activity, chest indrawing, seizures, jaundice in first 24 hours, should warrant detailed evaluation and specific management.

Parental Counseling

Every effort should be made to ensure implementation of thermal wellbeing, breastfeeding, cleanliness, and infection prevention practices throughout the neonatal period, and vaccination, recognition by parents and timely reporting by them for danger signs to the healthcare provider, and follow-up at scheduled time.

POTENTIAL HARMFUL PRACTICES IN DELIVERY ROOM

- Routine passage of naso- or orogastric catheter or feeding tube, to diagnose esophageal atresia with or without trachea esophageal fistula should not be done in lieu of poor sensitivity of the procedure. Only in babies with antenatal suspicion of esophageal atresia, associated congenital malformation, polyhydramnios in the mother, and excessive oral secretions in the newborn, should this be done.
- Routine gastric lavage for babies born through meconium-stained amniotic fluid is also not recommended.
- Routine suction of mouth and throat is not recommended for the potential hazards of trauma, infection, mucosal injury, pain, vagal nerve stimulation, and apnea. Suction is restricted to obvious obstruction to spontaneous breathing or for infants requiring positive-pressure ventilation.
- In nonvigorous babies born with meconium stained amniotic fluid, routine intubation for tracheal suction is not recommended. However, endotracheal intubation for suction of the airway may be used as needed on a case to case basis, for ensuring adequacy of oxygenation and ventilation.
- An examination of the placenta and cord is desirable.

SUGGESTED READING

1. Dempsey E, Pammi M, Ryan AC, et al. Standardised formal resuscitation training programs for reducing mortality and morbidity in newborn infants. Cochrane Database Syst. Rev. 2015;(9):CD009106.
2. Saugstad OD. Delivery room management of term and preterm newly born infants. Neonatology. 2015;107(4): 365-71.
3. Schmölzer GM, Kumar M, Pichler G, et al. Non-invasive versus invasive respiratory support in preterm infants at birth: systematic review and meta-analysis. BMJ. 2013;347:f5980.
4. Singh Y, Oddie S. Marked variation in delivery room management in very preterm infants. Resuscitation. 2013;84(11):1558-61.
5. Wyckoff MF, Aziz K, Escobedo MB, et al. Part 13: Neonatal Resuscitation: 2015. American Heart Association Guidelines Update for Cardiopulmonary Resuscitation and Emergency Cardiovascular Care. Circulation. 2015;132(18 Suppl 2):S543-60.
6. Wyllie J, Bruinenberg J, Roehr CC, et al. European Resuscitation Council Guidelines for Resuscitation 2015: Section 7. Resuscitation and support of transition of babies at birth. Resuscitation. 2015;95:249-63.

CHAPTER 27

First Evaluation in Outpatient Department

LS Deshmukh

Newborn exams have remained unchanged for years, just the diagnoses have improved to protect the innocent.

KEY POINTS

- History taking remains an active element of the neonatal examination. Without it, the clinical validity of the examination itself could indeed be negligible.
- Parental concern during the examination should be addressed.
- The history profile must be factual, accurate, concise, informative, and relevant.
- The baby should be examined within a thermal neutral environment, postfeed, and observed lying quietly in the supine position.
- The exact sequence in which the newborn is examined is not important. What is important is that all aspects of the newborn are examined at some stage and that the entire infant is observed.
- Maximum information is gained by observation. Initial impressions of the infant in a quiet state should be recorded followed by a systematic examination.

EQUIPMENT REQUIRED

- Stethoscope
- Measuring tape
- Infantometer
- Spatula
- Ophthalmoscope
- Appropriate growth charts.

Follow the art of clinical examination:
- Look (inspection)
- Feel (palpation)
- Listen (auscultation)
- Tap if necessary (percussion).

FIVE STEPS OF EVALUATION

1. *Preparation*:
   - Wash and warm hands
   - Gather equipment
   - Read case notes
   - Listen to mother/caretaker.
2. *Observations*:
   - Listen to the baby
   - Listen to the mother
   - Watch baby's behavior.
3. *Examination*:
   - Baby dressed
   - Baby undressed.

CHAPTER 27
First Evaluation in Outpatient Department

4. *Explanation*:
   - Findings conveyed and discussed with the mother.
5. *Documentation*:
   - Examination and action documented.

IMPORTANT CONSIDERATIONS IN HISTORY

- Family history
- Maternal medical problems
- Maternal blood tests
- Fetal scan results
- Antenatal details
- Risk factors for infection
- Details of labor
- Social history.

Check baby's notes for:
- Resuscitation details
- Birth weight
- Condition of baby since birth (i.e. feeding, passed urine/meconium).

What must be Considered and Examined during Examination of the Newborn?

Problems Anticipated from the History

- The antenatal booking visit presents an opportunity to elicit specific issues in the family history relevant to the new baby as well as those relevant to the mother and the pregnancy. For example, a family history of hearing impairment, cardiac abnormality, developmental dysplasia of the hips, or developmental problems in sibling are all risk factors.

Problems Arising in the Current Pregnancy

- Issues may have arisen during the pregnancy which require special consideration following the birth, for example, poor fetal growth.

Problems Arising at Birth

- Some issues, which are potential risk factors for the baby, may arise in labor.

SEQUENCE OF EXAMINATION

- The sequence in which the various features of the examination are assessed is not that important. Emphasis should be on a thorough evaluation. Regardless of the system used, it is best to assess observations by the amount of disturbance they produce.

  Infant evaluations that cause the least disturbance should be done first. The examiner may then proceed to the more disturbing maneuvers that are not so dependent on a quiet state for accurate interpretation.

Important: Before undressing the baby, concentrate on the exposed parts of the body.

Inspection without Contact

- A considerable amount of information is available by simply looking at an infant (Table 1).

Table 1: Observing the newborn.

Size	Preterm, term, small or large, IUGR
Color	Pink, pale, plethora, jaundice, cyanosis
Cry	High pitched, ill sustained, weak, absent, lusty
Activity	Spontaneous, induced, symmetry
Breathing	Regular, shallow, indrawing, grunt
Posture	Normal, hypotonia, hypertonia
Urine/Stool	Color, odor
Anomaly	Clefts, dysmorphism, absence or hypoplasia, swelling
Breastfeeding	Attachment, adequacy
Sounds	Grunt, stridor, gurgling
Umbilical cord	Moisture, dryness, smell, discharge, swelling

(IUGR: intrauterine growth restriction)

- When first approaching the infant, the examiner should not abruptly place a stethoscope on the infant's chest before doing anything else.
- The infant's overall size, color, and contour are immediately apparent, as is the relative size of the head, extremities, and trunk.
- Initial visual inspection can be of value in obtaining information about the intrauterine environment. The small term suggests hypertonicity. If only one arm is consistently straight and the infant does not flex that extremity, brachial plexus injury must be considered.
- Breech presentations are often identified by the characteristic positions of the lower extremities (discussed later).
- A number of features of the skin are immediately obvious. If cyanosis is present, its distribution is of great importance; generalized cyanosis is significant, but acrocyanosis is not.
- Jaundice, pallor, rash, bleeding from any site and evidence of trauma may be discernible.
- Abnormal facies should be appreciated or preterm infant's hair is sparse, whereas the postmature infant's hair is very dense.
- Furthermore, in postdate pregnancies the cord may be thin; this condition may also be observed in mature infants who are small for dates. Meconium staining may only be evident in the umbilical cord, or the cord may be the only site where it is visible, particularly when meconium is passed shortly before delivery. Fingernails are often long in postdate infants.
- Microcephaly or cranial enlargement is frequently obvious. If hydrocephalus is present, the forehead is often prominently protrusive (bossing).
- The cranial vault appears large in relation to the face. A thin trunk often causes a normal head to appear enlarged.
- The amount of subcutaneous fat is assessable at a glance.
- The abdomen is either distended, flat, or scaphoid, or it may bulge on one side because of a mass.
- The baby's posture is also informative. Normal flexion of the extremities indicates good muscle tone. Lack of flexion is associated with hypertonicity whereas excessive flexion indicates hypotonicity.
- Spontaneous movements can be evaluated only if the infant is undisturbed.
- At rest, sporadic, well-coordinated movements are the rule, but they are not symmetrical. Bilaterally identical, repetitive movements of the extremities are suggestive of seizure activity. Facial and eyelid twitches are also suggestive of convulsions. The infant who moves little or not at all is usually flaccid as well. Absent or diminished movement of one extremity when the others are used normally is indicative of paresis or paralysis.
- Information about respiration is first obtainable by simple inspection. Retractions are obvious and grunting and stridor are audible to the naked ear.
- Increased anteroposterior diameter of the chest (barrel chest) usually indicates an over-expanded lungs, which may be due to meconium aspiration.
- If one side of the chest appears larger than the other, pneumothorax, chylothorax, or diaphragmatic hernia is suggested. If the left side of the chest is larger, cardiomegaly associated with congenital heart disease is an additional possibility.

These diverse signs are described to emphasize the value of a careful visual inspection. Once visual assessment is completed, the examiner may proceed to the more manipulative aspects of the physical examination.

Table 2: Physical examination.

	Look for	Note
Skin	Texture, hydration, and color	Birthmarks, bruises, rash, pigmentation, anomaly
Head	Size, shape, symmetry, hair, fontanels, and sutures	Micro-macrocephaly, molding, craniosynostosis, tense anterior fontanel (AF), and swelling
Eyes	Size, shape, position, and slant	White reflex, asymmetry, discharge, and redness
Ears	Shape, size, and position	Low set, tags, pits, and malformation
Mouth	Shape, position, and symmetry	Tongue, gums, tooth, and swelling
Palate	Anterior/posterior palate	Cleft
Limbs	Symmetry, movements	Poly-, syn-, clinodactyly, malformation, and palmar crease
Genitalia	*Boys:* Penile size, urethral opening, scrotal symmetry, rugosity, and testis in scrotum *Girls:* Labia majora-minora, clitoris, and urethra-vagina	Penis <1 cm, chordee, hypospadias, epispadias, absent scrotal rugosity, empty scrotum, and asymmetric scrotum. Hymenal tags, discharge per urethra-vagina
Back-spine	Spine curvature	Defect, tufts of hair, dimple, and pits
Hips	Thigh crease symmetry, Barlow–Ortolani	Asymmetry, leg shortening

Table 3: Occult anomaly search.

Eyes	White reflex, clouding, asymmetry, and color
Mouth	Cleft palate
Umbilical cord cut section	Umbilical vessels
Pulse	Femoral
Hips	Developmental dysplasia of hip
Spine	Sinus tract
Cardiac	Single second heart sound
Pulse oximetry	Differential hypoxia

Undress the baby to complete the remainder of the examination while maintaining a warm environment (Tables 2 to 6).

Danger Signs
- Hypothermia
- Hyperthermia
- Cyanosis
- Chest indrawing
- Grunt
- Seizures
- Decreased feeding
- Decreased activity.

Cardiovascular System
- This includes feeding history, color, heart rate, and femoral pulse volume as well as listening to the heart for a murmur.
- The parasternal and epigastric area should be palpated for evidence of an overactive heart.
- The cardiovascular assessment should also include palpation of the abdomen to identify any organomegaly.
- Absence of a murmur does not, however, guarantee, there is no cardiac anomaly, other markers include cyanosis and poor pulses.
- Early investigation of cardiac murmurs, preferably by echocardiogram can clarify if there is a significant cardiac anomaly.

Respiratory System
- Respiratory effort (in conjunction with other signs of respiratory problems, such as

SECTION 2
Care of Well Newborn

Table 4: Evaluation and interpretation of vital signs.

Look	Well	Unwell
Temperature	36.5–37.5°C	Cold stress, hypothermia, core-axillary mismatch or fever
Appearance	Alert	Drowsy, lethargic, nonresponsive, persistent irritability, abnormal movements, ear discharge
Breathing	Rate 40–60/min, regular, no audible sounds	Rate <40 or >60/min, apnea, gasping, chest indrawing, grunt
Color	Pink	Pallor, plethora, icterus, cyanosis
Pulse oximeter	>95% after 24 hours of age	UL and LL difference of >5, SpO_2 <90%
Rationale	No active intervention	Hospitalize, stabilize, identify the cause, and treat the cause

Table 5: Physiological signs.

- Caput succedaneum
- Clear eye discharge
- Umbilical hernia
- Erythema toxicum
- Hypo- and hyperpigmented marks
- Miliaria
- Acne
- Tongue tie
- Hydrocele
- Epstein's pearl
- Capillary hemangioma
- Vaginal bleed
- Mongolian spots
- Peeling of skin
- Lanugo
- Subconjunctival hemorrhage
- Squint
- Breast engorgement

Table 6: Newborn examination in a nutshell.

Ask	Look
• Parental concerns • Maternal, antenatal, perinatal, and family history • Feeding and activity • Urine and stool pattern • Vaccination	• Appearance (posture, activity) • Breathing • Color (cry)

Examine	Document
• Vitals • Head to toe: Normal variations, anomalies, spine and genitals • Gestational age • DDH, neonatal reflexes • Systemic exam • Danger signs	• Age in hours (for first week) • Risk factors • Anthropometry on growth chart • Abnormal findings • Specific instructions/tests

tachypnea at rest, retraction, grunting, and nasal flaring) can be assessed at the same time as the cardiovascular assessment.
- Observe the rate and pattern of chest movement.
- Listen to the air entry to check for crackles and stridor.
- Crackles may indicate underlying infection and heart failure. Stridor may indicate airway obstruction.

Clavicles and upper limbs: Observation, palpation, and examination to identify any abnormalities, for example, Erb's palsy.

Abdomen

- Observe color and shape and palpate to identify any organomegaly.
- The condition of the umbilical cord can be included at this time. Information on the number of cord vessels should be included in the case records.
- *Renal area*—although with antenatal ultrasound examination now many suspected renal abnormalities are detected prior to birth, it has been shown that palpation performed bimanually does detect additional renal anomalies.
- *Genitalia and anus*—assess gender and appearance of genitalia. Patency of anus is examined.
- The femoral pulses must be palpated at this time if not already done.
- *Spine*—with baby prone inspect for completeness of bony structures and skin. Observe the coccygeal area, checking for incurving reflex and note any abnormal pigmentation and sacral dimple.

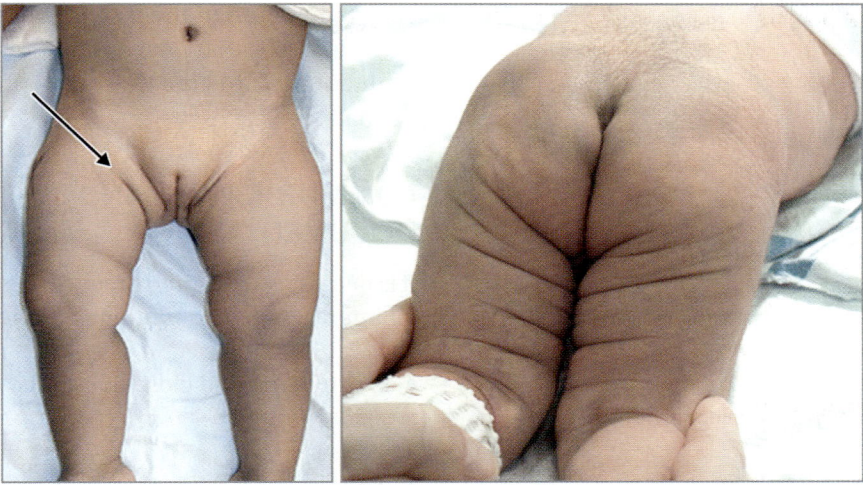

Fig. 1: Asymmetry of thigh creases.

- *Skin*—while examining other aspects of the baby any skin lesions should be identified and discussed with parents.
- *Reflexes*—the Moro, grasp, rooting, and sucking reflexes are assessed.

Throughout the examination, the baby's behavior and posture can be noted to complete the assessment of the central nervous system.

Hips

- Historically this examination is carried out toward the end of the assessment, but hip instability is best detected when the baby is least disturbed.
- The proportions and symmetry of the lower limbs and skin folds are examined before testing hip stability (Figs. 1 and 2).
- It is important to view the skin creases from the posterior aspect of the thigh and to look for any skeletal skew.
- Following gentle abduction the hips are tested using both the Barlow and Ortolani tests to ensure they are neither dislocated nor dislocatable (Fig. 3).

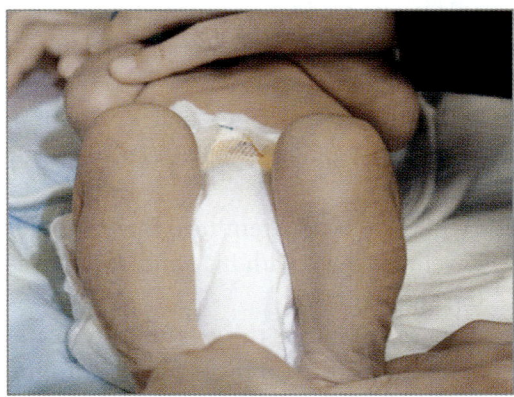

Fig. 2: Asymmetry of knees (Galeazzi's sign).

- *Feet*—observe and examine to identify postural abnormalities, for example, talipes.
- *Cry*—noting aspects of the baby's cry (weak, hoarse, lusty, absent) can indicate possible underlying conditions which require investigation and/or treatment.

Clinical Tips

- If the infant is disturbed by manipulations beforehand, adequate evaluation of the abdomen is difficult or impossible.

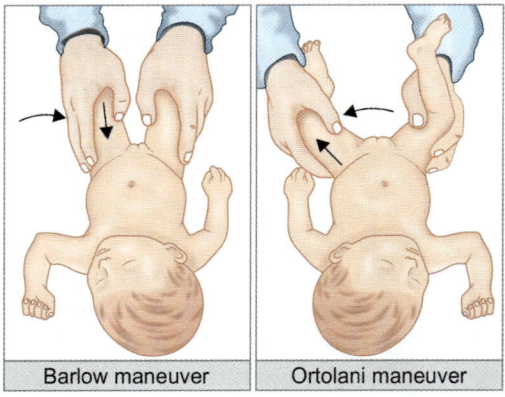

Fig. 3: Examination for DDH.

- The examiner's fingertips must be gently placed and held on the abdomen without exerting any downward pressure. Deep palpation should then proceed gradually.
- The neonate is easily agitated by abrupt manipulations.
- In conjunction with cardiac evaluation, the femoral and brachial pulses are gently palpated.
- To palpate the extremities, the examiner envelopes them with his hand and moves the joints gently.
- After completing the evaluation of the extremities, the infant is pulled into the sitting position by his or her wrists to evaluate head lag.
- Crying caused by the disturbance is of little concern, because the resultant deep inspirations and the noise of crying are helpful in auscultation of the lungs.
- With one hand holding a flashlight, the eyelids are gently separated with the examiner's index finger and thumb. Light is shined tangentially into the eyes to rule out corneal lesions and visible cataracts and the examiner should ensure that a red reflex is seen bilaterally.

Examination of the mouth and throat is performed as the last maneuver of the physical evaluation as it is the most agitating to the neonate.

COMMUNICATION AND DOCUMENTATION

It is necessary to use and practice these during all interactions with mothers and healthcare staff:
- Use of open and close questions, listening skills
- Praise
- Simple words while providing information and counseling
- Use of nonverbal means of communication (gestures)
- Discuss the findings with the parents and answer any questions or queries
- Ensure that the findings of the examination are appropriately and accurately recorded.

NEONATAL SCREENING

- Screening for congenital hypothyroidism, phenylketonuria, cystic fibrosis, etc. and the universal neonatal hearing screening is offered in the neonatal period.
- Rapid assessment to identify if the newborn is well or unwell.
- All unwell babies need detailed evaluation, workup, and treatment of the underlying cause.

SUGGESTED READING

1. Gooding JR, McClead RE Jr. Initial assessment and management of the Newborn. Pediatr Clin North Am. 2015;62(2):345-65.
2. Rennie JM. Examining the normal neonate. Curr Opin Paediatr. 2004;14(4):361-5.

CHAPTER 28

Growth Monitoring

Shamsher Singh Dalal

INTRODUCTION

Growth monitoring is an essential component of evaluation of well and sick newborns. Gestational age is taken into consideration while evaluating growth. Corrected age is used during first 2 years of life while evaluating preterms. The target weight gain expected is 10–20 g/kg/day (15–20 g/kg/day for infants <1,500 g) in weight, approximately 1 cm/week in length, and 0.5–1 cm/week in head circumference.

Growth monitoring involves serial measurements of anthropometry (weight, length, and head circumference) and plotting the values on appropriate growth chart. This helps in early detection of abnormal growth patterns. A trend helps to identify the growth trajectory.

While monitoring growth of preterm neonates we need to make adjustments for the degree of prematurity. Three types of age definitions used for premature infants are:
1. *Chronologic or birth age*: Time since birth.
2. *Postconceptional age (PCA)*: Estimated time since conception.
3. *Corrected age*: Age corrected for prematurity. It is equal to chronological age minus term gestational age, i.e. 40 weeks. It is used to monitor growth and development once the preterm infant reaches PCA of 40 weeks.

For preterm infants, till first 2 years, corrected age is used. After 2 years of age, a standard growth chart for chronologic age may be used. Catch-up growth is possible in appropriate for gestational age (AGA) infants. This usually takes place not later than 2 years of age. Those who are small for age (SGA) do not show catch-up growth.

Preterm growth charts: For monitoring the growth of preterm infant's three types of growth charts are commonly used.
1. *Fetal-infant growth charts*: Initial parts of the curves, till PCA of 40 weeks, are based on the size of healthy fetuses at birth (intrauterine growth) followed by curves based on the growth of term infants who have not had the growth depressing effect of prematurity. These charts depict the ideal growth trajectory which a preterm infant should follow. Drawback of these charts is that they do not show the change in weight that occurs after birth. In real life scenario most of the preterm infants in best of the neonatal centers around the world undergo some degree of weight loss after birth followed by slow catch-up

growth. For example, Babson and Benda fetal-infant chart (26 weeks of gestational age until 1 year of age after "term" has been reached) and Fenton fetal-infant chart (weight, length, and head circumference curves are given from 22 weeks to 50 weeks postmenstrual age). In Fenton charts preterm growth curves, based on intrauterine growth, were harmonized with the new World Health Organization (WHO) Growth Standard.

2. *Longitudinal postnatal growth chart*: These growth charts are based on the postnatal growth trajectory of a sample of healthy preterm infants showing the pattern of initial weight loss after birth followed by subsequent growth. Advantage of these charts is that they show the actual growth pattern of preterm infants. Their disadvantage is that they are not based on the ideal growth standard for preterm infants, that is, on fetal growth or intrauterine growth. Therefore, they do not show an infant's growth velocity or catch-up growth relative to the fetus or the term infant. Further, the curves on a longitudinal growth chart are highly influenced by the medical and nutritional care of the sample infants. Growth patterns may change with innovations and improvement in medical and nutritional care. Examples include growth chart by Dances et al., Wright et al., and those developed by the (National Institute of Child Health and Human Development (NICHD).

- Combined use of both fetal-infant and longitudinal charts together provide a more accurate assessment of growth of preterm infants.

3. *INTERGROWTH-21st Preterm Postnatal Growth Standards:* The criteria idea that the growth of preterm infants should match the growth of healthy fetuses is not substantiated by data and seldom achieved in practice, especially for very preterm neonates. To overcome these limitations INTERGROWTH-21st study has produced prospective, longitudinal, postnatal growth standards specifically for preterm infants from 27 weeks' gestation. Infants included in these standards were born to healthy mothers with well-dated pregnancies and with no intrauterine growth restriction as assessed by serial ultrasound scans from <14 weeks' gestation. These preterm neonates received up-to-date medical and feeding counseling and were followed up by using rigorous, standardized methodology for anthropometric measurement, feeding pattern, and neurodevelopment until 2 years of age. For correct comparator for assessing the growth of preterm neonates it is now recommended by WHO to use the INTERGROWTH-21st Preterm Postnatal Growth Standards. These standards can be used to assess preterm infants until 64 weeks' postmenstrual age (6 months' corrected age), the time at which they overlap with the WHO Child Growth Standards for term newborns. Centiles for weight, length, and head circumference, with corresponding z scores, are available in paper, Web-based, and smart-phone formats for the follow-up of preterm infants from hospital care to outpatient clinics and family care.

TERM GROWTH CHARTS

WHO 2006 growth charts for boys and girls for weight, head circumference, and length are used for term infants. Once the preterm reaches term equivalent age their growth is monitored on WHO charts. These charts are eligible up to 5 years of age regardless of ethnicity, socioeconomic status, and type of feeding. WHO reference 2007 for boys and girls are used for 5–19 years.

CHAPTER 28
Growth Monitoring

MEASURING GROWTH

During neonatal intensive care unit (NICU) stay weight should be monitored daily while length and head circumference should be monitored weekly. After discharge, the growth parameters should be monitored monthly for first 3 months and subsequently every 2 months till 1 year of age.

Weight

Postnatal growth varies from intrauterine growth in that it begins with a period of weight loss, primarily through the loss of extracellular fluid. The typical loss of 5–10% of birth weight for a full-term infant may increase to as much as 15% of birth weight in infants born preterm. During the first week of life, weight loss of 10–15% of birth weight is expected because of changes in body water compartments. Preterm infants regain their birth weight slower (2–3 weeks) than term infants (7–10 days). Weight gain generally begins by the second week of life. In preterm infants goal should be to limit the degree and duration of initial weight loss and to facilitate regain of birth weight within 10–14 days of life. Average daily weight is 1–2% of body weight/day.

Length

An infantometer is used to record length. Average length gain in preterm infants is 0.8–1.0 cm/week, whereas term infants average 0.69–0.75 cm/week.

Head Circumference

The expected increase is 0.5–0.8 cm/week. An increase >1.25 cm/week is pathological and associated with hydrocephalus or intraventricular hemorrhage.

TARGET GROWTH PARAMETERS

Optimum growth of preterm infants is considered to be equivalent to intrauterine rates. Goal of neonatal nutrition should be gain of 10–20 g/kg/day (15–20 g/kg/day for infants <1,500 g) in weight, approximately 1 cm/week in length, and 0.5–1 cm/week in head circumference. Common causes to be looked for poor weight gain in preterm neonates are inadequate nutritional intake, hypothermia, anemia of prematurity, unrecognized systemic illness, and hyponatremia.

Growth charts	
• Preterms	Babson and Benda chart, Fenton's chart, and Wright's chart INTERGROWTH-21st
• Term • Preterm on reaching term equivalent age	WHO 2006 charts for boys and girls (up to 5 years age)
• Frequency	During all vaccination visits, high risk follow-up visit and when there are parental or clinical concerns

SUGGESTED READING

1. Babson SG, Benda GI. Growth graphs for the clinical assessment of infants of varying gestational age. J Pediatr. 1976;89(5):814-20.
2. Dancis J, O'Connell JR, Holt LE Jr. A grid for recording the weight of premature infants. J Pediatr. 1948;33(11):570-2.
3. Fenton TR, Kim JH. A systematic review and meta-analysis to revise the Fenton growth chart for preterm infants. BMC Pediatr. 2013;13:59.
4. Wright K, Dawson JP, Fallis D, et al. New postnatal growth grids for very lowbirth weight infants. Pediatrics. 1993;91(5):922-6.

Newborn Metabolic Screening

Asim Kumar Mallick

INTRODUCTION

Newborn metabolic screening is a simple test to screen all asymptomatic newborns between D3-D7 for a genetic or metabolic disorder. The aim is to make an early diagnosis of inborn error of metabolism in the subclinical phase to help improve outcomes. *Screening tests results are not a final diagnosis but a pointer to perform specific tests to confirm a diagnosis.* Treatment is initiated based on confirmation tests and not screening results.

Newborn screening (NBS) is of proven public health value. It is best known and most widely used genetics-related preventative pediatric public health initiative. There is a need for universal NBS in phased manner for all newborns in India.

COMPONENTS OF NEWBORN SCREENING

Newborn screening is much more than merely a testing activity (Fig. 1). It has six components:
1. Education and counseling of the parents/the public about the need and benefit of doing NBS, so that they agree, participate, and permit NBS.
2. Screening of the well babies, by collecting the sample, transferring to a central laboratory, performing screening tests on the sample, and storing specimen.
3. Diagnosis involves interpreting the test, result by skilled and trained individuals.
4. Informing the report to the parents or the doctor, immediately. If the results are abnormal, appropriate counseling of parents is done.
5. If the results are abnormal, the test is repeated and a definitive confirmatory test is done [e.g. biochemical or deoxyribonucleic acid (DNA) analysis] to finalize the diagnosis.

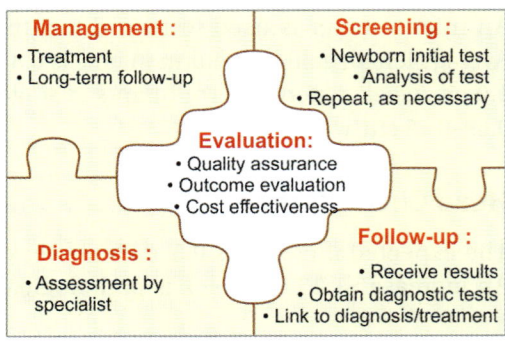

Fig. 1: Components of newborn screening.

6. Following diagnosis, parents are involved in decision making, treatment, follow-up of the infant.

The World Health Organization (WHO) has often recommended that genetic services should be introduced in countries with an infant mortality rate (IMR) less than 50. If we apply this criterion, the urban areas in all states should introduce NBS and genetic services as the IMR is less than 50.

BASIC PRINCIPLES OF SCREENING

- Condition should be a major health problem.
- Treatment should be available for the recognized disease.
- The diagnosis should be confirmed by specific tests and specific treatment advised.
- The condition should have a subclinical phase or an asymptomatic period.
- A test or examination should be available for the condition.
- The test should be acceptable to the study patients.
- The natural course of the condition from development from asymptomatic or preclinical stage to established or declared disease should be adequately known.
- There should be consensus on whom to initiate treatment for the condition.
- The screening test should be cost-effective in relation to expenditure on the disease treatment.
- Case-finding should be a continuous process and not one time event.

TYPES OF DISORDERS TO BE SCREENED

Newborn population can be categorized into three categories based on the battery of screening tests to be performed (Table 1).

Table 1: Priority screening tests.

	For all newborns	For high-risk newborns	For resource rich
Criterion	High incidence, delayed clinical diagnosis, definitive test, and definitive treatment	Unexplained disorder, suspected inborn errors of metabolism (IEM) or family history or sibling affection	Case-by-case basis
Conditions	<ul><li>Congenital hypothyroidism</li><li>Congenital adrenal hyperplasia</li><li>G6PD deficiency</li></ul>	<ul><li>Phenylketonuria</li><li>Homocystinuria</li><li>Alkaptonuria</li><li>Galactosemia</li><li>Sickle cell anemia and other hemoglobinopathy</li><li>Cystic fibrosis</li><li>Biotinidase deficiency</li><li>Maple syrup urine disease</li><li>Medium-chain acyl-CoA dehydrogenase (MCAD) deficiency</li><li>Tyrosinemia</li><li>Fatty acid oxidation defects</li></ul>	More than 100 plus disorders screened

SECTION 2
Care of Well Newborn

Table 2: Types of metabolic screening.

1st generation	2nd generation	3rd generation
Using filter paper	Using filter paper	Using cord blood and urine
Limited tests with a capillary heel prick	Expanded test but needs a capillary heel prick	Comprehensive and noninvasive
Uses metabolite/enzyme assay	Uses tandem mass spectroscopy (TMS). Increased sensitivity and specificity	Using combination of techniques like as chromatography/mass spectrometry (GC-MS), high-performance liquid chromatography (HPLC), enzyme-linked immunosor-bent assay (ELISA), and enzyme assay
Identifies few disorders	Identifies 29 disorders	118 conditions screened. Confirmatory testing not required for half the conditions (confirmed on same platform)
₹ 300/ per disorder	Approx ₹ 4,000/	Approx ₹ 5,000/

Types of Metabolic Screening (Table 2)

See Table 2.

IDEAL AGE FOR SAMPLE COLLECTION

Ideal time for collection from newborns is between 3 days and 7 days, preferably after two to three milk feeds so that amino acids and carbohydrate levels and their intermediate products of metabolism will be built up in the body. First day screening gives false positive and false negative results. Infants screened earlier than 24 hours of age need to be retested at 2 weeks of age.

Sample Collection, Transport, and Follow-up

- After proper cleaning the heel of the feet, allowing the area to be dry, with sampling done 3–7 days of age.
- A sharp prick by a lancet is done, the first drop of blood is wiped off and the second drop is taken on the filter paper. The

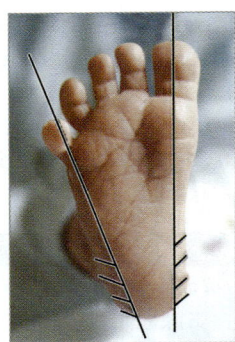

Fig. 2: Site of heel prick.

drop should be adequate to fill the circle (Figs. 2 to 4).
- Allow the sample to air dry. No special precautions to be taken. It should be stored at room temperature.
- Send the sealed envelope to the referral laboratory immediately with relevant baby's details (age of baby in hours, birth weight, gestational age, family history, and clinical status) (Fig. 5).

Report has to be collected as soon as possible from the laboratory and confirmatory tests are done if the screening test is positive.

CHAPTER 29
Newborn Metabolic Screening

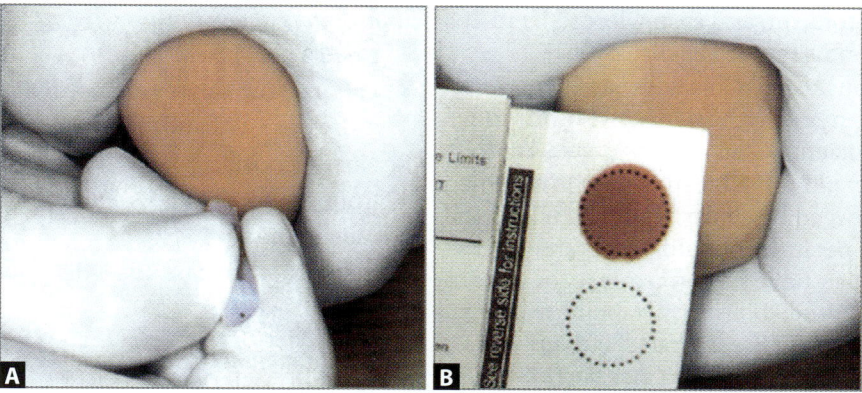

Figs. 3A and B: Sampling procedure.

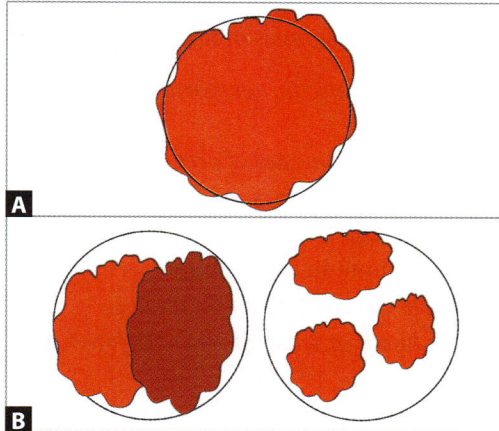

Figs. 4A and B: (A) Acceptable sample; (B) Unacceptable sample.

Fig. 5: Newborn screening filter paper.

This is followed by parental counseling, genetic counseling early dietary or other interventions.

PRACTICAL TIPS

- Sampling is done for all newborns, including sick newborns, prematurity, with or without feeding.
- Repeat tests at 36 weeks gestation for very premature babies.

SPECIAL CONSIDERATION

- *Prematurity or illness*:
  – If < 37 weeks or sick—collect specimen within 7 days
  – Associated with false +ve congenital hypothyroidism screens
- *Total parenteral nutrition (TPN)*:
  – May cause raised amino acids and organic acids
  – Indicate this on NBS card
- *Transfusion*:
  – Disorders may be missed
  – Ideally complete card before transfusion
  – Post-transfusion repeats at 72 hours (for phenylketonuria, congenital hypo-

thyroidism, and cystic fibrosis) and at 3 months (sickle cell disease)
- Transfusion of plasma may alter screens for hypothyroidism and biotinidase deficiency
- *Feeding*: If the NBS specimen is obtained before feedings have begun, an additional NBS specimen should be obtained, after feedings have begun, to test for inborn errors of metabolism (metabolite tests in an affected child B, e.g. phenylketonuria (PKU) and maple syrup urine disease (MSUD)—should become abnormal after feedings are begun.

Invalid or Incomplete Screening Test

- If a screening test is done before 48 hours of age and/or on protein supplementation.
- Incomplete or errors on information card.
- Inadequate sample or old sample (>10 days).

Interpreting Results

Screen positive means:
- Possibility of a disease and need for confirmation tests for complete diagnosis.
- It does not mean patient needs to start treatment now.
- Early referral for expert consult and tests are required.

Confirmation by specific metabolite measurement, molecular testing (DNA), sweat test, hemoglobin (Hb) electrophoresis, etc.

Limitations of newborn screening:
- Need a heel prick.
- Laboratory analyses are not 100% accurate (false positives and false negatives)
- Not diagnostic.
- Confirmatory testing required using separate method.
- May not detect late onset disorders.

Risks of screening:
- Parental anxiety (false positives)
- Missed diagnosis (false negatives)
- The right "not to know"
- Unanticipated outcomes
- Labeling—diagnosis of benign conditions

When should I discuss newborn screening with parents?
- *In the third trimester of pregnancy*:
  - Inform parents about blood spot screening
  - Recommend screening
  - Give them information leaflet
- *After birth, at least 24 hours before taking blood spots*:
  - Ensure parents have a copy of the leaflet
  - Discuss blood spot screening.

BIOCHEMICAL TECHNOLOGY AVAILABLE TO DETECT VARIOUS METABOLIC INHERITED DISORDERS (TABLE 3)

See Table 3.

Table 3: Biochemical technology available to detect various metabolic inherited disorders.

Detected by biochemical markers		• Galactosemia • Congenital hypothyroidism • Congenital adrenal hyperplasia • Glucose-6-phosphate dehydrogenase (G6PD) deficiency • Biotinidase deficiency • Cystic fibrosis
Disorders detected by TMS	Disorders of amino acid metabolism	• Aminoacidemias • Phenylketonuria • Maple syrup urine disease • Homocystinuria • Tyrosinemia
	Disorders of organic acid metabolism	• Propionic acidemia • Methylmalonic acidemia(s) • Isovaleric acidemia • Glutaric acidemia (type1) • Isolated 3-methylcrotonyl-CoA carboxylase deficiency • Hydroxymethylglutaric acidemia
	Disorders of fatty acid metabolism fatty acid oxidation disorders	• Short chain acyl-CoA dehydrogenase (SCAD) deficiency • Medium chain acyl-CoA dehydrogenase (MCAD) deficiency • Very long chain acyl-CoA dehydrogenase (VLCAD) deficiency • Long chain 3-hydroxy acyl-CoA dehydrogenase (LCHAD) deficiency • Mitochondrial trifunctional protein (TFP) deficiency • Glutaric academia type II • Carnitine palmitoyltransferase deficiency type II (CPT2)
Hormonal assay		• Thyroid-stimulating hormone (TSH) • 17OH progesterone
Enzyme assays		• Galactose-1-phosphate uridyltransferase (GALT) • Phenylketonuria (PKU)

SUGGESTED READING

1. Bijarnia S, Wilcken B, Veronica C, et al. Newborn screening for congenital hypothyroidism in very-low-birth-weight babies: the need for a second test. J Inherit Metab Dis. 2011;34:827-33.
2. Kacker SK. The scope of pediatric audiology in India. In: Deka RC, Kacker SK, Vijayalakshmi B (Eds). Pediatric Audiology in India, 1st edition. New Delhi: Otorhinolaryngological Research Society of AIIMS; 1997. p. 20.
3. Morton CC, Nance WE. Newborn hearing screening—a silent revolution. N Engl J Med. 2006;354:2151-64.
4. Mukhopadhyay K, Balachandran B. Universal newborn screening—Is it going to be a reality in India? Indian Pediatr. 2014;51:697-8.
5. Padilla CD, Krotoski D, Therrell BL Jr. Newborn screening progress in developing countries–overcoming internal barriers. Semin Perinatol. 2010;34:145-55.
6. Rama Devi AR, Naushad SM. Newborn screening in India. Indian J Pediatr. 2004;71:157-60.
7. Wilson JMG, Jungner G. Principles and practice of screening for disease; Public Health Paper No. 34. Geneva, Switzerland: World Health Organization; 1968.

CHAPTER 30

Vitamin K

C Aparna

INTRODUCTION

Vitamin K is an essential antihemorrhagic factor. It is required for the γ carboxylation of coagulation factors II (prothrombin), VII, IX, and X. Deficiency of vitamin K can result in the deficiency of these coagulant proteins and bleeding tendency.

Neonates are at risk of vitamin K deficiency due to the following factors: (A) Inadequate placental transfer of vitamin K, (B) Poor intestinal synthesis of vitamin K as the gut is sterile, and (C) Poor availability of vitamin K in breast milk (2 µg/L) as against the daily requirement of 3–5 µg/day.

ROLE OF PROPHYLACTIC VITAMIN K

Whom to Give?

All newborns—term and preterm.

When to Give?

- At birth, within 1 hour of birth but no later than discharge from health facility.
- At first contact, if no vitamin K given at birth.
- Infants with malabsorption (e.g. cystic fibrosis, alpha 1 antitrypsin deficiency) or cholestasis, weekly.
- Newborns on prolonged antibiotics (>7 days) weekly.

Strengths available: 1 mg/1 mL and 1 mg/0.5 mL.

Preparation: Vitamin K_1 or K_3.

Dose at Birth

- Birth weight 1,000 g or more: 1 mg.
- Birth weight less than 1,000 g: 0.5 mg.

For newborns on prolonged antibiotics: 1 mg, weekly.

For newborns with cholestasis: 5 mg, weekly.

Site and Mode of Administration

Anterolateral thigh, IM.

Precautions

- Follow safe injection practices
- Use 26 gauge needle and 1 mL syringe
- Do not aspirate before injecting
- Document administration of vitamin K on birth record or baby file.

ROLE OF THERAPEUTIC VITAMIN K

Deficiency of vitamin K leads to abrupt onset, spontaneous, profuse bleeding in an otherwise well-newborn.

Clinical Presentation

Depending on the postnatal age at presentation, Vitamin K deficiency bleeding (VKDB) is usually described in three forms.

Types of Vitamin K Deficiency Bleeding

Types of vitamin K deficiency bleeding (VKDB) are shown in Table 1.

Intracranial bleeding in late VKDB may cause seizures, developmental delay, or death. In some cases of late VKDB, an underlying disorder may be suggested by jaundice or failure to thrive.

Investigations

Prothrombin time (PT)/partial thromboplastin time (PTT): VKDB leads to prolonged PT and PTT with normal platelet counts and fibrinogen levels in the setting of bleeding. Mild forms of vitamin K deficiency may only result in prolonged PT, while severe vitamin K deficiency may be accompanied by both prolonged PT and PTT.

Normal adult concentrations of PT are achieved by 6 months of age. However, activated PTT shows it is similar to adult values.

Diagnosis is suggested by international normalized ratio (INR) ≥4 or a PT ≥4 control value. A deranged PT/PTT is not a predictor or diagnostic of vitamin K deficiency. It may be deranged due to variety of conditions.

Diagnosis is confirmed by return to normal values of deranged coagulation tests following vitamin K administration (within 2 hours).

Proteins induced in vitamin K absence (PIVKA): PIVKA-II is released into the circulation in vitamin K deficiency states and is normally undetectable (<0.02 ng/mL). The utility of this test for subclinical vitamin K deficiency is debated.

Proteins induced in vitamin K absence-II concentrations may be detected even days or weeks after correction of severe deficiency, due to long half-life (>60 hours) thus making it possible to make a retrospective diagnosis.

The normal values and the best technique to measure PIVKA-II is not known.

Table 1: Types of vitamin K deficiency bleeding.

	Postnatal age at presentation	Usual site of bleeding/clinical presentation	Risk factors/associated factors
Early	0–24 hours of life	Cephalic hematoma and gastrointestinal bleeds	Maternal intake of antagonist drugs (primidone, carbamazepine, barbiturates, phenytoin, warfarin, rifampicin, cephalosporins), maternal low vitamin K intake (<90 µg/day)
Classical	1–7 days of life	Gastrointestinal, cutaneous, nasal, umbilical bleeding and from circumcision site. Bleeding may be severe enough to require a blood transfusion	Lack of vitamin K administration at birth, low dietary intake (exclusive breast feeding)
Late	8 days to 6 months but typically 2–12 weeks	Intracranial (most common, up to 50%), cutaneous and gastrointestinal	Cholestasis, low dietary intake (exclusive breast feeding), fat malabsorption (e.g. cystic fibrosis), prolonged broad spectrum antibiotics

Measurement of serum vitamin K levels is not useful.

Management
- Head to toe physical examination and focused history gives clue to the cause of bleeding.
- Assist, support, and maintain temperature, airway, breathing, and circulation.

Treatment of VKDB
Administer vitamin K parenterally.

Preparation: Vitamin K_1 or K_3.

Dose: 1 mg.

Mode of administration: Intramuscular (IM) or intravenous (IV).

Strengths available: 1 mg/1 mL and 1 mg/0.5 mL:
- If bleeding is severe, transfusion with fresh frozen plasma may be required.
- If anemia develops, a packed cell transfusion may be required.

Vitamin K Supplementation
Vitamin K supplementation, see Table 2.

Table 2: Vitamin K supplementation.

Population	Dose and route of supplementation
All term neonates (at birth) and preterm (>1,000 g)	1 mg intramuscularly
Preterm neonates < 1000 gm (at birth)	0.5 mg intramuscularly
Malabsorption/Cholestasis	2.5–5 mg twice weekly to daily (unclear)
Prolonged parenteral antibiotics	1 mg weekly
Prior to major surgery	1 mg parenterally

Risks of Vitamin K
Potential problems with intramuscular vitamin K include local trauma, injury to vessels and nerves, and rarely, abscesses/osteomyelitis. Jaundice and hemolysis is not seen in the doses used now or with use of naturally occurring lipid soluble vitamin K_1. A possible increase in risk of childhood leukemia with parenteral administration of prophylactic vitamin K was refuted by studies.

Role of Oral Vitamin K
An alternative regimen comprising multiple doses of oral vitamin K has been advocated. It has disadvantages of poor absorption, short duration of effect, and uncertain efficacy. Oral vitamin K does not offer protection against late VKDB. Compliance also is an issue with multiple doses. Therefore, intramuscular route is preferred over oral vitamin K at present. Oral prophylaxis with repeat doses is practiced in Netherlands and in Germany.

Role of Antenatal Vitamin K
Administration of vitamin K to mothers during prenatal period of very preterm birth has not been shown to benefit in preventing periventricular hemorrhages postnatally.

APPENDIX: VITAMIN K FORMS
Based on the chemical structure, vitamin K is classified into three forms:
1. *Vitamin K_1 from plant sources*: Phytonadione (fat soluble).
2. *Vitamin K_2 from animal sources*: Menaquinone (fat soluble).
3. *Vitamin K_3 (synthetic)*:
   - *Fat soluble*: Menadione and acetomenaphthone.
   - *Water soluble*: Menadione sodium diphosphate/bisulfate.

Table 3: Vitamin K forms.

	Commercial preparations	Strength	Route
Vitamin K_1—Plant source (Phytonadione)	Injection Kenadion	10 mg/mL	IM/IV
	Injection Phytonadione	1 mg/0.5 mL vial	IM/IV
Vitamin K_3 (Menadione)	Injection Menadione Sodium bisulfate	10 mg/mL	IM/slow IV
		5, 10 mg tablets	Oral
	Acetomenadione	10 mg tablets	Oral
	Kapilin		

(IM: intramuscular; IV: intravenous).

Vitamin K_2 is not commercially available in India. The available preparations of vitamin K are as shown in Table 3.

Menadione and its water soluble salts can rapidly cause hemolysis in G6PD deficient neonates, in addition to competitively inhibiting glucuronide conjugation of bilirubin, potentially precipitating kernicterus in neonates.

Storage of Vitamin K

Injection vitamin K is thermostable in room temperature. It does not require refrigeration.

SUGGESTED READING

1. Hascoët JM, Picaud JC, Lapillonne A, et al. Vitamin K in the neonate: Recommendations update. Arch Pediatr. 2017;24(9):902-5.
2. McNinch A, Busfield A, Tripp J. Vitamin K deficiency bleeding in Great Britain and Ireland: British Paediatric Surveillance Unit Surveys, 1993-94 and 2001-02. Arch Dis Child. 2007;92(9):759-66.
3. Operational Guidelines. Injection Vitamin K Prophylaxis at Birth (In Facilities). Child Health Division, Ministry of Health and Family Welfare, Government of India. 2015. [online] Available form: http://nrhm.gov.in/images/pdf/programs/child-health/guidelines/Vitamin_K_Operational_Guidelines.pdf. [Accessed April, 2019].
4. Puckett RM, Offringa M. Prophylactic vitamin K for vitamin K deficiency bleeding in neonates. Cochrane Database Syst Rev. 2000;(4):CD002776.
5. Sankar MJ, Chandrasekaran A, Kumar P, et al. Vitamin K prophylaxis for prevention of vitamin K deficiency bleeding: a systematic review. J Perinatol. 2016;36(Suppl 1):S29-35.
6. Van Winckel M, De Bruyne R, Van De Velde S, et al. Vitamin K, an update for the paediatrician. Eur J Pediatr. 2009;168(2):127-34.
7. World Health Organization. Pocket Book of Hospital Care for Children: Guidelines for the Management of Common Childhood Illnesses, 2nd edition. World Health Organization; 2013. pp. 1-412.

CHAPTER 31

Not Passed Urine in the First 48 Hours

K Sankarnarayanan

INTRODUCTION

Oligoanuria is defined as no urine output noted by 48 hours of age or a diminished urine output (urine volume less than 1 mL/kg per hour over 8 hours on maintenance fluid). The presence of urine does not rule out acute kidney injury (AKI) since some infants are nonoliguric.

IDENTIFICATION, IMMEDIATE STEPS, AND POTENTIAL CONFOUNDERS

If a baby has not passed urine in the first 48 hours, many urgent and serious conditions need to be considered. Before beginning extensive investigations, consider the following:
- Is it possible that previous voiding has been missed? (Babies being looked after by relatives while mother is unwell may have missed previous voiding).
- Urine might have been mixed with stool.
- Even if a urine bag has been applied urine might have leaked round the bag.
- Urinary catheter might be blocked or displaced.
- Beware of highly absorbent diapers. Many babies who are suspected of having oligoanuria while wearing diapers actually have normal urine output.
- Always palpate for a distended bladder.

DIAGNOSIS OF OLIGOANURIA

- The main worry in the baby with oligoanuria is the possibility of AKI.
- Oligoanuria is defined as no urine output noted by 48 hours of age or a diminished urine output (urine volume less than 1 mL/kg/hr). However, the presence of urine does not rule out AKI since some infants are nonoliguric.
- An elevated or rising serum creatinine (>1.5 mg/dL) is an indicator of a reduction in glomerular filtration rate (GFR), which is the hallmark of AKI.

EVALUATION

The determination of the cause of the AKI is based on a combination of history, physical examination, and laboratory parameters.
Important history to be sought for:
- Oligohydramnios (could suggest antenatal onset renal problems).
- Polyhydramnios (could be a feature of Bartter's syndrome).
- Renal abnormality detected on antenatal ultrasound examination.
- Antenatal medications [Enalapril and other ACE (angiotensin-converting-enzyme) inhibitors taken by the mother could cause renal failure in the neonate].

- Neonatal conditions that may be associated with AKI include prematurity, perinatal asphyxia, respiratory distress syndrome, and sepsis [all these conditions could lead to diminished renal perfusion leading to prerenal failure and may also lead to acute tubular necrosis (ATN)].
- Umbilical artery catheterization (could lead to thrombosis in the aorta and renal arteries).
- Drug administration at or soon after birth (indomethacin and ibuprofen).
- Volume depletion (bleeding, hypotension, and shock lead to prerenal failure).
- Abnormal urine stream in males (could suggest the possibility of urinary obstruction).
- Family history should be obtained for conditions including congenital nephrotic syndrome, polycystic kidney disease, or any other renal disease.

PHYSICAL EXAMINATION

Findings on the physical examination that may be associated with AKI include:
- Edema or unexpected weight gain (because of fluid retention).
- High or low blood pressure.
- Enlarged or absent kidneys and an enlarged bladder.
- Dysmorphic features, e.g. meningomyelocele, anal atresia, and prune belly syndrome.
- Facial and limb deformities associated with oligohydramnios resulting from decreased fetal urine production (Potter facies).
- Signs of asphyxia, sepsis, blood loss, etc.

URINE ANALYSIS

The urinalysis is a very important noninvasive test in the diagnostic evaluation, since characteristic findings on microscopic examination of the urine sediment suggest certain diagnoses.

Table 1: Urinary sodium excretion.

Test	Prerenal	Intrinsic renal failure
Urinary sodium	<20–30 mEq/L	>30–40 mEq/L
Fractional excretion of sodium	<2%	>2.5–3%
Urinary osmolality	>400 mOsm/kg	<400 mOsm/kg

- The urinalysis is within normal limits with prerenal disease, obstructive tract obstruction, and some cases of ATN.
- Granular casts and epithelial cell casts are suggestive of ATN.
- Intrinsic renal disease is suggested by presence of red blood cells, tubular cells, and proteinuria.

Urinary Sodium Excretion

Several measurements which compare urinary sodium and urinary creatinine with serum levels are useful in distinguishing prerenal from intrinsic renal failure. However, these tests have several limitations. There is significant overlap in the values for these indices and interventions for renal failure like administration of fluid boluses and diuretics could alter the usefulness of these investigations. Some of these indices are listed in Table 1.

Urine specific gravity is very variable and not useful as a diagnostic marker.

Some investigators have used biomarkers as early indicators of AKI before other biochemical derangements happen. One of these biomarkers is neutrophil gelatinase-associated lipocalin. These biomarkers are still at an investigational stage and not routinely available or recommended.

RENAL ULTRASOUND

The abnormalities that can be identified on ultrasound are:
- Presence of single or multiple kidneys

- Kidney size and shape
- Echogenicity or cysts
- Identify signs of urinary obstruction like dilated posterior urethra, dilated ureters, and dilated renal pelvis
- Doppler examination can be helpful in identifying renal vein or renal artery thromboses.

MICTURATING CYSTOURETHROGRAM

Micturating cystourethrogram (MCUG) is helpful to evaluate an obstructed urinary tract, e.g. posterior urethral valves.

RADIONUCLIDE SCINTIGRAPHY

- Dimercaptosuccinic acid (DMSA) is helpful in identification of renal scar.
- Diethylenetriaminepentaacetic acid (DTPA) can be used to assess differential renal function.
- Mercaptoacetyltriglycine (MAG3) is helpful in identifying renal obstruction.

ETIOLOGY OF ACUTE KIDNEY INJURY IN NEONATES

The causes of AKI in newborns are prerenal failure, due to:
- Decreased renal perfusion—85%
- Intrinsic renal failure due to primary renal pathology—11%
- Postrenal failure, due to block in the conducting urinary system—3%.

Perinatal asphyxia is the leading cause of AKI in newborns. It occurs due to decreased renal perfusion due to hypovolemia or hypotension causing decreased glomerular filtration. The other common conditions causing prerenal disease or ATN are hypovolemia, hypoxemia, and septicemia.

Decreased renal perfusion can also be caused by drugs like indomethacin and other nonsteroidal anti-inflammatory drugs.

Bilateral renal vascular thrombosis leads to intrinsic renal failure as a complication of diarrhea, sepsis, perinatal asphyxia, polycythemia, administration of contrast media, congenital nephrotic syndrome, and infants of diabetic mothers.

Renal artery thrombosis secondary to umbilical artery catheter (UAC) placement at times leads to AKI.

Renal and urinary tract abnormalities leading to AKI are:
- Renal parenchyma malformation, e.g. renal dysplasia, renal agenesis, renal tubular dysgenesis, and polycystic renal diseases.
- Abnormalities due to embryonic migration, e.g. horseshoe kidney.
- Abnormalities of urinary collecting system, e.g. duplicate collecting systems, posterior urethral valves, and pelviureteric junction obstruction.

APPROACH TO A BABY WITH OLIGOANURIA

- Under aseptic techniques place a catheter in urinary bladder. This rules out obstruction of the lower urinary tract. The sample of urine is sent for analysis.
- Give a fluid challenge, with 10–20 mL/kg of normal saline over 1 to ensure normovolemia. If urine output improves to >1 mL/kg/hour, prerenal failure must be a strong consideration.
- Stop or discontinue potassium-containing medications.
- Adjust or stop all nephrotoxic medications.
- Obtain an urgent renal ultrasound to rule out urinary obstruction if there is no response to a fluid challenge.

- There is no role for routine use of furosemide merely to achieve a urine output (furosemide can cause ototoxicity and significant electrolyte abnormalities).
- There is no benefit for routine use of low dose dopamine in oliguric neonates. Dopamine infusion is helpful only if used to correct hypotension or cardiogenic shock.

MANAGEMENT (FLOWCHART 1)

The treatment of AKI depends upon the underlying type and severity of pathology. The general approach consists of:
- Maintain fluid and electrolyte balance
- Early recognition and treatment of serious electrolyte disturbances
- Ensure nutritional support
- Treat the underlying cause.

FLUIDS

Fluid administration should be limited to estimated insensible water losses plus the urine output.

Daily insensible loss in newborns is as follows:
- >2,500 g—15–25 mL/kg
- 1,500–2,500 g—15–35 mL/kg
- <1,500 g—30–60 mL/kg.

Fluid loss is more if the infant is under warmer. A 12 hourly weight is a very useful estimate of fluid status especially in resource limited settings.

HYPERKALEMIA

K >6 mEq/L is potentially life-threatening. Presence of electrocardiography changes is ominous and warrants urgent treatment, regardless of the degree of hyperkalemia.

Flowchart 1: Approach to a baby anuric at 48 hours.

Check
- Confirm true anuria
- Ensure airway, breathing, and circulation

Stop
- Stop potassium containing fluid,
- Stop or reduce nephrotoxic medications
- Catheterize bladder
- Administer fluid bolus

Investigate
- Obtain urgent renal ultrasound
- Obtain detailed history and perform thorough clinical examination

Beware
- Hypo-hyperkalemia and acidosis
- Hypocalcemia and hyperphosphatemia

Maintain
- Fluid and electrolyte status
- Nutrition

Consider
- Renal replacement

- Give 10% calcium gluconate [0.5–1 mL/kg intravenous (IV) over 5 minutes].
- Administer sodium bicarbonate (1–2 mEq/kg IV over 5–10 minutes).
- If above measures fail, consider continuous infusion of insulin (0.1 units/kg per hour with 2–4 mL/kg per hour of 10% dextrose in water).
- Salbutamol (4–5 mcg/kg IV over 20 minutes or 2.5 mg by nebulization)
- Kayexalate is an ion exchange resin, can be administered in a dose of 1 g/kg dissolved in saline for rectal administration or in 10% dextrose in water for enteral administration.
- Renal replacement therapy should be considered if these measures fail to correct hyperkalemia.

METABOLIC ACIDOSIS

- The most effective intervention for neonatal metabolic acidosis is treatment of the underlying cause.
- Sodium bicarbonate should not be used routinely to correct acidosis in preterm infants. If at all sodium bicarbonate is used, it should be infused slowly over 30 minutes.

HYPONATREMIA

- Hyponatremia is because of fluid retention and not because of sodium deficiency. Hence, the treatment is restricting free water. However, if there are neurological signs related to hyponatremia (S sodium <120 mEq/L) then hypertonic (3%) saline can be used to correct the hyponatremia.

NUTRITION

- Ensure caloric intake of atleast 100 kcal/kg/day.
- Ensure intake of atleast 1.50–2.0 gm/kg/day of protein.
- Very sick neonates will need parenteral nutrition.

RENAL REPLACEMENT

Consider for renal replacement therapy (e.g. hemodialysis, peritoneal dialysis, or hemofiltration) in a symptomatic infant if one or more of the following are present:
- Persistent acidosis, hyperkalemia, or hyponatremia.
- Fluid overload suggested by cardiac failure or pulmonary edema.

SUGGESTED READING

1. Jetton JG, Askenazi DJ. Update on acute kidney injury in the neonate. Curr Opin Pediatr. 2012;24(2):191-6.
2. Ringer SA. Acute renal failure in the neonate. NeoReviews. 2010;11(5);e243-51.

CHAPTER 32

Not Passed Stools in the First 48 Hours

Leslie Lewis

INTRODUCTION

Meconium is the first stool of the newborn, which is sticky, thick, and dark green. Passage of the first stool in full-term neonates within first 24 hours of life is a sign of well-being.

TIMING FOR FIRST PASSAGE OF MECONIUM

Majority of babies pass meconium in the first 24 hours (Fig. 1 and Tables 1 and 2).

Differential Diagnosis of Conditions Associated with Delayed Passage of Meconium

Medical causes:

- Maternal narcotics or magnesium sulfate supplementation
- Dehydration
- Electrolyte abnormalities—hypermagnesemia, hypokalemia, and hypercalcemia
- Hypothyroidism

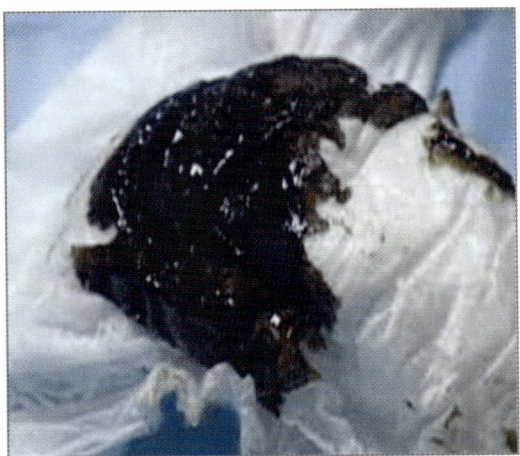

Fig. 1: Normal healthy meconium should be black, sticky and large quantity.

Table 1: Timing of passing meconium after birth.

Timing	Passage of first stool in percentage
First 8 hours	60
First 16 hours	91
First 24 hours	98.5
First 48 hours	100

Table 2: Gestational age and timing of meconium after birth.

Gestational age	Mean age at passage of first meconium
28–30 weeks	23.5 hrs ± 3.5 hrs
31–34 weeks	33 hrs ± 3.8 hrs
34–36 weeks	25.7 hrs ± 4.2 hrs
37 weeks or more	17.3 hrs ± 4.6 hrs

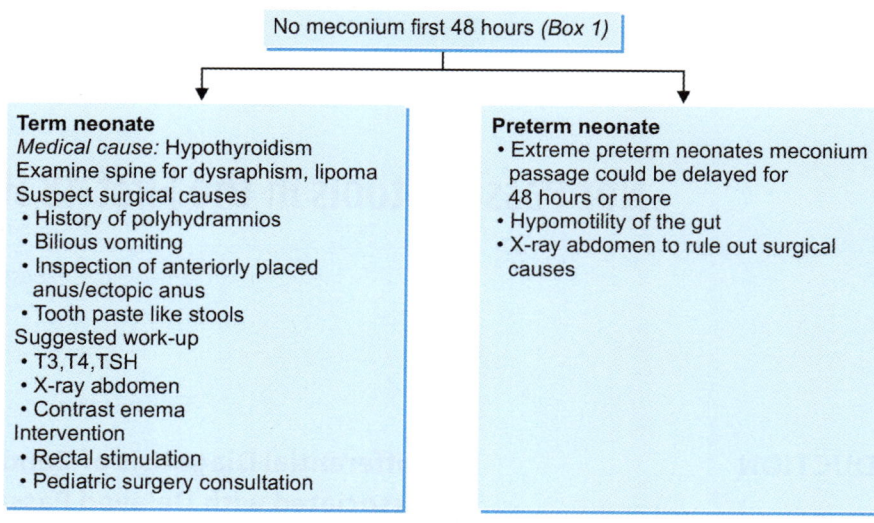

Flowchart 1: Approach and work-up for delayed passage of meconium.

(TSH: thyroid-stimulating hormone)

Table 3: Clinical clues.		
Clinical condition	Abnormal findings	Intervention
Hirschsprung's disease	Empty rectum	Surgery
Meconium plug syndrome	Meconium plugs	Rectal stimulation, glycerine enema
Meconium ileus	Abdominal distension	Intravenous fluids, enema surgery
Anorectal malformation	Absent/tight anus	Dilatation, surgery
Small left colon	Transition zone at splenic flexure	Enema, colostomy
Duodenal atresia	Polyhydramnios, bilious vomiting, abdominal distension	Surgery

- Sepsis
- Congestive heart failure.

Disorders of small intestine:
- Duodenal atresia
- Jejunoileal atresia
- Malrotation and volvulus
- Meconium ileus.

Disorders of large intestine:
- Meconium plug syndrome
- Anorectal malformations
- Hirschsprung's disease
- Small left colon syndrome.

Box 1

Red flags in delayed passage of meconium.

- Polyhydramnios
- Increased gastric aspirates at birth
- Bilious vomiting
- Absent/abnormal rectal opening
- Pellet/paste-like meconium
- Abdominal distension

Differential diagnosis of surgical conditions associated with failure to pass meconium has been shown in Flowchart 1 and Table 3.

SUGGESTED READING

1. Dillon PW, Cilley RE. Newborn surgical emergencies. Gastrointestinal anomalies, abdominal wall defects. Pediatr Clin North Am. 1993;40(6):1289-314.
2. Fitzgerald JF. Constipation in children. Pediatr Rev. 1987;8(10):299-302.
3. Haram-Mourabet S, Harper RG, Wapnir RA. Mineral composition of meconium: effect of prematurity. J Am Coll Nutr. 1998;17(4): 356-60.
4. Peña A. Imperforate anus and cloacal malformations. In: Ashcraft KW, Holder TM (Eds). Pediatric Surgery, 2nd edition. Philadelphia: Saunders; 1993. pp. 372-92.
5. Setu M, Mollah MA, Amin SK, et al. Duration of meconium passage in term and preterm infants. AKMMC J. 2013;4(1):6-9.

CHAPTER 33

Direct Jaundice

Sreeram S

INTRODUCTION

Conjugated or direct hyperbilirubinemia in a neonate is defined as a serum direct or conjugated bilirubin concentration greater than 1.0 mg/dL if the total serum bilirubin (TSB) is <5.0 mg/dL or >20% of TSB if the TSB is >5.0 mg/dL. Neonatal cholestasis is defined as direct hyperbilirubinemia due to diminished bile flow. It is important to remember that direct hyperbilirubinemia is always pathological.

CLINICAL FEATURES

Direct jaundice can manifest at any age in a neonate. It can present as a rapidly deteriorating entity over few days or as a chronic entity progressing gradually over days to weeks. The common mode of presentation would be a prolonged jaundice.

Babies with neonatal cholestasis especially due to obstructive etiology like extrahepatic biliary atresia (EHBA) usually present as prolonged jaundice with pale colored stools and dark yellow urine. Pale stool is very specific and relatively sensitive sign. EHBA babies are usually born at term, are active and appear well at presentation. Late presentation is common in our country due to under recognition.

Babies with neonatal cholestasis due to sepsis (usually bacterial), viral infections like cytomegalovirus (CMV), herpes simplex viruses (HSV), metabolic conditions like tyrosinemia, galactosemia, and neonatal hemochromatosis are sick looking at presentation and may present early in life. These entities present as acute liver cell failure. Catastrophic presentation due to large intracranial bleed is also known.

Facial dysmorphism, eye signs like cataracts, chorioretinitis, cherry red spot, cardiac murmurs, are some of the pointers to specific etiological diagnosis (Table 1). Presence of ascites and bleeding manifestations indicates liver cell failure. Endocrine causes like hypothyroidism, hypopituitarism can present with neonatal cholestasis. Other rare genetic/metabolic causes include Dubin Johnson syndrome, cystic fibrosis, arginase deficiency, glycogen storage diseases, fatty acid oxidation defects, mitochondrial respiratory chain disorders, cholesterol synthetic defects, bile acid synthetic defects, and peroxisomal disorders.

INVESTIGATIONS (TABLE 2)

Investigating a baby with direct jaundice should be considered as semi-emergency.

Table 1: Clues to etiology in neonatal cholestasis.

Clues	Possible etiology
Signs of hemolysis, high indirect jaundice initially followed by direct; ABO/RH/minor blood group incompatibility	Inspissated bile syndrome
Presence of facial dysmorphism	Trisomy 13, 18, 21, Allagille syndrome, Zellwegar
IUGR, hepatosplenomegaly, chorioretinitis, intracranial calcifications	CMV, toxoplasmosis
Palpable mass per abdomen, intermittent cholestasis	Choledochal cyst
Splenomegaly, cherry red spot, fetal ascites	Niemann-Pick disease
Acute presentation—acute liver cell failure	Bacterial sepsis Viral—entero, HSV, CMV Tyrosinemia Galactosemia Hemochromatosis
Low or normal GGT	PFIC I and II, bile acid synthetic defect
Recurrent cholestasis	Choledochal cyst, benign recurrent intrahepatic cholestasis PFIC
Pulmonary stenosis, facial dysmorphism	Alagille syndrome
Meconium ileus, recurrent infections, metabolic alkalosis	Cystic fibrosis

(CMV: cytomegalovirus; GGT: gamma glutamyl transferase; HSV: herpes simplex virus; IUGR: intrauterine growth restriction; PFIC: progressive familial intrahepatic cholestasis)

Table 2: Investigations.

First-line investigations	
Test	Rationale
Total and direct bilirubin	To define degree and severity of jaundice.
T3, T4, TSH	Congenital hypothyroidism
SGOT/SGPT	Acuity of liver disease
Serum alkaline phosphatase/GGTP	Obstructive etiology
Urine for nonglucose reducing substances	Galactosemia
Ultrasound of liver	Hepatobiliary obstruction
Urine routine and culture	Occult infection
Sepsis screen and blood culture	Suspected bacterial infection

(GGTP: gamma-glutamyl transpeptidase; TSH: thyroid-stimulating hormone; SGPT: serum glutamic pyruvic transaminase; SGOT: serum glutamic oxaloacetic transaminase)

Treatable entities should be investigated and ruled out initially.

Ultrasound of the abdomen is preferably done in preferred state to look for gallbladder status. Absence or small gallbladder, triangular cord sign suggest EHBA. Presence of gallbladder does not rule out EHBA.

Hepatobiliary iminodiacetic acid (HIDA) scan is available and it can be used to look for the patency of bile duct. Priming with phenobarbitone for at least 5 days yields better results, however this can be the limitation for those presenting late. Presence of tracer in the intestine rules out EHBA. Nonvisualization of tracer in the intestine can occur in both obstructive and hepatocellular causes of neonatal cholestasis.

If the above investigations are inconclusive, liver biopsy can be helpful. The characteristic histopathology features of EHBA are bile duct proliferation, bile plugs in ducts, fibrosis, and lymphocytic infiltrates in the portal tracts. Liver biopsy can also reveal other etiologies like bile duct paucity (Alagille and PFIC), CMV inclusion bodies, alpha-1 antitrypsin deficiency. Intraoperative cholangiography remains the gold standard for diagnosis of EHBA.

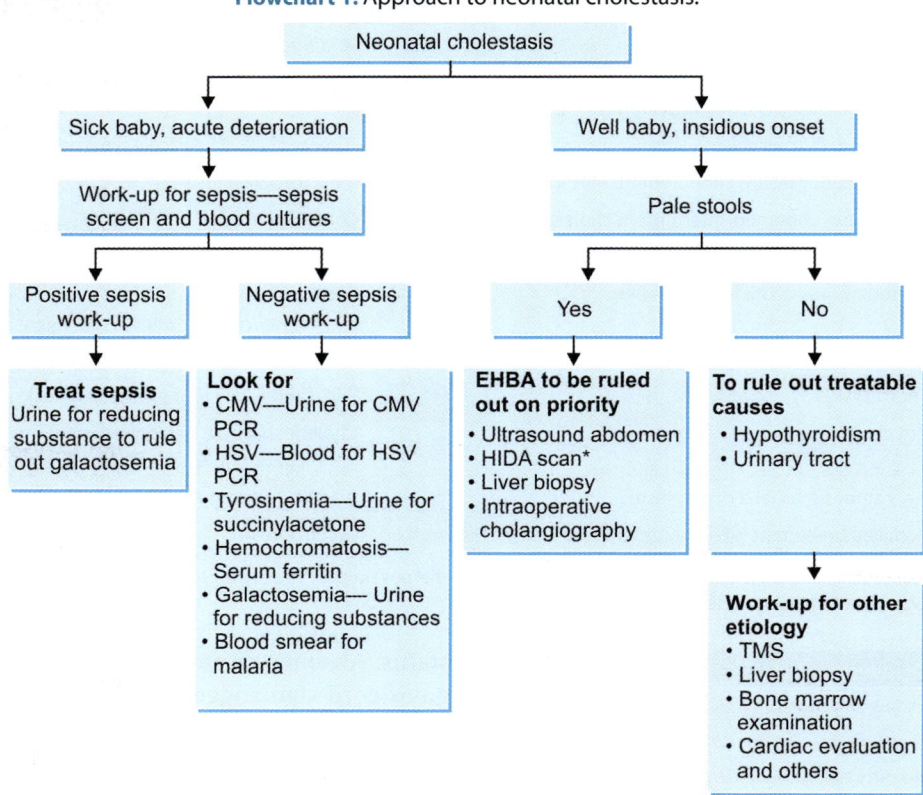

Flowchart 1: Approach to neonatal cholestasis.

*HIDA scan—if available and baby presents within 6 weeks.
(CMV: cytomegalovirus; HIDA: hepatobiliary iminodiacetic acid; HSV: herpes simplex virus; PCR: polymerase chain reaction; TMS: tandem mass spectrometry)

Serum ferritin, tandem mass spectrometry (TMS), urine for succinylacetone, PCR for CMV, HSV, hepatitis B, C markers, bone marrow examination, cardiac evaluation, may help in elucidating other causes of neonatal cholestasis (Flowchart 1).

MANAGEMENT

General

Neonates with cholestasis need additional calories to meet the metabolic demands. They need 125% of the recommended daily allowance (RDA) of calories. Protein should be at least 2–3 g/kg/day. Medium chain triglyceride (MCT) is the preferred fat as it does not require bile acids for absorption. MCT oil can be given to breastfed infants at a dose of 1–2 mL/kg/day (Table 3).

Specific Management

Medical: Specific management depends on the etiology (Table 4).

Surgical

Kasai's portoenterostomy is the standard procedure for EHBA. The success rate depends upon the age at the time of the surgery. Best results are seen if surgery is performed within

Table 3: Medical management of cholestasis.

Drug	Dose/day	Note
Vitamin A	5000 IU	3 months postcholestasis resolution
Vitamin D3	800–5000 IU	
Vitamin E	100 mg	
Vitamin K	2.5–5 mg, twice	No IM if INR abnormal
Zinc sulfate	1 mg/kg	Till resolution of cholestasis
MCT	1–2 ml/kg	
Calcium	100 mg/kg	
Phosphorus	50 mg/kg	
Ursodeoxycholic acid	20 mg/kg	

Table 4: Specific management in neonatal cholestasis.

Etiology	Specific management
Hypothyroidism	Thyroxine supplementation
Galactosemia	Lactose-free formula
Tyrosinemia	Nitisinone, tyrosine-restricted diet
Fructosemia	Avoid fructose
Bile acid synthetic defect	Ursodeoxy cholic acid or cholic acid supplementation
Bacterial infections	Antibiotics
Viral—CMV HSV Toxoplasmosis	Ganciclovir acyclovir pyrimethamine, sulfadoxine, and folinic acid

(CMV: cytomegalovirus; HSV: herpes simplex virus)

6 weeks, hence the need for investigating the cause of EHBA on a semiurgent basis. Choledochal cyst is surgically correctable and has good outcome.

PROGNOSIS

Only 20% of children after successful Kasai's procedure enter their adulthood with their native liver. Pediatric liver transplant is now a reality in our country. Most of the children with progressive forms of neonatal hepatitis/cholestasis will need liver transplant. Those presenting late or those presenting with signs of decompensated liver cell failure should be referred to liver transplant center.

SUGGESTED READING

1. Bhatia V, Bavdekar A, Matthai J, et al. Management of neonatal cholestasis: consensus statement of the Pediatric Gastroenterology Chapter of Indian Academy of Pediatrics. Indian Pediatr. 2014;51(3):203-10.
2. Feldman GA, Sokol RJ. Neonatal cholestasis: Neoreviews. 2013;14:e63-73.

CHAPTER 34

Congenital Hydronephrosis

Jaikrishan Mittal, Manish Mittal

INTRODUCTION

Fetal hydronephrosis (HN) (dilatation of the renal pelvis with or without dilation of the renal calyces) is a common, readily diagnosed finding on antenatal ultrasound (US) examination and can be detected as early as the 12th–14th week of gestation. Although renal pelvic dilatation is a transient, physiologic state in most cases, urinary tract obstruction and vesicoureteral reflux (VUR) are also causal. These conditions can be a result of abnormal renal development and/or causes renal injury. However, the majority of cases of antenatal HN are not clinically significant and therefore, excessive concern may lead to unnecessary testing of the newborn baby and anxiety for patients and healthcare providers.

The goal of postnatal management of infants with antenatal HN is to identify those with significant congenital anomalies of the kidney and urinary tract (CAKUT) while avoiding unnecessary testing in patients with physiological or clinically insignificant hydronephrosis.

In children in whom HN does not resolve during follow-up, it takes approximately 30 months for maximal US improvement in HN (Table 1).

PHYSICAL EXAMINATION

The physical examination of the newborn can detect abnormalities that suggest genitourinary abnormalities associated with antenatal HN. These include in Table 2.

Table 1: Chance of resolution of antenatally diagnosed hydronephrosis.

Grade I	50%
Grade II	36%
Grade III	16%
Grade IV	3%
Grade V	0%

Classification of hydronephrosis

Grade I: Pelvic anteroposterior diameter (APD) is 1 cm and the calyces are normal
Grade II: Pelvic APD is 1–1.5 cm but the calyces remain normal
Grade III: Pelvic APD is >1.5 cm and there is slight caliectasis
Grade IV: Pelvic APD is >1.5 cm with moderate caliectasis
Grade V: APD is >1.5 cm with severe caliectasis and thinning of the renal cortex (<2 mm thick)

Table 2: Clinical clues.

Finding on examination	Significance
Abdominal mass	Enlarged kidney due to obstructive uropathy or multicystic dysplastic kidney (MCDK)
Palpable bladder in a male infant especially after voiding	Suggest posterior urethral valves
Deficient abdominal wall musculature and undescended testes in male neonate	(Prune Belly syndrome)–Look for presence of associated congenital anomalies of the kidney and urinary tract (CAKUT)
Outer-ear abnormalities	Increased risk of CAKUT
Single umbilical artery	Increased risk of CAKUT, particularly vesicoureteral reflux
Spinal and/or lower extremity abnormalities	Suggests a neurogenic bladder, which may result in hydronephrosis and dilated ureters
Failure to void within first 48 hours	Obstructive uropathy, such as posterior urethral valves or urethral atresia

Table 3: Causes of antenatal hydronephrosis and ultrasound characteristics.

	Ipsilateral ureter	Bladder
UPJO	Normal	Normal
VUR	Dilated/Normal	Dilated/Normal
Ectopic ureter	Often dilated	Normal
PUV	Often dilated (bilateral)	Thick wall, increased Postvoid residual
Multicystic kidney	Normal	Normal
Primary obstructive or nonrefluxing Nonobstructing megaureter	Dilated	Normal
Urethral atresia	Dilated (bilateral)	Thick wall, not emptying (oligohydramnios)
Retrocaval ureter	Dilated proximal and normal distal	Normal

RADIOLOGIC STUDIES

Ultrasonography

Examination should be avoided in the first 2 days or 3 days after birth because HN may not be detected because of extracellular fluid shifts that will underestimate the degree of HN. However, infants with bilateral HN and those with a severe hydronephrotic solitary kidney require more urgent evaluation within 48 hours of birth because of the increased likelihood of significant disease and a possible need for early intervention (Table 3). For unilateral HN without antenatal bladder pathology, postnatal sonogram may be done at 1–4 weeks after birth.

Voiding Cystourethrogram

A voiding cystourethrogram (VCUG) is performed to detect vesicoureteral reflux (VUR) and in boys, to evaluate the posterior urethra.

For this procedure, a urinary catheter is inserted into the bladder and contrast material is instilled. Fluoroscopic monitoring is performed while the bladder is filling and during voiding. Although the duration of fluoroscopy is minimized, the gonads, especially the ovaries, are exposed to radiation.

Diuretic Renography

Diuretic renography (renal scan and the administration of a diuretic, typically furosemide) is used to diagnose urinary tract obstruction in infants with persistent HN, usually ordered after a VCUG has demonstrated no VUR. It measures the drainage time from the renal pelvis and assesses total and each individual kidney's renal function.

The test requires insertion of a bladder catheter to relieve any pressure that can be transmitted to the ureters and kidneys. Intravenous access is needed for hydration and the administration of the radioisotope and diuretic. The preferred radioisotope is technetium-99m-mercaptoacetyltriglycine (Tc99mMAG3), which is taken up by the renal cortex, filtered across the glomerular basement membrane to the renal tubules, and excreted into the renal pelvis and urinary tract.

A number of factors can affect the accuracy of the diuretic renogram. This includes the state of hydration of the infant, the functionality of the bladder catheter, the timing of diuretic administration, the accuracy of physically outlining the renal tissue in the presence of severe HN, and background effect from the liver and spleen. As a rule of thumb, a 5% change in spilt renal function is unlikely to be clinically significant.

Magnetic Resonance Urography

Magnetic resonance urography (MRU) in children is becoming more commonly used in the diagnosis and management of congenital uropathies, such as ureteropelvic junction obstruction. MRU is especially useful in the management of obstructed kidneys that have rotation or ascent anomalies, or are solitary. MRU can more clearly define the anatomy and delineate the proper surgical approach (i.e. retroperitoneal versus transperitoneal). The disadvantage of MRU is that the study often requires a general anesthesia or heavy conscious sedation in children. Furthermore, the contrast agent gadolinium can only be used if the renal function is normal (requiring a preprocedure serum creatinine test) because of reports of irreversible renal fibrosis in patients with renal insufficiency. Newer MRU technology may even define obstruction, eliminating the need for diuretic renal scans.

APPROACH

The risk of renal and urinary tract abnormality increases with the severity of HN, persistence of HN into the third trimester, bilateral involvement, and the presence of oligohydramnios.

Step I: Is it unilateral or bilateral hydronephrosis?

Step II: Confirmation by US at 4–7 days of life.
- *Unilateral:*
  Ureter present: Yes: Do micturating cystourethrogram (MCU)
  No: Tc99DTPA renal scan with diuretic renography should be done to detect pelvic ureteric junction (PUJ) obstruction.
- *Bilateral:* As above + BUN/Serum creatinine.

Step III: Medical management:

Asymptomatic HN or HN which is mild to moderate and stable after USG within 3–7 days, with no obstruction (hydronephrosis due to VUR)
- Antibiotic prophylaxis not routinely recommended.
- Urine cultures may be necessary if fever occurs or clinical suspicion of urinary tract infection (UTI).
- Diuretic renography, MCU are recommended at 1–2 months after antibiotics.
- USG after a year.

If VUR is detected:
- Dimercaptosuccinic acid (DMSA) renal scan to detect renal scars.

Table 4: Indications for surgical evaluation.	
Initially at diagnosis	**On follow up**

PUJ obstruction
1. At initial diagnosis–
   a. Symptomatic HN (UTI, renal mass, growth failure)
   b. Solitary kidney with impaired function
   c. Bilateral severe HN
2. Relative renal function of obstructive kidney <30%.
	1. 10% decline in relative renal function on DTPA renal scan when repeated after 6–12 weeks
	2. Increasing HN
	3. Post urethral valves, ureteroceles
	4. VUR Grade IV–V persisting beyond infancy
	5. New renal scars or recurrent UTI despite antibiotic prophylaxis

PUJ: pelvic ureteric junction; HN: hydronephrosis; UTI: urinary tract infection; DTPA: diethylenetriamine pentaacetic acid; VUR: vesicoureteral reflux)

- Surgery may be needed if scars are present or there is presence of Grade IV–V VUR.
- Repeat MCU/diuretic venography at 2 years to decide about resolution of VUR.
- DMSA renal scan should be done every 2–3 years if scars are persistent or to detect presence of new scars.
- Blood pressure (BP), growth monitoring, serum creatinine/BUN, USG should be done yearly till 15–20 years.

Step IV: Surgical management (Tables 4 and 5)
Antibiotic prophylaxis: Routine prophylactic antibiotics are no longer recommended for all infants with antenatal HN (APD ≥5 mm). Families should be counseled on signs and symptoms of UTIs.

Normal Postnatal Ultrasound

Infants with a normal postnatal examination (defined as a renal pelvic diameter ≤ 7 mm without any evidence of calyceal or ureteric dilatation, or signs of renal dysplasia or anomalies) require no further evaluation. Many studies recommend a repeat US at 4–6 weeks of age.

Table 5: Clinical parameters to indicate surgical intervention.
- Reduced differential function, less than 40% - Deterioration of differential function greater than 5% - Sustained or increased HN - Unilateral gross HN, greater than 50 mm - Severe HN in solitary kidney - Severe bilateral HN, greater than 30 mm - Febrile breakthrough infection or symptoms.

Prognosis

The outcome is based on—(i) renal function, (ii) bladder function, and (iii) presence/absence of other anomalies, such as high-grade reflux or a nonfunctioning kidney.

SUGGESTED READING

1. Cohen JN, Ringer SA. Congenital kidney abnormalities: Diagnosis, management, and palliative care. Neo Reviews. 2010;11(5):e226-35.
2. Fefer S, Ellsworth P. Prenatal hydronephrosis. Pediatr Clin North Am. 2006;53(3):429-47, vii.
3. Liu DB, Armstrong WR 3rd, Maizels M. Hydronephrosis prenatal and postnatal evaluation and management. Clin Perinatol. 2014;41(3):661-78.

CHAPTER
35

Common Problems in Newborn in Outpatient Department

Nishad Plakkal

DIAPER RASH

Diaper dermatitis is commonly an irritant contact dermatitis but can be complicated by candida or bacterial infections. It can be considered the price paid (by the baby) for the convenience (of the family more than the baby) of using diapers, since maximizing diaper-free time is an effective, albeit inconvenient, way of preventing and treating diaper rash (Fig. 1). The spectrum of diaper dermatitis can vary from mild localized erythema to widespread erosions and ulceration.

Clinical pearl: Irritant dermatitis typically spares the folds and involves convex surfaces of the thighs and buttocks, while a candida rash can be identified by beefy red plaques with satellite lesions and involvement of the folds (Fig. 2).

Treatment
- Minimizing skin contact with the etiological factors, i.e. wet diaper, stools, and urine
- Parents can be requested to check the diaper frequently and change them promptly when wet
- Avoid tight-fitting diapers or "nonbreathable" diapers with plastic backing
- Barrier preparations like zinc oxide paste also help

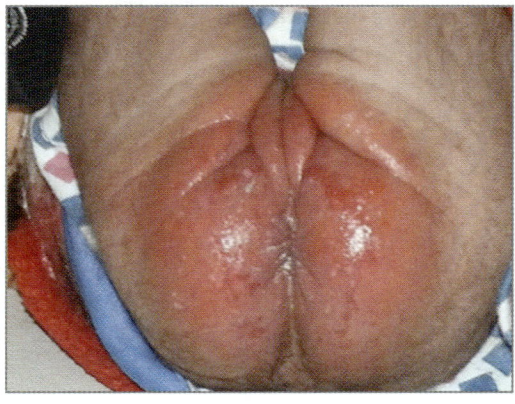

Fig. 1: Diaper dermatitis.

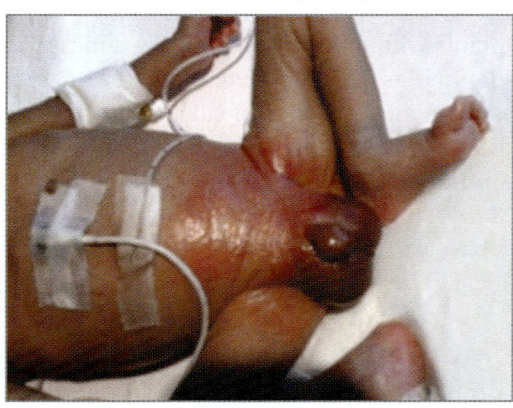

Fig. 2: Candida dermatitis.

- Parents can be instructed to gently clean the affected areas with lukewarm water and dry by patting (as opposed to vigorous wiping)
- If a candida infection is suspected, topical clotrimazole (or other azoles, nystatin or ciclopirox) can be prescribed for a week. In severe cases, a mild steroid like 1% hydrocortisone can be applied. It is better to obtain a dermatology consultation if the rash does not respond to these measures.
Tip: Occasionally, seborrheic dermatitis can be mistaken for diaper dermatitis. Suspect this if there are seborrheic dermatitis lesions elsewhere on the infant's skin or if there is poor response to treatment.

COLIC: THE CRYING INFANT

Infantile colic is traditionally defined by the "rule of three": Crying for more than three hours per day, for more than three days per week and for longer than three weeks in an otherwise well infant.

Clinical pearl: A baby who is otherwise well in between the crying episodes, gains weight, has no localization on physical examination and is exclusively breastfed, does not need further evaluation.

Practice tip: It is impossible to examine a baby adequately during a bout of crying, so a repeat examination should be done when the infant is quiet. A cursory examination might miss clues regarding the etiology of crying, which might be as simple as a shed eyelash irritating the conjunctiva.

NOT ENOUGH MILK!

The first question that begs an answer is if there is a genuine problem, or if it is merely the perception of the infant's mother (or sometimes the aunt or the father or the grandmother).

In many cases, the infant is *thriving well* and growth charting shows growth along the appropriate centile lines. Even in these cases, where the infant's milk intake is likely normal, it is worthwhile finding out why the mother perceives that she has less milk. The case is often that all crying on the infant's part is attributed to he or she being hungry and not satisfied with the mother's milk output. Reassurance and if needed, lactation counseling are usually all that are required.

But when the infant's growth is faltering, there may be a problem with the mother's milk output (Fig. 3). Carefully examine the infant for retrognathia, cleft palate, severe tongue tie, or systemic illnesses that may be responsible for poor feeding and weight loss. Examine the mother's breast for abnormalities like inverted nipples.

Successful lactation is dependent on the physical and mental well-being of the mother and true lactation failure is probably rare, so an in-depth discussion with the mother (rather than a metoclopramide prescription, no questions asked) may help to identify the hurdles to breast feeding. None of the galactogogues has been studied for long-term use. Herbal preparations should not be prescribed.

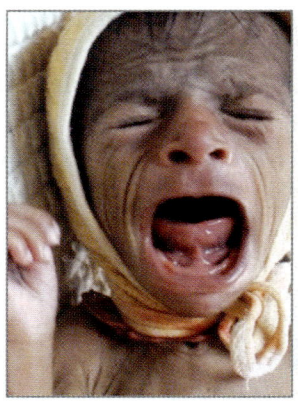

Fig. 3: Loss of subcutaneous fat.

Practice tip: When a galactogogue is indicated, domperidone may be preferable to metoclopramide in view of a better adverse effect profile including extrapyramidal effects, with similar augmentation of milk output.

HEALTH SUPPLEMENTS

Currently for term breast-fed and formula-fed neonates, vitamin D supplementation is recommended by World Health Organization (WHO). Exclusive breast-feeding for the first 6 months is still the gold standard. Preterm infants should receive vitamin D, multivitamins, iron and calcium phosphorous.

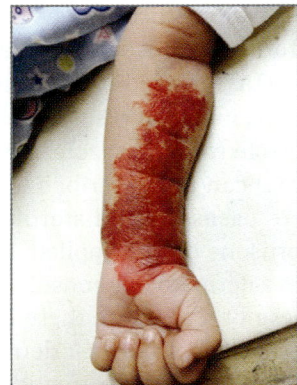

Fig. 4: Capillary hemangioma.

HEMANGIOMAS

Strawberry hemangiomas can be present at birth but are usually not prominent in the first days and weeks of life. The typical history is of an enlarging swelling on the skin and examination shows a red or purplish, soft and compressible mass on the skin, most commonly in the head and neck region (Figs. 4 to 6). After increasing in size during infancy, they involute and often disappear completely, but sometimes leave behind scars, skin atrophy or hypopigmentation. Parents can be told that 50% of these lesions will disappear by 5 years of age and 90% by 10 years. Unless they involve the eyes or airway or are extensive, they can be left alone. Parents can be instructed to seek medical care in case of ulceration or bleeding.

Treatment is indicated if there is loss of function or the hemangioma is likely to be life threatening. Propranolol has emerged as the treatment of choice in recent years. The typical dose is 2 mg/kg/day in 3 divided doses (mean duration of treatment is around 6 months). Steroids are useful, but are much less commonly used after propranolol was found to be effective.

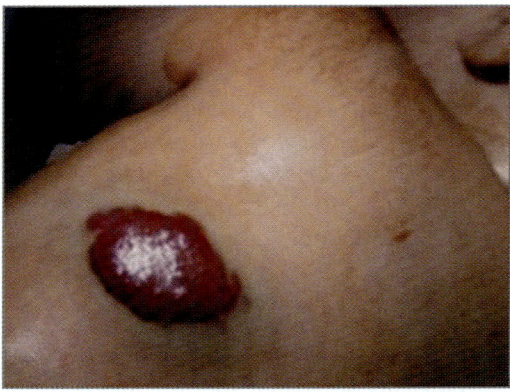

Fig. 5: Cavernous hemangioma.

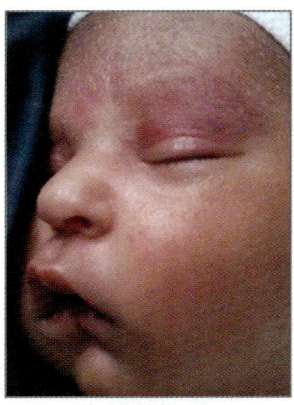

Fig. 6: Stork bites.

JAUNDICE

Assessment and management of the neonate with jaundice is covered in detail elsewhere in this book, but with the increasing tendency towards early hospital discharge of infants born vaginally (typically within 24 hours), more neonates can be expected to present with clinically important jaundice to the outpatient department. A few practice points are to be noted when evaluating jaundice on an outpatient basis (Fig. 7).

- A transcutaneous measurement or serum bilirubin must be obtained when possible, rather than relying solely on clinical assessment. Hour-specific nomograms are very helpful, but the commonly used American Academy of Pediatrics (AAP) (American) and National Institute for Health and Care Excellence (NICE) (British) nomograms are not validated for Indian infants. Hence, it may be the best to err on the side of caution if the values are borderline.
- Assessment of risk factors is important in all cases but is especially relevant if the jaundice is being assessed only clinically. Major risk factors (as identified by the AAP) include:
  - Predischarge bilirubin value in the high-risk zone.
  - Jaundice observed in the first 24 hours.
  - Blood group incompatibility with positive DCT (direct Coombs test) or other hemolytic disease (like G6PD deficiency).
  - Late preterm infant (34–36 weeks).
  - Previous sibling received phototherapy
  - Cephalhematoma or significant bruising.
  - Exclusive breastfeeding (especially with excessive weight loss).
- If screening for hypothyroidism is not routinely done as part of neonatal screening in your institution, a low threshold should be kept for sending thyroid function tests. This is especially true if the jaundice is prolonged and breast-milk jaundice is the diagnosis being considered.

Clinical pearl: Remember that infants who had phototherapy for ABO or Rh incompatibility can have ongoing hemolysis due to maternal antibodies in their blood for weeks. These infants may present to the OPD with anemia and not with jaundice (by then the liver and gastrointestinal system have often matured enough to handle the bilirubin load).

BREAST DISCHARGE

Both male and female infants can have swelling of the breast tissue under the influence of maternal estrogens, sometimes with small quantities of fluid leaking from the breast (Fig. 8). This usually happens in the first week of life and resolves by the second week. Parents should be reassured and sometimes expressly instructed not to attempt to squeeze out the fluid or handle the breast. Injury to the breast tissue may result from unnecessary handling, leading to infection and neonatal mastitis.

NATAL/NEONATAL TEETH

Natal teeth are present at birth and neonatal teeth appear in the first month of life (Fig. 9).

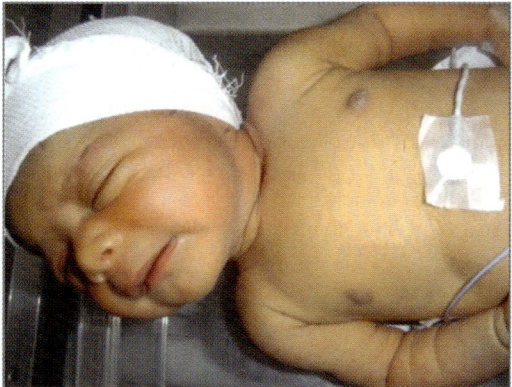

Fig. 7: Jaundice.

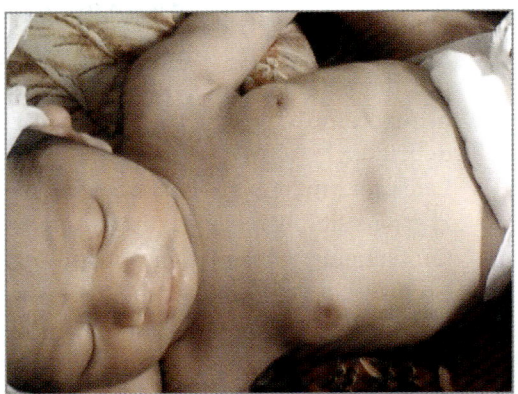

Fig. 8: Breast engorgement.

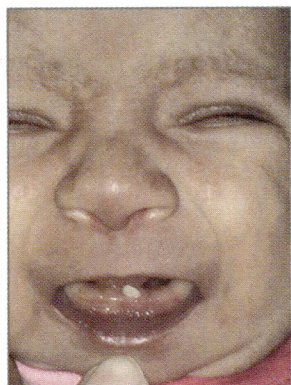

Fig. 9: Natal tooth.

They are usually poorly formed, conical and often hypermobile, unlike regular teeth. If they are left alone, traumatic injury and ulceration of the tongue can result, interfering with feeding. Because these teeth are very mobile, there is also a possibility that the infant may swallow or aspirate the teeth. A dental consultation and planned extraction is the usual treatment. Radiographic examination can help confirm that the tooth is supernumerary and not of normal dentition (which are usually preserved). If nonmobile, no intervention is required.

Clinical pearl: Remember to check if vitamin K has been administered prior to dental extraction.

ORAL THRUSH

Oropharyngeal candidiasis is caused by *Candida albicans (Fig. 10)*. In majority it is a benign condition. Presence of diarrhea, recurrent infections, failure to thrive, hepatosplenomegaly or other symptoms may be a subtle indication for underlying immunodeficiency. Diagnosis is usually made by visual inspection alone. If in doubt, a simple Gram stain will show gram-positive yeast.

1% clotrimazole drops are easily available, inexpensive and do not stain clothes or mucous

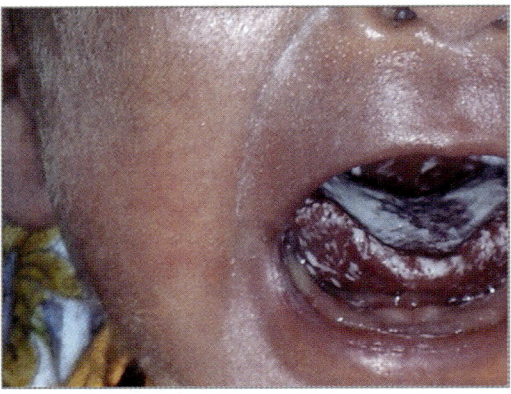

Fig. 10: Oral thrush.

membranes, unlike gentian violet. Two drops can be applied to the mouth thrice a day for a week. Alternatively, nystatin or miconazole can also be used where available. It is not necessary to spread the medication around the oral cavity with a finger or swab.

> *Tip:* A coated tongue, as in an infant who has just fed, is not thrush. The plaques in oral thrush are difficult to remove with the wooden spatula that is commonly used for examining the oral cavity and bleeding spots are noted when the plaques are removed.

PHIMOSIS

The foreskin is nonretractable at birth in most neonates due to adhesions between the prepuce and the glans and this phimosis can therefore be considered physiological. However, this can be a source of anxiety for parents. It is physiological during first year of life.

SEBORRHEIC DERMATITIS/ CRADLE CAP

A common complaint raised by mothers is the presence of unsightly scaly plaques on the scalps of their infants (Fig. 11). Less commonly, the rash is around the eyebrows, eyelids, ears or on other areas. The greasy, crusty scales are typical of the condition and no diagnostic testing is required. *Malassezia furfur* has been associated with seborrheic dermatitis.

The condition is self-limited and parents can be reassured. Application of oil followed by gentle combing a few hours later will dislodge the scales. This can be repeated daily or as necessary. Lotions or shampoos containing ketoconazole or selenium sulfide may be safe (low systemic absorption) but are better avoided since the condition is harmless. 1% hydrocortisone preparations are also effective; surface area of application should be limited to minimize the risk of systemic absorption and adrenal suppression.

TRANSITIONAL STOOLS/DIARRHEA

True infective diarrhea is rare in exclusively breastfed infants. Transitional stools are often mistaken for diarrhea and the typical time of onset (around the third or fourth day of life) and character of the stool (greenish, liquid stool, sometimes with yellowish curds) should be enough to reassure both the pediatrician and the parent. These infants are also well-looking and there are no signs of dehydration. By the end of the first week, a breastfed infant should be typically passing bright yellow, seedy stools. If the loose stools are of later onset or last longer than 4–5 days, especially in a bottle-fed infant or an infant with fever, dehydration or other symptoms, diarrhea is probable. If still in the neonatal period, these infants should be admitted to the hospital for further evaluation and treatment.

Clinical Pearl: Watery stools, blood or mucus in the stool should not be ignored.

UMBILICAL DISCHARGE/BLEEDING

Discharge and bleeding from the umbilical stump are common complaints in the neonatal period (Fig. 12). The etiology can vary from

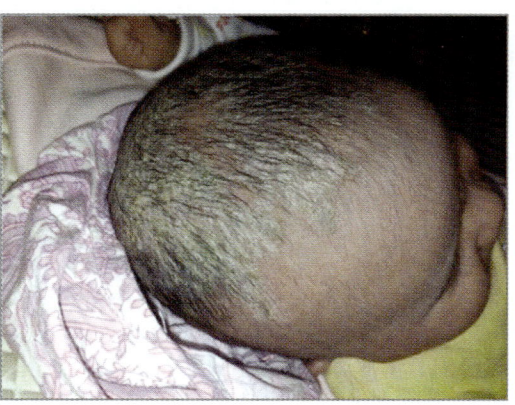

Fig. 11: Seborrheic dermatitis.

Box 1: Normal findings mistaken as abnormal.

- Dehydration fever
- Transitional stool
- Setting sun sign
- Sutural separation
- Cortical thumb
- Erythema toxicum
- Phimosis
- Umbilical granuloma/hernia
- Red spot in eye
- Sternomastoid tumor
- Jitteriness
- Palpable kidneys

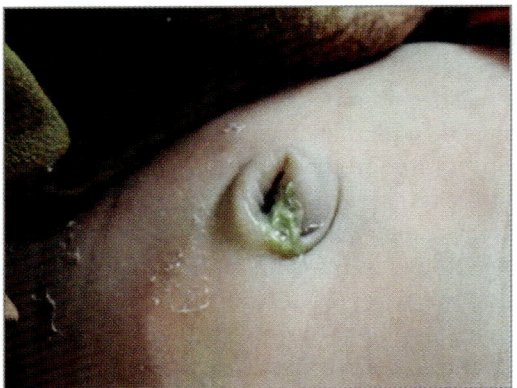

Fig. 12: Umbilical discharge.

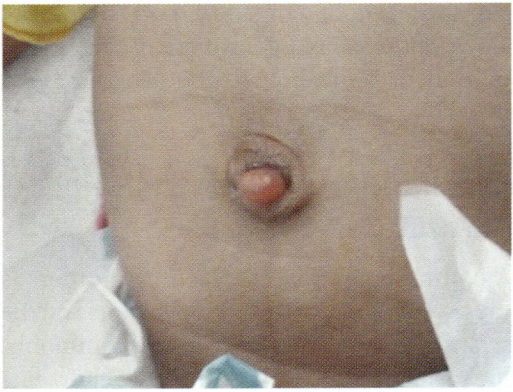

Fig. 13: Umbilical granuloma.

potentially life-threatening conditions like omphalitis to more benign conditions like umbilical granulomas or the presence of omphalomesenteric remnants.

Umbilical granulomas are a common cause of both discharge and bleeding from the umbilicus and result from persisting granulation tissue at the base of the umbilicus (Fig. 13). They are pink, friable and typically less than a centimeter across. When symptomatic, they can be treated with salt application. Cauterizations with copper sulfate or silver nitrate are other options. If cauterization is done, care must be taken to protect surrounding normal skin with Vaseline® or other occlusive material to prevent burns. If these measures fail, especially with large granulomas, surgical excision is done.

Persistent omphalomesenteric remnants can result in the presence of polyps or cysts. A polyp is often redder than a granuloma because it arises from gastric/intestinal mucosa. While it is sometimes mistaken for a granuloma, it does not respond to topical therapy and will need to be removed by the pediatric surgeon.

The presence of urachal remnants like a patent urachus, sinus or cyst can also result in umbilical discharge and when the patent urachus is connected to the bladder, urine may be seen draining from the umbilicus. These also need surgical removal.

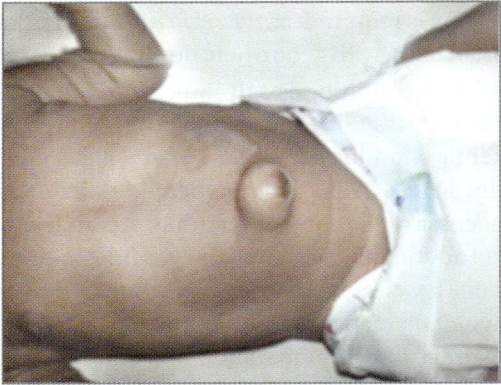

Fig. 14: Umbilical hernia.

UMBILICAL HERNIA

An umbilical hernia results when the anterior abdominal wall underlying the umbilicus is defective and is a common neonatal finding (Fig. 14). In majority, the condition is self-limiting and benign. The rate of complications is less than 1%. Many umbilical hernias close spontaneously in the first year of life and most before 4–5 years of life.

It is important to differentiate them from paraumbilical hernias which arise from above the umbilicus and do not close spontaneously. In general, parents can be reassured and surgical closure is only indicated if complications occur or for cosmetic reasons in school-age children (after 4–5 years).

VAGINAL BLEEDING

Vaginal bleeding in female neonates can be very worrying to parents (Figs. 15 and 16).

This bleeding is related to withdrawal of maternal estrogens and is most common in the first week of life, typically starting around 3–5 days after birth and lasting 2–3 days, with passage of a few drops of blood.

If the bleeding persists beyond a week or is copious, a bleeding disorder or coagulopathy has to be ruled out and vitamin K administration status should be checked. Trauma and abuse, although very rare, have to be kept in mind when evaluating any bleeding female neonate.

BATHING/SKIN CARE OF THE PRETERM INFANT AT HOME

Given the limited evidence regarding best practice recommendations for bathing preterm or VLBW (very low birth weight) infants at home, it is prudent to err on the side of caution. In general, it is best to advise parents that the baby be given a bath indoors in lukewarm water to prevent hypothermia. Bath time can be restricted to around 5 minutes, following which the baby can be quickly dried and clothed.

The use of soap or other cleansers is not routinely recommended for preterm infants because of concerns about interference with skin barrier function and skin integrity. If, however, a soap is used to wash the diaper region or for a bath, a pH-balanced soap or liquid cleanser, or a syndet-based (syndets are synthetic detergents and are used in commercial products like Dove® and Cetaphil®) product is probably the best option.

If skin emollients are used, especially during winter months, coconut oil is the best choice, since it is time-tested, economical and easily available.

The use of powders for skin care should be discouraged, since they have no proven benefits and can cause skin irritation or be accidentally inhaled.

EYE DISCHARGE

The most common cause is nasolacrimal duct obstruction. If there is no redness or swelling of the eye, the mother can be advised to massage the inner angle of the eye with her finger, after cutting her fingernails and taking care to keep away from the white of the eye. If the discharge persists for more than a year, probing by an ophthalmologist may be required.

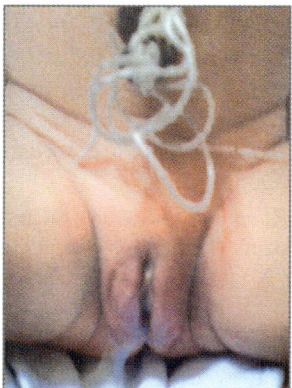

Fig. 15: Vaginal discharge.

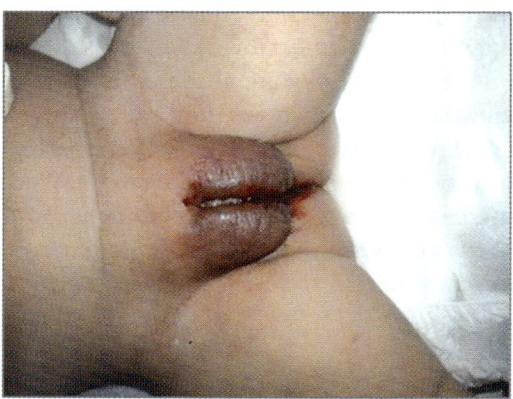

Fig. 16: Vaginal bleed.

Practice tip: If the eye is red and edematous in a neonate, start antibacterial eye drops and consult an ophthalmologist.

REGURGITATION

Feed regurgitation is common and is due to overfeeding. This is usually mistaken as vomiting by the mother. A newborn who gains weight, is active and appears calm and composed postfeed does not need further evaluation. Altered cry, activity, and poor or static weight is a cause of worry. Assurance to parents and not medications is the mainstay.

CONSTIPATION/INFREQUENT STOOLS

Some newborns pass infrequent stools, at times once in 10 days. The infant is otherwise active, playful, gaining weight with abdomen soft and no localization. This physiologic variation, if not realized, can lead to unnecessary investigations or interventions, viz. enema, laxative, soap or oil instillation which is potentially harmful. Assurance and allaying anxiety is indicated.

NEONATAL SLEEP MYOCLONUS

Some newborns develop sudden jerky body movements especially during sleep which may affect the trunk, arms or legs to disappear on their own. They are absent when awake and the newborn shows no localizing signs and appears well and active. The classical history and clinical status is diagnostic. Work up on seizures is negative including an EEG (electroencephalogram). The benign nature of the condition should lead to assurance to the parents to allay their anxiety. No treatment is required and anticonvulsive therapy is not indicated. The condition disappears by 6 months in majority with no neurologic consequences.

Box 2: Abnormal findings mistaken as normal.
- Excess weight gain
- Quiet baby
- Fullness of dorsum of hand and feet
- Murmur
- Cyanosis relieved on crying
- Cyanosis exacerbated on crying

Box 3: Danger signs.
- Decreased/Poor feeding
- Decreased activity
- Excessive crying
- Lethargy
- Ear discharge
- Convulsions
- Fever (>37.5°C)
- Hypothermia (<36.5°C)
- Not passed urine (24 hours), not passed stool (48 hours after birth)
- Bleeding from any site
- Cyanosis

SUGGESTED READING

1. Barreto L, Khan AR, Khanbhai M, Brain JL. Umbilical hernia. BMJ. 2013;347:f4252.
2. Cunha RF, Boer FA, Torriani DD, Frossard WT. Natal and neonatal teeth: review of the literature. Pediatr Dent. 2001;23(2):158-62.
3. Lawn JE, Davidge R, Paul VK, et al. Born too soon: care for the preterm baby. Reprod Health. 2013;10 Suppl 1:S5.
4. Martin RJ, Fanaroff AA, Walsh MC (Eds). Fanaroff and Martin's Neonatal-Perinatal Medicine, 9th Edition. 2011.

CHAPTER 36

Optimizing Breastfeeding in a Normal Newborn

Anu Thukral

Breast milk is the most optimum nutrition for the newborn baby. WHO recommends exclusively breastfeeding for the first 6 months. Complementary food needs to be introduced while continuing breastfeeding for 2 years or beyond.

BREASTFEEDING INITIATION AND MAINTENANCE

When?

As early as possible, in the delivery room.

Why?

Early breastfeeding initiation increases milk production and infant weight gain.

How?

Immediately after birth a normal newborn should be placed skin-to-skin and mother-infant dyad should be helped in initiation of breastfeeding. Allow some time to the neonate for licking. Ensure optimal latch. Shift to other breast once the infant stops swallowing from the breast. This leads to stimulation of breast milk. The infant may not feed but it is important that he be put to the other breast.

Focus on?

Good positioning and good attachment.

Key Position during Breastfeeding

The key points of good positioning are as follows (Figs. 1 and 2):
- Head in line with the body.
- Whole body well supported.
- Baby turned toward the mother.
- Baby's abdomen touching the mother's abdomen.

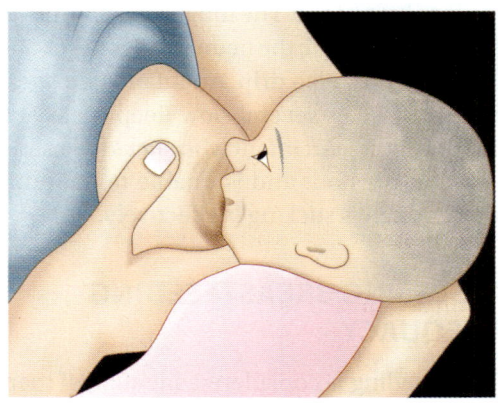

Fig. 1: Good positioning.

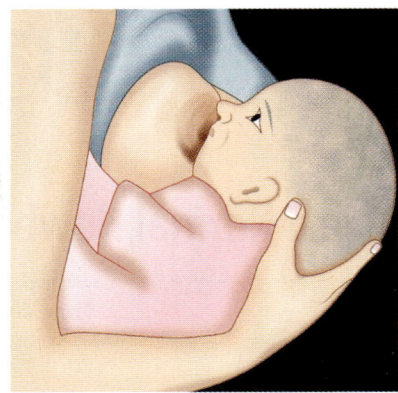

Fig. 2: Football positioning for breastfeeding.

Key Points of Attachment during Breastfeeding

The four signs of good attachment are:
1. More areola visible above the baby's mouth than below it.
2. Baby's mouth is wide open.
3. Baby's lower lip is turn outward.
4. Baby's chin is touching the mother's breast.

Breastfeeding Cues

A newborn opens eyes, seeks breast, turns the head back slightly and open the mouth when ready to breastfeed. The tongue usually moves down and forward; the neonate tries to lick and the saliva may also drip. An infant who sucks effectively takes several slow deep sucks and then swallows. An infant who sucks for a short time but tires out and is unable to continue long enough is sucking ineffectively.

ASSESSING BREASTFEEDING ADEQUACY

Breastfeeding is considered adequate if there is softening of breast after a feeding session and the neonate sleeps well between the breastfeeding sessions, passes urine at least 6–8 times in a day, crosses birth weight by 2 weeks and gains at least 25–30 g per day after the initial 7–10 days.

ISSUES/CONCERNS FOR BREASTFEEDING IN THE FIRST FEW DAYS AND THEIR MANAGEMENT

Managing Anatomical Nipple Variations in the Early Neonatal Period

Amongst the problems of anatomical variation, flat nipple is by far the most common. Very rarely one may see inverted nipple as well.

Flat/Inverted Nipple

This nipple can be everted with a nipple everter which is made from a plastic syringe. It is applied over the nipple to help make the nipple prominent making it easier for the infant to latch on the breast.

To use syringe method (preparation of syringe depicted in Figures 3A to D) for flat nipple: ask the mother to apply the plunger and gently pull back applying suction over a count of 10 to the nipple. This is done prior to each feeding or repeated between feedings as required. Breast pump may be used to apply gentle pressure prior to feedings to assist eversion of nipple and ease babies latch-on.

Note: Nipple shield should not be used in the first few days of breastfeeding.

At every point of contact, breastfeeding needs to be assessed for positioning and attachment.

Managing a Frantic Baby

- The characteristics of a fussy baby include a baby who continuously demands feeds, is irritable making the mother exhausted.
- One should check position and attachment, promote skin-to-skin contact and help mother to identify feeding cues. One can express colostrum and apply it over breast

CHAPTER 36
Optimizing Breastfeeding in a Normal Newborn

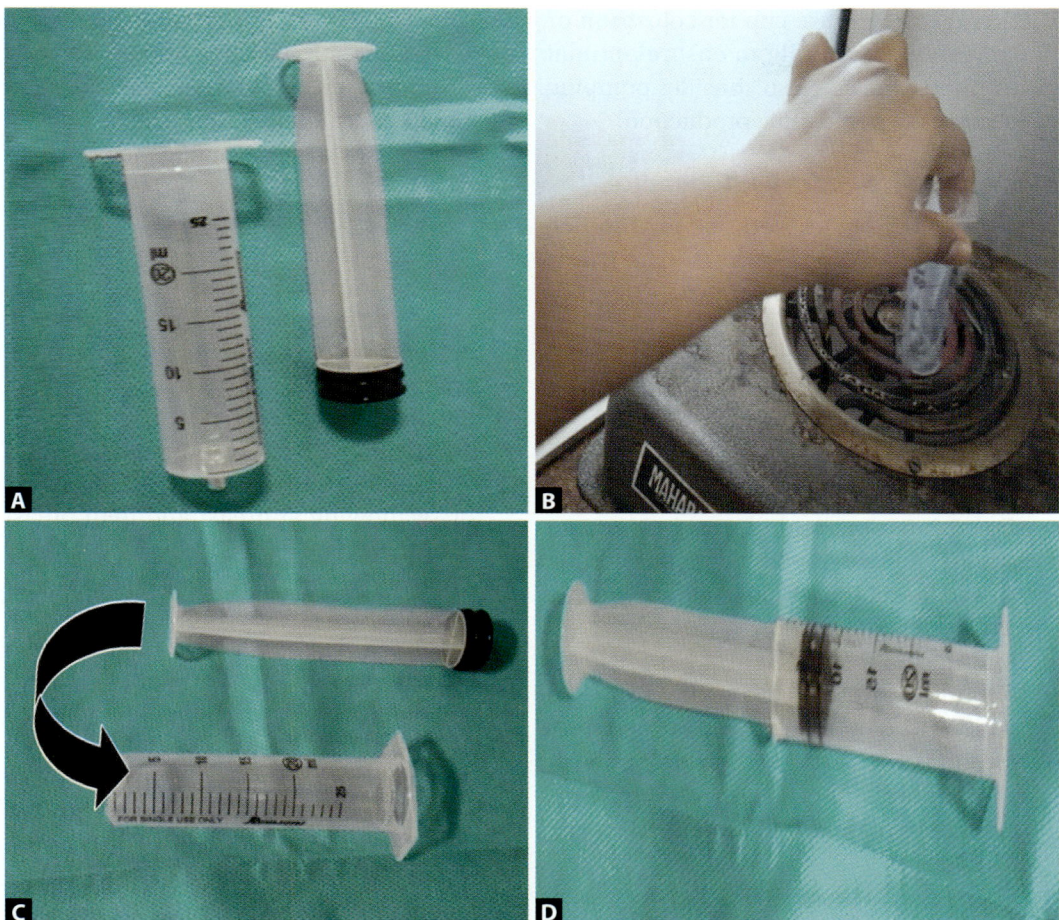

Figs. 3A to D: Preparation of syringe for flat nipple. (A) The plunger is removed from the syringe, (B) The tip of the syringe is heated over hot plate so that the plastic melts and can be easily cut with the blade, (C) The plunger is put into the syringe through the cut end, (D) The syringe method for flat nipple is ready.

to promote latch on. At times cup feeding after attempt to breastfeed helps. This problem may require pumping to stimulate earlier milk production.
- The mother has to be reassured that the baby will quieten once the volume of milk increases.

Managing a Sleepy Newborn
- The characteristics of a sleepy newborn include having difficulty in waking for feeds, the baby latching but not feeding vigorously, having weight loss or inadequate voids and stools.
- This newborn needs assessment and optimization of position and attachment. Skin-to-skin contact needs to be promoted. Mother should be taught about feeding cues. The mother should stimulate the newborn by tickling or tapping ensuring the baby stays awake at breast.
- Encourage mother to wake the baby to feed every 3 hours after 24 hours of age.

- Alternative is to use cup for colostrum or expressed breast milk to ensure optimal nutrition. One can also consider pumping to stimulate earlier milk production.

Managing a Newborn with Jaundice

Newborns have increased risk of jaundice due to inherent known factors. One needs to increase the frequency of effective breastfeeding.

Indications for Supplementation in the Hospital Setting

- Supplemental feedings are not indicated routinely. In cases of maternal infant separation, maternal illness, inadequate mother's milk, asymptomatic hypoglycemia or need for contraindicated medication one may need to use them.
- Bottle feeding should be avoided as it leads to nipple confusion. Every effort must be made to feed by syringe, paladai, or cup.
- Potential concerns with supplementation include decreased milk output, engorgement, and perceived breast milk insufficiency.

Managing Sore Nipples

- The most common cause of sore nipples in a breastfeeding mother is poor attachment, which means a poor latch or improper placement of the mouth on the mother's breast.
- Very rarely the underlying cause may be candidiasis. Treatment includes ensuring proper positioning and attachment.
- The mother can apply hind milk to the sore nipple after breastfeeding the infant.
- However, if the nipple is very sore and the mother has unbearable pain one can consider pumping for 24–48 hours; however, ensuring proper latch during breastfeeding is the single most important maneuver to prevent sore nipples. In addition, frequent washing of the nipple with soap and water should be avoided. Bathing once a day in sufficient for a breastfeeding mother.

Breast Engorgement

- Mother should be assessed for breast swelling, warmth, redness, throbbing pain, fever. The neonate should be assessed for difficulty in latching to the breast; the swelling may make nipple and the areola taut and less everted.
- The staff should ensure optimum latch and position, increase frequency of feeds, assess for swallowing at breast and help breast compressions.
- Teaching the mother optimal latch and assessment of adequate intake needs to be reinforced. The mother should do a brief massage prior to breastfeeding.
- Application of warm moist heat prior to breastfeeding helps increase milk flow.
- The mother can also hand pump milk or use a breast pump. Gentle circular massage from the periphery toward the nipple area will stimulate let-down. For severe engorgement, heat and massage are used simultaneously till the breasts are emptied. Breastfeeding frequently helps prevent engorgement in the breast. The breasts should be completely emptied.
- Every attempt must be made to ensue that the baby finishes suckling on the breast and then is moved to the other breast. This helps relieved discomfort as it leads to complete emptying of breast.
- Cabbage leaves are home remedy for engorgement. To use them either cool them in the fridge or use dry leaves leaving them inside the bra. The crumpled leaves are replaced by fresh ones. Engorgement is relieved by 8 hours of application.

Mastitis

- Breastfeeding mothers with mastitis complain of sudden onset localized lump with intense localized pain. On examination, redness may appear in a wedge-shaped area on the breast which is pink or red, hot, tender, and swollen. Mother has flu-like symptoms and fever. The infant may be "fussy" during feeding because of decreased flow of milk from affected area.
- Apply heat to the affected breast area to promote breast drainage. Mother should be advised warm showers, hot water packs, a heating pad, or a hot water bottle between breastfeeding sessions.
- Massage to the affected area when it is warm, in a gentle but firm circular motion also helps relieve discomfort.
- Following warmth application and massage mother may feed or express milk. Getting the milk to flow while the breast is still warm will help to thoroughly drain affected area.
- Frequent breastfeeding is necessary to ensure adequacy of milk flow. If a bra is used the size should be larger or one that has a different cut or style. This prevents any pressure on the affected area.
- Ensue appropriate attachment and supervise feeds.

Inadequate Milk Supply

- It is to be considered: (a) If the neonate is losing weight after the first week or (b) the neonate does not regain birth weight by two weeks or (c) the weight loss is greater than 10% of birth weight. One must evaluate if there is enough milk or if the baby is not taking enough milk.
- Signs of dehydration are rare and indicate a search for pathological cause.
- Mother needs to be evaluated for why she is not getting enough milk—viz. stress, illness, pain, false perception, infertility, lack of support, top feeds, and maternal medication (including oral contraceptives and antihypertensives).
- If baby is not having a good suck it leads to progressive milk decrease. The milk production needs to be stimulated, increased, or maintained by frequent expression of milk, galactogogues, or using back massages.

SUGGESTED READING

1. Agostoni C, Braegger C, Decsi T, et al.. Breastfeeding: A commentary by the ESPGHAN Committee on Nutrition. J Pediatr Gastroenterol Nutr. 2009;49(1):112-25.
2. Demirtas B. Strategies to support breastfeeding: a review. Int Nurs Rev. 2012;59(4):474-81.
3. Quigley MA, Kelly YJ, Sacker A. Breastfeeding and hospitalization for diarrheal and respiratory infection in the United Kingdom Millennium Cohort Study. Pediatrics. 2007;119(4):e837-42.
4. WHO Collaborating Centre for Training and Research in Newborn Care. Facility Based Newborn Nursing, 3rd edition. New Delhi: All India Institute of Medical Sciences; 2014-15.
5. World Health Organization (WHO). 10 Facts on Breastfeeding. 2012. [online] Available from: http://www.who.int/features/factfiles/breastfeeding/en/. [Last accessed Apr., 2019].

CHAPTER

Golden Hour Care for Preterm

Ashwani Singal

INTRODUCTION

The first minutes of life are decisive and actions during these minutes and the first hour of life will have an influence later on. All preparations in the delivery room are similar as for term infants. Following are special preparations needed for anticipated preterm delivery.

PREPARATION PRIOR TO BIRTH

High-risk pregnancies should be referred, when possible, to high-risk perinatal centers.
- *Personnel:* Added skilled personnel should be available. The emphasis is on team work during resuscitation.
- *Equipment:*
  - Equipment of various sizes for varied gestational age should be available and in functional order
  - For extremely low birth weight (ELBW) babies (<1,000 g), special care to maintain temperature may be required which includes the use *of plastic bags* or exothermic mattress
  - Use of compressed air and *blender* for oxygen delivery titration is desirable
  - Use of signal extraction technology (SET) based *pulse oximeter* is preferred for oxygen assessment of heart rate and oxygenation
  - For preterm babies less than 32 weeks, availability of *delivery room* continuous positive airway pressure (CPAP) is desirable should the baby have respiratory distress soon after birth
  - Prophylactic *surfactant* may be used in babies less than 26 weeks but sterilization and resuscitation always is a priority.
- *Counseling:* Prenatal counseling should include anticipated problems in nursery and need for neonatal intensive care unit (NICU) care. Anticipated problems in first few days with potential treatments, costs involved, likely outcome (based on unit data) should be informed.

CARE OF PRETERM AT BIRTH

The resuscitation of preterm and term births follows the standard resuscitation guidelines with following preterm specific interventions to optimize the outcome:
- *Thermal care:*
  - *How:* Ensure room temperature of 26°C. Receive the infant from the delivery table in a preheated sterile towel. Place the infant (especially <28 weeks gestation) in

food-grade plastic sheet without drying, covering the body below the shoulders. This is used in conjunction with skin-temperature probes and servo control of radiant-warmer output. Cover the head with a loose cap. Exothermic mattress may also be used. The temperature should be monitored.
  - *Rationale:* All resuscitation efforts yield the best results when the newborn is normothermic. Iatrogenic hyperthermia should be avoided. For every 1°C below 36°C on admission temperature, neonatal mortality increases by 28%.
- Cord clamping:
  - *How:* Delay in umbilical cord clamping for at least 1 minute (30 seconds to 3 minutes) is recommended for infants not requiring resuscitation.
  - *Rationale:* Infants have improved iron status through early infancy, better blood pressures during stabilization, a lower incidence of intraventricular hemorrhage, and receive fewer blood transfusions.
  - *Risk:* Slightly increased need for phototherapy.
- Position:
  - *How:* The infant should be placed on a firm, flat surface. The head should be in neutral position. The head may be kept in slightly elevated position. Head-low position should be avoided.
  - *Rationale:* Cerebral blood flow is altered when the newborn head is not kept midline and elevated.
- Positive-pressure ventilation:
  - *How:* T-piece resuscitator provides consistent delivery of peak inspiratory pressure (PIP), positive end-expiratory pressure (PEEP), and inspired oxygen fraction (FiO_2) compared to self-inflating bag. Every effort should be made to avoid hyperventilation. A pressure gauge maybe used for consistent delivery of pressures.
  - *Rationale:* Even few excessive pressure breaths are known to trigger an inflammatory lung response.
- *Delivery room CPAP:*
  - *Rationale:* Use of CPAP leads to decrease in the requirement for intubation, days on mechanical ventilation and use of postnatal steroids.
  - *When:* Is considered for preterms with spontaneous respiration but labored breathing or persistent cyanosis after initial steps of resuscitation.
  - *How:* Using a flow-inflating bag or a T-piece resuscitator.
- *Oxygen administration*:
  - *When:* If the minute specific oxygen saturation is low or as adjunct with chest compression (100%).
  - *How:* Free-flow oxygen by face mask, nasal catheter, blended oxygen via self-inflating bag or T-piece resuscitator or flow inflating bag.
  - *Technique:* Initiate resuscitation with air or a blended oxygen (30–40%) and titrating the oxygen concentration to achieve a SpO_2 in the target range as described using pulse oximetry. If blended oxygen is not available, resuscitation should be initiated with air.
  - Target SpO_2 (Table 1).

Table 1: Normal oxygen saturation immediately after birth.

Time	Acceptable preductal SpO_2
2 minutes	60%
3 minutes	70%
4 minutes	80%
5 minutes	85%
10 minutes	90%

- *Using pulse oximeter:*
  - *Which:* Signal extraction technology-based pulse oximeter is preferred for heart rate and oxygen assessment.
  - *When*: (i) When resuscitation can be anticipated; (ii) when positive pressure is administered for more than a few breaths; (iii) when cyanosis is persistent; or (iv) when supplementary oxygen is administered.
  - *How:* Attach probe to preductal site.
  - Connect probe to oximeter. Provides reliable readings within 1-2 minutes following birth. Should be used in conjunction with and should not replace clinical assessment of heart rate.
- *Discontinuing resuscitation:* If available and feasible, electrocardiogram (ECG) electrodes are better for a reliable measure of heart rate compared to auscultation or pulse oximetry.

  In a newly born baby with no detectable heart rate, it is appropriate to consider stopping resuscitation if the heart rate remains undetectable for 10 minutes. Infants with gestation <23 weeks are a contraindication to resuscitation. Every unit must have a policy for noninitiation and discontinuation of resuscitation.

STABILIZATION IN NURSERY

- *Position:* Keep the head in midline. Avoid flexion or extension of the neck. A small roll placed under the shoulders can help maintain the airway in optimal sniffing position. U-shaped boundaries should be maintained around the infant to maintain his/her extremities in a flexed position, with knees and hands supported toward midline.
- *Thermal care:* Apply the thermal sensor over the abdomen. Using a servo-control mode ensure the temperature is set at 36.5°C. A plastic shield may be applied on the panels of the warmer to prevent evaporative losses. A double-walled incubator may also be used. Providing a 70-90% relative humidity level is an additional technique that can minimize fluid loss.
- *Monitor:* The newborn should be placed on continuous multichannel monitor to display heart rate, oxygen saturation, and blood pressure. Ensure the oxygen saturation limits are kept at 90-95%. Set alarm limits for heart rate and blood pressure. A trend in measurements displayed is more informative then an isolated value.
- *Oxygen:* If the minute specific oxygen saturation is low, initiate oxygen to titrate saturations to 90-95%.
- *Venous access:* For ELBW infants, it is desirable to secure umbilical venous lines. If facilities exist, umbilical arterial access for blood pressure monitoring and blood gas sampling may be used.
- *Labs and sugars:* Basic investigations include complete blood count (CBC), blood group, and blood sugar on admission. If antibiotics are initiated a blood culture must be drawn.
- *Perfusion:* Assess for sensorium, heart rate, pulse volume, respiration, blood pressure, urine output, skin color, and temperature and capillary refill time. None of the above parameters in isolation suggest shock. More the parameters deranged more are the chances of shock. The mean blood pressure should be at least the infant's gestational age in weeks.
- *Urine output:* Urine output should be at least 0.5 mL/kg/hour on the first day of life and rise to 1-2 mL/kg/hour.
- *Skin care:* A preservative-free, water-miscible, petrolatum-based emollient can also be used to keep the skin moist and free from drying, fissures, or flaking. Minimal handling and gentle handling is the key.

Remove adhesives using saline soaked gauze. Rotate the site of venous access every 48 hours. Ensure change in probe position every 4–6 hours. Be vigilant for loss of integrity of skin and monitor religiously.
- *Fluids and electrolytes:* Fluids are provided to ensure hydration avoiding under or over hydration. Dextrose only fluids in the first 24–48 hours followed by dextrose-electrolyte fluid is preferred. Dextrose content is assessed by glucose infusion rate (GIR). Every attempt is made to keep blood glucose between 50 mg/dL and 150 mg/dL by frequent glucose monitoring. Electrolytes are checked every 2–3 days to titrate fluid therapy.
- *Asepsis:* All disposables should be single use and sterile. Strict attention to daily housekeeping and hand hygiene is must. NICU cleaning and disinfection protocols should be in place.
- *Nutrition:* For stable infants, minimal enteral feeding or trophic feeding (12–24 mL/kg/day) should be considered. Breast milk is the preferred substrate. For sick or ELBW infants, total parenteral nutrition (TPN) should be the goal. Starting TPN on day 1 with proteins at 3–4 g/kg/day and lipids at 3–3.5 g/kg/day has been shown to improve short-term growth in ELBW infants (titrated up as triglyceride levels indicate tolerance of less than 200 mg/dL).
- *Antibiotics:* There is no role for prophylactic antibiotics. Presence of risk factors or clinically suspected sepsis should warrant an antibiotic with gram-positive and gram-negative coverage. Blood cultures should be sent prior to starting the antibiotic. Exit criterion should be laid down to stop antibiotics taking into consideration the clinical course, sepsis screen, and blood culture reports.
- *Respiratory support:* All preterms should be assessed for respiratory status. Presence of respiratory distress should be objectively evaluated by serial Silverman Anderson score. A score of 3 or more for CPAP. Intubation should be restricted to apneic infants, failure of CPAP, and with respiratory failure.
- *Surfactant:* In a preterm with respiratory distress, a FiO_2 requirement of 0.4 or more or respiratory distress not stabilizing on CPAP, should merit natural surfactant administration. Inutbate-Surfactant-Extubate (INSURE) technique is the preferred mode of surfactant delivery with ongoing CPAP support. Prophylactic surfactant usage is restricted to infants <28 weeks with no antenatal steroids to mother, on case by case basis.
- *Parental support:* Parents must be given a realistic understanding of the infant status on day-by-day basis. Anticipated problems, present problems, response, and therapeutic end points should be discussed. All queries should be addressed. Parents should have access to the newborn. Mother should be counseled for breast milk pumping and provided support to ensure lactation.

SUGGESTED READING

1. Sharma D. Golden 60 minutes of newborn's life: Part 1: Preterm neonate. J Matern Fetal Neonatal Med. 2016;1:1-12.
2. Vento M, Nuñez A, Cubells E. Updating the management of preterm infants in the 1st minute after birth. J Clin Neonatol. 2014;3(3):133-8.
3. Wyllie J, Perlman JM, Kattwinkel J, et al. Part 7: Neonatal resuscitation: 2015 international consensus on cardiopulmonary resuscitation and emergency cardiovascular care science with treatment recommendations. Resuscitation. 2015;95:e169-201.

CHAPTER 38

Colic

Rhishikesh Thakre

INTRODUCTION

Infantile colic is characterized by episodic, incessant, abrupt onset crying episodes in a well-appearing infant. It is a diagnosis of exclusion. The role of clinician is to identify or rule out a pathological cause, provide options of treatment, and counsel family about its benign nature. Infantile colic is self-limiting disorder with no adverse effects on health.

DEFINITION

"Rule-of-three" is used for definitive diagnosis. This involves: (i) crying for more than 3 hours/day; (ii) for more than 3 days/week; and (iii) for longer than 3 weeks in an infant who is well-fed and otherwise healthy.

Identify "Danger Signs"

- Poor weight gain
- Poor or decreased feeding, change in behavior, vomiting, alternating drowsiness, decreased urination, or bloody stools
- Decreased responsiveness
- Documented fever
- Inconsolable cry for 2 or more hours.
- Crying as a result of postinjury or fall
- Abnormal movements
- Bruises or swelling over the body
- Turns blue, mottled, or very pale
- History—vague, evolving, contradictory, or changing—not consistent with clinical findings, delay in seeking care, or inappropriate parental behavior.

ETIOLOGY OF COLIC

The underlying cause of infantile colic is unknown. The possible pathological causes of excessive crying are given in Table 1.

Table 1: Organic causes of excessive crying in infants.

Central nervous system (CNS)
• CNS abnormality (Chiari type I malformation) • Infantile migraine • Subdural hematoma
Gastrointestinal
• Constipation • Gastroesophageal reflux • Lactose intolerance • Rectal fissure
Infection
• Meningitis • Otitis media • Urinary tract infection • Viral illness
Trauma
• Abuse • Corneal abrasions • Foreign body in the eye • Fractured bone • Hair tourniquet syndrome

CLINICAL FEATURES

Episodes of irritability and crying are normal during first months of life. Colic typically *starts abruptly by 2 weeks of age to resolve spontaneously by 4 months of age.* Crying occurs during evening, with prolonged bouts, spontaneous in onset. There do not appear to be any trigger factors. The infant cannot be quieted even by feeding or carrying. Such episodes, in addition, have flushed face, furrowed brow, and clenched fists. The legs may be pulled across the abdomen. As much as the onset so dramatic so also is the termination of colic. In between the episodes, the infant is playful and active.

Infantile colic leads to significant parental suffering and, at times, sleep deprivation. Stress in the parents alters the relationships with the infant. This may lead to earlier stoppage of breast milk and early weaning blaming inadequate milk, maternal milk, or not getting enough milk.

DIAGNOSIS

History should focus on time of onset of cry, duration, and infant's behavior between episodes. The red flag signs are thermal instability, lethargy, poor skin perfusion, and tachypnea. A poor weight gain suggests systemic pathology and requires further workup. The infant is examined naked head-to-toe for localizing signs. Presence of break in the continuity of bones, unexplained fracture, multiple lesions of varying age may indicate abuse.

No investigations are required in majority especially if the infant is gaining weight and has no clues on physical examination.

MANAGEMENT OF COLIC (FLOWCHART 1)

Option 1: General Measures

- *Breastfeeding*: Offer a breastfeed. Majority of cry is due to hunger or thirst. A hungry baby suckles quickly onto breast and calms down easily.
- *Environmental temperature*: Too hot or too cold ambient temperature causes discomfort to the baby.
- *Talk, hold, or rock the baby*: Cry due to boredom responds to just being held, talked, or being in vision. Use toys to distract the attention of the baby. Holding the baby or gently rocking while walking or in swing or in a rocking chair may provide relief.
- *Music*: Regular beat or rhythmic music may be soothing to baby crying due to boredom.
- *Clothing*: Ensure the clothes are not too tight. An overwrapped baby may feel discomfort and unwrapping in plain cotton cloth may be helpful.

Flowchart 1: Approach to crying infant.

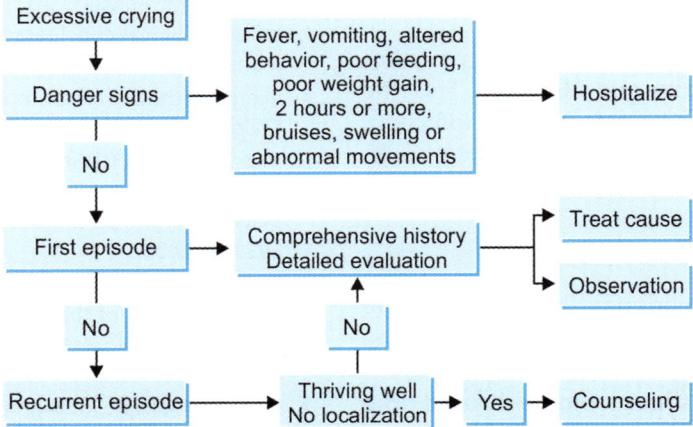

- *Change diapers*: Wet or soiled diapers may irritate the baby and changing them may provide relief. When cloth diapers are used, look for diaper pins that have become loose or loose threads that have become tightly wrapped around fingers or toes. Diaper rashes also can be uncomfortable.
- *Burping/nurse prone*: Burping or nursing the baby prone may help relieve gas and discomfort.
- *Carrying*: Carrying the infant in arms, sling, or a motor ride can decrease the infant's crying and parents' anxiety.
- *Counseling*: The parents must be informed about the well-being of the infant as evidenced by growth pattern. Parents at times feel frustrated, angry, exhausted, guilty, and helpless because of their infants crying. These feelings are normal, and they must be made to realize that this does not indicate that they are incapable or unworthy of caring for their child.
- *Nasal drops*: Blocked nose gets relieved with normal saline drops instantly.

Option 2: Observation

At times, the infant appears normal on initial evaluation only to deteriorate sometimes later. Onetime assessment may not give a clue. When in doubt or where the parents are anxious, the child should be kept under observation and re-evaluated periodically.

Option 3: Specific Treatment

Continued crying of unknown etiology requires extensive evaluation and admission. Treat the underlying cause—e.g. fever, pain, infection, injury, abnormal heart rhythm, surgical cause, or heart failure.

ROLE OF MEDICATIONS

There is little evidence that the available medicines are effective. They may serve as placebo.
- *Simethicone* is most commonly used drug for decreasing intraluminal gas. Despite its clinical use during colicky episodes, studies indicate no benefits.
- Dicyclomine is contraindicated for use in first 6 months of life due to adverse effect profile.

Summary of Evidence-based Guidelines for Management of Infantile Colic

- May be beneficial
  - Dicycloverine (dicyclomine)
- Unknown effectiveness
  - Soya-based infant feeds
  - Casein hydrolysate milk
  - Low lactose milk
  - Sucrose solution
  - Herbal tea
  - Advice to reduce stimulation
  - Car ride simulation
  - Counseling
  - Cranial osteopathy
  - Infant massage
  - Spinal manipulation

SUGGESTED READING

1. Barr RG. Changing our understanding of infant colic. Arch Pediatr Adolesc Med. 2002;156:1172-4.
2. Garrison MM, Christakis DA. A systematic review of treatments for infant colic. Pediatrics. 2000;106(1 pt 2):184-90.
3. Harley LM. Fussing and crying in young infants. Clinical considerations and practical management. Clin Pediatr. 1969;8:138-41.
4. Illingsworth RS. Three-months' colic. Arch Dis Child. 1954;29:165-74.
5. Metcalf TJ, Irons TG, Sher LD, et al. Simethicone in the treatment of infant colic: a randomized, placebo-controlled, multicenter trial. Pediatrics. 1994;94:29-34.
6. Parkin PC, Schwartz CJ, Manuel BA. Randomized controlled trial of three interventions in the management of persistent crying of infancy. Pediatrics. 1993;92:197-201.
7. Reust CE, Blake RL Jr. Diagnostic workup before diagnosing colic. Arch Fam Med. 2000;9:282-3.

SECTION 3

Care of Preterm/Low Birth Weight/High Risk Newborn

SECTION OUTLINE

39. Kangaroo Care
40. Low Birth Weight Feeding
41. Nutritional Supplementation
42. Discharge Planning
43. Retinopathy of Prematurity Screening
44. Hearing Screening
45. Follow-up of the High-Risk Newborn
46. IVH and PVL Screening and Classification
47. Developmental Supportive Care
48. Antenatal Corticosteroids
49. Breast Milk Storage and Handling
50. Immunization in Low Birth Weight Infants

CHAPTER 39

Kangaroo Care

Suman Rao, Balla Kalyan Chakravarthy

INTRODUCTION

Kangaroo mother care (KMC) is now regarded as a standard of care for low-birth weight (LBW) infants with strong evidence supporting its implementation. It can prevent nearly half of the deaths among infants less than 2,000 g.

DEFINITION

Early prolonged and continuous skin-to-skin contact between the mother and her low-birth weight infant, both in hospital and after discharge with exclusive and frequent breastfeeding.

COMPONENTS OF KANGAROO MOTHER CARE

- *Kangaroo position*: Continuous skin-to-skin contact between mother and baby.
- *Kangaroo feeding policy*: Exclusive breastfeeding.
- *Kangaroo discharge*: Early discharge and continuation of KMC at home.

This natural form of human care stabilizes temperature, decreases hypoglycemia, promotes breastfeeding, prevents infection, and other morbidities.

Skin-to-skin contact at birth should not be confused with kangaroo care, which is for all stable babies irrespective of weight, for providing warmth and initiation of breastfeeds. Kangaroo care implies sustained prolonged skin-to-skin contact in stable low-birth weight babies.

ADVANTAGES OF KANGAROO MOTHER CARE (TABLE 1)

Kangaroo mother care simulates in utero environment and facilitates physiological stability. It is the most holistic form of developmentally supportive care providing multimodal stimulation satisfying all the six senses in the right way.

PROCEDURE

- Start KMC for babies less than 2,500 g as early as possible—after stabilization. Flowchart 1 discusses the time of initiation of KMC. Under close supervision, KMC can also be provided to babies on respiratory support in a unit where KMC is well-established and nurses are confident in KMC.

Table 1: Benefits of kangaroo mother care.

Benefits in the neonatal period:
- Improved survival
- *Temperature regulation*: Reduced hypothermia
- *Physiologic stability*: Heart rate, oxygenation
- Reduced apnea, crying
- Reduced nosocomial sepsis
- Pain reduction
- Sleep organization
- Improved growth
- Improved breastfeeding

Benefits to the mother:
- Increased confidence, satisfaction
- Better bonding
- Empowerment
- Better milk production
- Early discharge
- Lower stress
- Lower postpartum depression

Benefits in infancy and childhood:
- Growth
- Neurodevelopment
    - Increased intelligence quotient (IQ)
    - Better executive functions
- Physiologic organization
- Lower stress
- Better parent–infant interaction
- Lower admission rate

PREPARATIONS FOR THE KANGAROO MOTHER CARE PROVIDER

Though close adult family members such as father, grandmother, or aunt can provide KMC, the best KMC provider is the mother. The full spectrum of benefits due to KMC is seen when the mother is the main KMC provider.
- The KMC provider must be willing, in good health, free from serious illness.
- She should maintain hygiene including hand washing, daily bath, clipped fingernails, tied up hair, and clean clothes.
- Jewelry, watches, and sacred threads must be removed as they may be a barrier to maintain hygiene and might cause injury to the newborn.
- Mother should preferably wear a culturally acceptable front open loose dress.
- Encourage the mother to keep the baby in KMC for as long as possible during the day and night.

PREPARATIONS FOR THE BABY (FIG. 1)

- Dress the baby in a soak-proof diaper, woolen cap, and socks.
- Baby may be placed in a KMC bag. KMC bag is an Indian innovation for a KMC binder and promotes continuous KMC.

THE "KANGAROO MOTHER CARE POSITION" (FIG. 2)

- Place the baby between the mother's breasts in skin-to-skin contact.
- Secure the baby to the mother by a binder—long piece of cotton cloth/dupatta/KMC bag/KMC lycra bag.
- Ensure the baby is in upright position to prevent aspiration. Even when the mother sleeps, she should be inclined at an angle of at least 45°.

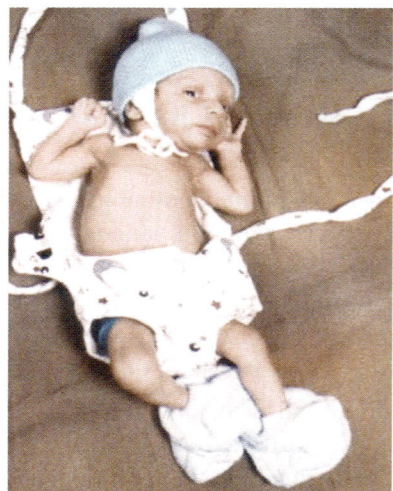

Fig. 1: Low-birth weight baby in kangaroo mother care (KMC) bag.

- The head should be turned to one side with slight extension—this keeps the airway open and allows eye-to-eye contact between mother and baby.
- The hips should be abducted in a frog position and arms should be flexed.
- The baby's abdomen should be at the level of the mother's abdomen.

DURATION OF KANGAROO MOTHER CARE (TABLE 2 AND FIG. 3)

- Every KMC session should last at least 1 hour to prevent frequent handling of the baby.
- The duration of each KMC session should be gradually increased for as long as the mother can comfortably provide KMC.
- Breastfeeding can be continued in KMC position. Feeding duration should be about 2–3 hourly.

The mother carrying an infant in the KMC position can walk, stand, sit, or engage in different activities.

Table 2: Duration of kangaroo mother care (KMC).*

Short	4 hours daily
Extended	5–8 hours daily
Long	9–12 hours daily
Continuous	>12 hours daily

*Documented on 2 consecutive days or more prior to discharge. Duration to be counted as cumulative completed hours during a 24-hour period.

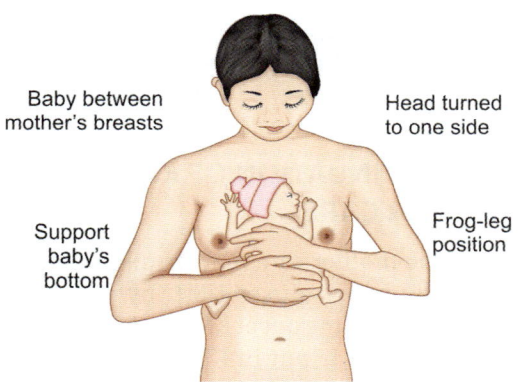

Fig. 2: Kangaroo mother care (KMC) position.

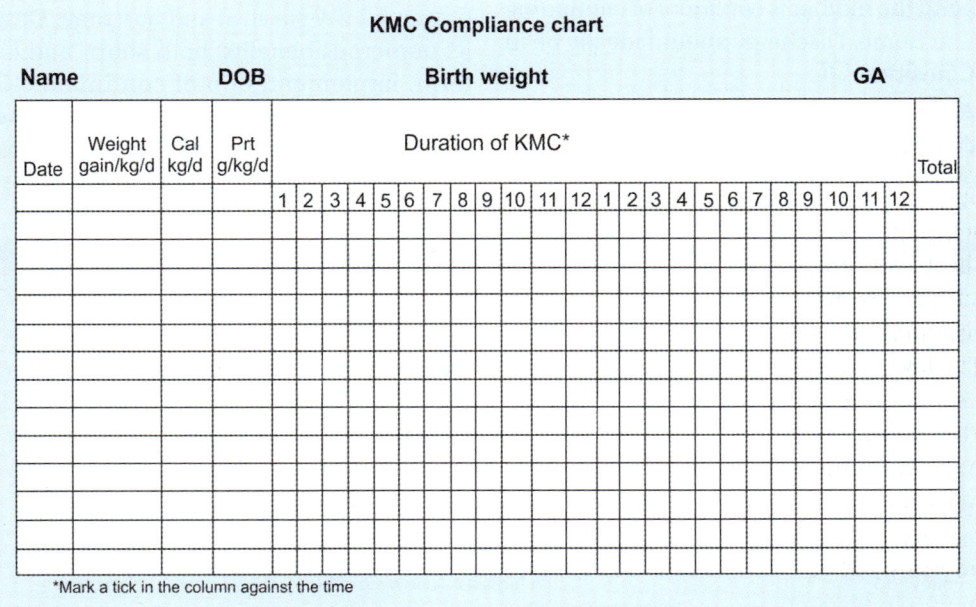

Fig. 3: Kangaroo mother care (KMC) chart—for compliance with KMC.

MONITORING A BABY IN KANGAROO MOTHER CARE (TABLE 3)

- The mother and the nursing personnel should continue to monitor the baby.
- Continue to monitor the vital parameters: Heart rate, respiration, glucose.
- The mother should be educated about the danger signs and trained to monitor her baby in KMC.
- The mother's compliance with KMC should be monitored (as shown in Fig. 3).
- The mother should be taught the "touch technique" of temperature assessment. She should be able to feel the baby's breathing and recognize apneic episodes, if any.
- Advise the mother to continue to provide KMC at home.

DISCHARGE AND FOLLOW-UP

The KMC baby is ready for discharge if she/he is stable, free of illness, off parenteral medication, accepting oral feeds, gaining weight at 15–20 g/day for at least 3 consecutive days and the mother is confident of continuing KMC at home. Discharge should ideally be in KMC position.

Adequate follow-up is an essential criterion of KMC. First follow-up should be at 1 week, followed by fortnightly follow-ups till next two visits. Additional follow-up visits may be done until she/he reaches 40 weeks of postconception age or achieves a weight of 2,500 g.

DON'TS OF KANGAROO MOTHER CARE

- Do not bathe till infant weighs 2,500 g, sponging may be done
- Do not handle infant too frequently
- Do not give bottle feed
- Do not allow infant to be in contact with sick people.

DISCONTINUATION OF KANGAROO MOTHER CARE

Kangaroo mother care may be discontinued when the baby refuses KMC by excessive crying or wriggling out of KMC or fusses every time the baby is put in KMC. This usually occurs by about 37–40 weeks.

Kangaroo mother care is a low cost, easy, evidence based, high impact intervention to promote LBW survival and outcome. Despite its numerous benefits, both short- and long-term, implementation of continuous KMC and scale up of KMC has not been successful. Barriers and bottlenecks need to be overcome for successful KMC programs.

Table 3: Monitoring in kangaroo mother care.

	What to monitor?	How to monitor?	Who monitors?
T	Temperature	Axillary temperature/touch technique	Nurse/mother
A	Airway, apnea, breathing	*Clinically*: Respiratory efforts and apnea, KMC position/pulse oximeter	Nurse/mother
B	Breastfeeding	Exclusivity and adequacy of breastfeeding	Nurse/mother
C	Compliance with kangaroo care	KMC compliance chart	Nurse/mother
D	Danger signs	Clinically	Mother
E	Education and emotional support to mother	Counseling	Nurse/family
F	Follow-up	In high-risk follow-up clinic	Doctors
G	Growth	Postnatal growth charts	Nurse/doctors

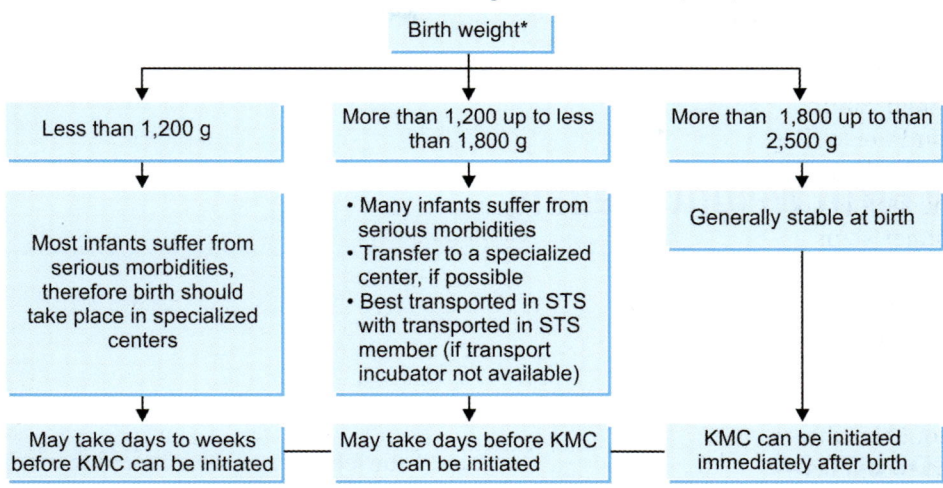

Flowchart 1: Initiation of kangaroo mother care (KMC).

*Cut-off birth weight for KMC has been based on Operational Guideline of facility-based Newborn Care

OVERCOMING BOTTLENECKS IN KANGAROO MOTHER CARE IMPLEMENTATION

System Changes

- *Kangaroo mother care ward*: Where growing preterm babies can be cared for in KMC by the mothers. Recreation and education of the mothers can be provided by appropriate audiovisual aids
- *Comfortable reclining chairs*: Back pain is one of the most frequent barriers for KMC acceptance
- *Extra pillows*: For maintaining 45° position while providing KMC during sleep
- Improve KMC knowledge and skills among health care personnel.

Improving Acceptance to Kangaroo Mother Care

- In-hospital KMC adaptation for the KMC mother: Detailed counseling to educate her about the numerous benefits of KMC.
- Involve the family in KMC counseling. Family support is essential for successful KMC implementation and for continuous KMC.
- Provide plenty of educative material including video films in local language.
- Create KMC mother support groups.

SUGGESTED READING

1. Kangaroo Mother Care and Optimal Feeding of the LBW: Operational Guidelines. Publication by Child Division, Ministry of Health and Family Welfare, Govt. of India; 2014.
2. Rassaily R, Ganguly KK, Roy M, et al. Community based kangaroo mother care for low birth weight babies: a pilot study. Indian J Med Res. 2017;145:51-7.
3. Seidman G, Unnikrishnan S, Kenny E, et al. Barriers and enablers of kangaroo mother care practice: a systematic review. PLoS One. 2015;10(5):e0125643.
4. World Health Organization. Department of Reproductive Health and Research. Kangaroo Mother Care: A Practical Guide. Geneva: World Health Organization; 2003.

CHAPTER 40

Low Birth Weight Feeding

Sandeep Kadam

INTRODUCTION

Nutritional management of low birth weight (LBW) babies influences immediate survival as well as their subsequent growth and development. Nutritional needs of these infants vary based on gestational age, metabolic state, and physiological complications (Table 1).

When to start feeding a low birth weight baby? (Box 1 and Table 2)
- All stable LBW infants should be put on their mothers' breast in the delivery room.
- Preterm infants born before 34 weeks or infants who are unstable (Box 1) are initiated on intravenous (IV) fluids. Once they are stable, tube feeds with mother's own milk are gradually introduced and volume is increased gradually (Flowchart 1).
- Tube feeding may be initiated immediately after birth in stable preterm infants of less than 34 weeks gestation.
- If the LBW infant is unstable in addition to IV fluids, trophic feeds or minimal enteral

Box 1: When not to feed?
- Unstable infant, e.g. circulatory or respiratory instability
- Evidence of intestinal obstruction/perforation or paralytic ileus
- Feed intolerance
- On inotropes
- Bile-stained vomiting
- Infants scheduled for surgical or anesthetic procedures
- Active necrotizing enterocolitis
- Small for gestational age with absent or reversed diastolic blood flow
- Preterm with gestation less than 28 weeks at birth

Table 1: Maturation of oro-motor skills and choice of initial feeding method.

Gestational age	Maturation of feeding skills	Initial feeding method
<28 weeks	• No proper sucking efforts • Inadequate peristalsis	Intravenous fluids
28–31 weeks	• Immature sucking efforts	Orogastric/nasogastric tube feeding
32–34 weeks	• Slight mature sucking pattern • Suck, swallow coordination present	Spoon/paladai/cup feeding
>34 weeks	• Mature sucking pattern • Good suck, swallow, and breathing coordination	Breastfeeding

CHAPTER 40
Low Birth Weight Feeding

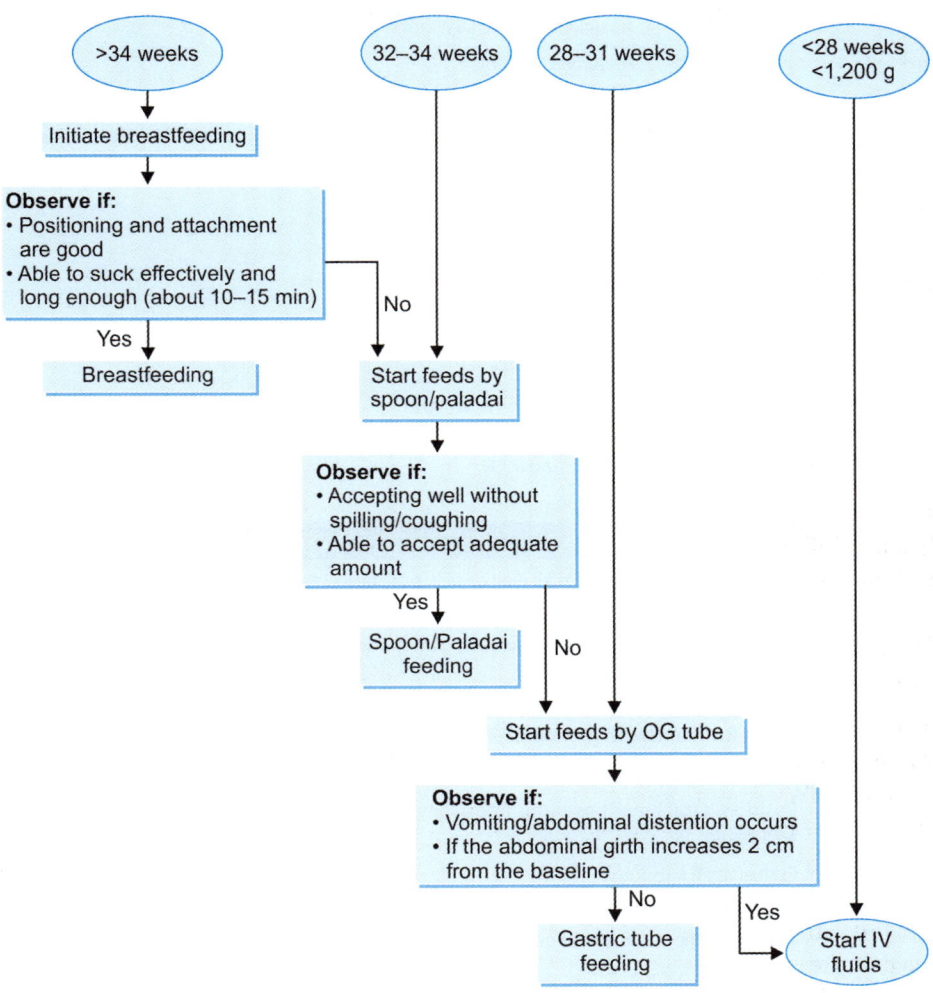

Flowchart 1: Feeding in sick and unstable babies.

(IV: intravenous; OG: orogastric)

Note: For sick infants start with IV fluids and gradually progress to oral feeds.

feeds are started. These are minimal volumes of milk feeds (10–15 mL/kg/day) with no increments and are given to all sick babies (Table 2).

Which milk to feed?
- Low birth weight infants, who are able to breastfeed, should be put to the breast as soon as possible after birth (within 1st hour) or when they are clinically stable and should be exclusively breastfed until 6 months of age (Table 3).

- In case mother's own milk is not available, then the next best choice is expressed donor milk from other lactating mothers obtained from human milk bank.
- When breast milk is not available to meet the needs of LBW infant, preterm formula milk may be given with proper preparation and hygiene.
- Cow or buffalo milk is unsuitable and inferior alternatives and avoided as far as possible.

SECTION 3
Care of Preterm/Low Birth Weight/High Risk Newborn

Table 2: Tropic feeding practices/minimal enteral nutrition (MEN).

Indications	All sick but stable LBW not on enteral feeds
Timing	As early as feasible
What to give	Expressed mother milk or donor mother milk
How much	10–20 cc/kg/day
Increments	None
How to give	Bolus feeds via naso-/orogastric tube
Contraindication	Hemodynamic instability
Transition to enteral feeding	On clinical stability
Adverse effects	None
Monitor	Feed intolerance

(CPAP: continuous positive airway pressure; LBW: low birth weight)

Practical tip: Commercial formulas are best avoided for MEN. Mechanical ventilation, CPAP, indomethacin, and/or use of umbilical catheters are not contraindication to using MEN.

Table 3: Optimizing the use of human milk in low birth weight (LBW).

Whom to give	Preferred choice of feed for all well or sick, but stable LBW irrespective of gestation
How to give	• Breastfeeding (>34 weeks) • By expressed milk in (32–34 weeks, wati spoon) • By tube feeding (<32 weeks)
When to give	As early as feasible in unstable (as trophic feeds) and in delivery room (putting to mothers' breast for infants with gestation >34 weeks)
How frequently	On demand in well babies. Every 2–3 hourly in sick babies (as indicated)
Monitor	Position, attachment, weight, frequency and color of urine/stool, maternal concerns, and well-being
How long	Exclusive till 6 months
Disadvantage	A subset of <32 weeks (<1,500 g) may have slower growth on unsupplemented breast milk. The implications for slower growth are unclear
Contraindication	Infants with galactosemia, maple syrup urine disease, phenylketonuria, mother on cytotoxic drugs, radioactive compounds, or maternal severe illness like psychosis, sepsis

STRATEGIES TO OPTIMIZE BREAST MILK IN MOTHERS WITH LOW BIRTH WEIGHT BABY

Education

- Provide written educational information addressing common concerns, such as insufficient breast milk, expressing breast milk, colostrum, and benefits.
- Consistent message about the importance of human milk from all neonatal intensive care unit (NICU) clinicians.
- Educate new staff to support breastfeeding
- Placing infant in skin-to-skin contact with the mother immediately after delivery.

Mother and Infant Bonding

- Communicate and involve mother in day-to-day NICU baby care
- 24-hour visitation and access to infant
- Daily skin-to-skin holding in the NICU
- Initiating and providing kangaroo mother care (KMC)

- Comfortable, supportive chairs for mothers at the bedside

Expression of Milk and Sustain Milk Supply

- Aim for the first oral feedings to be at the breast
- Encourage milk expression 8–10 times/day
- Use of expression of breast milk at infant's bedside
- Responding to maternal concerns, stress, or anxiety
- Promote non-nutritive feeding (suckling at emptied breast), regardless of infant weight and gestation
- No free formula samples or other promotion of artificial feeding
- Use hospital-grade breast pump and collection kit and storage containers
- Managing breast/nipple problems such as retracted or cracked nipple and breast engorgement.

How to start and grade up feeds? (Table 4)

Feeding small for gestational age (SGA) babies with/without history of absent or reversed end-diastolic flow (AREDF)—If the abdominal examination is normal, start feeding within 24 hours of life, but advance slowly with volumes at the lowest end of the range. Advance feeds extremely slowly in the first 10 days among preterm SGA babies with gestation <29 weeks and AREDF. Make every effort to feed human milk, especially in SGA babies with AREDF and gestation <29 weeks.

Which route to use in feeding?

Route to use in feeding is given in Table 5.

When to start oral feeding from tube feeds?

As an infant's feeding ability develops, he or she should progress from the initial method through the intermediate steps to feeding exclusively from the breast directly. An infant given oral feeds with spoon or paladai should be given opportunity to suckle on the breast, so as to enhance progression to breastfeeding which is the ultimate goal (Flowchart 2).

How often and how much to feed? (Table 6)

- Semi-demand feeding is more suitable for preterm infants than demand feeding. With semi-demand feeding, the infant is assessed every 3 hours for behavioral signs of hunger. If the infant wakes up and demonstrate hunger signs before the 3 hours are over, the feeding can be provided earlier. The amount

Table 4: How to start and grade up feeds?

Weight (kg)	Initial feed (per day)	Increment (per day)
<1	15–20 cc/kg	15–20 cc/kg
1–1.5	20 cc/kg	20 cc/kg
>1.5	30 cc/kg	30 cc/kg
Intrauterine growth restriction	10–15 cc/kg	15–20 cc/kg

Table 5: Which route to use in feeding?

Weight	Clinical status	Initial feeding
Term or preterm (LBW)	• Unstable	• IV fluids, nil by mouth
	• Potentially unstable	• Trophic feeds, IV fluids
2–2.5 kg	Stable	Breastfeeding
1.5–2 kg	Stable	Breastfeeding and/or supervised oral feeding by spoon, syringe, cup, or paladai
1–1.5 kg	Stable	Tube feeding
<1 kg	Stable	IV fluids, enteral feeds, and parenteral nutrition

(IV: intravenous; LBW: low birth weight)

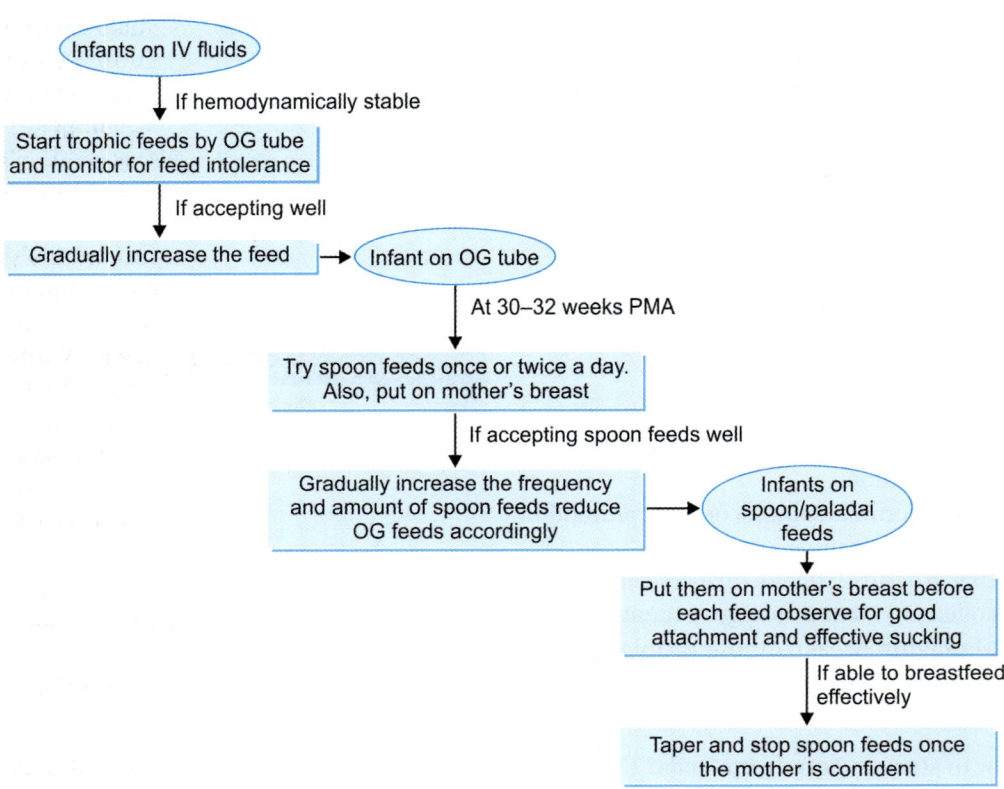

Flowchart 2: Progression of feeding in low birth weight babies.

(IV: intravenous; OG: orogastric; PMA: postmenstrual age)

of each feed volume is calculated on the basis of daily fluid requirements.
- It is usual clinical practice to provide LBW infants of 1,500 g or more about 60 mL/kg fluids on the 1st day of life. Infants less than 1,500 g are usually given about 80 mL/kg fluids on the 1st day of life. The feeds/fluids are increased by 15–30 mL/kg/day to a maximum of 150 mL/kg/day by the end of the 1st week of life.
- Eight feeds per 24 hours are required, which does not necessarily mean that they be at 3 hourly interval. Infants feeding every 2–2.5 hours during the day may stretch night feed intervals to 4 hours, allowing more rest for the mother-infant dyad. However, infants less than 2.5 kg should be awake every 3 hours during the day for feeds and should not sleep for more than 4 hours consecutively without a feed. After 2.5 kg, these intervals may stretch to 5 hours to allow more rest for the dyad.

When to start breast milk fortification?

The objective of fortification is to increase the concentration of nutrients to such levels that at the customary feeding volumes, infants receive amounts of all nutrients that meet the requirements. Multicomponent fortification of human milk result is short-term increase in weight gain, linear growth, and head circumference but long-term neurodevelopmental and growth outcomes are not different.

Table 6: Feed volume.

Day of life	Fluid requirement (± 20 mL/kg)	
	>1,500 g	<1,500 g
1	60	80
2	75	95
3	90	110
4	105	125
5	120	140
6	135	150
7	150	150

- Fortification can be started when enteral intake reaches 100 mL/kg/day
- Discontinue fortification when the baby reaches 1,800 g or start taking direct breastfeeding
- One sachet of human milk fortifier (HMF) available in Indian market is to be added in 25 mL of breast milk, it increases the calorie density of breast milk from 20 kcal/oz to 24 kcal/oz
- No role of single component fortification like medium-chain triglyceride (MCT) oil or coconut oil.

How to assess feed intolerance?

Symptoms
- Vomiting (altered milk/bile or blood-stained)
- *Systemic features*: Lethargy and apnea.

Signs
- Abdominal distension (with or without visible bowel loops)
- *Increased gastric residuals*: >2 mL/kg or any change from previous pattern
- Abdominal tenderness
- Reduced or absent bowel sounds
- *Systemic signs*: Cyanosis and bradycardia.

Practical Tips
- Do not check gastric residuals routinely. Check pre-feed gastric residual volume (GRV) only after a minimum feed volume (per feed) is attained. We suggest the following thresholds—<500 g: 2 mL, 500–749 g: 3 mL, 750–1,000 g: 4 mL, and >1,000 g: 5 mL.
- Do not check abdominal girth routinely.
- Isolated green or yellow residuals are unimportant. Vomiting bile may indicate an intestinal obstruction or ileus. Withhold feeds in case of hemorrhagic residuals, as hemorrhagic residuals are significant.
- If the problem of residual volumes persists despite slow bolus feeds, consider decreasing the feed volume to the last well-tolerated feed volume.
- Use the smallest volume syringe for checking residuals. Take care to aspirate gently.
- After a feed, nurse the baby in the prone position for half an hour.

What and when to supplements? (Details in Chapter on Nutritional Supplementation)

How do we monitor growth and nutrition?
Adequacy of nutrition is ensured by:
- Frequency of urine (8–12 times/day)
- Weight gain (15–20 g/day). Most LBW infants lose weight in the first few days of life. Usually, this loss would not exceed 10–15% of the birth weight. They regain their birth weight by about 2 weeks and then start gaining weight at the rate of 1.0–1.5% of body weight per day. For small infants below 1,500 g (less than 32 weeks), it is advisable to use a postnatal growth chart to plot weight every day until they are of 40 weeks postmenstrual age (PMA) or 2,500 g.
  - From birth until 40–50 weeks corrected age (CA), use the Fenton growth chart

> **Box 2: Adjunct strategies to optimize nutrition.**
> - *Antenatal steroids*: Maturation of small intestinal motor patterns and reduce risk of necrotizing enterocolitis (NEC)
> - *Restrictive fluid intake strategy*: Reduce risk of NEC
> - *Non-nutritive sucking*: Accelerates maturation of sucking reflex
> - Kangaroo mother care
> - *Prebiotics and probiotics*: Potential to reduce risk of NEC
> - *Infant position*: Left lateral position reduces gastroesophageal reflex
> - Standardized feeding regimen

- From term to 24 months CA, use the World Health Organization (WHO) growth charts
- After 24 months, use the Centers for Disease Control and Prevention (CDC) growth charts.

What other strategies can promote nutrition?

The strategies, which can promote nutrition, are described in Box 2.

DEVELOPMENTAL ORIGINS OF HEALTH AND DISEASE

Adequate nutrition and optimal catch-up growth of LBW infants are critical for better neurodevelopmental outcome. However, excessive rate of catch-up growth may also have adverse consequences for long-term health. These concerns arise from newly emerging research in the area of "developmental origins of health and disease" (DOHaD) or "fetal programming", which has linked LBW infants with intrauterine compromise to be vulnerable to the development of chronic disease in later life. The combination of poor growth in the womb with rapid catch-up growth may further enhance the risk of chronic disease in later life.

SUGGESTED READING

1. Cleminson JS, Zalewski SP, Embleton ND. Nutrition in the preterm infant: what's new? Curr Opin Clin Nutr Metab Care. 2016;19(3):220-5.
2. Ditzenberger G. Nutritional support for premature infants in the neonatal intensive care unit. Crit Care Nurs Clin North Am. 2014;26(2):181-98.
3. Harding JE, Cormack BE, Alexander T, et al. Advances in nutrition of the newborn infant. Lancet. 2017;389(10079):1660-8.
4. World Health Organization (WHO) (2011). Guidelines on optimal feeding of low birth-weight infants in low-and middle-income countries. [online] Available from https://www.who.int/maternal_child_adolescent/documents/9789241548366.pdf?ua=1. [Last accessed May, 2019].

CHAPTER 41

Nutritional Supplementation

VC Manoj

INTRODUCTION

Birth of a preterm is a potential nutritional emergency. The goal of nutrition is to achieve optimal growth. Newborns should be consistently feeding well before discharge. Attention must be given to newborns who continue to lose weight after day 7 of life or who are not back to birth weight by 2 weeks of age.

ROLE OF HUMAN BREAST MILK

Human milk is the preferred source of enteral nutrition for all newborns, including preterms. It is safe and appropriate, because of its better digestion and absorption, improve host defense, and improve neurodevelopmental outcomes (Table 1 and Box 1).

SUPPLEMENTATION IN PRETERM BREASTFED INFANTS

Breast milk at full enteral intake (200 mL/kg/day) provides sufficient calories and most of macronutrients to meet the nutritional needs of preterm babies. However, it is deficient in calcium-phosphorus, vitamins, and iron, which needs to be supplemented

Table 1: Optimizing use of human milk in preterm.	
Whom to give	Preferred choice of feed for all well or sick, but stable preterms irrespective of gestation
How to give	Breast feeding (>34 weeks), by expressed milk in (32–34 weeks, wati-spoon), by tube feeding (<32 weeks)
When to give	As early as feasible in unstable (as trophic feeds) and in delivery room (putting to mothers breast for >34 weeks)
How frequently	On demand in well babies. Every 2–3 hourly in sick babies (as indicated)
Monitor	Position, attachment, weight, frequency and color of urine/stool, maternal concerns, and well-being
How long	Exclusive till 6 months
Disadvantage	A subset of < 32 weeks (<1,500 g) may have slower growth on unsupplemented breast milk. The implications for slower growth are unclear
Contraindication	Infants with galactosemia, maple syrup urine disease, phenylketonuria, mother on cytotoxic drugs, radioactive compounds or maternal severe illness like psychosis, and sepsis
Note	Discourage prelacteals (water, honey, ghutti, etc.)

SECTION 3
Care of Preterm/Low Birth Weight/High Risk Newborn

Box 1: Best practices to maintain lactation in preterm mothers separated from their babies.

- 24 × 7 access to infant
- Uniform message regards breast milk or feeding
- Parental involvement in care of the newborn
- Breast milk be the first feed for newborn, well or sick
- Teach and help mother to express breast milk
- Early and ongoing skin-to-skin care
- Frequent emptying of breasts at least 8–10 times per day
- Assess and support for concerns, stress, or anxiety
- Easy and comfortable chairs for mothers
- Support for expression and storage of breast milk
- Written parent education material about breast feeding issues
- Educate new doctors, nurses about breast milk feeding
- Advocate, support, and promote non-nutritive feeding (suckling at emptied breast) for all babies
- Discourage formula samples or promotions of nonbreast milk

Table 2: Target intake in preterm infants.

	Target	Breast milk (200 mL/kg/day)
Calorie/kg	120–130	134
Proteins (g/kg)	2.5–3.5	2.0
Fat (g/kg)	6.0–8.0	7.8
CHO (g/kg)	10–14	13.2
Vitamin A (IU/kg)	1,000	780
Vitamin D (IU)	400–1,000	4
Vitamin E (IU/kg)	6–12	2.0
Ca (mg/kg)	150–175	50
P (mg/kg)	90–105	26
Fe (mg/kg)	2–4	0.2

(Table 2). Donor human milk is available as an alternative feeding option, if breast milk is unavailable or mother cannot breastfeed, and needs same supplementations.

The following options can be used for the preterm infants to compensate for the nutritional deficiency of breast milk.

Breast Milk Fortification

The aim of fortification is to raise the concentration of nutrients of breast milk so that at the customary feeding volumes nutrients requirements are met.
- Multicomponent fortification of human milk by adding human milk fortifier (HMF) to the expressed breast milk (EBM) result is short-term increases in weight gain, linear growth, and head circumference but long-term neurodevelopmental and growth outcomes are not different. The following two approaches can be followed in the unit:
    1. Universal fortification of all babies <1,500 g. Fortification can be started when enteral intake reaches 100 mL/kg/day.
    2. Selective fortification of very low birth weight (VLBW) babies, if weight gain is inadequate or discharge weight is below 10th centile for the postmenstrual age.
- Discontinue HMF when the baby reaches 1,800 g or start taking direct breastfeeding. One sachet of HMF available in Indian market is to be added in 50 mL of EBM, which increases the calorie density of breast milk from 67 kcal/100 mL–81 kcal/100 mL. On HMF, vitamin D 800–1000 IU/day and iron 2–3 mg/kg/day supplementation is needed (Table 2).
- No role of single component fortification like medium-chain triacylglycerols (MCT) oil or coconut oil.

Individual Micronutrient Supplementations

- Preterm infant on unfortified breast milk or direct breastfeeding needs individual supplementation of calcium-phosphorus, multivitamins, vitamin D, and iron (Table 3).

Table 3: Nutrition supplements for preterms.

Nutrient	Timing	Dose	Duration	Comment
Multi vitamins (A, C, B_1, B_2, B_6, folic acid, and niacin)	On full enteral feeds	Vitamin A 1,000 IU/day	3 months–1 year	0.5–1 mL of most of multivitamin preparation suffice
Vitamin D	On full enteral feeds	800–1,000 IU/day	Till 1 year	Avoid "combo" packs containing multimineral, antioxidants, iron, micronutrients, amino acids, etc.
Iron	On full enteral feeds earliest by 2–3 weeks of postnatal age	2–3 mg/kg/d	Till 1 year	Use ferrous form. Avoid combo supplement packs
Calcium-phosphorus (2:1)	On full enteral feeds	150/75 mg/kg/day	Till 40 weeks PMA	Use in isolation and not as part of combo supplement
Human milk fortifier	On full enteral feeds with inadequate weight gain	1 sachet per 50 mL of EBM, as required	Till weight of 2,000 g	Need iron and vitamin D supplements. Multivitamin and calcium-phosphorous not required

(EBM: expressed breast milk; PMA: postmenstrual age).

SUPPLEMENTATION IN FORMULA/ANIMAL MILK FED PRETERM INFANTS

- Preterm formula (PM, 80–81 kcal/100 mL) is formula of choice for feeding preterm infants in hospital when breast milk is not available. It contains adequate calorie and all the macronutrients as well as micronutrients to meet the needs of preterm infants and no extra supplementation is not required.
- Postdischarge special formula (PDF, 73–74 kcal/100 mL) is formula of choice in feeding preterm infants in the postdischarge period till 40–52 weeks of postmenstrual age. Preterm infants being fed on this formula need no extra supplementation.
- Term formula (TF, 67 kcal/oz) should be used only when PT or PDF are not available. Preterm infant on term formula needs calcium-phosphorus, multivitamin, vitamin D, and iron as outlined in Table 2.
- Animal milk like cow or buffalo milk is not recommended during the first year of life. They are inferior alternatives to mother's milk.

APPENDIX: NUTRITIONAL SUPPLEMENTATION IN LBW BABIES *(ESPGHAN)*, 2010

Recommended intakes for macro- and micronutrients expressed per mg/kg/day and per 100 kcal unless otherwise denoted.

Min–max	Per kg/day	Per 100 kcal
Fluid, mL	135–200	
Energy, kcal	110–135	
Protein, g <1 kg body weight	4.0–4.5	3.6–4.1
Protein, g 1–1.8 kg body weight	3.5–4.0	3.2–3.6
Lipids, g (of which MCT <40%)	4.8–6.6	4.4–6.0

Contd...

Contd...

Min–max Per kg/day Per 100 kcal		
Linolenic acid, mg*	385–1540	350–1400
α-linolenic acid, mg	>55 (0.9% of fatty acids)	>50
DHA, mg	12–30	11–27
AA, mg∞	18–42	16–39
Carbohydrate, g	11.6–13.2	10.5–12
Sodium, mg	69–115	63–105
Potassium, mg	66–132	60–120
Chloride, mg	105–177	95–161
Calcium salt, mg	120–140	110–130
Phosphate, mg	60–90	55–80
Magnesium, mg	8–15	7.5–13.6
Iron, mg	2–3	1.8–2.7
Zinc, mg±	1.1–2.0	1.0–1.8
Copper, μg	100–132	90–120
Selenium, μg	5–10	4.5–9
Manganese, μg	<27.5	6.3–25
Fluoride, μg	1.5–60	1.4–55
Iodine, μg	11–55	10–50
Chromium, ng	30–1230	27–1120
Molybdenum, μg	0.3–5	0.27–4.5
Thiamin, μg	140–300	125–275
Riboflavin, μg	200–400	180–365
Niacin, μg	380–5500	345–5000
Pantothenic acid, mg	0.33–2.1	0.3–1.9
Pyridoxine, μg	45–300	41–273
Cobalamin, μg	0.1–0.77	0.08–0.7
Folic acid, μg	35–100	32–90
L-ascorbic acid, mg	11–46	10–42
Biotin, μg	1.7–16.5	1.5–15
Vitamin A, μg RE, 1μg ~ 3.33 IU	400–1000	360–740
Vitamin D, IU/day	800–1000	
Vitamin E, mg (α-tocopherol equivalents)	2.2–11	2–10
Vitamin K$_1$, μg	4.4–28	4–25
Nucleotides, mg		<5
Choline, mg	8–55	7–50
Inositol, mg	4.4–53	4–48

(AA: arachidonic acid; DHA: docosahexaenoic acid; IU: international unit; MCT: medium-chain triacylglycerols). Calculation of the range of nutrients expressed per 100 kcal is based on a minimum energy intake of 110 kcal/kg.
*The linoleic acid to α-linolenic acid ratio is in the range of 5–15:1(wt/wt).
∞The ratio of AA to DHA should be in the range of 1.0–2.0 to 1 (wt/wt), and eicosapentaenoic acid (20:5n-3) supply should not exceed 30% of DHA supply.
±The zinc to copper molar ratio in infant formulae should not exceed 20.

SUGGESTED READING

1. Agostoni C, Buonocore G, Carnielli VP, et al. Enteral nutrient supply for preterm infants: Commentary from ESPGHAN Committee on Nutrition. J Pediatr Gastroenterol Nutr. 2010; 50:85-91.
2. Bai-Horng Su. Optimizing nutrition in preterm infants. Pediatr Neonatol. 2014;55:5-13.
3. Embleton ND. Optional protein and energy intakes in preterm infants. Early Hum Dev. 2007;83:831-7.
4. Greer FR. Postdischarge nutrition: what does the evidence support? Semin Perinatol. 2007;31:89-95.
5. Tsang R, Uauy R, Koletzko B, et al. Nutrition of the Preterm Infant, Scientific Basis and Practical Guidelines, 2nd edition. Cincinnati, Ohio: Digital Educational Publishing Inc.; 2005.

CHAPTER

Discharge Planning

VC Manoj

INTRODUCTION

A discharge plan tailored to the individual baby ensure a smooth transition from the neonatal intensive care unit (NICU)/nursery to home and probably brings about best reductions in hospital length of stay and readmission rates for these high-risk neonates.

TIMING OF DISCHARGE

- When the infant demonstrates necessary physiologic maturity (in the case of the preterm infant)
- Discharge planning and arrangements for follow-up and home care if any, have been completed
- Parents have learned essential knowledge and skills for taking care of high-risk baby at home.

PLANNING

- Prior to discharge, a detailed discharge summary should be prepared mentioning all the events during the stay of the infant in NICU that may have a bearing on the long-term prognosis
- Unresolved medical problems should be identified and plans for follow-up monitoring and treatment instituted
- An individualized home-care plan should be developed with input from all concerned disciplines.

Following important factors which must be considered while planning discharge:

1. *Infant readiness for discharge*: It is useful to have a checklist for planning discharge. An infant is considered ready for discharge if the points given in Table 1 have been accomplished.
2. *Readiness of the physician: Development of a comprehensive follow-up plan:*
   - A suitable plan for follow-up of each high-risk neonate should be developed and mentioned in the discharge summary to be handed over to the parents at the time of discharge (Table 1).
   - There should be clarity regarding the management of issues likely to be faced by the infant especially regarding the unresolved medical problems.
3. *Parent education and readiness for discharge:*
   - Involve the parents while planning discharge and develop a comprehensive home care plan in consultation with the parents. Ensure readiness of family and home environment

Table 1: Discharge planning.		
Criteria	Checklist	Remarks
• Temperature stability	• Study the temperature chart	Maintaining normal body temperature fully clothed in an open bed with normal ambient temperature
• Growth assessment	• Weight, length, and OFC plotted in the Fenton's chart	Weight gain for at least ≥3 consecutive days. Cutoff weight for discharge varies from center to center
• Feeding capability and nutrition	• Supervision of feeding by mother	Feeding by breast or paladi without cardio-respiratory compromise. Full breastfeeding prior to discharge is not a prerequisite, provided the baby is able to suck strongly. However, the mothers should be aware of the need to continue to monitor progress once further feeding changes are made at home, i.e. a switch from complementary to fully breastfeeding, etc. Nutritional risks should be assessed and therapy and dietary modification instituted if indicated.
• Screening prior to discharge:		
– Clinical	• Pallor, jaundice, cyanosis • Skin injury, abscess, rash, neurocutaneous markers, hemangioma • Skull shape, AF, PF, dysmorphism • Eye discharge • IU infection markers • Cardiac apex, abnormal sounds, murmur • Hepatosplenomegaly, hernia evaluation, genitalia, hips • Respiratory status • Tone, reflexes, primitive reflexes, etc.	Physiologically mature and stable cardiorespiratory function should be documented for a sufficient duration. Detailed head to toe examinations should be carried out and presence of any major congenital anomaly should be ruled out.
– Pulse oximetry	• Pulse oximetry reading of right hand and one foot	It is mandatory to do a detailed cardiac evaluation/functional echocardiography before discharge in all babies who do not have saturation levels greater than 95% in either extremity with <3% absolute difference between upper and lower extremity
– Laboratory investigations	• Hb, PCV • Na levels • Calcium, phosphorus, alkaline phosphatase	Anemia of prematurity growing preterm babies may develop hyponatremia due to immature sodium reabsorption and less sodium in breast milk, osteopenia of prematurity
– Hearing	• ABR and OAE tests	
– Eye	• ROP screening	Funduscopic examinations should be completed, as per the unit protocol
– Neuroimaging	• Cranial ultrasound • MRI scan if required	For early detection of IVH and PVL
– Neurodevelopmental assessment	• Amiel Tison angles • Hammersmith short screening chart	

Contd...

Contd...

Criteria	Checklist	Remarks
– Thyroid function	• TSH, T4	Thyroid screening should be done to rule out congenital hypothyroidism
– Metabolic screening	• Heel prick sample collected in a filter paper and sent for Tandem mass spectrometry according to unit protocol	Neonatal screening for genetic, endocrine and metabolic disorders should be ideally done 24 hours to 7 days of life (baby should have received at least one feed prior to sample collection). Early detection, diagnosis and intervention can prevent mortality and morbidity in neonates.
• Immunization	• Routine (Inj BCG, Inj HBV, OPV) • Special vaccines for preterm infants	Appropriate immunizations should be administered prior to discharge

(ABR: auditory brainstem response; BCG: Bacillus Calmette–Guérin; IVH: intraventricular hemorrhage; MRI: magnetic resonance imaging; OAE: otoacoustic emissions; OFC: occipitofrontal circumference; OPV: oral polio vaccine; PCV: packed cell volume; PVL: periventricular leukomalacia; ROP: retinopathy of prematurity; TSH: thyroid-stimulating hormone)

- Ensure education of mother/parents about feeding, temperature management at home, prevention of infections and danger signs
- Address the main concerns of parents like development, recognition, and management of illness at home, safety issues, emotional support, and role integration. Availability of written information on these issues is very helpful.

SUGGESTED READING

1. Hospital discharge of the high-risk neonate: committee on fetus and newborn. Pediatrics. 2008;122(5).
2. Merritt TA, Pillers D, Prows SL. Early NICU discharge of very low birth weight infants: a critical review and analysis. Semin Neonatol. 2003;8(2):95-115.
3. Shepperd S, Lannin NA, Clemson LM, et al. Discharge planning from hospital to home. Cochrane Database Syst Rev. 2013:(1):CD000313.

CHAPTER 43

Retinopathy of Prematurity Screening

Snehal Thakre

INTRODUCTION

Retinopathy of prematurity (ROP) is a preventable but leading cause of blindness affecting both eyes of premature infants. With improving survival of very low-birth weight infants in India, ROP is emerging as a significant problem with approximately 18,000 infants projected to become blind per year. In low/middle income countries, ROP affects babies with higher birth weights and gestational age.

Why to Screen for Retinopathy of Prematurity?

- It is an important preventable cause of childhood blindness.
- Premature babies are not born with ROP, but develop it after birth. Timely screening and appropriate treatment if necessary can arrest its development.
- Retinopathy of prematurity, if not detected in time, it may lead to *ocular morbidity like myopia, strabismus, visual impairment, and permanent blindness due to retinal detachment.* This retinal detachment will be diagnosed only at such a time, when little or nothing can be done to salvage vision.
- Retinopathy of prematurity is a reflector of quality of care provided to preterm newborns.

INDICATIONS

- All preterm infants ≤34 weeks of gestational age
- All babies with birth weight <2,000 g
- Gestational age between 34 weeks and 36 weeks but with risk factors such as:
  - Cardiorespiratory support
  - Prolonged oxygen therapy
  - Respiratory distress syndrome
  - Chronic lung disease
  - Fetal hemorrhage
  - Blood transfusion
  - Neonatal sepsis
  - Exchange transfusion
  - Intraventricular hemorrhage
  - Apneas
  - Poor postnatal weight gain
- Infants with an unstable clinical course who are at high risk (as determined by the neonatologist or pediatrician).

Timing of Screening

- First screening at 4 weeks of birth
- Infants with period of gestation less than 28 weeks (gestation age) or less than 1,200 g birth weight should be first screened at 2–3 weeks after delivery

- Follow-up examinations are recommended by the screening ophthalmologist based on retinal findings.

Prerequisite for Screening

The ophthalmologist should be trained in ROP screening and treatment. The neonatologist and the ophthalmologist should coordinate the ROP screening and treatment.

As per the Rashtriya Bal Surakhsa Karyakram (RBSK), it has been suggested that the pediatrician in charge of the newborn intensive care unit (NICU) are responsible for identifying infants to be screened, ensure timely screening and follow-up, and provide support during screening.

Preparation for Screening

- Counsel the parents for screening
- Admitted babies should always be examined under a radiant warmer in the neonatal unit. Discharged and stable babies may be examined in the ophthalmologist's outpatient department (OPD)
- Feed the baby half an hour prior to the examination
- After confirming the time with ophthalmologist, baby is prepared for examination by dilating the pupil
- Infant can be swaddled, made to suck on a swab soaked in sucrose during screening to reduce the pain.

Eye Preparation for Retinopathy of Prematurity Examination

To dilate the pupil, a commercially available preparation of tropicamide 0.8% + phenylephrine HCl 5% is diluted in 1:1 ratio with a tear substitute (methyl cellulose). These drops are instilled at an interval of 5 minutes for three times. Pupil dilatation is confirmed. Topical anesthetic eye drops (proparacaine) and tear substitutes are kept ready to use through the screening.

If pupils are not dilating despite administration of adequate mydriatic drops, severe or advanced ROP should be suspected.

Screening Procedure

Screening is done by the ophthalmologist with an indirect ophthalmoscope and a hand-held 20D lens after dilating the pupil (Fig. 1) or if available with a handheld fundus visualizing device. Scleral depressor is used to visualize the peripheral retina.

How to Classify Retinopathy of Prematurity?

The Revised International Classification of ROP (2005) is being used to describe the acute phase of ROP by the four parameters (Table 1): Location, extent, severity by stage, and plus disease.

When to Treat?

Definitions of Retinopathy of Prematurity for Treatment

The ETROP@ demonstrated a statistically significant benefit to earlier treatment, particularly for eyes with the most posterior disease.

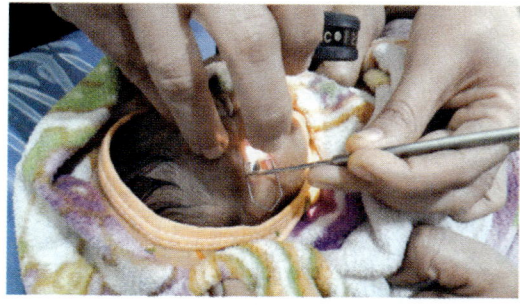

Fig. 1: Technique of retinopathy of prematurity (ROP) screening.

CHAPTER 43
Retinopathy of Prematurity Screening

Table 1: Classification of retinopathy of prematurity (ROP).	
Location (expressed in zones)	
Zone I	An imaginary circle with optic nerve at center and a radius of twice the distance from optic nerve to macula (innermost zone)
Zone II	From edge of zone I to the nasal ora serrata
Zone III	The residual crescent of retina anterior to zone II
Extent (recorded as hours of the clock or as 30° sectors)	
Severity (expressed stage looking at the vessels)	
Stage 1	*Demarcation line*: Presence of thin white line separating the avascular retina anteriorly from vascular retina posteriorly
Stage 2	*Ridge*: Line, has height and width and extends above the plane of the retina. Small isolated tufts of neovascular tissue lying on the surface of the retina, commonly called "popcorn" may be seen posterior to ridge
Stage 3	Extraretinal fibrovascular proliferation or neovascularization extends from the ridge into the vitreous
Stage 4	*Partial retinal detachment*: 4A: Extrafoveal—not involving macula, 4B: Foveal—involving macula
Stage 5	Total retinal detachment
Plus disease (this indicates a severe stage where a urgent action has to be taken)	
Plus disease	Vascular dilatation and tortuosity are present in at least two quadrants of the eye and may include iris vascular engorgement, poor papillary dilatation (rigid pupil), and vitreous haze. A "+" symbol is added to the ROP stage number to designate the presence of plus disease
Preplus disease	Vascular abnormalities of the posterior pole that are insufficient for the diagnosis of plus disease but that demonstrate more arterial tortuosity and more venous dilatation than normal. May progress to frank plus disease
Aggressive posterior ROP (AP-ROP)	This is a rapidly progressing severe form of ROP. If untreated, it usually progresses to stage 5 ROP. The characteristic features of this type of ROP are its posterior location, prominence of plus disease, and the ill-defined nature of the retinopathy. It is observed most commonly in zone I, but may also occur in posterior zone II
	This rapidly progressing retinopathy has been referred previously as "type II ROP" and "Rush disease," but was not specifically included in International Classification of Retinopathy of Prematurity (ICROP). Aggressive, posterior ROP seems to be the most appropriate term since the diagnosis can be made on a single visit and it does not require evaluation over time. Another important feature of AP-ROP is that it usually does not progress through the classic stages 1–3 (Fig. 2)

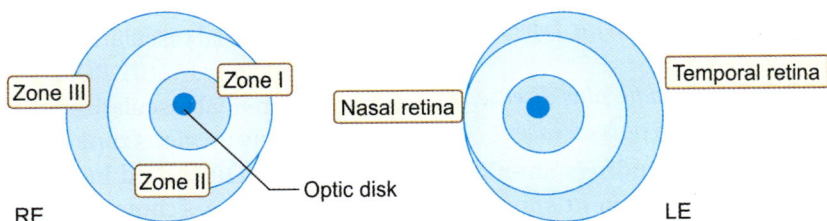

Fig. 2: Zones—As per International Classification of Retinopathy of Prematurity (ICROP) in which retinopathy of prematurity (ROP) is described and staged.
(RE: right eye; LE: left eye)

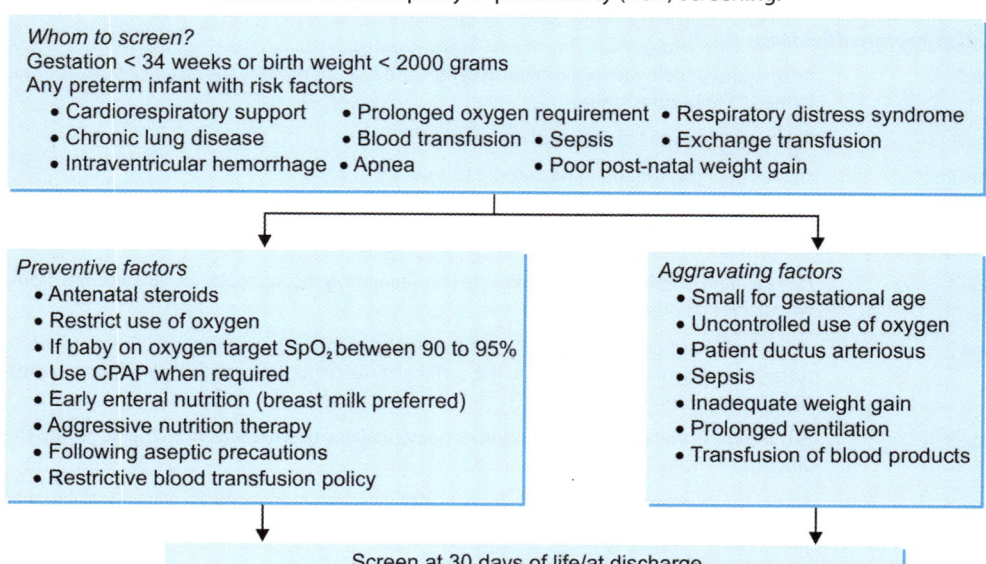

Flowchart 1: Retinopathy of prematurity (ROP) screening.

The clinical algorithm recommended peripheral retinal ablation should be considered for any eye with Type I ROP, defined as:
- Zone I, any stage ROP with plus disease, or
- Zone I, stage 3, with or without plus disease, or
- Zone II, stage 2 or 3 ROP, with plus disease.

Plus disease is defined as dilation and tortuosity of the posterior retinal blood vessels in at least two quadrants.

Treatment should also be considered for eyes showing signs of Aggressive Posterior Retinopathy of Prematurity or APROP.

Serial examinations (a "watch and wait" approach) were recommended for Type II ROP, defined as:
- Zone I, stage 1 or 2 with no plus disease, or
- Zone II, stage 3 with no plus disease.

Any eye with these findings should be followed closely and treatment should be considered when progression to type 1 status occurs.

What are the Treatment Modalities?

- Laser therapy *(Gold Standard)*
- Cryotherapy
- Intravitreal injection of anti-VEGF drug (specific indications— AP ROP, stage 3 ROP in Zone I or Posterior Zone II).

How to Follow-up?

It depends upon the retinal findings (Table 2).

When to Stop Examinations?

Zone III retinal vascularization without previous zone I or II ROP.
1. Zone III retinal vascularisation without any previous zone I/II/III ROP
2. Zone III retinal vascularization with regression of any previous zone I/II/III ROP
3. Treated ROP should be followed up till there are signs of complete resolution of the disease/vascularization of the retina/no signs of recurrence seen (especially in eyes

CHAPTER 43
Retinopathy of Prematurity Screening

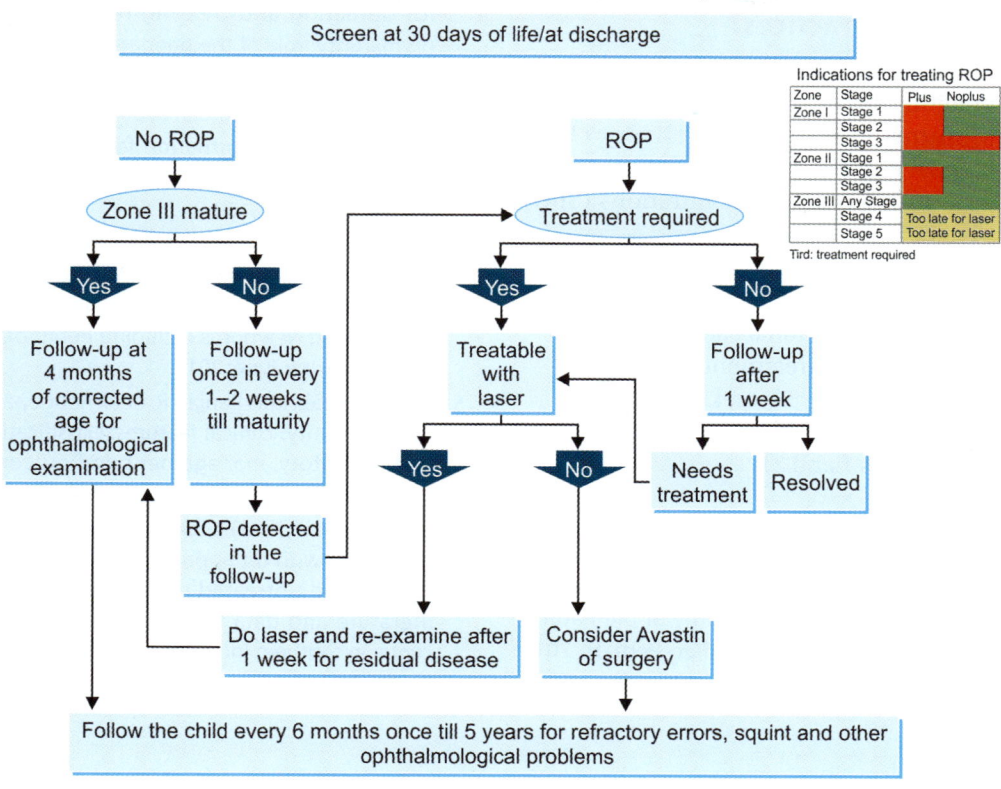

Flowchart 2: Algorithm for retinopathy of prematurity (ROP) care.

Table 2: When to follow-up repeat retinopathy of prematurity (ROP) examination.	
Retinal findings	**Follow-up schedule**
Stage 1 or 2 ROP: Zone I Stage 3 ROP: Zone II	1 week or less
Immature vascularization: Zone I—no ROP Stage 2 ROP: Zone II Regressing ROP: Zone I	1–2 weekly
Stage 1 ROP: Zone II Regressing ROP: Zone II	2 weekly
Immature vascularization: Zone II—no ROP Stage 1 or 2 ROP: Zone III Regressing ROP: Zone III	2–3 weekly

treated with intravitreal anti-VEGF) maybe as long as 60 weeks post conceptional age or even longer.

Eye Complications in babies with Retinopathy of Prematurity

- Visual disability
- Refractory errors
- Strabismus
- Cataract
- Glaucoma
- Late retinal detachment.

All babies with ROP should have yearly eye evaluation till school age.

What are Potentially Best Preventive Practices?

- Antenatal steroids to mother with threatened preterm labor
- Monitoring of oxygen delivery (FiO_2, blender)
- Monitoring of oxygen saturations (SpO_2: 91–95%)
- Judicious use of blood transfusion
- Early enteral nutrition (human breast milk)
- Aggressive nutritional care
- Prevention and treatment of sepsis
- Use of caffeine (<32 weeks gestation)
- Timely screening and treatment of ROP (Flowcharts 1 and 2).

SUGGESTED READING

1. Blencowe H, Moxon S, Gilbert C. Update on blindness due to retinopathy of prematurity globally and in India. Indian Pediatr. 2016; 53(Suppl 2):S89-92.
2. Grover S, Katoch D, Dogra MR, et al. Programs for detecting and treating retinopathy of prematurity: role of the neonatal team. Indian Pediatr. 2016;53(Suppl 2):S93-9.
3. Mariam S, Kumar P, Katoch D, et al. Retinopathy of prematurity: information for parents and frequently asked questions. Indian Pediatr. 2016;53(Suppl 2):S100-2.
4. Rashtriya Bal Swasthya Karyakram (RBSK). Ministry of Health and Family Welfare Government of India. Guidelines for Universal Eye Screening in Newborns including Retinopathy of Prematurity; June; 2017.
5. Shah PK, Prabhu V, Ranjan R, et al. Retinopathy of prematurity: clinical features, classification, natural history, management and outcome. Indian Pediatr. 2016;53(Suppl 2):S118-22.
6. Vijayalakshmi P, Kara T, Gilbert C. Ocular morbidity associated with retinopathy of prematurity in treated and untreated eyes: a review of the literature and data from a tertiary eye-care center in southern India. Indian Pediatr. 2016;53 (Suppl 2):S137-42.

CHAPTER 44

Hearing Screening

Chetana Naik

INTRODUCTION

Inability to hear impairs communication and hinders development of speech and language. No child is born mute. It is the deafness at birth or later on which render a child to become mute. Hence, even though deafness cannot be prevented, but, mutism is totally preventable. A clinician's ignorance should not delay the diagnosis of deafness and add to lifelong mutism in a child.

IMPORTANCE OF HEARING SCREENING

- The incidence of bilateral congenital deafness is 1.5–6 per 1,000 live births in our country. Half of these are genetic in origin and other half due to conditions like prenatal rubella (Box 1), ototoxic drug intake during pregnancy, etc. Many are childhood acquired deafness like postmeningitis, neonatal jaundice, Alport syndrome, etc. However, substantial proportion may have no risk factors.
- Symptoms and signs of hearing loss are subtle because infants with hearing loss demonstrate high degree of environmental vigilance (appear to respond to sound but actually respond by perceiving visual or other sensory input).
- The critical age for language learning is from birth to 3.5 years of age. A child, who is born deaf or partially hearing impaired, cannot perceive sounds and thus, fails to learn speech if the remedial measures for the hearing defect are not taken early. Later on, this may result in lower education level and employment opportunities.

In most of the advanced countries, it is mandatory by law for every child born to go through the neonatal screening for hearing (universal hearing screening). Though universal hearing screening is ideal, it is probably not possible in most centers in our

Box 1: Risk factors for hearing impairment.

- In utero infections like rubella, cytomegalovirus
- Herpes, toxoplasma
- Use of ototoxic drugs during pregnancy
- Alcohol intake during pregnancy
- Prolonged labor
- Babies admitted to NICU for more than 5 days
- Babies hospitalized for 48 hours or more within first 4 weeks
- Lowbirth weight babies <1,500 g
- Apgar score <4 at 1 min, <6 at 5 min of birth
- Syndromes like Down, Treacher Collins syndrome
- Family history of sensorineural hearing loss
- Craniofacial anomalies
- Consanguineous marriage

(NICU: neonatal intensive care unit)

country. Thus, it becomes imperative that we take the initiative to screen at least high-risk babies (selective hearing screening) as enlisted in Box 1.

In addition to these, the International Joint Committee on infant hearing screening has further recommended that in between age of 4 weeks and 2 years, a screening test should be done in cases of parental doubt, delayed milestones, postnatal infections like meningitis, hyperbilirubinemia, head trauma, and otitis media with effusion.

HEARING LOSS

Hearing loss is defined based on the degree of loss, measured in logarithmic decibels, at frequencies between 125 Hz (low-pitch sounds) and 8,000 Hz (high-pitch sounds). It can be sensorineural, conductive, or mixed. Severity of hearing loss is categorized and shown in Box 2.

HEARING TESTS TO IDENTIFY DEAFNESS IN A CHILD

To identify any deafness in a child, different objective and subjective tests are carried out. Both are essential to have a good idea of child's hearing status. These tests have high sensitivity (92%) and specificity (98%) in early neonatal period itself. A battery of tests is necessary, just doing a stray brainstem evoked response audiometry (BERA) or free-field audiometry is no good (Table 1).

Box 2
Severity of hearing impairment.

Degree of hearing impairment hearing threshold (dB)
- Normal hearing: 0–20
- Mild: 20–40
- Moderate: 40–60
- Severe: 60–80
- Profound: >80

The best way for early identification of deafness is neonatal screening, i.e. when the baby is born. Evoked otoacoustic emission test (EOAE) can be done in a new born. It is noninvasive, quick, sensitive and does not require highly trained personnel. If the baby fails this test, a confirmatory test of BERA is carried out. Comparison of newborn hearing tests is given in Table 2.

Two types of neonatal hearing screening are practiced. Most effective is the universal neonatal hearing screening program which has 100% specificity and no child is missed as all live births are screened within 48 hours of birth (Flowchart 1). The other is the "high-risk neonatal hearing screening program" in which only babies from high-risk conditions (Box 1) undergo screening. This reduces the cost and manpower involved. High-risk category can be identified in few easy steps by physician. Firstly, through mother's interview by a questionnaire enquiring about her obstetric history, family history of any deafness and any

Table 1: Tests for hearing assessment.

Objective tests	Subjective tests
Brainstem evoked response audiometry (BERA)	Free-field audiometry
Evoked otoacoustic emissions (EOAE)	Visual response audiometry
Auditory steady state response (ASSR)	

Table 2: Comparison between EOAE and BERA.

	EOAE	BERA
Expertise	Trained personnel	Audiologist
Time	Few minutes	30 min
Sedation	Not required	Required
Failure rate	Higher	Lower
Motion artifacts	No	Yes

(BERA: brainstem evoked response audiometry; EAOE: evoked otoacoustic emissions)

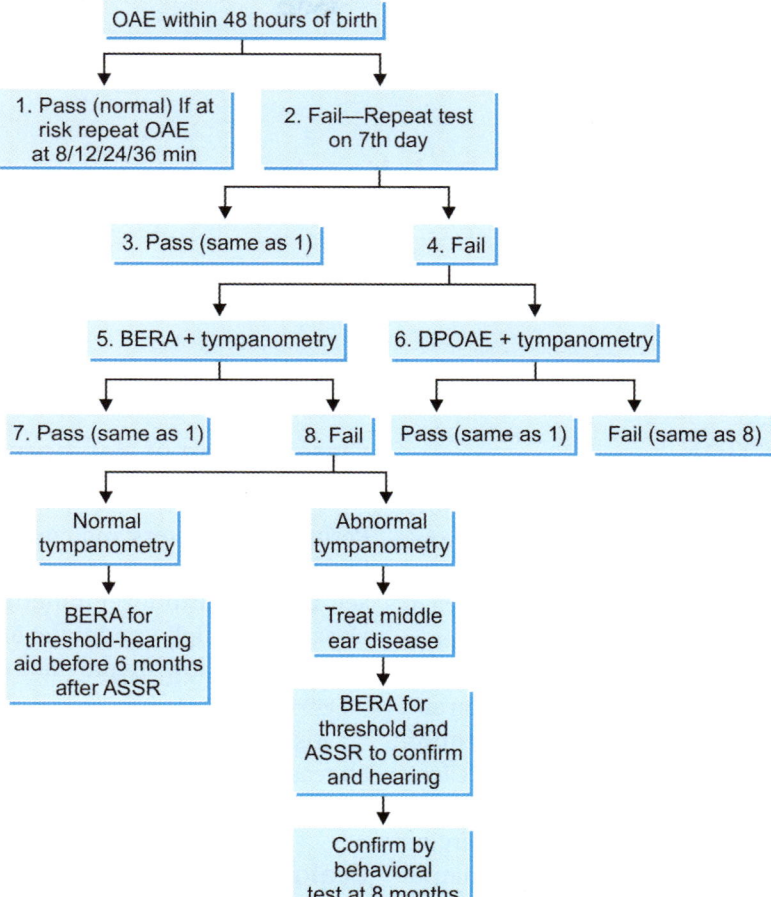

Flowchart 1: Neonatal hearing screening.

(ASSR: auditory steady state response; BERA: brainstem evoked response audiometry; OAE: otoacoustic emission; DPOAE: distortion product otoacoustic emissions)

medical illness and by physical examination of the neonate for congenital defects.

EARLY MANAGEMENT

Once the hearing defect is confirmed rehabilitative measures in the form of good hearing aids at an early age or even cochlear implants and supportive speech therapy will help the child lead a life on par with his "normal" counterparts. Cochlear implants are considered in case of severe to profound hearing loss only if there is inadequate response to hearing aids.

SUGGESTED READING

1. Biswas A. Clinical Audio-Vestibulometry for Otologists and Neurologists, 5th edition. New Delhi: Bhalani Publishing House; 2017.
2. Nagapoornima P, Rames A, Srilakshmi, et al. Universal hearing screening. Indian J Pediatr. 2007;74:545-9.
3. Northern JL. Hearing in Children, 4th edition. Baltimore, MD: Williams and Wilkins; 1991.
4. US Preventive Services Task Force. Universal screening for hearing loss in newborn: US Preventive Service Task Force, Recommendation Statement. Pediatrics. 2008;122:143-8.

CHAPTER

Follow-up of the High-Risk Newborn

Archana Kadam

INTRODUCTION

Advances in perinatal intensive care have resulted in improved survival of extreme preterm and sick neonates. These neonatal intensive care unit (NICU) graduates are at risk of developmental disabilities, incidence of which increase with decreasing birth weight and gestation. A method of early detection and thereby early and appropriate intervention can modify these future disabilities. Close monitoring of development together with coordination of treatment for any emerging problems is referred to as developmental follow-up. The ultimate aim of follow-up is to ensure early appropriate intervention that gives better functional outcome for at risk neonates if started before 2 years of age.

Components of Developmental Surveillance

- Identifying risk factors and high-risk infants.
- Documenting and maintaining developmental history.
- Eliciting and attending to parents' concern regarding the child's development.
- Make accurate observations of the child.
- Maintaining accurate record of findings.
- Identifying protective factors.

Classification of Newborns as per Risk (Table 1)

Perinatal risk factors and course of neonatal illness define a group of neonates at increased risk of neurodevelopmental disability, classified as high, moderate, and mild risk. The type of follow-up provided is then based on severity.

Risk factors are likely to be additive, with increased risk of adverse outcomes as number of risk factors increase.

Evaluation at Discharge for High-Risk Newborn (Tables 2 and 3)

- Clinical evaluation for well being
- Anthropometry: Weight, head circumference, length
- Neurologic evaluation to assess tone and reflexes
- Screening for developmental dysplasia of hip (DDH)
- Document a hematocrit if not recently done
- Screen for hearing and vision
- USG cranium at 36 weeks and 40 weeks of post-menstrual age (PMA)
- Appointment for follow-up
- Counseling for follow-up and danger signs.

Table 1: Classifications of newborns as per risk.

Mild risk	Moderate risk	High risk
Preterm	Preterm <33 weeks	<28 weeks
Weight 1,500–2,500 g	Weight 1,000–1,500 g	Weight <1,000 g, small for gestational age (SGA), large for gestational age (LGA)
Hypoxic ischemic encephalopathy (HIE) grade I	HIE moderate	Apgar's < 3 at 5 min and or HIE
Transient hypoglycemia	Hypoglycemia (blood sugar <25 mg/dL)	Persistent prolonged hypoglycemia
Suspect sepsis	Sepsis	Meningitis, shock needing Inotropes/vasopressor support
Neonatal jaundice needing phototherapy	Neonatal jaundice serum bilirubin >20 or needing exchange	Neonatal bilirubin encephalopathy
Grade I IVH	IVH grade 2	Major morbidities intraventricular hemorrhage (IVH), periventricular leukomalacia (PVL)
		Abnormal neurology on discharge, seizures
	Twins or triplets	Twin-to-twin transfusion
		Failed newborn hearing screening
		Ventilation more than 24 hours, bronchopulmonary dysplasia (BPD)
	Suboptimal home environment	Surgical conditions, major malformations
		Hypocalcemia
		Inborn errors of metabolism and or genetic disorders
		Infant of human immunodeficiency virus (HIV) positive mother
Care by pediatrician	Care by neonatologist/developmental pediatrician	

Table 2: Clinical outcomes of high-risk newborns.

Morbidity	Clinical manifestations
Developmental delay	Delayed milestones, speech delay, academic underachievement
Motor deficits	Delayed motor milestones, tone abnormalities, cerebral palsy, visuomotor integration issues, sensory processing difficulties, speech clarity issues
Sensory impairment	Vision impairment
	Sensorineural hearing loss
Learning difficulties	Dyslexia, dysgraphia, dyscalculia
Behavioral issues	ADHD, autism, others
Epilepsy	

(ADHD: attention deficit hyperactivity disorder)

Table 3: High-risk baby follow-up schedule.

Who will follow-up	*High-risk team
Where	High-risk clinic
When	**4 months, 8 months, 1 year and yearly till 6 years

*High-risk team: Neonatologist, developmental pediatrician, physiotherapists, speech and language therapists, psychologists, dieticians, social workers, ophthalmologist, Ears, Nose and Throat (ENT), orthopedician and neurologist.

**Age: Age used for follow-up is calculated as corrected age. Corrected age is the sum of chronologic age in weeks minus the difference between 40 weeks of gestation and gestational age at birth. The correction is to be considered till 2 years of age.

COMPONENTS OF THE DEVELOPMENTAL FOLLOW-UP (TABLE 4)

- Cognitive development (Flowchart 1)
- Neuromotor development (Flowchart 2)
- Growth
- Neurosensory
- Behavior

Cognitive Development Follow-up (Table 5)

Developmental Screening

Its purpose is to identify children who are in need of further evaluation. If the results of a screening test suggest developmental delay, the

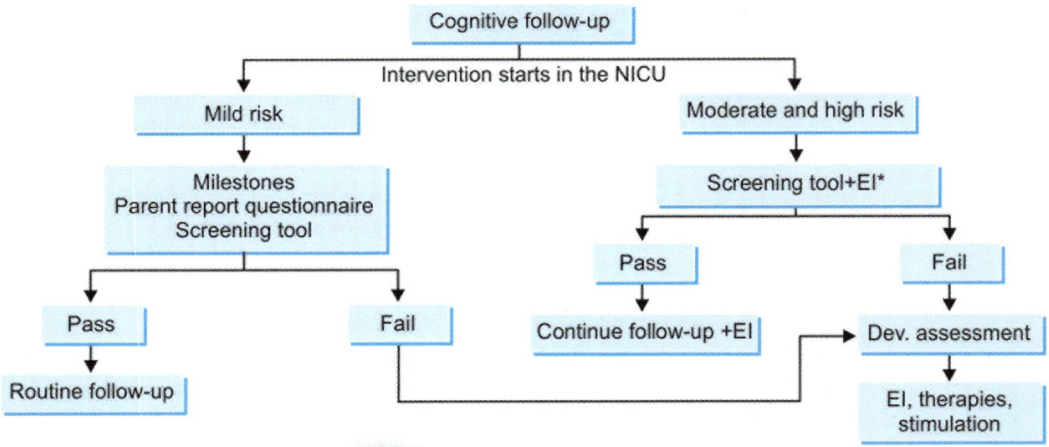

Flowchart 1: Cognitive follow-up algorithm.

*EI—early Intervention; Dev: developmental
Note: Early intervention reduces the impact of the disability and improves functional outcomes.

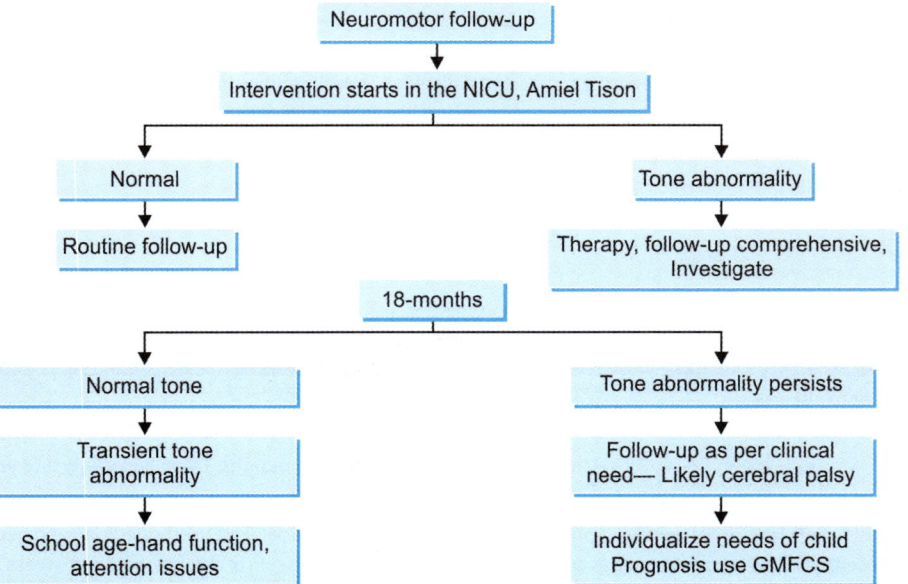

Flowchart 2: Algorithm for neuromotor follow-up.

(GMFCS: gross motor function classification system; NICU: neonatal intensive care unit)

Table 4: Ages when deficits become apparent.

Gross motor deficits: By 2 years of age
Language deficits: In preschool age
Behavioral or learning problems: In school age

Table 5: Developmental screening tools.

Parent report questionnaires	Screening tool
Form for parents: use any of the below tool	Administered: Use any of the below tool
Use in mild risk	Use in moderate and high risk
Ages and Stages Questionnaires (ASQ)	Trivandrum Development Screening Chart (TDSC)
Child Development Inventories (CDI)	Denver Developmental Screening Test (DDST II)
Parents' Evaluation of Developmental Status (PEDS)	

Table 6: Red flag signs for vision.

Age	Check
0–3 months	Not following face from side-to-side
	Not smiling at your face
3–6 months	Holding objects closer
	Nystagmus
	Head tilt
	Strabismus

child should be referred for a developmental assessment (Tables 6 to 8).

Developmental Assessment

A developmental evaluation is an in-depth assessment used to create a profile of the child's strengths and weaknesses in all developmental areas. Its results are used to plan intervention (Tables 9 to 11).

Neuromotor Follow-up

Amiel Tison

- It is a neurodevelopmental assessment in the first year done at corrected 3 months, 6 months, 9 months and 1 year of age.
- It assesses tone, primitive reflexes, postural reactions, and deep jerks.

Gross Motor Function Classification System

- It is used for assessment of severity of motor disability and function after 2 years.

Note:
- Serial comprehensive assessments by trained observers give an idea whether tone abnormalities are transient or persistent.

Table 7: Red flag signs for hearing.

Receptive	Age	Expressive	Age
No turn sound	6 months	No babble, gesture need	12 months
No 1 step command	12 months	No bye or three words	15 months
No locate or point 5 objects	15 months	No join words	2.5 years
No point body parts	2 years	No simple sentences	3 years
No 2 step commands	3 years	Conversation not clear	4 years
	Loss of language at any age		

Table 8: Development observation chart (DOC).

Age	Milestone: If not achieved refer for developmental assessment
2 months	- Social smile
4 months	- Head holding
8 months	- Sit alone
12 months	- Stand alone
	- Make sure the baby can see, hear, and listen

Table 9: Developmental assessment tools for children.

Cognitive tests	DQ	DQ	IQ
	DASII: Developmental Assessment Scales for Indian Infants	BSIDIII: Bayley Scale of Infant Development III	Wechsler Intelligence scale, Stanford Binet test
Use till	0–2.5 years	0–3.5 years	Above 2.5 years
	Indian adaptation of Bayleys	Revision of Bayleys II	
Results	Motor and mental scales	Motor, mental, language, socioemotional adaptive scales	Performance and verbal IQ
When	If fails screen or yearly	If fails screen or yearly	Yearly
Delay	DQ < 70	DQ < 70	IQ < 70
			Borderline: 70–85

Table 10: Implications of DQ scores.

DQ	Implications
>85	Considered as within normal limits
<70	In two or more streams is considered as global developmental delay
<70	In any stream warrants serious consideration of the cause and early intervention
<50	Evaluate for organic etiology

Note:
- In the Indian context, the DASII is the best cognitive developmental assessment tool till 2.5 years of age.
- For children with DQ of 75 and less, in any area then a center-based program is advised. For a child with a DQ between 76 and 85, a home program is given with regular review and follow-up.

Table 11: Major neurodevelopmental disabilities in the high-risk newborn.

Cerebral palsy
DASII score < 70 on Mental and Motor Scale
Blindness in one or both eye
Hearing impairment warranting assistive devices in one or both ears

- A diagnosis of cerebral palsy (CP) is generally evident if the neurological signs persist by 18–24 months.
- Loss of abnormal neurological findings by 12 months is associated with better outcomes.
- Deep tendon reflexes are not very helpful in the diagnosis of CP in the first 6 months of life as the reflexes are normally brisk during this period.
- At school age, assess hand function and coordination.

Growth and Nutrition Follow-up (Table 12)

- While monitoring growth, use corrected age till 2 years.
- *In preterm <40 weeks gestation*: Use intrauterine growth charts Fenton, Infant Health and Development Program (IHDP), Casey P, Wrights, Gairdner, and Pearson (Castlemead), Modified Babson Brenda charts.
- Later postnatal growth charts by World Health Organization (WHO) can be used.

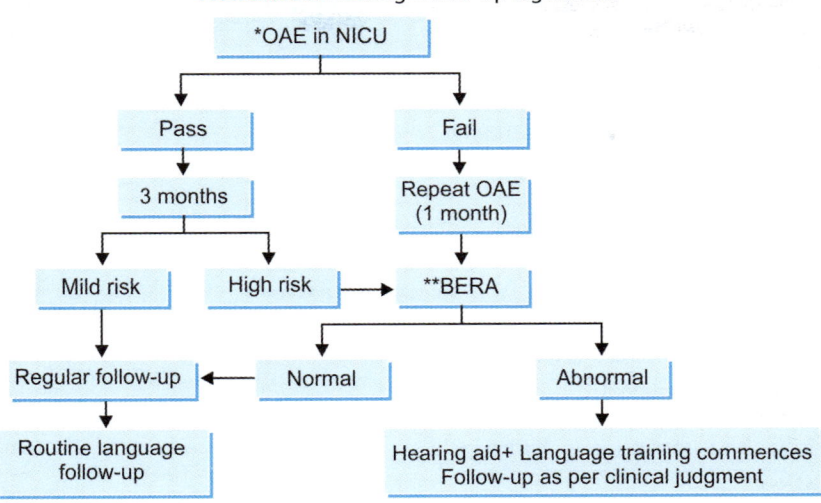

Flowchart 3: Hearing follow-up algorithm.

*Screen—OAE: otoacoustic emission; **Assessment—BERA: brainstem evoked auditory response; NICU: neonatal intensive care unit.
Note: Infants with permanent hearing loss who receive intervention services prior to 6 months of age have significantly better language outcomes.

Table 12: Red flag signs for growth.	
Weight	<20 g/day
Head circumference	<1 cm/week
Height	<1 cm/week

Table 13: Red flag signs for Autism.	
Age	Note
12 months 16 months 24 months	• No babbling, pointing, or other gestures • No single words • No two words spontaneous phrases • Any loss of any language or social skills at any age

Neurosensory

- Vision screening for retinopathy of prematurity: Details in ROP Chapter.
- Hearing follow-up (Flowchart 3)

Behavioral (Table 13)

- There is high incidence of behavioral problems in the high-risk newborn.
- Pediatrician monitoring follow-up must probe for attention issues in social settings and its effect on learning.
- With the rise in incidence of autism, administering a simple screen like the M-CHAT-R, follow-up at 18 months may help identify children with autistic features earlier.

Duration of Follow-up

Components of follow-up are depicted in Table 14. Ideally follow-up should continue till late adolescence as many cognitive, learning, and behavioral problems more common in at risk newborn may only become apparent on longer follow-up.

SECTION 3
Care of Preterm/Low Birth Weight/High Risk Newborn

Table 14: Checklist for high-risk newborn follow-up.

Components +	1.5 m	2.5 m	3.5 m	6 m	9 m	12 m	18 m	24 m
Parental concerns	At every visit							
Medical problems	At every visit							
Vaccination	As per IAP schedule (2018–19)							
Anthropometry@	At every visit (Wt~, HC*, TL) Use WHO Growth charts (for boys/girls, separate)							
Nutrition								
• Diet	Exclusive breastfeeding			Complimentary nutrition	Home diet			
• Vitamin D	400 IU, daily							
• Iron	For preterm only			For term	For preterm		—	Yearly
• Cal/PO$_4$	For preterm only			For term	—	—	—	Yearly
• Formula: Shift to term formula at 3 kg weight								
Neurologic exam #	At every visit							
Development test^	Screening at each visit	Formal testing		Screening at each visit		Behavioral assessment (MCHAT)	—	Formal testing
Eye evaluation	Retinopathy of prematurity (ROP) screening at 1 month age (All < 2 kg)				For vision, squint, optic atrophy	—	—	For vision, squint, optic atrophy
Hearing	Otoacoustic emissions (OAE) at discharge. Brainstem evoked response audiometry (BERA) for testing or confirmation at 3 m. Screen at each visit							
Computed tomography (CT) or magnetic resonance imaging (MRI) brain, USG brain (!)	As clinically indicated (!) At 36–40 weeks corrected age							
Language	—	—	—	—	LEST	—	LEST	—
Counseling	At every visit							
Biochemical screen	—	—	—	—	Hb, urine	—	Hb	Hemoglobin (Hb), urine, blood pressure (BP)

+Correction for gestational immaturity at birth should be done till 24 months age for all preterms. Use corrected age for complimentary feeding and milestone screening. Use postnatal age for vaccination.
Note: Follow-up every 2 weeks until a weight of 3 kg. Then follow as per above schedule.
~ Use Fenton's chart till 40 weeks gestation for preterm. Thereafter, use World Health Organization (WHO) growth chart as for term infants.
*Interpret head circumference with total length till 12 months of age. (HC = TL/2 + 9.5 + 2. 5 cm).
#Amiel Tison till 12 months of age.
^Screening tests = History + TDSC (Trivandrum development screening chart) OR DOC (Development observation card). Formal testing – DASII (Developmental assessment scale for Indian infants).
LEST: language evaluation scale Trivandrum, behavioral assessment: CBCL (Achenbach child behavior checklist), pediatric symptom checklist.
Formal cognitive development, IQ is tested by 3 years of age.

SUGGESTED READING

1. Doyle LW, Anderson PJ, Battin M, et al. Long term follow up of high risk children: who, why and how? BMC Pediatr. 2014;14:279.
2. Follow up care of high risk infants. Pediatrics. 2004;114:1377-97.
3. How you can implement the AAP's new policy on developmental and behavioral screening. Contemporary Pediatrics Archive, April 2003.
4. Illingworth R. The Development of the Infant and Young Child: Normal and Abnormal, 10th edition. New Delhi: Harcourt India; 2012.

5. Pandit A, Mukhopadhyay K, Suryawanshi P, et al. Follow up of high risk newborns. In: Kumar P (Ed). National Neonatal Forum. Clinical Practice Guidelines. New Delhi: NNF India; 2010. pp. 217-52.
6. Poon JK, La Rosa AC, Pai GS. Developmental delay timely identification and assessment. Indian Pediatr. 2010;47:415-22.
7. Sujatha R, Jain N. Prediction of neurodevelopmental outcome of preterm babies. Using Risk Stratification Score. Indian J Pediatr. 2016;83(7):640-4.
8. Vohr BR. Long Term Follow up of Very Low Birth Weight Infants. Neurology Neonatal Questions and controversies, 2nd edition. pp. 325-40.

CHAPTER 46

IVH and PVL Screening and Classification

Pradeep Suryawanshi

INTRAVENTRICULAR HEMORRHAGE

Definition

- Germinal matrix hemorrhage (GMH) or intraventricular hemorrhage (IVH) is the most common type of intracranial hemorrhage and is classically seen in preterm infants.
- Characteristically originates from the fragile involuting vessels of the subependymal germinal matrix, located in the caudothalamic groove. The vascularized subependymal germinal matrix lacks the supporting basement membrane and there is an increased amount of fibrinolytic activity in the germinal matrix region that predisposes to the development of IVH. This germinal matrix is most vulnerable for bleeding between 24 weeks and 32 weeks and incidence is 15–20% in infants born at <32 weeks' gestation. It is uncommon in term neonates.

Causative Mechanisms

Intravascular factors	Ischemia or reperfusion (e.g. volume infusion after hypotension)
	Increase in cerebral blood flow (e.g. with hypertension, anemia, and hypercarbia)

Contd...

Contd...

	Increase in cerebral venous pressure (e.g. with high intrathoracic pressure, usually from ventilator, and pneumothorax)
	Platelet dysfunction with coagulation disturbances
Vascular factors	Tenuous, involuting capillaries with large luminal diameter
Extravascular factors	Deficient vascular support
	Excessive fibrinolytic activity

Whom to screen?

- All newborns less than 32 weeks' gestation or less than 1,500 g, irrespective of clinical signs.
- Preterm infants more than 32 weeks or more than 1,500 g, if they are ill or have risk factors such as perinatal asphyxia, tension pneumothorax, ventilation, or abnormal neurologic signs.

When to screen?

- Up to half of hemorrhages occur during the first 24 hours of life. Less than 5% of infants develop IVH after the 4th or 5th day of life. Therefore for stable preterm infant's first cranial ultrasound (CUS) should be done at age 4–7 days and later repeated around day 30 and corrected age 36–40 weeks. Besides grade of IVH, presence or absence of ventricular dilatation and evidence of white matter injury on CUS have important prognostic value. For very sick extremely low birth weight (ELBW) infants, first screening should be performed on day 1 as this will aid in counseling and decision making.

NICU and/or <32 weeks GA and/or birth weight <1,500	High care and ≥32 weeks GA and ≥1,500 g
<24 hours after birth	
On the third day	On the third day
Biweekly until the second week	
Weekly until discharge	Weekly until discharge
Around term	
More frequently in the case of (suspected) abnormalities	More frequently in the case of (suspected) abnormalities

Classification of GM/IVH

- *Volpe's classification (Volpe 1989):*

Grade 1	Germinal matrix hemorrhage with no or minimal IVH (<10% of ventricular area on parasagittal view)
Grade 2	IVH (10–50% of the ventricular area on parasagittal view)
Grade 3	IVH (>50% of the ventricular area on parasagittal view; usually distends to the lateral ventricle at the time of diagnosis)
Separate notation	Concomitant periventricular echodensity (location and extent), referred to as "IPE" (intraparenchymal echodensity), periventricular hemorrhagic parenchymal infarction, or venous infarction

- *Classification of GM/IVH by Papille et al.:* Grading system of Papille and colleagues is the most widely used system for describing IVH.

Grade 1 (Figs. 1A and B)	A small hemorrhage confined to the germinal matrix and without effect on adjacent parenchyma
Grade 2 (Figs. 2A and B)	Hemorrhage originating within the germinal matrix where small amount of blood has leaked into the lateral ventricle, but no ventricular dilatation
Grade 3 (Figs. 3A and B)	Hemorrhage originating into germinal matrix where large amount of blood has leaked into ventricular system leading to acute ventricular dilatation
Grade 4 (Figs. 4A and B)	Larger hemorrhage into germinal matrix along with evidence of venous infarction of the adjacent periventricular white matter

How to identify IVH?

- Ultrasound scan of brain is the preferred choice for diagnosis and screening of IVH. It can identify all degrees, severity, and extent of hemorrhage.
- Anterior fontanelle is usually used as an ultrasonographic "window" and real-time images are visualized using sequential coronal and parasagittal projections. The posterior fontanelle provides anatomic details of periventricular white matter or the presence of blood in the lateral ventricles.
- In the coronal views, GM/IVH appears next to the concave curve of lateral wall of the lateral ventricle (Fig. 5).
- In the sagittal plane, GM/IVH is seen along the inferior border of ventricle anterior to caudothalamic notch (Fig. 6).

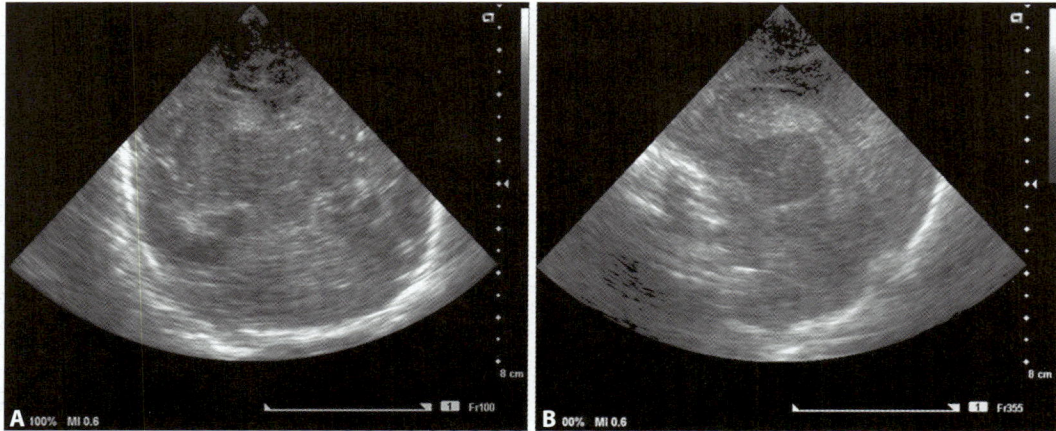

Figs. 1A and B: Grade 1 intraventricular hemorrhage (IVH), confined to the germinal matrix at the caudothalamic notch.

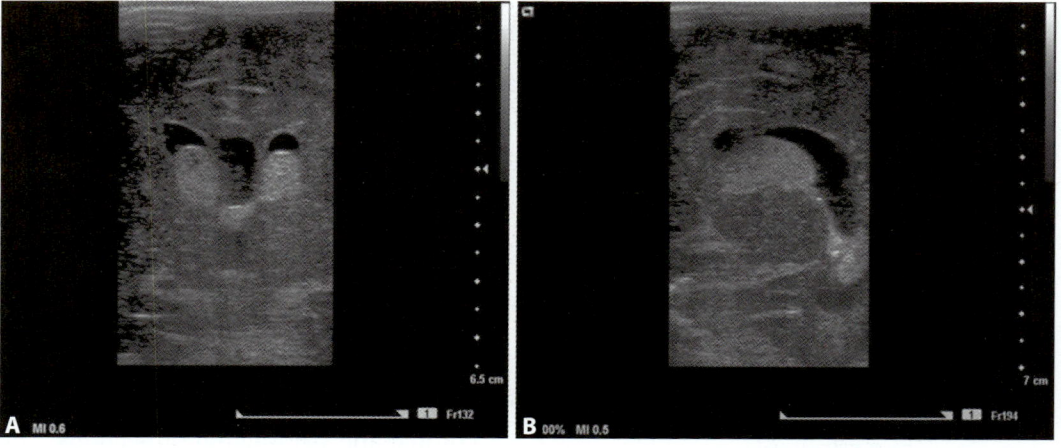

Figs. 2A and B: Grade 2 IVH on right side. Note presence of blood within the lateral ventricle.

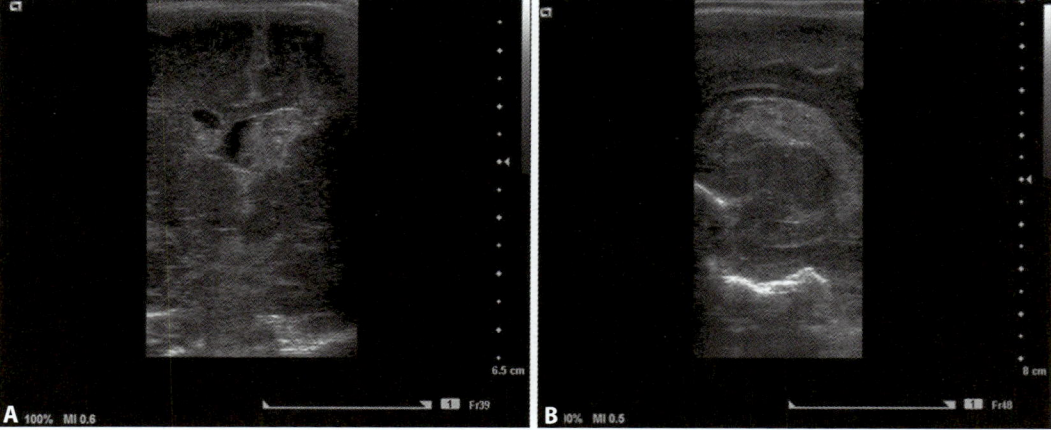

Figs. 3A and B: Presence of blood within the lateral ventricles forming a cast of lateral ventricle. Note acute dilatation of lateral ventricle (Grade 3 IVH).

CHAPTER 46
IVH and PVL Screening and Classification

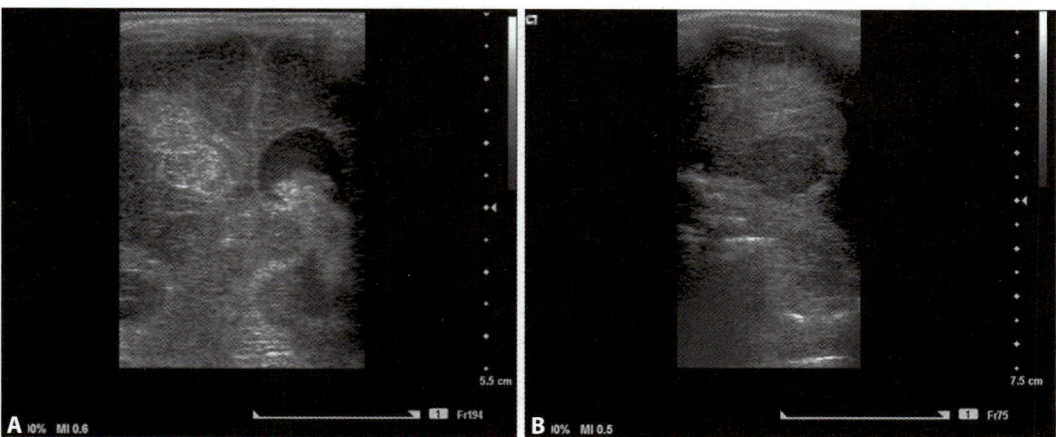

Figs. 4A and B: Presence of periventricular hemorrhagic infarction (Grade 4 IVH).

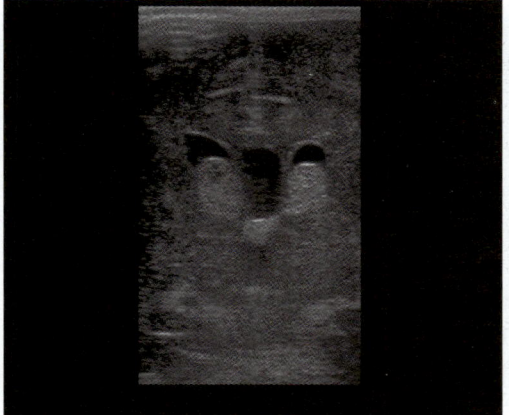 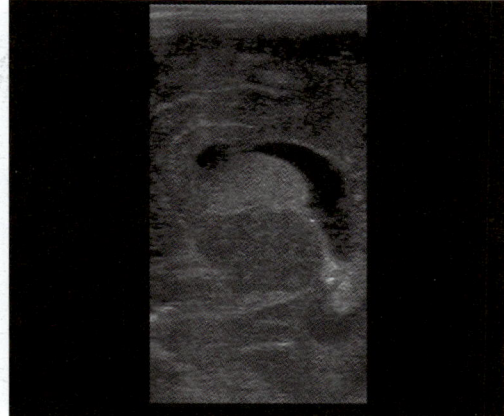

Fig. 5: Coronal view of brain at the level of foramen of Monro. Note hyperechogenic lesions (IVH) on the lateral wall of the lateral ventricle.

Fig 6: Sagittal view of lateral ventricles. Note presence of hyperechogenic lesions (IVH) at the caudothalamic notch.

Prediction of Long-term Outcome

Severity of hemorrhage	Ventricular dilatation	Outcome and neurodevelopmental outcome
Grade I	0%	Resolve and good outcome
Grade II	5%	Resolve and good outcome
Grade III	20–55%	Mortality—10–20%
		Cognitive and motor—30–40%
Severe with apparent periventricular hemorrhagic infarction	80%	Mortality—50–80%
		Neurological impairment—80–90%

- Presence of ventriculomegaly on the CUS at corrected age of term has direct correlation with long-term neurologic impairment, likely because mild ventriculomegaly represents white matter injury that results in decreased cerebral volume.
- Infants with IVH complications (e.g. periventricular hemorrhagic infarction and progressive ventricular dilatation) have much higher risk of neurologic impairment than those with IVH alone.

Potentially Best Preventive Practices

- *Prenatal:*
  - Prevent premature births
  - In utero transport of premature deliveries to perinatal center
  - Antenatal steroids
  - Avoid prolonged labor and difficult deliveries
- *Postnatal:*
  - Gentle newborn resuscitation practices
  - Vitamin K at birth
  - Minimal handling protocols
  - Avoid hypotension and blood pressure fluctuations
  - Gentle ventilation strategies
  - Early use of surfactant therapy
  - Minimal and gentle endotracheal suction practices
  - Avoid pneumothorax
  - Prophylactic indomethacin may be used.

PERIVENTRICULAR LEUKOMALACIA

Definition

- Periventricular leukomalacia (PVL) is necrosis or softening of white matter in a characteristic distribution, i.e. in the white matter dorsal and lateral to the external angles of the lateral ventricles and less severe injury to the white matter peripheral to these focal necroses. The lesions are usually bilaterally symmetric. It has two components:
  1. Focal necrosis evolving to cystic PVL
  2. Diffuse gliosis evolving to noncystic PVL.
- Most important brain lesion of premature infants determining the neurodevelopmental outcome.

Clinical Correlates

Site of lesion	Neonatal manifestation	Long-term sequelae
Periventricular white matter including descending motor fibers, optic radiation, deficit of cerebral cortex, basal ganglia, thalamus, and cerebellum	Lower limb weakness	Spastic diplegia Motor deficit Cognitive deficits Behavioral/attention deficit

Classification of Periventricular Leukomalacia

According to de Varies et al. (1992):
- *Grade I*—transient periventricular echo densities persisting for >7 days
- *Grade II*—transient periventricular echo densities evolving into small, localized frontoparietal cysts
- *Grade III*—periventricular echo densities evolving into extensive periventricular cystic lesions
- *Grade IV*—densities extending into the deep white matter evolving into extensive cystic lesions.

Ultrasonography Findings

- Sonographically, PVL initially appears as a highly echogenic area in the parietal lobe adjacent to the lateral ventricles or in the

frontal lobes. There are two phases of the evolution of PVL:
1. *Early acute phase:* The acute insult takes place during the late antenatal or early postnatal period. Hence, findings may be noted during the end of 1st week till 10 days.
2. *Late chronic changes:* Noted as "swiss-cheese" multicystic appearance. This evolves over a period of first 6 weeks.

- *The most significant sequel of PVL:* The cystic change occurs weeks later than the initial insult. Severe PVL leads to cystic encephalomalacia and porencephaly, and is a cause of developmental delay and refractory seizures.
- *Grade I PVL (Fig. 7):* Note the venous congestion or "peritrigonal blush". Echogenicity greater than that of the choroid plexus is significant. A "peritrigonal blush" is normally seen around frontal horns and the parieto-occipital junction of the lateral ventricles. Persistence of "flare" beyond 7–14 is pathological.
- *Grade II PVL:* Limited (focal) cystic PVL (Figs. 8A and B)—note the white matter

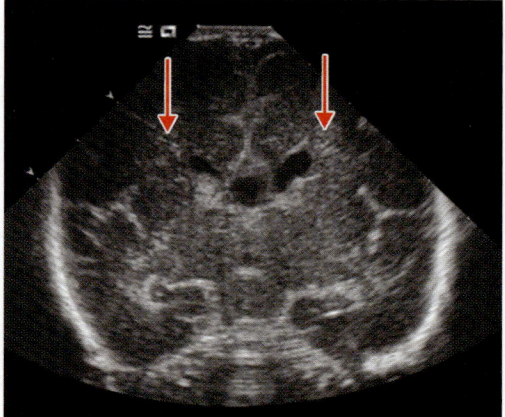

Fig. 7: Grade I periventricular leukomalacia (PVL): Flaring.

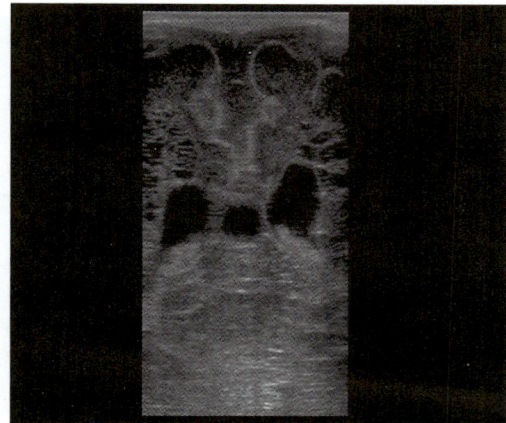

Fig. 9: Grade III PVL—coronal view—diffuse and cystic lesions.

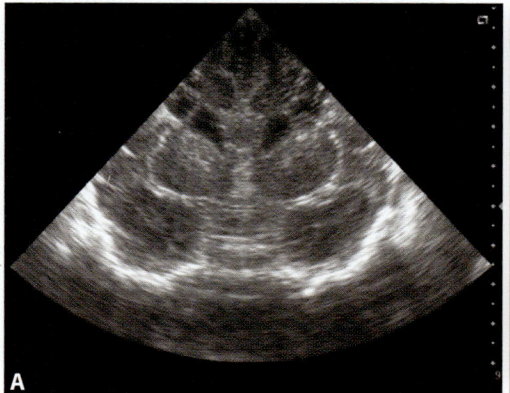 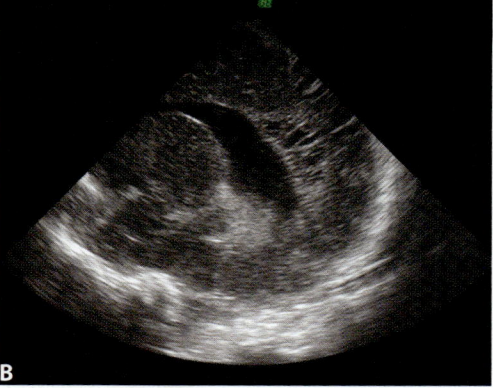

Figs. 8A and B: Grade II PVL: Cystic PVL—lesions near lateral ventricle.

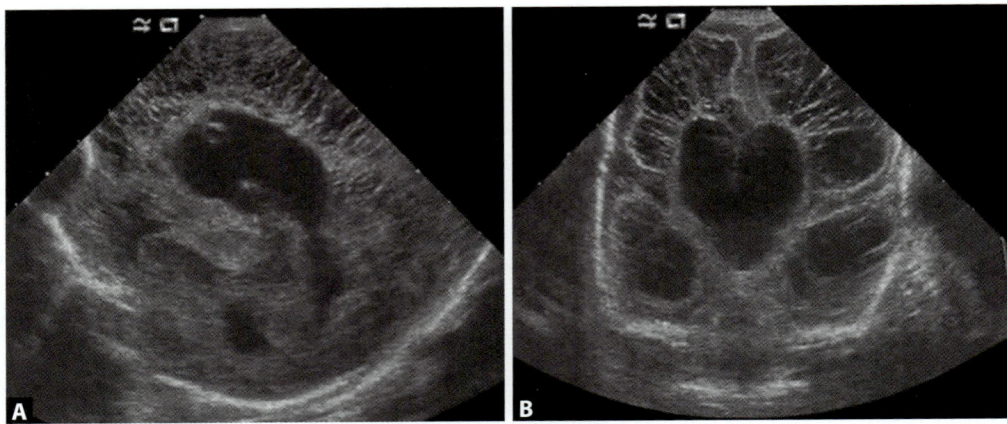

Figs. 10A and B: Grade IV PVL.

cysts within the flare near the frontoparietal white matter.
- *Grade III extensive cystic PVL (Fig. 9):* When there are cyst formations at the fronto-parieto-occipital region, they are referred to as grade III PVL. The cystic zone is smaller than the hyperechoic zone.
- *Grade IV: Subcortical leukomalacia (Figs. 10A and B):* This is rarely seen and is restricted to more mature neonates and postasphyxial term neonate where periventricular and cortical cysts develop.

Whom to screen?
- All babies < 32 weeks' gestation or < 1,500 g.
- Preterms ≥ 32 weeks or ≥ 1,500 g, if they are sick or have risk factors such as perinatal asphyxia, hypotension, tension pneumothorax, ventilation, or abnormal neurologic signs.

When to screen?
- One ultrasound cranium at 1–2 weeks of life.
- Repeat at 36–40 weeks of postconceptional age.

SUGGESTED READING

1. Bassan H. Intracranial hemorrhage in the preterm infant: understanding it, preventing it. Clin Perinatol. 2009;36(4):737-62.
2. Routine screening cranial ultrasound examinations for the prediction of long-term neurodevelopmental outcomes in preterm infants. Canadian Pediatric Society Statement. Paediatr Child Health. 2001;6(1):39-43.
3. Sarkar S. Screening Cranial Imaging at Multiple Time Points Improves Cystic Periventricular Leukomalacia Detection. Am J Perinatol. 2015; 32(10):973-9.
4. Volpe J. Neurology of Newborn, 5th edition. Philadelphia: Saunders Elsevier; 2008.

CHAPTER 47

Developmental Supportive Care

Rhishikesh Thakre

INTRODUCTION

The newborn intensive care unit (NICU) environment is an additional stress to the preterm and sick newborn. In addition to the handicaps of prematurity, weight and underlying illness the environment may add to injury of the "vulnerable" newborn causing double jeopardy.

STEPS FOR DEVELOPMENTAL SUPPORTIVE CARE IN NURSERY

Consistency of Caregiving

- All NICU staff should be aware and geared to provide consistent supportive care in addition to ongoing acute care.
- Each baby should have an "individualized" plan.
- There should be involvement of the family in care of the newborn.
- The "care plan" should be assessed every day based on the response and modified during daily rounds.
- The parental concerns, anxiety and suggestions should be addressed and acknowledged.

Assist Infants in Transition State

1. Ensure the newborn is clinically stable.
2. Reach for the newborn in slow and gentle manner. Place hands on the newborn and watch for the response.
3. Unclothe the baby if covered.
4. Allow the newborn to respond and settle.
5. Provide calming measures, if the newborn appears distressed.
6. Practice during and following procedure till at least 10 minutes till the newborn has settled down.

Calming measures:
- Ensuring boundaries for extremity support.
- Allowing clasping of hands.
- Supporting by placing hand on head or back.
- Allowing feet in flexion posture.
- Using a pacifier.
- Use of cloth for swaddling or creating an artificial "nest"
- Promoting hand to mouth support.
- Talking gently
- Using music which is soothing.

Infant Assessment

1. Over a period of 24 hours observe the newborn for cry, activity, posture, breathing, color, and symmetry.

2. Note the changes with feeding and procedures.
3. Note and document signs of stress, cues for engagement and disengagement.
4. Based on physiologic parameters and behavioral cues modify the care giving.
5. Responses that are beneficial or cause stress should be documented.

> **Signs of stress behavior:**
> - *Change in color:* Pale, mottling, dusky, or cyanosis.
> - Periodic breathing, apnea, variability in heart rate (HR), and respiratory rate (RR).
> - Hiccoughs, sneeze, yawns, vomiting, or regurgitation.
> - Tremors, twitching, irritability, back arching, and frowning.
> - Truncal hypotonia.
> - Paucity of spontaneous movement.

Family Involvement

- Parents should be involved in patient care.
- Parents should be made aware of infant behavior. They should be alerted to infant cues.
- Parents should be encouraged to express their concerns and observations.
- Parental participation, interaction with infant should be noted. At times inter parent relationship may be stressed which may come in the way.
- Parents should be informed about the stress increasing and decreasing behaviors and how to recognize it.

INTERVENTIONS FOR DEVELOPMENTAL SUPPORTIVE CARE IN NICU

Assist infant to maintain organized behavior by:
- Bringing hand to mouth.
- Clustering and timing care to provide undisturbed rest and sleep periods.
- Introducing cycled lights for the preterm infants.
- Decreasing noise levels around the infant at all times.
- Bringing infant to a more alert state prior to initiating procedures.
- Providing "purposeful" touch.
- Offering a swaddle bath.
- Encouraging alert state during wakeful periods by enfacement, elevating infant's head and shading eyes—extending the time as tolerance develops.
- Supporting infant after procedures or care to assist infant in regaining physiological stability through containment and gentle, "purposeful" touch.
- Helping infant to console him/herself.

Clustering of Activities

- Procedures should be scheduled so ensuring infant has uninterrupted sleep.
- Vital signs should be noted while the neonate is sleeping and awake.
- Neonates should be monitored for all stressful behavior. Calming measures should be initiated with stress.
- Procedures and care taking measures should be modified based on infant cues.
- Family should be involved in infant care. Tasks should be scheduled with parental visits.
- Avoid nonemergency interventions during the night—e.g. bathing and weighing.

Positioning of Infant

- Neonate's posture should be altered every 3–4 hours.
- Prone position if often preferred. The ideal position has flexion of the arms and the legs with the body. Place the infant between rolls on either side or around the flexed legs to provide boundaries (Fig. 1).

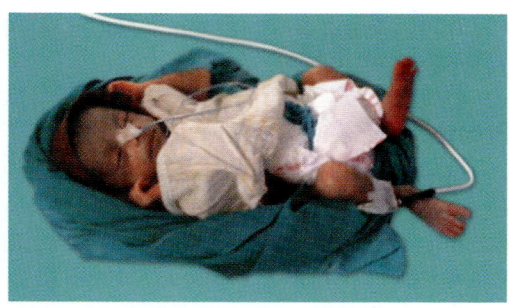

Fig. 1: Cocooning.

- Swaddling and nesting ensure containment, reserved energy, calmness, and sense of security to the infant.
- Using supports and placements must be to promote flexion position.
- Ensure the infant has a stable midline posture.
- Small rolls below the head may be placed to avoid flattening and promote molding.
- Endotracheal tubes should be secured with rolls, devices to ensure smooth posture change.
- If an infant has laid down its own boundaries (e.g. hand across the bassinet), do not intervene.

NICU Environment

- *Noise:* Interventions to decrease environmental noise include:
  - Padded doors
  - Rubber on rim cans
  - Move telephone out of nursery
  - Have discussion rounds outside nursery
  - Use incubator doors gently
  - Minimize talking in nursery
  - Place covers over incubator to absorb noise
  - Do not place any equipment on incubator
  - Promote everyday "quiet time" periods
  - Empty trash cans outside the nursery
  - Adjust alarm limit volumes and keep beep volume to minimum
  - Acoustic floors, walls, windows and ceilings
  - Avoid loud talks.
- *Light:* Interventions to decrease bright lighting include:
  - Cover incubator and cribs with a cloth.
  - Graded lightning which is individualized.
  - Allow natural light as far as possible. Avoid overhead direct light focus.
  - Promote day night cycle.

Promote Oromotor Competency

- Offering pacifier or infant's fingers to suck on during OG or NG feedings or on a fixed schedule, if receiving parenteral nutrition or continuous feeding.
- Introducing taste and smell by placing a drop or two of formula or breast milk on lips or tongue during feedings.
- Holding infant during feedings, when conditions permit.
- Stroking cheeks and supporting chin
- Providing oral sucrose before performing painful procedures.

Facilitate and Promote Motor Development

- Providing a support for legs and feet against which the infant can press.
- Placing infant on his/her abdomen on a folded blanket, with arms and legs close to his/her body, in a manner that prevents external rotation.
- Providing vestibular stimulation by holding and rocking.
- Placing in sitting position a few moments each day, increasing as tolerated.

- Performing range of motion exercises and stretching activities
- Providing infant massage as tolerated for infants > 32 weeks gestation.

Facilitate and Promote Language, Vision and Hearing Development

- Placing black/white/red, or high-contrast pictures and objects in line of vision 8–15 inches from face as long as infant remains relaxed and focused.
- Providing auditory stimulation such as tapes of mother's and father's voices, music boxes, and classical music when infant is quiet, alert, relaxed, and appears interested.
- Talking or singing to infant when providing care or holding and touching him/her, using different pitches or volume in voice.
- Allowing for face-to-face interaction with infant with or without talking, depending on infant's developmental level.

Facilitate Social and Behavioral Development

- Encouraging parental or caregiver to participate in care when possible.
- Encouraging parents or caregivers to participate in Kangaroo Care when possible.
- Placing family pictures and mementos on bed.
- Calling infant by first name.
- Encouraging parents or caregivers to attempt to gain eye contact with infant.
- Consoling infant with cuddling, swaddling, rocking, or pacifier.
- Encouraging parents or caregivers to participate in feeding infant.

Promoting Family-centered Care

- Support groups for parents.
- Round the clock access to parents
- Educate parents infant behavioral cues and stress relieving interventions.
- Educate parents to be involved in appropriate care for the newborn.
- Provide teaching material to parents, viz. videos, leaflets, and supervised handling.
- Ensure kangaroo care as much as possible.
- Involve parents in developmental planning and implementation.
- Ask parents for their fears and concerns.
- Involve parents in daily rounds.

DOCUMENTATION

- Implementation of developmental care of the preterm/ill infant.
- Assessment findings.
- Interventions and patient responses or outcomes.
- Patient or caregiver teaching and level of understanding.

SUGGESTED READING

1. Vandenberg KA. Individualized developmental care for high risk newborns in the NICU: a practice guideline. Early Hum Dev. 2007;83; 433-42.
2. White RD. The newborn intensive care unit environment of care: how we got here, where we're headed, and why. Semin Perinatol. 2011;35:2-7.

CHAPTER 48

Antenatal Corticosteroids

Rhishikesh Thakre

INTRODUCTION

Preterm birth is the second most common cause of death among children under 5 years of age. The majority of preterm births develop respiratory distress syndrome (RDS) due to surfactant deficiency, which is gestational age specific. Antenatal steroids are a simple, effective, evidence-based, and low cost intervention to help accelerate the lung maturity of fetus, thereby decreasing the risk of RDS.

IMPACT OF ANTENATAL STEROIDS ON PRETERM OUTCOME

- Reduction in RDS (34%)
- Reduction in intraventricular hemorrhage (IVH) (46%)
- Reduction in necrotizing enterocolitis (NEC) (54%)
- Reduction in mortality (31%).

Other benefits include reduction in the incidence of patent ductus arteriosus (PDA), reduction in systemic infections, decreased need for respiratory support and therefore, reduced length of hospital stay, lower intensive care admissions, and reduced cost of care.

INDICATIONS

- All mothers expected to deliver between 24 weeks and 34 weeks of gestation.
- Preterm labor between 34 weeks and 36 weeks of gestation (not a uniform recommendation).

Which drug to give?

Dexamethasone [intramuscular (IM)] course is given to a pregnant woman in preterm labor (Table 1).

What is the recommended dose of IM dexamethasone?

6 mg, 12 hours apart for four doses.

Why betamethasone is not preferred over dexamethasone in India?

In India, the salt betamethasone acetate + phosphate, which requires only two doses

Table 1: Dexamethasone.

Dose	6 mg each
Number of injections	4
Interval between injections	12 hours
Complete course	24 mg (four doses)
Storage	Room temperature
Repeat courses	No

at 12-hourly intervals, is not available. The available salt is betamethasone phosphate, which has properties similar to dexamethasone with no added benefit. Also, dexamethasone is in the essential drug list and is available at all primary health centers.

ONSET AND DURATION OF ACTION

Action following steroid therapy is seen 24 hours after the first dose and lasts till 7 days. Partial effect is evident within a few hours before steroid administration and is worth it.

ADVERSE EFFECTS

Long-term follow-up of survivors from randomized trials of antenatal corticosteroid therapy through childhood to adulthood (up to 20 years of age) shows no definite adverse effects.

Should the course of steroid be repeated if there is no preterm delivery?

No. Repeated courses/more frequent doses are not useful. Multiple courses in fact could have harmful neurodevelopmental effects on the baby.

What are contraindications for prenatal steroids?

Frank chorioamnionitis is an absolute contraindication for prenatal steroids. Presence of the following confirms chorioamnionitis:
- History of fever and lower abdominal pain
- Foul smelling, vaginal discharge, tachycardia, and uterine tenderness
- Fetal tachycardia.

What is the role of steroids in maternal diabetes, preeclampsia, or preterm prelabor rupture of the membranes?

It is safe to give steroids to mothers with these conditions.

Is there a role for steroids in the era of surfactant?

Infants who received both antenatal steroids and surfactant had significant reductions in mortality, severity of respiratory distress, and frequency of air leaks compared with infants who received neither treatment, or only antenatal steroids, or only surfactant. The effects of antenatal steroids and surfactant are, thus, synergistic and additive improving mortality and clinical outcomes. The nonrespiratory benefits of steroids and very low cost make steroids an essential intervention for all mothers with threatened preterm labor irrespective of availability of surfactant.

What is the utility of antenatal steroids in late preterm births?

Mothers who received antenatal corticosteroids at 34 0/7 to 36 6/7 weeks had a significantly lower incidence of transient tachypnea of the newborn [relative risk (RR), 0.72; 95% confidence interval (CI), 0.56–0.92], severe RDS (RR, 0.60; 95% CI, 0.33–0.94), and use of surfactant (RR, 0.61; 95% CI, 0.38–0.99). Routine administration of antenatal steroids to all mothers with preterm labor at this gestation is still not a uniform recommendation.

SUGGESTED READING

1. Ministry of Health and Family Welfare. (2014). Use of Antenatal Corticosteroids in Preterm Labour (Under Specific Conditions by ANM): Operational Guidelines. [online] Available from http://www.nrhmorissa.gov.in/writereaddata/Upload/Documents/Operational%20Guidelines-Use%20of%20Antenatal%20Corticosteroids%20in%20Preterm%20Labour.pdf. [Last accessed May, 2019].
2. Saccone G, Berghella V. Antenatal corticosteroids for maturity of term or near term fetuses: systematic review and meta-analysis of randomized controlled trials. BMJ. 2016;355:i5044.

CHAPTER 49

Breast Milk Storage and Handling

Rhishikesh Thakre, Srinivas Murki

INTRODUCTION

Human milk needs to be stored in a designated refrigerator/freezer or container.

PROCEDURE

- Infant's name, case number, and date is labeled on the pumped milk jar.
- Store pumped milk small aliquots equivalent to feed requirement after pumped by the mother. All jars are clubbed together for each infant together.
- Every time the jar is used for infant feeding, ensure the correct name and record number matches the infant.
- Postpumping the mother's milk is refrigerated or frozen at earliest. Priority is given to fresh milk, if not available, frozen milk is used.
- Fresh milk can be used within 4 hours postpumping kept at room temperature.
- All refrigerated milk should be utilized within a day of collection.
- Frozen milk is stored at 0°C in freezer and can be kept for 6 months.
- Thawing involves placing the milk cup with warm water around. After defrosting, the milk is to be labeled and date/time of thawing noted.
- Ensure thawed milk is kept in the refrigerator. It should be used within 24 hours of thawing.
- Refrigerator temperature should be kept between 33°F and 45°F. Freezer temperature should be kept at −20°C or lower.

TRANSPORTING BREAST MILK

A packed cooler without ice is used to transport milk within the hospital. Clean towel, newspaper, or freezer gel packs are used to fill the dead space. Ice may cause thawing as it is warmer than frozen milk. Chilled state is required for transporting non-frozen breast milk. Milk may be refrozen if partial thawing of half the milk container occurs during transport.

THAWING BREAST MILK

Ensure hand hygiene before handling breast milk. Allow cool running water to thaw frozen milk. Avoid dipping the jar in water. The thawed milk must have date, time of thawing, and expiry date (24 hours) written on it. Thawed milk is not refrozen.

WARMING BREAST MILK FOR FEEDING

Ensure hand hygiene. Place milk container in warm water or running warm water. Avoid dipping or immersing in hot or boiling water. Do not use microwave for warming. Overheating leads to loss of nutrients and may reduce the anti-infective factors. Use warmed milk within one hour.

SUGGESTED READING

1. Ottawa (ON): Canadian Agency for Drugs and Technologies in Health; CADTH Rapid Response Reports. Storage, Handling, and Administration of Expressed Human Breast Milk: A Review of Guidelines; 2016.
2. Peters MD, McArthur A, Munn Z. Safe management of expressed breast milk: a systematic review. Women Birth. 2016;29(6):473-81.

CHAPTER 50

Immunization in Low Birth Weight Infants

Rhishikesh Thakre

BASIC PRINCIPLES

- Birth weight and gestational age should not be taken into consideration for deciding about routine vaccination newborns (except for hepatitis B vaccine).
- All routine vaccines have been found to be safe for use in preterm/low birth weight (LBW) infants.
- The risk and incidence of common adverse events appear to be similar in both full-term and preterm/LBW.
- There is adequate antibody concentration postvaccination in LBW infants though the immunogenicity may be less.

TIMING

- All well preterm/LBW infants should receive routine vaccines as per National Immunization Schedule based on chronologic age.
- Hepatitis B vaccination should be modified in infants less than 2 kg based on maternal hepatitis B status (Table 1).

DOSING

- Vaccine dosages should not be reduced or divided when given to preterm/LBW infants.
- Majority of preterm infants produce adequate vaccine-induced immunity against the disease with standard dose.

VACCINE ADMINISTRATION

- The preferred site for intramuscular vaccines to preterm/LBW infants is the anterolateral thigh.
- The needle length is decided based on available muscle mass of the preterm/LBW infant for intramuscular administration.

SCHEDULE FOR HEPATITIS B VACCINATION FOR PRETERM/LOW BIRTH WEIGHT BABIES

Breastfeeding and Vaccination

- All vaccines given to lactating woman are safe and do not affect the infant.
- Breastfeeding does not interfere with uptake of vaccine and all vaccines can be given safely to breastfed infants. There are no adverse effects to mother.

Combination Vaccines

- Only combination vaccines approved by the licensing authority should be used.

Table 1: Hepatitis B immunoprophylaxis scheme for preterm/LBW infants.

Maternal status	Infant ≥2,000 g	Infant <2,000 g
Hepatitis B surface antigen (HBsAg) positive	Hepatitis B vaccine + hepatitis B immune globulin (HBIG) (within 12 h of birth)	Hepatitis B vaccine + HBIG (within 12 h of birth)
	Immunize with three vaccine doses at 0, 1, and 6 months of chronologic age	Immunize with four vaccine doses at 0, 1, 2–3, and 6–7 months of chronologic age
	Check anti-HBs and HBsAg at 9–15 months of age	Check anti-HBs and HBsAg at 9–15 months of age
	If infant is HBsAg and anti-HBs negative, reimmunize with three doses at 2-month intervals and retest	If infant is HBsAg and anti-HBs negative, reimmunize with three doses at 2-month intervals and retest
HBsAg status unknown	Hepatitis B vaccine (by 12 h) + HBIG (within 7 days) if mother tests HBsAg positive	Hepatitis B vaccine + HBIG (by 12 h)
	Test mother for HBsAg immediately	Test mother for HBsAg immediately and if results are unavailable within 12 h, give infant HBIG
HBsAg negative	Hepatitis B vaccine at birth preferred	Hepatitis B vaccine dose one at 30 days of chronologic age if medically stable, or at hospital discharge if before 30 days of chronologic age
	Immunize with three doses at 0–2, 1–4, and 6–18 month of chronologic age	Immunize with three doses at 1–2, 2–4, and 6–18 month of chronologic age
	May give hepatitis B-containing combination vaccine beginning at 6–8 weeks of chronologic age	May give hepatitis B-containing combination vaccine beginning at 6–8 weeks of chronologic age
	Follow-up anti-HBs and HBsAg testing not needed	Follow-up anti-HBs and HBsAg testing not needed

Extremes of gestational age and birth weight no longer a consideration for timing of HBV doses.
Some experts prefer to perform serologic testing 1–3 months after completion of the primary series.
(LBW: low birth weight).

- Individual vaccines must never be given separately as per schedule. Mixing of vaccine is done only if cleared by licensing authority.
- Use of licensed combination vaccines is preferred over separate injection of their equivalent component vaccines.

THIOMERSAL ISSUE

Studies indicate no evidence of harm caused by low levels of thiomersal in vaccine. However, it is recommended that vaccines be thiomersal free as a precautionary measure.

VACCINATION IN BLEEDING DISORDER INFANT

All vaccines should be administered as per schedule unless there is likely to be harm based on clinical status of the infant. A small gauge needle (≤23 gauge) should be used for the vaccination. This should be followed by local firm pressure, with no rubbing, for at least few minutes. The family should be informed about possibility of hematoma formation at the site.

IMMUNOCOMPROMISED INFANT

Live vaccines are not indicated in immunocompromised infants. Inactivated, recombinant, subunit, polysaccharide, and conjugate vaccines and toxoids can be safely given. Studies suggest a suboptimal response in immunocompromised.

Antibody containing products (intravenous immune globulin, specific hyperimmune globulin (for example: hepatitis B immune globulin, tetanus immune globulin, varicella zoster immune globulin), whole blood, packed red cells, plasma, and platelet products) and vaccines

Antibody-containing products and inactivated antigen can be administered simultaneously provided different sites are used. They can be administered with no time restriction between the doses. Antibody-containing products and live antigen are not to be administered at the same time. Antibody-containing products are administered after 2 weeks of live antigen administration.

SUGGESTED READING

1. Hogue MD, Meador AE. Vaccines and immunization practice. Nurs Clin North Am. 2016;51(1):121-36.
2. Shah SI. Immunization issues in preterm infants: pertussis, influenza, and rotavirus. Neo Rev. 2014;15(10):e439.
3. Whittaker E, Goldblatt D, McIntyre P, et al. Neonatal immunization: rationale, current state, and future prospects. Front Immunol. 2018;9:532.

SECTION 4

Neonatal Dilemmas

SECTION OUTLINE

51. Cryptorchidism
52. Baby Born to HIV Positive Mother
53. Baby Born to HBsAg Positive Mother
54. Baby Born to Mother having Tuberculosis
55. Baby Born to Mother with Chickenpox
56. Baby Born to VDRL Positive Mother
57. Breastfeeding and Medications
58. Stem Cell Banking: Scope and Practice
59. Declaring Newborn Death

CHAPTER 51

Cryptorchidism

Rhishikesh Thakre, Srinivas Murki

INTRODUCTION

Cryptorchidism is the most common congenital genitourinary abnormality in male infants.

Cryptorchidism (hidden testis): An undescended testis is defined as one that is absent in the scrotum and cannot be manipulated into scrotum.

Ectopic testis: Descended testis is one which is located below the external inguinal ring but at an abnormal location.

Retractile testis: A testis which stays out of the scrotum but can be manipulated into the scrotum, where it remains without tension. It retracts into the upper scrotum owing to a hyperactive cremasteric reflex.

Gliding testis: A form of cryptorchidism in which the undescended testis can be manipulated into the upper scrotum but retracts immediately when tension on it is released.

AT RISK GROUPS

- Preterm infant
- Neural tube defects
- Abdominal wall defects
- Congenital dislocation of hip.

RETRACTILE TESTIS

- Most common in children at ages at 5–6 years.
- Infants develop cremasteric reflex by 3 months of age. The condition manifests thereafter during infancy.
- The testis moves freely from its intrascrotal location due to hyperreactive cremasteric reflex.
- Retractile testes normally descend by puberty.
- Once in the scrotum, a retractile testis should not retract when released.

ECTOPIC TESTIS

An ectopic testis may be located in one of the following areas: Opposite scrotum, suprapubic area, superficial inguinal pouch, femoral canal, or the perineum.

CRYPTORCHIDISM (FLOWCHART 1)

- Normal testis and cryptorchid testes appear identical histology till 1 year of age. Soon

Flowchart 1: Algorithm for undescended testis.

```
High index of suspicion
(Neonates, preterm, neural tube defects, abdominal wall defect)
                │
                ▼
Examine
Supine and squatting position
Scrotal fullness, rugosity, inguinal area, urethral opening.
Position/size/consistency of the testicle in relation to opposite testicle
Two-handed technique
Start at the hip and gently sweep along the inguinal canal.
Palpate with the other hand
         │                              │
         ▼                              ▼
Testis palpable                  Testis not palpable
Testis can be brought down       USG abdomen
and stay down in scrotum         Karyotyping
but retract on cremasteric reflex Serum electrolyte
(Retractile testis)              Serum testosterone
Testis cannot be brought         Serum LH/FSH/MIS
down to scrotum                  Serum cortisol/thyroid assay
(Ectopic testis)
         │                              │
         ▼                              ▼
Re-evaluate at                   Bilateral cryptorchidism:
3 and 6 months                   Normal LH/FSH
in doubtful                      Anorchia: High LH/FSH
retractile vs ectopic testis              │
(Retractile testis : Assurance)           ▼
                                 Surgical exploration
                                 Orchidopexy
```

(FSH: follicle stimulating hormone; LH: luteinizing hormone; MIS: Müllerian inhibiting substance)

thereafter, the cryptorchid testis begins to deteriorate.
- If there is bilateral undescended testis one must rule out anorchia, female adrenogenital syndrome, and hypothalamic-pituitary insufficiency.
- Infertility is most common issue. Up to half the patients with unilateral cryptorchidism and majority with bilateral cryptorchidism develop infertility.
- The malignant transformation is most commonly seen in abdominal location of testis.
- Long-term follow-up of the patient after orchiopexy is important because of the potential for infertility and tumorigenesis.

PHYSICAL EXAMINATION

Look for:
- *Scrotum*: Development, rugosity, palpate testicle. Impalpable testes are present in 20% of cryptorchidism cases.
- *Inguinal fullness*: Ninety percent of cryptorchid testes are associated with the presence of an indirect inguinal hernia.
- *Urethral opening*: Hypospadias with cryptorchidism has a 62% chance of having an intersex disorder.

MANIPULATIONS

- With patient supine, place a finger at the top of both hemiscrotum and at the

base of penis. This will trap a normal and retractile testis. If the scrotum is still empty, apply gradual pressure medial to the iliac crest and palpate the scrotum with the other hand. This maneuver may reduce intracanalicular testis.
- Ask the patient to take squatting position. Most retractile testes will spontaneously descend into the scrotum but not the ectopic testis.

DIAGNOSTIC TECHNIQUES

- Ultrasonography is a good screening tool.
- Abdominal laparoscopy is preferred method and is indicated for localizing nonpalpable testes.
- Hormonal evaluation is indicated with bilateral nonpalpable testis. Baseline luteinizing hormone (LH) and follicle-stimulating hormone (FSH) levels in males, if elevated, suggest anorchia and, if normal, suggest cryptorchidism.

MANAGEMENT

Surgical management of undescended testis is indicated between 6 months and 24 months of age.

Clinical Pearls

- All newborns at first visit should undergo evaluation for testes in the scrotum. Most undescended testicles are present at birth.
- Cryptorchidism is a common disorder of sexual development and in the majority resolve spontaneously by 3 months of age. Retractile testis does not require surgical management.
- If a testis has to descend it does so latest by 6 months of age and rarely thereafter.
- Hypospadias with an undescended testis should warrant chromosomal testing to rule out an intergender disorder.
- Surgery may serve to diagnose and possibly treat nonpalpable testicle.
- Treatment for the undescended testis is recommended in early infancy and definitely not beyond age of two.

SUGGESTED READING

1. Kollin C, Ritzén EM. Cryptorchidism: a clinical perspective. Pediatr Endocrinol Rev. 2014;11(Suppl 2):240-50.
2. Mau EE, Leonard MP. Practical approach to evaluating testicular status in infants and children. Can Fam Phys. 2017;63(6):432-5.

CHAPTER 52

Baby Born to HIV Positive Mother

Hemasree Kandraju, Venkat Kallem

INTRODUCTION

The most common form of acquiring human immunodeficiency virus (HIV) in infants and children is by vertical transmission from an infected mother. The transmission can occur during pregnancy, labor, delivery, or breastfeeding and is called mother-to-child transmission (MTCT). The most common time to acquire infection is during labor.

Multiple factors aggravate the risk of HIV transmission from mother to infant (Table 1).

RISK OF TRANSMISSION

In the absence of any intervention, MTCT occurs from 15% to 45%. This transmission can be effectively decreased by appropriate measures taken during pregnancy, labor, delivery, and during breastfeeding.

INTERVENTIONS FOR PREVENTION OF MOTHER-TO-CHILD TRANSMISSION

Prenatal Intervention

World Health Organization (WHO) recommends all pregnant women detected to be HIV positive during the prenatal period be initiated on antiretroviral therapy (ART). This is to be continued during pregnancy, labor, with breastfeeding, and preferably lifelong.

Table 1: Factors increasing risk of human immunodeficiency virus (HIV) transmission.

Maternal factors	Intrapartum factors	Postnatal factors
• Low CD4+ lymphocyte count • High viral load • Primary infection during pregnancy • Advanced acquired immunodeficiency syndrome (AIDS) • Preterm delivery • Chorioamnionitis • Presence of p24 core antigen	• Instrumental delivery • Use of fetal scalp monitor • Fetal scalp pH measurement • Suctioning • Artificial rupture of membranes • Rupture of membranes for longer than 4 hours	• Breastfeeding • Mastitis or nipple lesions • Maternal seroconversion during pregnancy

Interventions in the Delivery Room

- Antiretroviral therapy is continued as per regular schedule during labor and delivery.
- Cesarean section (CS) is recommended only for obstetric indication. For prevention of MTCT, CS is not indicated.
- If the mother is not on ART but requires emergency CS, ART is given prior to the surgery and continued thereafter.
- Standard/universal precautions.
- There is no role of artificial rupture of membranes.
- Vaginal examination are performed by aseptic techniques and kept to minimum.
- Avoid invasive procedures (e.g. fetal blood sampling, fetal scalp electrodes).
- Avoid instrumental delivery, if possible.
- Avoid routine episiotomy, if possible.
- Emphasis is on good observation for bleeding, following of surgical fascial planes during surgery and rational use of electrocautery.
- During CS, it is preferred to keep the membranes intact until the head is delivered through the surgical incision. The cord is clamped immediately after delivery.

Postnatal Interventions

All infants are started on antiretroviral (ARV) prophylaxis to reduce HIV transmission. Nevirapine (NVP) is the drug of choice (Table 2).

- **ARV prophylaxis for infants born to women presenting in active labor**

  All infants should be started on daily NVP prophylaxis at birth and continued for at least 6 weeks. Ideally, they should receive for 12 weeks as mother has not been on regular ART. However, early infant diagnosis (EID) should be carried out at 6 weeks as per guidelines.

- **ARV prophylaxis for infants born to women who did not receive any ART (home delivery)**
  - Infant should be started on daily NVP prophylaxis at the earliest, during the first contact with healthcare services.
  - NVP prophylaxis should continue for at least 12 weeks, by which time the mother should be linked to appropriate ART services.

- **ARV prophylaxis for infant born to mother with HIV-2 infection**

  The infants have to be started on Zidovudine instead of Nevirapine. The dose is as shown in the Table 3.

- **ARV prophylaxis for infant born to mother with HIV-1 and HIV-2 infection**

  The infants have to be given prophylaxis with Nevirapine similar to HIV-1 infection.

Table 2: Nevirapine (NVP) prophylaxis.

Birth weight (g)	NVP daily dose (mg)	NVP daily dose (mL*)	Duration
<2,000	2 mg/kg once daily	0.2 mL/kg once daily	Up to 6 weeks irrespective of whether breastfed or exclusively replacement fed. May be extended to 12 weeks, if mother has not received antiretroviral therapy (ART) for adequate duration, i.e. at least 24 weeks
2,000–2,500	10 mg once daily	1 mL once a day	
>2,500	15 mg once daily	1.5 mL once a day	

*Considering the content of 10 mg nevirapine in 1 mL suspension.

Table 3: Dose of AZT (Zidovudine) for infants of mother with HIV-2 infection.

Birth weight (g)	Dosage	Duration (weeks)
<2,000	5 mg/dose twice daily	6
2,000–2,500	10 mg/dose twice daily	6
>2,500	15 mg/dose twice daily	6

PRINCIPLES OF INFANT FEEDING FOR HUMAN IMMUNODEFICIENCY VIRUS EXPOSED INFANTS

- Exclusive breastfeeding for the first 6 months is the preferred choice. Mothers known to be HIV-infected, if insist on opting for exclusive replacement feeding which is contrary to the WHO/NACO guidelines of giving exclusive breastfeeds for first 6 months, are doing so at their own risk.
- If breastfeeding cannot be done (maternal death or terminal illness) or if the parents wish, then replacement feeding may be considered only if the Acceptable, Feasible, Affordable, Sustainable, and Safe (AFASS) criteria for exclusive replacement feeding is fulfilled (Table 4).
- Antiretroviral therapy reduces the risk of postnatal HIV transmission in the context of mixed feeding. Although exclusive breastfeeding is recommended, practicing mixed feeding is not a reason to stop breastfeeding in the presence of ARV drugs and shorter durations of breastfeeding of less than 12 months are better than never initiating breastfeeding at all.
- For breastfeeding infant diagnosed HIV negative, breastfeeding is recommended until 12 months of age ensuring the mother is on ART as soon as possible.
- For HIV positive breastfeeding infants, pediatric ART is recommended with continuation of breastfeeding.
- Breastfeeding should *NOT be stopped abruptly*.
- Exclusive breastfeeding is recommended for at least 6 months. Complementary feeding is introduced at 6 months irrespective of infant's HIV status.
- Once the infant is on adequate foods, breastfeeding can be stopped.

CARE DURING POSTPARTUM PERIOD

- Nevirapine prophylaxis should be started immediately after birth.
- Early skin-to-skin care and early (<1 hour) breastfeeding is recommended.
- Advice is given to parents about how to give NVP prophylaxis.

CARE AND FOLLOW-UP OF THE INFANTS BORN TO HUMAN IMMUNODEFICIENCY VIRUS POSITIVE MOTHER (TABLE 5)

At 6 weeks/first immunization visit, all following issues need to be addressed:
- Compliance to NVP prophylaxis for the past 6 weeks.
- Extend NVP prophylaxis for another 6 weeks if mother was detected during delivery or if she has taken ART for less than 24 weeks
- Start co-trimoxazole prophylactic therapy (CPT) at 6 weeks of age for all HIV exposed infants (irrespective of breastfeeding or replacement feeding practice). Discontinue CPT when HIV infection has been ruled out at 18 months (Table 6).
- Early infant diagnosis (EID)-deoxyribonucleic acid/polymerase chain reaction (DNA/PCR) as per National Guidelines.

CHAPTER 52
Baby Born to HIV Positive Mother

Table 4: Acceptable, Feasible, Affordable, Sustainable, and Safe (AFASS) criteria.

Affordable	The mother or the caregiver should be able to *afford* the complete replacement feeding to support normal growth and development
Feasible	It should be *feasible* for them to maintain the supply of replacement feeding without compromising the growth and nutrition of the infant
Acceptable	It should be *accepted* by the family and they should not force breastfeeding at any point of time within the first 6 months of age
Safe	*Safe* water and sanitation should be assured at the household and the community level and can prepare clean feeds
Sustainable	The mother should be able to *sustain* the supply and the safe practices for at least first 6 months of life, so that there is lower risk of malnutrition or diarrhea

Table 5: Follow-up plan for a human immunodeficiency virus (HIV) exposed child ≤18 months.

Visit	Birth	6 Weeks	10 Weeks	14 Weeks	6 Months	9 Months	12 Months	18 Months
Co-trimoxazole prophylactic therapy (CPT) prophylaxis		Start CPT from 6 weeks for all HIV-exposed infants. Continue CPT for all babies up to 18 months irrespective of early infant diagnosis (EID) status and thereafter if confirms positive						
Counseling for feeding	Exclusive breast-feeds (BF) for first 6 months	✓	✓	✓	BF + Complementary feeds	✓	If EID is −ve stop BF, continue till 2 years if +ve	✓
Growth monitoring	✓	✓		✓	✓	✓	✓	✓
Developmental assessment	✓	✓		✓	✓	✓	✓	✓
Clinical assessment	✓	✓		✓	✓	✓	✓	✓
HIV testing		✓ Deoxyribonucleic acid/polymerase chain reaction (DNA/PCR)			✓ (Rapid test + DNA/PCR)		✓ (Rapid test + DNA/PCR)	✓ Only Rapid test No DNA/PCR

- For *exclusively breastfed infants* whose mothers are not taking ART:
  - Check for breastfeeding concerns, position, and attachment.
  - Ensure monthly follow-up of the infants.
  - Counsel mothers for need for life-long ART.
- For infants *on exclusive replacement feeding*:
  - Emphasis good hygiene, use of clean boiled water, handwashing.

Table 6: Co-trimoxazole prophylaxis.

Weight (kg)	Syrup 5 mL (40 mg TMP/200 mg SMX)	Dispersible tablet (20 mg TMP/100 mg SMX)
<5	2.5 mL	1 Tablet
5–10	5 mL	2 Tablets
10–15	7.5 mL	3 Tablets
15–22	10 mL	4 Tablets

- The vaccination dose, schedule is as per National Schedule of Immunization. If the infant is diagnosed HIV positive, the live vaccines should be avoided.
- All HIV-exposed infants should be followed-up monthly till first year and every 3 months thereafter.
- *Any infant* should be tested for HIV if there are any clinical suspicions.
- All HIV exposed infants must have a confirmatory HIV test at 18 months using three rapid antibody tests, even if the first rapid test is negative.
- Dried blood spot (DBS)/whole blood specimen, i.e. WBS (DNA/PCR) testing is not recommended at or after 18 months.

CARE OF HUMAN IMMUNODEFICIENCY VIRUS POSITIVE INFANT

- All infants with HIV DNA/PCR positive results must follow-up at ART center.
- Confirmation with WBS test is carried out at ART center.
- All infants/children less than 2 years of age with a confirmed WBS positive status at ART center should be initiated on pediatric ART (irrespective of CD4 percentage).
- Co-trimoxazole prophylactic therapy should be continued beyond 18 months.
- All HIV-exposed infants should be followed-up monthly during first year and every 3 months thereafter.

SUGGESTED READING

1. Updated Guidelines for Prevention of Parent to Child Transmission (PPTCT) using Multi-drug Antiretroviral Regimen in India, NACO, 2013.
2. World Health Organization, United Nations Children's Fund. Guideline: Updates on HIV and Infant Feeding: The Duration of Breastfeeding, and Support from Health Services to Improve Feeding Practices among Mothers Living with HIV. Geneva: World Health Organization; 2016.

CHAPTER 53

Baby Born to HBsAg Positive Mother

Giridhar Sethuraman

INTRODUCTION

India has a 2–7% prevalence rate for hepatitis B surface antigen (HBsAg) seropositivity, whereas the prevalence in pregnant women is between 0.9% and 11.2%. Mother-to-child transmission (MTCT) of hepatitis B virus (HBV) leads to development of chronic hepatitis B infection. Transmission can occur in utero, at birth (most common), or after birth.

FACTORS ASSOCIATED WITH HIGH RATE OF MOTHER-TO-CHILD TRANSMISSION

1. High maternal serum HBV deoxyribonucleic acid (DNA) level > 200,000 IU/mL (≥6 log copies/mL)—most significant risk factor for MTCT.
2. HbeAg positivity in mother.
3. Duration of first stage of labor > 9 hours.
4. Premature rupture of membranes and threatened preterm labor.
5. Prior child with passive active immunoprophylaxis failure.

Note: 1 and 2 can be associated with high risk of MTCT in spite of active–passive immunoprophylaxis

CLINICAL MANIFESTATIONS AND TREATMENT

- There are no clinical signs, symptoms, or biochemical derangements at birth.
- Majority present with minimal or persistent elevated liver enzyme at 2–6 months of age.
- No specific drug therapies are recommended for antigenemia in the neonatal period.

Prevention of Mother-to-Child Transmission (Table 1)

Table 1: Prevention of mother-to-child transmission.

Antepartum (suggested in mothers with high viral load)	
Antiviral drugs: Treatment should be started preferably 6–8 weeks before delivery to allow enough time for hepatitis B virus (HBV) deoxyribonucleic acid (DNA) levels to decline. Tenofovir is preferred because of least resistance potential.	
Intrapartum (suggested in mothers with high viral load)	
Elective lower segment cesarean section (LSCS) performed before the onset of labor or before the rupture of membranes in settings of high viral load.	
Postpartum	
Hepatitis B surface antigen (HBsAg) positive mother:	Clean neonate's eye and non-intact skin with water as soon as possible after birth. Administer a bath with mild soap solution, once medically stable. Vaccinate.

Contd...

	Postpartum
	Hepatitis B vaccine and hepatitis B immuno globulin (HBIG) (0.5 mL) intramuscular (IM) ≤12 hours of birth.
Term baby or preterm baby ≥ 2 kg	Repeat vaccine doses at 1 month/6 weeks and 6 months (85–95% efficacy). The final dose in the vaccine series should not be administered before age 24 weeks (164 days). If patient cannot afford HBIG, administer vaccine first dose ≤12 hours of birth with repeat doses at 1/6 weeks, 2 months/10 weeks, and 9–12 months (70–75% efficacy).
HBsAg positive mother: Preterm baby < 2 kg	Same as previous scenario. Initial vaccine dose (birth dose) should not be counted as part of the vaccine series. Three additional doses of vaccine (for a total of four doses) should be administered at 1/2/6 months.
HBsAg status unknown	Ensure administration of vaccine ≤12 hours of birth. If mother turns out to be HBsAg positive later, administer HBIG as soon as possible within 7 days of birth. Repeat vaccine doses are given as per schedule.

PRACTICE POINTS

- The HBsAg positive mother may continue to breastfeed her infant upon delivery irrespective of newborn vaccination. Avoid breastfeeding if antiviral drugs started during pregnancy for high maternal viral loads, are continued after delivery.
- HBIG is commercially available in strengths of 100 U/mL, 200 U/mL, 180 U/mL. In low birth weight infants, if using 100 U/mL of HBIG, split as 0.5 mL aliquots and administer in both thighs.
- Hepatitis B immunoglobulin should be given immediately after birth (within 12 hours of birth and not later than 48 hours) as its efficacy decreases markedly if given more than 48 hours after birth.
- Monovalent hepatitis B vaccine is given to the infant preferably within 24 hours of birth, and not later than 7 days.

- Postvaccination testing for anti-HBs and HBsAg can be performed after completion of the vaccine series, between 9 and 18 months. Testing should not be performed before age of 9 months or before 4 weeks of the last vaccine dose.
- If the infant is HBsAg-negative and has anti-HBs levels ≥10 mIU/mL, no further medical management is provided. If the infant is HBsAg-negative infants with anti-HBs levels <10 mIU/mL, a second 3-dose series of vaccination should be performed and antibody levels rechecked 1–2 months after the final dose of vaccine.

MANAGEMENT (FLOWCHART 1)

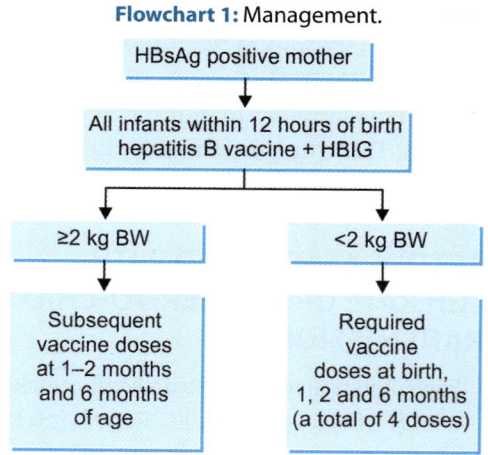

Flowchart 1: Management.

(BW: body weight; HBIG: hepatitis B immunoglobulin; HBsAg: hepatitis B surface antigen)

SUGGESTED READING

1. Mast EE, Margolis HS, Fiore AE. CDC Advisory Committee on Immunization and Practices: a comprehensive immunization strategy to eliminate transmission of hepatitis B virus infection in the United States. MMWR Recomm Rep. 2005;54(RR-16):1-31.
2. Vashishtha VM. IAP Guidebook on Immunization 2013-14. New Delhi: CBS Publishers and Distributors; 2014.

CHAPTER 54

Baby Born to Mother having Tuberculosis

Rajesh Kumar

IDENTIFY THE PROBLEM

Neonate can get infected with tuberculosis from mother either by vertical transmission (congenital tuberculosis) or horizontal transmission after birth (acquired postnatal tuberculosis). Criterion for diagnosis of congenital tuberculosis in the presence of proven tuberculous disease and at least one of the following (Cantwell et al.):
- Lesions in the newborn baby during the first week of life
- A primary hepatic complex or caseating hepatic granuloma
- Tuberculous infection of the placenta or the maternal genital tract
- Exclusion of the possibility of postnatal transmission by investigation of contacts, including hospital staff.

Postnatally transmission through breast milk for tuberculosis does not occur.

IDENTIFY SEVERITY/RED SIGNS

Mothers with extrapulmonary, miliary, and meningeal tuberculosis increase the risk for congenital tuberculosis in newborn. Untreated mothers are more likely to transmit the disease to the newborn compared to treated mothers.

IDENTIFY CAUSE—HISTORY, PHYSICAL EXAMINATION

A high index of suspicion is required to make a diagnosis. Placenta examination for histopathology in suspected cases is the earliest clue to the diagnosis. Household contact screening helps identify the source of infection. The median age of presentation of congenital TB is 24 days (range: 1–84 days).

CLINICAL FEATURES

Clinical manifestations are nonspecific and mimic sepsis. No single sign or symptom predicts tuberculosis. Presence of unexplained hepatomegaly, splenomegaly, abdominal distension, respiratory distress, or lymphadenopathy should raise suspicion of tuberculosis.

LABORATORY INVESTIGATIONS

Microscopy	From gastric aspirate (3 consecutive days), tracheal aspirate (if ventilated), ear discharge, ascitic fluid, CSF, and pleural fluid
PCR	From bronchoalveolar lavage (BAL) fluid, CSF
Biopsy	Lymph node, percutaneous liver biopsy
Mantoux test (MT)	May be negative on admission but a repeat test is positive 4 weeks later suggesting TB; a negative test does not rule out TB
Chest X-ray	Abnormal in all cases. Miliary shadows (50% cases) are very suggestive of tuberculosis

(CSF: cerebrospinal fluid; PCR: polymerase chain reaction)

NEWER TESTS

- Light-emitting diode (LED) fluorescence microscopy
- Liquid-based mycobacteria growth indicator tube (MGIT)
- QuantiFERON-TB Gold assay
- Gene Xpert [real time polymerase chain reaction (PCR)].

MANAGEMENT: GENERAL OR SPECIFIC

- *Indications for isoniazid (INH) prophylaxis:* INH prophylaxis is advisable to the newborn, if the mother is on treatment for less than 2 weeks, or despite treatment of more than 2 weeks the mother has sputum smear positive. Dose of INH for prophylaxis is 10 mg/kg/day (IAP).
- Treatment protocol for congenital tuberculosis (See Table 1).
- *Bacillus Calmette-Guérin (BCG) vaccination:* BCG vaccination is given at birth to all neonates after excluding congenital tuberculosis. INH prophylaxis is not a contraindication. Special INH-resistant BCG is not required.
- *Breastfeeding:* Breastfeeding should not be stopped. Mother and infant should stay together. Use of face mask should be advised for the mothers with open case of tuberculosis. Pyridoxine is suggested, if the mother is taking INH. If the mother is on rifabutin or fluoroquinolones then it is not recommended.
- *Follow-up:* For the babies who are on INH prophylaxis, Mantoux test should be done at the age of 3 months. If MT is negative, prophylaxis is discontinued. Antituberculosis treatment is started if MT is positive and evidence for disease is found. In Mantoux positive neonates with no evidence for disease, INH is given for another 6 months. In HIV positive cases

Table 1: IAP RNTCP guidelines 2019.

Types of patient[a]	Regimens
New microbiologically confirmed pulmonary TB	2HRZE+ 4HRE[b]
New clinically diagnosed pulmonary TB	
New microbiologically confirmed extrapulmonary TB	
New clinically diagnosed rifampicin sensitive extrapulmonary TB	
Drug sensitive previously treated TB[c] (recurrence, treatment after loss to follow-up, treatment after failure)	

[a] Molecular testing shall be done in all new cases in children with suspected TB at diagnosis.
[b] In case of Neuro and spinal TB, the continuation phase is extended to 8 months
[c] All these category of children shall be evaluated as DR TB suspects and evaluated as per DR TB Algorithm. DST based treatment shall be followed. In case they are found to be drug sensitive they shall be started on the above regimen as for a new case. This group was earlier treated with CAT II regimen which is now withdrawn from RNTCP.

CHAPTER 54
Baby Born to Mother having Tuberculosis

Table 2: Management of HIV-TB co-infection in infants and children.

Patients' details	Timing of ART in relation to initiation of TB treatment	ART recommendations
HIV infected Infants, children and adolescents co-infected with all forms of TB	• Start ART regardless of the CD4 count • Start ATT first, initiate ART as soon as TB treatment is tolerated (between 2 weeks and 2 months) • HIV-TB co-infected patients with CD4 count < 50 cells/cmm (in children aged >5 years of age), need to be started on ATT first and then ART within 2 weeks with strict clinical monitoring	Appropriate ART regimen*

* Efavirenz is the preferred drug, whenever children are being treated with Rifampicin containing drug regimen for TB co-infection.

However, in children aged < 3 years and in children weighing < 10 kg, Efavirenz is not recommended; Superboosted Lopinavir/ritonavir must be given.

Table 3: Management of HIV-TB co-infection in infants, children and adolescents in relation to age groups and bodyweight.

Age group/ Bodyweight	ART regimen
Age< 3 years and Bodyweight < 10 kg	Zidovudine + Lamivudine + Super boosted Lopinavir/ritonavir; Preferred for children with Hb > 9 g/dL Abacavir + Lamivudine + Super boosted Lopinavir/ritonavir; Preferred for children with Hb < 9 g/dL

prophylaxis is continued for another 9 months (See Tables 2 and 3).

INDICATIONS FOR SEPARATION OF INFANT BORN TO MOTHER WITH TB

- Mother is ill enough to require hospitalization.
- Mother has been or is expected to become non-adherent to her treatment, or
- Mother is infected with a drug resistant strain of *M. tuberculosis*.

ALGORITHM

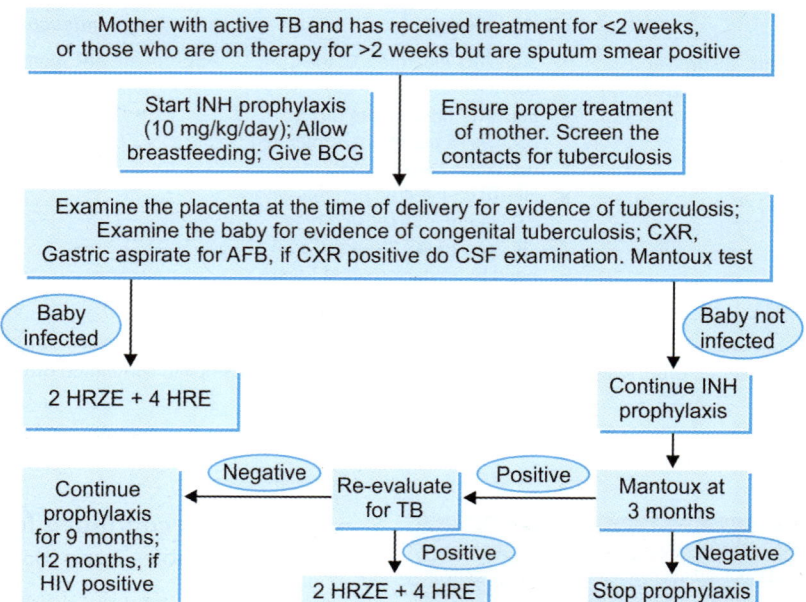

Note: Chemoprophylaxis not recommended in MDR TB contacts.

SUGGESTED READING

1. American Academy of Pediatrics. Tuberculosis. In: Pickering LK (Ed). Red book: 2012 report of the committee on infectious diseases, 29th ed. Elk Grove Village, IL: American Academy of Pediatrics; 2012. pp. 736-56.
2. Cantwell MF, Shehab ZM, Costello AM, et al. Brief report: congenital tuberculosis. N Engl J Med. 1994;330:1051-4.
3. Kumar A, Gupta D, Nagaraja SB, et al. Updated national guidelines for pediatric tuberculosis in India, 2012. Indian Pediatr. 2013;50:301-6.
4. Mittal H, Das S, Faridi MMA. Management of newborn infant born to mother suffering from tuberculosis: Current recommendations & gaps in knowledge. Indian J Med Res. 2014;140:32-9.
5. RNTCP Updated Pediatric TB Guidelines 2019 Developed by Revised National Tuberculosis Control Program and Indian Academy of Pediatrics, Guidance Document, 4 Feb 2019, Central TB Division, Ministry of Health and Family Welfare, New Delhi, India.
6. World Health Organization. Treatment of tuberculosis guidelines, 4th edition. Geneva: WHO; 2009. WHO/HTB/TB/2009.420.

CHAPTER 55

Baby Born to Mother with Chickenpox

Rhishikesh Thakre

TIMING OF CHICKENPOX INFECTION

If a newborn develops chickenpox in the initial 10 days of life, it is secondary to *transplacental* transmission. If the newborn develops chickenpox between day 10 and 28, it is due to *postnatal* transmission.

RISK OF TRANSMISSION

The risk of transmission of chickenpox to a susceptible is 3 days before appearance of lesions and up to 5 days after (or until lesions have crusted). The incubation period is 10–21 days.

MANAGEMENT OF NEWBORNS WITH MATERNAL CHICKENPOX DURING DELIVERY (TABLE 1)

Severe chickenpox in the newborn is most likely, if born within a week of onset of the mother's rash. If mother has chickenpox 1–4 weeks prior to delivery, there is a 50% chance of newborn affection with 25% chance of clinical disease. Such a newborn is at risk for severe chickenpox, lung involvement (e.g. pneumonia), and liver involvement (e.g. fulminant hepatitis).

- If there is contact with chickenpox, no intervention is required, if the mother had past history of chickenpox.
- During hospital stay a mother and/or infant with lesions should stay together but isolated from other patients. Newborns with the congenital varicella syndrome are not infectious and need not be isolated.
- Breastfeeding is continued. If the lesions affect the nipple, expression of breast milk is done.
- Observe the newborn for signs of development of infection (14–16 days).
- If the newborn is sick or develops rash hospitalization and isolation is indicated.
- Zoster immune globulin (ZIG) is indicated as soon as possible after birth or onset of maternal illness within 72 hours if:
  - Mother is chickenpox seronegative.
  - Mother has no history of chickenpox or the serostatus cannot be determined.
  - Newborn is < 28 weeks gestation or < 1 kg weight
  - If mother develops chickenpox 1 week before or after delivery, ZIG is indicated in the newborn.

The ZIG dose, regardless of weight, is 2 mL (= 2000 IU) intramuscular (IM) for newborns.

SECTION 4
Neonatal Dilemmas

Table 1: Management of newborn with chickenpox.

Mother	Chickenpox exposure	Chickenpox infection
Past history of chickenpox	• No intervention is required in postnatal ward or at home. • ZIG if < 1000 g or < 28 weeks • In nursery, ZIG within 24 hours + isolate from day 7–21 following exposure or till crusts are formed	Acyclovir
No past history or indeterminate history or seronegative	ZIG within 72 hours Give acyclovir, (i) If ZIG not received within 24 hours. (ii) Mother develops chickenpox 4 days before to 2 days after delivery. Infants should be closely monitored for signs of infection for 14–16 days.	Acyclovir
Isolate mother and baby from others. Do not isolate baby from mother. Continue breastfeeding unless lesions affect the nipple. Hospitalize and isolate newborn, if develops chickenpox or is sick		

(ZIG: zoster immune globulin)

Role of Acyclovir

Acyclovir is given to infants *who develop chickenpox* and/or:
- Did not receive ZIG prophylaxis within 24 hours
- Are immunocompromised
- Are premature (less than 28 weeks gestation at birth)
- In infants, whose mothers develop chickenpox 4 days before to 2 days after birth. Despite varicella zoster immune globulin (VZIG) prophylaxis, the infection is likely to be fatal.

There is no data for oral acyclovir in neonatal period. There is no role for routine acyclovir prophylaxis with ZIG. Intravenous (IV) acyclovir is given 20 mg/kg every 8 hours as infusion over 1 hour for 7 days or there are no new lesions over 2 days

Acyclovir should be administered to a nursing mother with caution and only when indicated. Acyclovir cream or ointment is not recommended in chickenpox.

CHICKENPOX EXPOSURE DURING POSTNATAL WARDS OR AT HOME FROM SIBLINGS

If the mother has had past chickenpox, the risk from siblings with chickenpox is practically none. If mother has had no chickenpox in the past, ZIG is indicated in newborn. Newborn baby needs not be isolated from its siblings with chickenpox, irrespective of the ZIG status.

CHICKENPOX EXPOSURE WITHIN THE NEONATAL UNIT

- Isolation in a separate room is must for infected babies and those requiring respiratory support.
- Hand hygiene helps reduce spread of infection.
- All newborns below 28 weeks' gestation or less than 1,000 g with should be given ZIG regardless of the results of serological testing of the mother.

- All staff with exposure to index case should have serological tests done, if there is no past history of chickenpox or vaccination. If they are VZV antibody negative, they should be relieved from work from days 7 to 21 after exposure (days 7–28; if they receive ZIG)
- Quarantine of cases should continue (7–28 days) till lesions have crust formation.

IMPLICATIONS FOR PRACTICE

- If possible, delivery should be delayed until 5 days from onset of maternal chickenpox to allow for passive transfer of antibodies.
- The risk to newborn is highest, if the mother has chickenpox 5 days before or 2 days after delivery.
- Varicella zoster immune globulin has no role with onset of chickenpox. Its role is in prevention and not treatment.
- Acyclovir is indicated in newborn with chickenpox and when the mother develops chickenpox 4 days before or 2 days after birth.

SUGGESTED READING

1. Lipton SV, Brunell PA. Management of varicella exposure in a neonatal intensive care unit. JAMA. 1989;261:1782-4.
2. Nathwani D, Maclean A, Conway S, et al. Varicella Infections in pregnancy and the newborn. A review prepared for the UK Advisory Group on Chickenpox on behalf of the British Society for the Study of Infection. J Infect. 1998;36 (Suppl 1):59-71.

CHAPTER 56

Baby Born to VDRL Positive Mother

Naveen Bajaj

INTRODUCTION

The evaluation for an infant born to venereal disease research laboratory (VDRL) positive mother should include the following:
- Physical examination for evidence of congenital syphilis (CS)
- *Nontreponemal test:* VDRL or rapid plasma reagin (RPR)
- Pathologic examination of placenta or umbilical cord
- Dark-field microscopic examination or direct fluorescent antibody testing of body fluids.

PHYSICAL EXAMINATION FOR EVIDENCE OF CONGENITAL SYPHILIS

The clinical manifestations are variable. The infant may have nonspecific signs, have multiorgan dysfunction, or have only laboratory or radiographic abnormalities. The earlier the infection during pregnancy and absence of treatment, more is the risk of spontaneous abortion, preterm delivery, or stillbirth.

Majority of infants are asymptomatic at birth. The clinical features develop manifestations of over several months or years later, if left untreated.

The spectrum of CS is classified as:
- *Early* CS—onset of symptoms any time in first 3 months of age. Presence of unexplained hydrops fetalis or placentomegaly should raise suspicion of CS.
- *Late* CS—features are secondary to initial lesions of early CS or reactions to persistent on-going inflammation. Beyond 2 years, a persistently positive treponemal serologic test may be the only clue.

MAJOR FINDINGS IN EARLY CONGENITAL SYPHILIS

Evaluate	Finding
Appearance	Preterm, SGA, irritable on handling, quietens down when left alone
Mucocutaneous	Snuffles, shiny palms and soles, desquamation, blistering and crusting of soles and palms, mucous patches (palate, perineum), and condyloma lata (perioral-perianal)
Reticuloendothelial	Generalized nontender lymphadenopathy, anemia, leukopenia or leukocytosis, thrombocytopenia, and hepatosplenomegaly

Contd...

Contd...

Evaluate	Finding
Skeletal	Symmetric lesions in long bone (lower > upper), metaphyseal osteochondritis, Wimberger's sign, osteitis, and dactylitis
Neurologic	Suggestive of abnormal CSF, VDRL +ve CSF, untreated may lead to cranial nerve palsy, infarcts, and hydrocephalus
Ocular and others	Salt and pepper chorioretinitis, glaucoma, uveitis, nephritic syndrome, and myocarditis

(CSF: cerebrospinal fluid; SGA: Small for gestational age; VDRL: venereal disease research laboratory)

CLINICAL MANIFESTATIONS OF LATE CONGENITAL SYPHILIS

Teeth	Hutchinson teeth, mulberry molars
Eye	Interstitial keratitis, healed chorioretinitis, secondary glaucoma (uveitis), and corneal scarring
Ear	Eighth nerve deafness
Nose and face	Saddle nose, protuberant mandible
Skin	Rhagades
Central nervous system	Mental retardation, arrested hydrocephalus, convulsive disorders, optic nerve atrophy, juvenile general paresis, and cranial nerve palsies
Bones and joints	"Saber shins", Higoumenakis sign, and Clutton joints

SEROLOGIC AND DIAGNOSTIC TESTS

A high index of suspicion is needed to make a clinical diagnosis.

The two types of serologic tests for syphilis (STS) are the nontreponemal (nonspecific) antibody tests and the treponemal (specific) antibody tests.

Type	Detects	Tests
Nontreponemal (nonspecific)	IgG and IgM against lipoidal cellular antigens (cardiolipin)	VDRL RPR
Treponemal (specific)	IgG and/or IgM against *Treponema pallidum*	TP-PA FTA-ABS

(FTA-ABS: fluorescent treponemal antibody absorption; RPR: rapid plasma reagin; TP-PA: *Treponema pallidum* particle agglutination; VDRL: venereal disease research laboratory)

Nontreponemal (nonspecific) antibody tests: In the original test described by Wassermann, syphilitic tissue was used as antigen to detect the presence of antibody (reagin), which is induced by *Treponema Pallidum*. In the commercial tests available today, cardiolipin (diphosphatidylglycerol), a component of normal cell membranes in mammalian tissue, and lecithin are used as antigens; and these tests measure immunoglobulin G (IgG) and immunoglobulin M (IgM) antibodies. The RPR titer is more than one to two dilutions of the titer obtained using the VDRL test.

Interpretation of VDRL for diagnosis of CS in infants:
- Only serum and cerebrospinal fluid (CSF) are appropriate specimens for the VDRL tests.
- A fourfold rise of titer suggests an active disease, whereas a fourfold decrease suggests response to therapy.
- The patient usually becomes seronegative within 2 years even if the initial titer was high or the infection was congenital
- A reactive VDRL test on CSF, free of blood or other contaminants, usually suggests past or present syphilis infection of the central nervous system.
- *Biologic false-positive (BFP) of VDRL:* These can result from laboratory error and also from serum antibodies that are unrelated to

syphilis infection. These reactions have <1:8 titers and a negative specific treponemal test. They are classified as either acute (<6 months) or chronic BFP results.
- *Acute BFP*: Epstein-Barr virus, varicella, measles, malaria, tuberculosis, brucellosis, mumps, lymphogranuloma venereum, and hepatitis.
- *Chronic BFP:* Autoimmune diseases and chronic inflammatory processes (e.g. systemic lupus erythematosus, polyarteritis nodosa, antiphospholipid syndrome, chronic liver disease, and endocarditis), and pregnancy itself.

Treponemal (specific serologic) tests: These are used to confirm the validity of a positive nontreponemal test and to diagnose late stages of syphilis. These tests are unlikely to revert to a nonreactive state after treatment of the patient.

Fluorescent Treponemal Antibody Absorption

- Detects treponemal antibody by fluorescein-labeled antihuman antibody
- Uses lyophilized Nichols strain organisms as antigen and measures IgG and IgM antibodies.
- The presence or absence of antibody is determined by fluorescent microscopy.

Microhemagglutination Tests (*T. pallidum* Particle Agglutination)

- It is the most efficient specific test for antibody to *T. pallidum*.
- It involves passive hemagglutination of erythrocytes or latex particles that have been sensitized with Nichols strain *T. pallidum*.

Seroreactivity of Common Tests for Untreated Syphilis

Test	% Positive			
	Primary stage	Secondary stage	Latent stage	Tertiary stage
VDRL or RPR	80–85	95–98	75	<66
FTA-ABS, TP-PA	75–85	100	100	100

(FTA-ABS: Fluorescent treponemal antibody absorption; TA-PA: *T. pallidum* particle agglutination)

Other Serologic Tests

IgM Tests
- These tests are not yet commercially available
- Detect IgM antibody in the fetal or neonatal serum, which would indicate antibody production in the fetus due to active fetal infection and hence, differentiates passive transplacental transfer from active infection.

Polymerase Chain Reaction
- Polymerase chain reaction (PCR) has been used on neonatal blood and CSF for establishing the diagnosis of CS
- The sensitivity and specificity of PCR on CSF was 65–71% and 97–100%.

Situations where radiology and lumbar puncture is warranted:
- If infant or child has signs or symptoms of CS.
- If there is no documented treatment in pregnancy.
- If the mother was treated within 4 weeks of delivery.
- If maternal treatment was inadequate or inadequately documented.
- A fourfold decline in titer following therapy was not documented.

CHAPTER 56
Baby Born to VDRL Positive Mother

TREATMENT OPTIONS

WHO recommends that treatment of CS in developing countries should be based on the following:
- Identifying maternal syphilis (by RPR) during pregnancy and/or at time of delivery
- Identifying whether an infant is clinically symptomatic.

FOLLOW-UP

- *Infants with diagnosis of* CS—STS every 2-3 months until negative or decreased fourfold. Nontreponemal test titer should fall fourfold within 6 months of treatment and be nonreactive by 6-12 months. If test remains reactive ≥12 months after treatment, consider reevaluation and

Patient status	Protocol	Alternative
Symptomatic infants	Crystalline penicillin, 50,000 U/kg, IM or IV, every 12 hours for first 7 days of life and then every 8 hours after 7 days of life for 10–14 days	Procaine penicillin, 50,000U/kg, single dose, IM, for 10–15 days
Symptomatic infants at least 4 weeks of age or older	Aqueous Penicillin G 50,000 U/kg/dose, every 6 hours, IV for 10–14 days	-
In asymptomatic neonates born to PRP positive mothers	Single IM dose of benzathine penicillin G, 50,000 U/kg	-

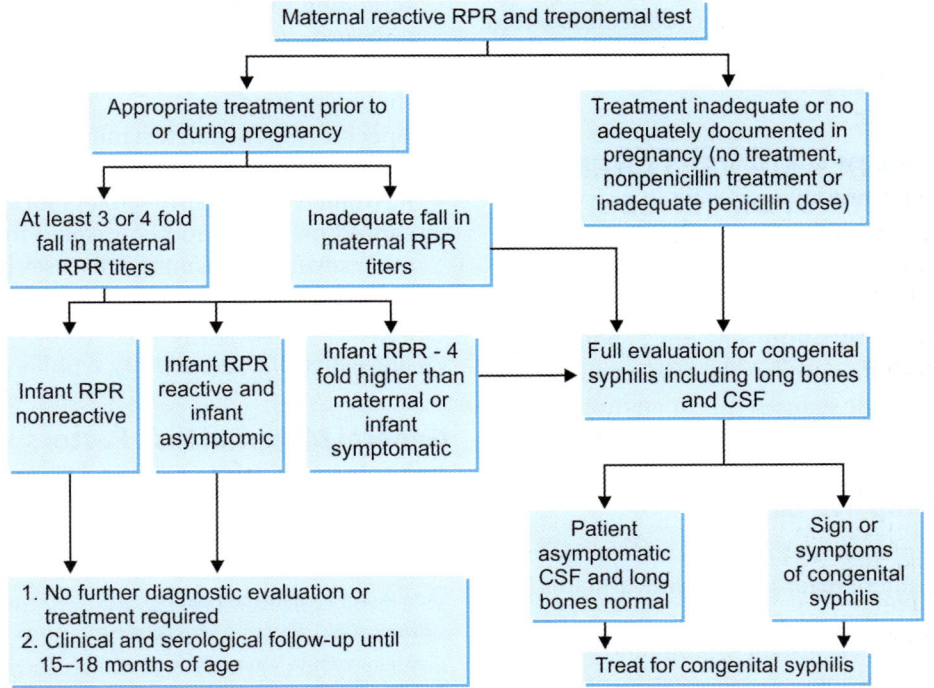

(*Source:* Phiske MM. Current trends in congenital syphilis. Indian J Sex Transm Dis AIDS. 2014;35(1):12-20.)

retreatment. If nontreponemal test titer increases fourfold, full reevaluation and retreatment for proven disease are required. CSF study if abnormal or if there are CNS signs, CSF study should be repeated every 6 months till a normal CSF is documented. If CSF analysis is abnormal and not due to intercurrent illnesses, infant should be treated again. Assessment of development, vision, and hearing should be done on follow-up.

- *Infants who received treatment in utero or at birth because of maternal syphilis*—Serologic test should be done at birth and repeated every 3 months until negative result; specific tests are done after 15 months of age.
- *Woman who received treatment for syphilis during pregnancy*—STS testing monthly till delivery, then every 6 months until negative result or titer reduced fourfold; repeat treatment anytime if there is fourfold rise in titers.

APPENDIX 1: SURVEILLANCE CASE DEFINITIONS FOR CONGENITAL SYPHILIS

Confirmed Case

Confirmation of presence of *T. pallidum* by dark-field microscopy, fluorescent antibody or other specific stains in specimens from lesions, placenta, umbilical cord, or autopsy material.

Presumptive Case

- An infant born to mother with partial or no treatment regardless of clinical status (or)
- Any infant or child who has a reactive treponemal test for syphilis and any one of the following:
  - Clinical evidence of CS on examination
  - Presence of X-ray changes suggestive of CS on long bones
  - Reactive CSF VDRL
  - Raised CSF cell count or protein (without other cause)
  - Quantitative nontreponemal serologic titers with fourfold higher titers than the mothers (both collected at birth)
  - Reactive test for IgM antibody by an approved method.

APPENDIX 2: SCREENING AND TREATMENT OF PREGNANT WOMEN FOR SYPHILIS

Screening of pregnant women must include:
- All women must be screened with a nontreponemal test at first prenatal visit
- A repeat test in high-risk pregnancies at 28–32 weeks and at the time of delivery be carried out.
- If a woman had no prenatal visits or no screening for nontreponemal test during delivery, a nontreponemal test of the mother followed by screening of neonate should be done.
- Specific treponemal test must be done for all positive nontreponemal tests.
- All women with positive serology for syphilis should be tested and counseled for HIV, other sexually transmitted diseases (STDs)
- A lumbar puncture is done during the late stages of syphilis, if eye or brain involvement suggestive of active tertiary syphilis.

General Maternal Risk Factors Associated with Increased Rates of Early Syphilis in Pregnancy

Infection with HIV
Adolescent or unmarried status
History of sexually transmitted disease
Substance abuse, especially cocaine
Inadequate or absent prenatal care
Sex workers
Poor communication among medical personnel regarding maternal/infant status

Table 1: Maternal therapy for Syphilis.		
Early syphilis: • Primary • Secondary • Early latent	Benzathine penicillin G IM Single dose	50,000 U/kg (maximum 2.4 million U)
Late latent syphilis	Benzathine penicillin IM Weekly × 3 doses	150,000 U/kg (maximum 7.2 million U)
Neurosyphilis	Crystalline penicillin G IV Every 4 hours × 10–14 days OR Penicillin G, IM, od × 10–14 days + probenicid (PO), 6 hourly	3–4 million U 2.4 million U + 500 mg
Use of erythromycin, azithromycin, or nonpenicillin treatment for pregnancy is unreliable and not recommended.		

Treatment of Pregnant Women for Syphilis

All mothers with a confirmed diagnosis of syphilis should be treated with penicillin-based therapy, regardless of the stage of pregnancy (Table 1).

SUGGESTED READING

1. American Academy of Pediatrics. In: Baker CJ (Ed). Red Book Atlas of Pediatric Infectious Diseases, 2nd ed. United States: American Academy of Pediatrics; 2013.
2. Dobson SR, Sanchez PJ. Syphilis. In: Feigin RD, Cherry JD, Demmler-Harrison GJ, Kaplan EL (Eds). Feigin & Cherry's Textbook of Pediatric Infectious Diseases, Vol 1 6th ed. Philadelphia: Elsevier Saunders; 2009.
3. Kollmann TR, Dobson SR. Syphilis. IN: Remington JS, Klein JO, Wilson CB, Nizet V, Maldonado YA (Eds). Infectious Diseases of the Fetus and Newborn, 7th ed. Philadelphia: Elsevier Saunders; 2011.
4. World Health Organization. The National Strategy & Operational guidelines towards Elimination of congenital syphilis. New Delhi: World Health Organization; 2015.

CHAPTER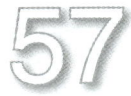

Breastfeeding and Medications

Anjali Kulkarni, Kiran Sathe

INTRODUCTION

Almost all medications consumed by the mother eventually get secreted in breast milk although in variable proportions. Numerous studies clearly show that most medications can be safely administered during lactational period without any major untoward action on the baby if we adhere to certain simple principles and practices as outlined here. Only under exceptional circumstances as directed by the doctor, breastfeeding may have to be avoided to avoid damage to the neonate.

COMMON MEDICATIONS DURING PREGNANCY

The common medications, which may be used during pregnancy, are discussed in Table 1.

Drug	Pharmacokinetic properties (Summary of Various Parameters)	Comments	Category: Compatible with breastfeeding/caution/contraindicated
Analgesics			
Opioid analgesics: Codeine, fentanyl, methadone morphine	• Low transfer in maternal milk • High first pass metabolism		Compatible
Meperidine	Low transfer in maternal milk	Neurobehavioral side effects from retained metabolites	Caution
Nonsteroidal anti-inflammatory drugs: Paracetamol, ibuprofen, mefenamic acid, indomethacin, ketorolac, naproxen, sumatriptan, propoxyphene	Low transfer in maternal milk		Compatible
Aspirin	Low transfer in maternal milk	Risk of Reye's syndrome	Caution

Contd...

Contd...

Drug	Pharmacokinetic properties (Summary of Various Parameters)	Comments	Category: Compatible with breastfeeding/caution/contraindicated
Antibiotics			
Penicillins, cephalosporins, macrolides	Low transfer in maternal milk	Alteration in newborn bowel flora, allergic sensitization	Compatible
Aminoglycosides			Compatible
Fluoroquinolones	Attain higher concentrations in maternal milk	Risk of arthropathy in newborn's joints	Contraindicated
Sulfonamides	Low transfer in maternal milk	Unsafe in hyperbilirubinemia and G6PD deficiency	Caution
Nitrofurantoin			
Metronidazole	High transfer in maternal milk		Caution
Tetracyclines	Low transfer in maternal milk	Risk of affecting bone growth and dental staining	Caution
Antifungals			
Fluconazole	High transfer in maternal milk	Unsafe in presence of neonatal renal failure	Caution
Ketoconazole	Low transfer in maternal milk		
Antivirals			
Acyclovir	Low transfer in maternal milk		Compatible
Anthelminthic			
Mebendazole, pyrantel embonate	Poor gastrointestinal (GI) absorption		Compatible
Antimalarial: Chloroquine	Low transfer in maternal milk		Compatible
Anticoagulants			
Heparins [unfractionated and low molecular weight (MW)]	High MW, do not enter in maternal milk		Compatible
Warfarin	Low transfer in maternal milk	Need to monitor newborn's prothrombin time	Compatible
Anticonvulsants			
Phenytoin, carbamazepine, sodium valproate, topiramate	Low transfer in maternal milk		Compatible
Phenobarbitone	High transfer in maternal milk	Phenobarbitone-induced sedation and infantile spasms in neonate	Caution
Lamotrigine			
Antidepressants			
Selective serotonin reuptake inhibitors (SSRI): Paroxetine, alprazolam	Low transfer in maternal milk		Compatible

Contd...

Contd...

Drug	Pharmacokinetic properties (Summary of Various Parameters)	Comments	Category: Compatible with breastfeeding/caution/contraindicated
Fluoxetine	Accumulation of metabolites in maternal milk	Side effects in neonate common	Caution
Citalopram, sertraline, venlafaxine	High transfer in maternal milk	Need to monitor the infant	Caution
Moclobemide	Low transfer in maternal milk		Compatible
Antihistaminics			
Promethazine, chlorpheniramine, diphenhydramine, loratadine, fexofenadine	Low transfer in maternal milk		Compatible
Benzodiazepines			
Midazolam	Low transfer in maternal milk		Compatible
Diazepam	High transfer in maternal milk	Lethargy, poor sucking in neonate	Caution
Decongestants			
Pseudoephedrine	Low transfer in maternal milk	Topical medications preferred	compatible
Acid suppressants			
Famotidine, Omeprazole	Low transfer in maternal milk	Tendency to accumulate	Compatible / Compatible
Ranitidine	Active transport in milk		Compatible
Cimetidine	Active transport in milk		Caution
Antiemetics			
Domperidone, metoclopramide	Low transfer in maternal milk	Use low dose	Compatible
Hormonal preparations			
Levonorgestrel, medroxyprogesterone norethisterone, prednisolone	Low transfer in maternal milk	Use low dose <20 mg/day	Compatible / Compatible
Cardiovascular drugs			
Nifedipine, diltiazem, verapamil, captopril, enalapril, propranolol, metoprolol, labetalol, methyldopa, digoxin, chlorothiazide	Low transfer in maternal milk	Monitor infant for hypotension, changes in heart rate, gynecomastia and other related side effects wherever applicable	Compatible
Amiodarone, atenolol	High transfer in maternal milk		Caution
Oral antidiabetic agents			
Metformin	Low transfer in maternal milk		Compatible

Contd...

Contd...

Drug	Pharmacokinetic properties (Summary of Various Parameters)	Comments	Category: Compatible with breastfeeding/caution/contraindicated
Sulfonylurea, biguanides, glucosidase inhibitors, thiazolidinediones		Risk of hypoglycemia in infant	Caution
Immunosuppressant			
Cyclosporine	Low transfer in maternal milk	Monitor for nephrotoxicity, hyperkalemia in infant	Contraindicated
Tacrolimus	Low transfer in maternal milk		
Mycophenolate sodium			
Methotrexate			
Cyclophosphamide	Secreted in milk	All immunosuppressant agents are potentially harmful to the infant	
Radioactive agents		Harmful to infant	Contraindicated
Social/recreational agents			
Ethanol, cannabis	High transfer in maternal milk	Impaired neonatal neurodevelopment	Contraindicated
Caffeine	High transfer in maternal milk	Irritability in neonate	Caution
Nicotine (smoking)			Contraindicated
Herbal medications	Lack of data on transfer in maternal milk		Caution

BREASTFEEDING AND MEDICATIONS

The breastfeeding and medications are described in Table 2.

WAYS TO MINIMIZE INFANT DRUG EXPOSURE

- Avoid unnecessary medication usage in breastfeeding mothers. Avoid over the counter usage of drugs during lactational period without doctor's consent.
- Wherever possible, delay the medication usage till baby is weaned-off breastfeeding.
- Refer to the drug literature regarding compatibility during breastfeeding prior to use.
- Select drugs which are poorly secreted in maternal milk.
- Preferably use lowest effective drug dosage and lesser frequent administration of drugs.
- Use alternative routes of medication usage, for example, topical analgesics may be preferred in place of oral analgesics.
- Depending on the T_{max}, avoid breastfeeding during the time interval corresponding to peak drug levels in breast milk.
- Preferably breastfeed the baby before administering the scheduled drug dose.
- Avoid drugs with long $t_{1/2}$ with potential to accumulate in breast milk.
- For less frequently administered drugs such as once daily dosing, schedule the dosing just prior to the longest sleeping phase of the infant so as to minimize frequency of breastfeeding for next couple of hours.
- For drugs which are actively secreted in breast milk, it would be advisable to express

Table 2: Safety of medications in mothers who are breastfeeding.

Medication	Safety recommendation	Possible effect on infant
Analgesics		
Acetaminophen, ibuprofen, opioids	Safe in commonly prescribed doses	—
High-dose aspirin	Second-line option	Platelet dysfunction; one case of metabolic acidosis
Meperidine, naproxen	Use with caution	Long half-life may lead to accumulation in infant
Antibiotics		
Aminoglycosides	Safe	—
Cephalosporins	Safe	—
Fluoroquinolones	American Academy of Pediatrics considers safe	Possible risk of arthropathy
Macrolides	• Use with caution • Concentrated in human milk	Erythromycin associated with increased incidence of pyloric stenosis
Metronidazole	Pump and discard breast milk during use and 24 hours after last dose	In vitro mutagen; no association with cancer seen in humans
Nitrofurantoin	Use with caution	Hemolysis in infant with G6PD deficiency
Penicillins	Safe	—
Sulfa drugs	Avoid use in first month	Elevates infant bilirubin levels
Tetracycline	Avoid prolonged use (greater than 3 weeks)	Tooth staining
Antihypertensives		
Angiotensin-converting enzyme inhibitors	Safe after 4–6 weeks	Possible renal toxicity in premature infants
Beta-blockers	—	—
Atenolol	Do not use	Cyanosis, bradycardia
Other beta blockers	Use with caution	Bradycardia
Calcium-channel blockers	Use with caution	—
Antidepressants		
Fluoxetine	Weigh risks versus benefits	May cause colic, irritability, feeding and sleep disorders, slow weight gain
Sertraline, paroxetine	Excreted in breast milk, but infant serum levels very low or undetectable	No reported effect
Combined oral contraceptives	Avoid until breastfeeding well-established (60–90 days); low dose preferred	May decrease milk supply

and discard the breast milk before nursing the infant.
- If the drug is to be consumed for a short course of time, it would be advisable to avoid breastfeeding during that duration. However, the mother needs to continue expressing breast milk to facilitate continued breast milk production.

SUGGESTED READING

1. Bhatt S, Parikh P, Kantharia N, et al. Knowledge, attitude and practice of post natal mothers for early initiation of breast feeding in the obstetric wards of a tertiary care hospital of Vadodara city. Nat J Comm Med. 2012;3(2):305-9.
2. Nice FJ, Luo AC. Medications and breast feeding: current concepts. J Am Pharm Assoc. 2012;52(1):86-94.
3. Nordeng H, Havnen G, Spigset O. Drug use and breast feeding. Tidsskr Nor Legeforen. 2012;132(9):1089-93.
4. Ostrea EM, Mantaring III JB, Silvestre MA. Drugs that affect the fetus and the newborn infant via placenta or breast milk. Pediatr Clin N Am. 2004;51:539-79.

CHAPTER 58

Stem Cell Banking: Scope and Practice

Femitha P

INTRODUCTION

Stem cells are characterized by ability to multiply and differentiate into specialized cells. Stem cells are hematopoietic progenitor cells (HPC) or hematopoietic stem cells (HSC). These cells can be sourced from embryo, fetus, cord blood, or adult tissues.

As of now, only umbilical cord, bone marrow, and peripheral blood have clinical applications.

UMBILICAL CORD BLOOD BANKING

Steps Involved

- *Recruitment*: Expectant parents are educated about the process, advantages, and cost incurred (for private banking) during antenatal visits
- Consent
- Collection is done by company recruited personnel or health workers at the birthing unit
- Transport to storage center
- Processing (at this stage itself, testing for viability, cell counts, screening, and typing may be done and units labeled)
- Cryopreservation in liquid nitrogen at −196°C
- Releasing cord blood unit to transplant center as need arises.

Advantages of Umbilical Cord Blood

- The procedure is painless to mother and baby
- Does not interfere with the birthing process
- Involves a simple technique with minimal training
- Can be utilized as early as 2 weeks after a patient requirement is identified.
- There is better tolerance of human leukocyte antigen (HLA) mismatches
- Lesser incidence of severe graft versus host disease (GVHD) (as low as 10%)
- Fewer risks of transmitted viral infections.

Drawbacks

- Repeat stem cell donation from the same donor is never possible in umbilical cord blood (UCB)
- Limited number of viable HSC within a given UCB unit
- There is often delayed engraftment.

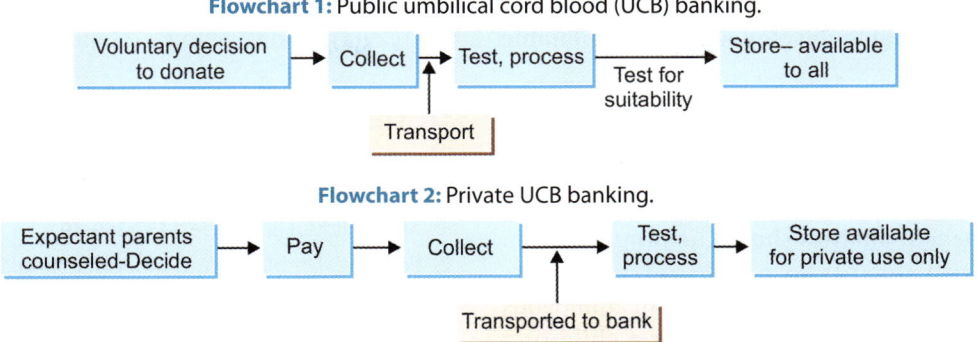

Flowchart 1: Public umbilical cord blood (UCB) banking.

Flowchart 2: Private UCB banking.

Types of Transplant

- *Autologous transplant*: Cord blood is collected at birth is used for same baby. A child's stem cells are not used to treat genetic, storage, or hemoglobinopathies
- *Allogenic transplant*: Stem cells can be used for others if there is good match between donor and recipient.

Indications

- Stem cell therapy is indicated in conditions where bone marrow transplant is the standard of care. Food and Drug Administration (FDA) has approved it in 80 conditions (e.g. malignancies like leukemia's, lymphoma, immune disorders (SCID), genetic hematological disorders like thalassemia, Fanconi anemia, sickle-cell anemia, pure red cell aplasia and metabolic disorders like MPS, osteopetrosis).
- To preserve stem cells from cord blood for autologous use (by the same child), or if the child goes on to develop a disease in future, especially with history of a family member (sibling or biological parents only) with a potentially treatable disease with an allogeneic hematopoietic stem cell.

TYPES OF CORD BLOOD BANKING

- *Public banks* promote allogenic altruistic donation in the real sense (similar to voluntary blood donation) (Flowchart 1). From the delivery room, the cord blood is sent to a central processing facility. It must meet strict laid down standards for donor screening and infection testing. Initial HLA typing of these units is done and entered into computerized registries so that when the need arises, a specific unit can be rapidly located for a patient.
- *Private banks* store stem cells from UCB for autologous use (by the same child), or if the child develops disease later in life (Flowchart 2). It is feasible to use these for matched siblings or family members also. There is a significant cost associated with sample processing and storage fee, charged annually, for these "for-profit" UCB banks. It is estimated that utility of autologous stem cells is as low as 1 in 200,000 individuals.

PRACTICE POINTERS

- Given the costs associated and current extremely low utility of banking for autologous use, private storage of cord blood as "biological insurance" is unwise.
- All the major governing bodies like Indian Council of Medical Research, American Academy of Pediatrics/ACOG, and Royal college of Obstetrics and Gynecology **do not recommend private cord blood banking for healthy neonates with no family**

members known to have or with the potential to develop a disease amenable to SCT.

- If expectant parents request information on UCB banking, they should be counseled regarding its advantages and disadvantages, myths and realities and a realistic cost benefit analysis should be properly given with regards to public versus private banking. The rare chance of an autologous unit of UCB being used for a child or a family member should be informed.
- *Delayed cord clamping versus UCB banking:* The collection should not be a priority and emphasis should be on timed umbilical cord clamping. Early umbilical cord clamping and collection for banking results in an artificial loss of these stem cells.
- Public banks in India include Jeevan Public Blood Bank (Chennai), Reliance Dhirubhai Ambani Life Sciences Center (Navi Mumbai), School of Tropical Medicine (Kolkata), StemCyte India (Gujarat), etc.

SUGGESTED READING

1. Elmoazzen H, Holovati JL. Cord blood clinical processing, cryopreservation and storage. Methods Mol Biol. 2015;1257:369-79.
2. Petrini C. Umbilical cord blood banking: from personal donations to international public registries to global bioeconomy. J Blood Med. 2014;5:87-97.
3. Sachdeva A, Gunasekaran V, Malhotra P, et al. Umbilical cord blood banking: consensus statement of the Indian Academy of Pediatrics. Guidelines on Umbilical Cord Blood Banking' Committee of Indian Academy of Pediatrics. Indian Pediatr. 2018;55(6):489-94.
4. Thornley I, Eapen M, Sung L, et al. Private cord blood banking: experiences and views of pediatric hematopoetic cell transplant physicians. Pediatrics. 2009;123(3):1011-7.

CHAPTER
59

Declaring Newborn Death

Rhishikesh Thakre, Srinivas Murki

WHEN NOT TO INITIATE NEWBORN RESUSCITATION?

- If the confirmed gestational age is <22 weeks (AAP) consider <25 weeks or less based on hospital NICU outcomes
- Birth weight <400 g
- Major chromosomal anomalies prenatally detected (e.g. trisomy 13 or trisomy 18)
- Anencephaly

Note: When in doubt, resuscitation should be initiated.

WHEN TO CONSIDER DISCONTINUATION OF RESUSCITATION IN A NEWBORN?

- An Apgar score of 0 at 10 minutes with ongoing resuscitation
- An Apgar score of 0 after 10 minutes of resuscitation, if the heart rate remains undetectable
- Resuscitation until 20 minutes in the absence of a clinically detectable heartbeat.

Note:
- Ensure resuscitation has been optimum. Examples of optimization include intubation before initiating chest compressions, administering intravenous rather than endotracheal epinephrine, assessment for reversible factors reversible factors particularly hypovolemic (and/or severe anemia) and tension pneumothorax
- Collect sample of cord blood for blood gas study and document pH
- When in doubt, the discontinuation of resuscitation decision should not be taken in delivery room. Ongoing care should be provided, and clinical and laboratory data be collected for informed decision making
- Consider decision making based on availability of advanced care (e.g. therapeutic hypothermia), perinatal events, and parental wishes.

WHEN TO DECLARE PATIENT DEAD AFTER INITIATING RESUSCITATION?

No heart rate, no spontaneous breathing, electrocardiogram (ECG) showing asystole, cyanosed, despite 50 minutes of resuscitation.

Note: During 50 minutes of resuscitation, inform parents every 15 minutes about the response to resuscitation.

DOCUMENTATION

- Document resuscitation using extended Apgar score (Table 1)
- Document ECG for asystole before declaring death
- Document cord blood gas pH, if feasible
- Document parents being informed and counseled
- For stillbirth "Stillbirth Declaration Form" will be filled by the Doctor X (two copies).

NURSING RESPONSIBILITY
During Resuscitation

- Document ECG before withdrawing resuscitation or declaring death.

After Death

- Nurse has to review the documentation which validates the death of the baby before starting the death care.
- Allow parents with baby for some time before starting the death care
- Give the death care to the baby in consultation with family member
- Remove all lines and tubes, give required pressure to stop the bleeding.
- Clean the baby, pack all orifices, and wrap in the white sheet (mortuary sheet).
- For stillbirth, "Stillbirth declaration form" will be filled by the Doctor X (two copies). One copy of Stillbirth form will be handed over to the parent along with baby and one

Table 1: Documentation of resuscitation using extended Apgar score.

Apgar Score				Gestational age_____weeks				
Sign	0	1	2	1 minute	5 minute	10 minute	15 minute	20 minute
Color	Blue or pale	Acrocyanotic	Completely pink					
Heart rate	Absent	<100 minute	>100 minute					
Reflex irritability	No response	Grimace	Cry or active withdrawal					
Muscle tone	Limp	Some flexion	Active motion					
Respiration	Absent	Weak cry; hypoventilation	Good, crying					
			Total					
						Resuscitation		
Comments:			Minutes	1	5	10	15	20
			Oxygen					
			PPV/NCPAP					
			ETT					
			Chest compressions					
			Epinephrine					

copy will be kept in the medical record department (MRD) file along with strip of flat ECG from the monitor.
- For death of preterm baby and full-term baby, death certificate will be filled by the doctor. One copy of death certificate will be handed over to the parents along with baby and one copy will be kept in the MRD record along with strip of flat ECG.
- Complete the documentation of entire sequence of resuscitation and death care in the nurse's note.
- Take signature of the parents in the death record for receiving the body as well as all reports. Notify the quality department by filling up the incident form for stillbirth. As a policy, all stillbirths will be discussed in the mortality and morbidity meeting.
- Hand over the baby and take signatures of the parents/in-charge relative.
- Handover the details of the patient summary and advice for follow-up appointment with the doctor for counseling.

Counseling is done by the duty doctor, preferably the same person, periodically. In the delivery room, a joint counseling by the obstetrics and pediatrician should take place. Counseling should include details of the current situation—what is the problem, what is being done, what is the response. Handle parents/relatives with empathy, genuineness, and compassion. Be non-judgmental.

Death declaration: Death will be declared by the most experienced duty doctor.

SUGGESTED READING

1. American Academy of Pediatrics Committee on fetus and newborn and American college of obstetricians and gynecologist committee on obstetric practice. The Apgar Score. Pediatrics. 2015;136:819.
2. Nakagawa TA, Ashwal S, Mathur M, et al. Guidelines for the determination of brain death in infants and children: an update of the 1987 task force recommendations: executive summary. Ann Neurol. 2012;71(4):573-85.
3. Perlman JM. Highlights of the new neonatal resuscitation program guidelines. Neo Rev. 2016;17:e435.
4. Wyckoff MH, Aziz K, Escobedo MB, et al. American Heart Association guidelines update for cardiopulmonary resuscitation and emergency cardiovascular care. Circulation. 2015;132(Suppl 2):S543-56.

SECTION 5

Specific Therapies

SECTION OUTLINE

60. Antibiotic Policy in Neonatal Intensive Care Unit
61. Surfactant Replacement Therapy
62. Continuous Positive Airway Pressure
63. INtubate, SURfactant, Extubate (INSURE) Procedure
64. Blood Component Therapy
65. Total Parenteral Nutrition
66. Oxygen Therapy
67. Chest Physiotherapy

CHAPTER 60

Antibiotic Policy in Neonatal Intensive Care Unit

Hemasree Kandraju

INTRODUCTION

The judicious use of antibiotics is an important means to limit the emergence of antibiotic resistant organisms (AROs). Antibiotic policy is one of the core elements of the antibiotic stewardship program, which includes accurately identifying patients who need antibiotic therapy, using local epidemiology to guide the selection of empiric therapy, avoiding agents with overlapping activity, adjusting antibiotics when cultures results become available, monitoring for toxicity, and optimizing the dose, route, and duration of therapy.

The signs and symptoms of sepsis in neonates are nonspecific and may represent the presentations of a noninfectious process; hence, identifying the infants who need antibiotics is crucial.

Conditions *where antibiotics are not indicated* are:
- Asymptomatic preterm needing admission
- Asphyxiated infants
- Severe jaundice
- Meconium aspiration syndrome
- Exchange transfusion
- Bacterial colonization.

Conditions *where antibiotics are indicated* are:
- Symptomatic infants with respiratory distress with no clear history
- Clinical suspicion of sepsis (presence of impaired perfusion, off-color, cold peripheries, fever, signs of shock, seizures, multiorgan involvement, sick neonate with no evident cause, etc.)
- Evidence of pneumonia on chest X-ray
- Asymptomatic infants with preterm premature prolonged rupture of membranes (PPROM)
- Presence of risk factors for infection in case of preterm infants
- Presence of risk factors along with positive septic screen in case of term infants
- Culture positive sepsis.

Note: In neonates with gestation less than 34 weeks, antibiotics should be started, with any duration of PPROM. In infants between 34 weeks and 36 weeks, a septic screen can be done after 6 hours of life and if positive, then antibiotics should be started.

Without exception, blood culture should be obtained before starting antibiotics.

SELECTION OF EMPIRIC ANTIBIOTIC THERAPY

- Depends on the local cumulative antibiograms over last 3–6 months duration or at least 30–40 culture reports

Table 1: Antibiotic choice in neonatal sepsis.

Mode and time of suspicion of infection	Appropriate empiric antibiotic
Within 24 hours of life (EOS), overwhelming signs of sepsis	Gram-negative cover
LOS, prolonged hospital stay, fever, evidence of abscess or pustules	Gram-positive cover
ELBW infants, multiple antibiotic usage, multiple invasive lines, and procedures	Fungal cover

(ELBW: extremely low birth weight; EOS: early onset sepsis; LOS: late onset sepsis)

- Unit specific antibiograms are most useful as the common organisms prevalent, the common drugs to which they are sensitive and ARO are different at each unit
- The first-line antibiotics chosen can have 70–80% sensitivity, the second-line with 80–90% and the third-line with more than 90% sensitivity (Table 1)
- Knowledge of outbreaks can inform the temporary modification in the empiric regimens
- Agents with overlapping spectrum of activity should be avoided.

To choose the antibiotic for empiric therapy, understanding of the different organisms causing early onset sepsis (EOS) or late onset sepsis (LOS), and their sensitivity to different antibiotics is necessary. The organisms and the antibiotics can be grouped into the following:
- Gram-negative organisms
  - Aminoglycosides (amikacin or gentamicin), cephalosporins, ampicillin, piperacillin, ciprofloxacin, meropenem, colistin
- Gram-positive organisms
  - Cloxacillin, vancomycin, teicoplanin, tigecycline
- Fungus
  - Fluconazole, amphotericin
- Anaerobic organisms
  - Penicillin, metronidazole.

Note: The EOS in our country is usually caused by gram-negative organisms compared to the west, where the group B streptococcal (GBS) is more prevalent. Hence, a monotherapy with any one of the above antibiotics would be sufficient instead of a combination therapy like ampicillin and gentamicin.

Depending on the time and mode of presentation of the infection, the appropriate empiric therapy can be initiated.

Note:
- Cephalosporins should be avoided as the first-line therapy, as there is an emergence of multidrug-resistant bacteria [especially extended spectrum beta-lactamase (ESBL)] with their extensive usage
- Anaerobic infections are rare in neonates.

RE-EVALUATING THE ANTIBIOTIC REGIME

The microbiology report with the antibiotic sensitivity testing is an invaluable tool to determine if antibiotics should be continued, modified, or discontinued.
- The body site from which the positive culture was isolated should be reviewed. Growth from nonsterile body sites (such as tracheal aspirates) may be colonizing flora, particularly when the clinical course is not suggestive of infection.
- Susceptibility results provide the opportunity to treat with a narrow spectrum, less toxic, and more efficacious antibiotic.

The minimum inhibitory concentration (MIC) can guide treatment for infections at sequestrated sites, such as lung or the central nervous system. At these sites, decreased antibiotic penetration is expected. Thus, the use of agents with MICs near the clinical breakpoint (the transition from susceptible to intermediate or resistant) would not be

recommended, as the adequate tissue levels may not be achieved.
- The date and time of the microbiology report, provide an opportunity for timely discontinuation of therapy when infection is not suspected. Nearly, all blood cultures with clinically meaningful bacterial growth will be positive within 48 hours.
- Cultures with growth after 48 hours are more likely to be contaminants or colonizing organisms as these microbes are generally present at a lower inoculum.
- If the blood culture is sterile after 48–72 hours of incubation, it is almost always safe and appropriate to stop antibiotics.

How to Upgrade or Downgrade Antibiotics?

Depending on the clinical improvement or based on the blood culture and sensitivity pattern, either we upgrade or downgrade the antibiotics. It is always better not to upgrade the antibiotics at least for 48–72 hours of starting if there is improvement. Our focus should also be on the supportive care, which would improve the outcome. It includes:
- Maintaining the temperature
- Proper adjustment of the fluid balance
- Correction of the electrolyte disturbances
- Acid base balance
- Use of inotropes for hypotension
- Ventilation or continuous positive airway pressure (CPAP) if needed
- Blood and blood products to correct anemia or the bleeding tendency.

There should be a unit policy for the hierarchy of the antibiotics to be used, i.e. from first-line to second-line. To modify from second- to third-line of antibiotics, the sensitivity report has to be considered or can be done when the infant is very sick, or when there is not much clinical improvement even after 72–96 hours of first-line of antibiotics and the supportive care.

How to Downgrade the Antibiotics?

- The antibiotics should be downgraded, when there is clinical improvement.
- If on clinical suspicion if multiple antibiotics (e.g. gram-negative and antifungal cover) have been started for a sick infant; after the susceptibility report, the antibiotics specific to the organism isolated has to be continued and the rest should be stopped.
- The antibiotic with narrow spectrum should be chosen; for instance, for gram-negative organism better to choose one among aminoglycosides, piperacillin, or ampicillin. For gram-positive organism, choose cloxacillin over vancomycin and for fungal cover prefer to use fluconazole over amphotericin.
- If the neonate has clinically improved, the same empirical antibiotics can be continued, even if there is in vitro resistance.
- If the organism isolated is *Staphylococcus* or *Pseudomonas*, it is always better to follow the susceptible antibiotic on the antibiograms.
- If meningitis is suspected, a drug which penetrates cerebrospinal fluid (CSF) has to be chosen (cephalosporins and penicillin would be preferable over aminoglycosides or quinolones for meningeal penetration).

MODIFICATION OF ANTIBIOTIC AFTER THE AVAILABILITY OF ANTIBIOGRAM

- Continue any one of the sensitive antibiotic.
- Any one of the narrowest spectrum should be chosen. For instance:
  - Ampicillin over meropenem
  - Piperacillin-taz obactam over levofloxacin
  - Fluconazole over amphotericin
  - Cloxacillin over vancomycin
- If the susceptible antibiotics are of intermediate sensitivity, two of them can be combined.

- If only aminoglycosides have to be used, its usage has to be restricted to 1 week duration, because of the nephrotoxicity and ototoxicity.

Antibiotic Stewardship Program

To rationalize the antibiotic usage and prevention of resistant bacteria, antibiotic stewardship program has to be followed. The core components include:
- Formulary restriction or optimal use of antibiotics
  - Restricting the use of antibiotics
  - Restricting the use of broad spectrum antibiotics
  - Monitoring the drug toxicity
- Prospective surveillance and auditing of cultures
- Protocol for antibiotic prescription
- Improving the infection control practices
- Education of the staff.

Formulary Restriction

- There is no role for prophylactic antibiotics
- The blood culture has to be considered to guide the continuation of antibiotics rather than the septic screen
- Minimize the duration of antibiotics
- The standard practice is to discontinue antibiotics as soon as blood cultures are confirmed negative (48–72 hours) and there are no clinical or hematologic signs of infection
  - *Suspect sepsis*: 3 days or less
  - *Culture positive sepsis*: 7–10 days for gram negative and 10–14 days for gram positive
  - *Pneumonia or screen positive sepsis*: 5–7 days
- There should be unit policy for upgrading of antibiotics and it should be strictly followed
- Antibiotics should be continued for symptomatic infants and those with positive blood culture
- The members of the antibiotic stewardship team should be involved in the use of restricted or broad spectrum or newer antibiotics.

Restricting the Use of Broad Spectrum Antibiotics

- Avoid cephalosporins as the first-line of antibiotics as their use will increase the incidence of drug resistant bacteria ESBLs
- Aminoglycosides or piperacillin are better choices as first-line empiric antibiotics
- Re-evaluate the antibiotics after the culture and stop the broad spectrum antibiotics, choose narrow spectrum
- Rotation of antibiotics is not recommended
- Audit of the antibiogram has to be done every 3–6 months.

Surveillance of the Cultures

Periodic cultures from the unit (surveillance swabs) should be taken, to understand the prevalence of organisms in the neonatal intensive care unit (NICU) environment
- The process measures should be audited, like:
  - The procedure of hand washing
  - Availability and usage of disinfectants in the baby care area
  - Audit of insertion and maintenance of central lines or peripherally inserted central catheter (PICC) lines [central line associated bloodstream infection (CLASBI bundle)]
  - Use of enteral nutrition
  - Compliance of ventilator-associated pneumonia (VAP) bundle
- Audit of the cultures is needed to know the type of organisms causing early onset or

CHAPTER 60
Antibiotic Policy in Neonatal Intensive Care Unit

late onset sepsis, the sensitivity pattern and to formulate the empiric use of first-line or second-line antibiotics.

Antibiotic Prescription Protocol

- Every unit should have a written antibiotic policy/protocol. Unit protocol should strictly adhere to restrict the use to 4–5 antibiotics in the unit
- Always document the initiation and change of antibiotic
- Upgrading of antibiotics, especially from the second-line to third-line, must be done under the supervision of the consultant or senior physician
- A blood culture has to be taken before any change in the antibiotic.

Protocol for Use of Commonly Used Drugs

The dose of the antibiotics would depend on the age, weight, and the renal function of the infant; also on the site of infection and simultaneous use of other interfering drugs.

Amikacin

- Dose and dosing interval is given on Table 2.
- Always given as infusion over 30 minutes
- Preferable as single daily dose and duration less than 5 days
- Nephrotoxicity may increase when used with frusemide, vancomycin or cefotaxime
- The peak level indicates efficacy and the trough level indicates toxicity.
- The usual therapeutic range is peak (µg/mL) of 20–30 and trough (µg/mL) of 2–5.
- The serum drugs levels > 10 mcg/L are nephrotoxic and >35 mcg/L are ototoxic.
- Optimum time to obtain levels is 30 minutes prior to next dose for trough levels, and 30 minutes after completion of IV infusion for peak levels.

Ampicillin

- The dosage depends on the gestational age and the postnatal day of life. For dosing interval, see Table 3.
- *Mild/moderate infection*: 50–100 mg/kg/dose IV
- *Meningitis:* 400 mg/kg/d ÷ q 8–12 hr IV (See Table 3 for dosing interval)
- Administer by IV push over 3–5 minutes
- Dosage adjustment should be done for renal impairment.
- Reconstituted solution must be used within 1 hour after mixing, due to loss of potency.
- Not compatible with parenteral nutrition, avoid mixing.
- Blunting of the peak aminoglycoside level if administered simultaneously, so always separate by a saline flush.
- May cause thrombocytopenia, rash or seizures with large doses

Table 2: Dosage and dosing interval for amikacin.

PMA (weeks)	Postnatal age (days)	Dose (mg/kg)	Interval (hours)
≤ 29	0–7	18	48
	8–28	15	36
	>28	15	24
30–34	0–7	18	36
	≥ 8	15	24
≥35	All	15	24

(PMA: postmenstrual age)

Table 3: Dosing interval chart for Cefotaxime and Ampicillin.

Gest. age (weeks)	Postnatal age (days)	Interval (hours)
< 29	0–28	12
	>28	8
30–36	0–14	12
	>14	8
≥37	0–7	12
	>7	8

Meropenem

- The use of meropenem is not well established in the neonates. The dose used for the infants more than 3 months of age was found to be effective.
- *Dose:* 10–20 mg/kg/dose q 8–12 hours. (In case of meningitis can increase to 40 mg/kg q 8 hourly). See Table 4 for dosing interval.
- Always given as infusion over 15–30 minutes. Can be reconstituted with dextrose or saline. The drug reconstituted with sterile water maintains its potency at room temperature (up to 25°C) up to 8 hours and under refrigeration for 48 hours.
- Can be used in resistant and difficult to treat gram-negative infections.
- It penetrates well into CSF.
- Most common adverse effects are diarrhea, nausea/vomiting and rash. May cause thrombocytopenia, leucopenia and anemia.

Piperacillin Tazobactam

- *Dose:* 50 to 100 mg/kg per dose q8–12 hourly IV or IM. See Table 5 of the dosing interval.
- The dosing depends on the postmenstrual age (PMA) and the postnatal age
- The reconstituted solution is stable for 24 hours at room temperature and 48 hours if refrigerated.
- Not to be used for meningitis due to poor CSF penetration.

Table 4: Dosing interval for meropenem.

Gestational age (weeks)	Postnatal age (days)	Interval (hours)
≤ 32	0–14	12
	>14	8
>32	0–7	12
	>7	8

Table 5: Dosing interval for piperacillin.

PMA (weeks)	Postnatal age (days)	Interval (hours)
≤ 29	0–28 days	12
	>28	8
30–36	0–14	12
	>14	8
37–44	0–7	12
	>7	8
≥45	All	6

Table 6: Dosing interval for vancomycin.

PMA (weeks)	Postnatal age (days)	Interval (hours)
≤ 29	0–14	18
	>14	12
30–36	0–14	12
	>14	8
37–44	0–7	12
		8
≥45	All	6

- May cause thrombocytopenia, azotemia, liver dysfunction, cholestasis and hypokalemia.

Vancomycin

- *Dose:* 10 mg/kg per dose—Bacteremia; 15 mg/kg/dose—Meningitis. See Table 6 for the dosing interval.
- Reconstituted solution is stable for 4 days if refrigerated.
- Always given as infusion over 1–2 hours.
- Rapid infusion can cause hypotension, red man syndrome and thrombophlebitis.

Lengthening the infusion time will eliminate the risk of hypotension for subsequent doses.
- NEVER give rapidly and no IM route.
- The usual therapeutic range is Peak (µg/mL) of 25–40 and trough (µg/mL) of 5–10.
- Optimum time to obtain levels is 30 min. prior to next dose for trough levels, and 30 minutes after completion of IV infusion for peak levels.
- Monitor the trough levels as it can cause ototoxicity and nephrotoxicity.
- Has interaction with amikacin, amphotericin, frusemide, indomethacin.

Amphotericin B
- *Dosage*: 1–1.5 mg/kg IV q24 hour infusion over 2- 6 hours.
- Incompatible with saline, hence always dilute with dextrose
- First dose to be given over six hours and the subsequent doses over 4 hours
- Reconstituted solution is stable for 24 hours at room temperature or 7 days in refrigerator.
- Conventional is preferred
- Liposomal can be used if there is intolerance to the conventional
- Decreases renal blood flow/GFR; Monitor renal/hepatic status closely.
- *Total dose*: 15–30 mg/kg
- Nephrotoxic and can cause hypokalemia, bone marrow suppression, thrombophlebitis and fever. Cardiac arrest can occur if 10 times the recommended dose is given.

Fluconazole
- *Invasive candidiasis*: 12–25 mg/kg loading dose, then 6–12 mg/kg per dose as IV infusion over 30 minutes.

Table 7: Dosing interval for fluconazole.

Gestational age (weeks)	Postnatal age (days)	Interval (hours)
≤29	0–14	48
	>14	24
30 and older	0–7	48
	>7	24

- *Prophylaxis (only in VLBW at high risk of invasive fungal disease)*: 3 mg/kg per dose via infusion twice weekly IV, or orally. A dose of 6 mg/kg per dose can be considered if targeting *Candida* strains with higher MICs (4 to 8 mcg/mL).
- *Thrush*: 6 mg/kg on Day 1, then 3 mg/kg per dose every 6 hours orally.
- For invasive Candidiasis dosing interval chart, see Table 7.
- Store at room temperature. Do not freeze.

Cefotaxime
- *Dose*: 50 mg/kg per dose as IV infusion over 30 minutes or IM. For dosing interval, see Table 3.
- Penetrates well across BBB and good for use in meningitis.
- Restricted use is recommended, to decrease the incidence of ESBLs.

SUGGESTED READING
1. Centers for Disease Control and Prevention's (CDC) Get Smart Campaign, www.cdc.gov/getsmart/healthcare/.
2. Patel SJ, Saiman L. Principles and strategies of antibiotic stewardship in neonatal intensive care unit. Semin Perinatol. 2012;36(6):431-6.
3. Tripathi N, Watt K, Benjamin DK Jr. Antibiotic use and misuse in neonatal intensive care unit. Clin Perinatol. 2012;39(1):61-8.

CHAPTER 61

Surfactant Replacement Therapy

Dinesh Chirla

INTRODUCTION

Surfactant replacement therapy is standard of care for management of respiratory distress syndrome (RDS) in preterm infants due to immense benefits (Box 1).

INDICATIONS OF SURFACTANT THERAPY

Preterm with respiratory distress with any one of the following:
- Fraction of inspired oxygen (FiO_2) > 3
- Continuous positive airway pressure (CPAP) > 6
- Who fails CPAP and needs ventilation
- Need intubation in delivery room.

Box 1 Benefits of surfactant replacement therapy.

- Decreased severity of respiratory distress syndrome (RDS)
- Decreased need for oxygen
- Decreased ventilatory support
- Decreased mortality
- Lowers the incidence of pneumothorax, pulmonary interstitial emphysema, and the combined outcome of death or bronchopulmonary dysplasia (BPD)
- No increase in adverse neurodevelopmental outcome

Nonrespiratory distress syndrome treatment indications include meconium aspiration syndrome, persistent pulmonary hypertension of the newborn, neonatal pneumonia, and pulmonary hemorrhage on *case-by-case basis.*

FACTORS INFLUENCING SURFACTANT THERAPY

- *Interfere with surfactant*:
  - Hypoxia, acidosis
  - Shock (infection)
  - Uncontrolled diabetes
  - Multiple births
  - Oligohydramnios
  - Hydrops fetalis.
- *Accelerate production*:
  - Placental insufficiency
  - Abruptio placentae
  - Premature rupture of membrane (PROM)
  - Pregnancy-induced hypertension (PIH)
  - Diabetes.

CHOICE OF SURFACTANT

There are several different surfactant preparations that have been licensed for use in neonates with RDS (Table 1). Natural

CHAPTER 61
Surfactant Replacement Therapy

Table 1: Comparison of surfactant preparations.

	Beractant (Survanta)	Poractant (Curosurf)	BLES (Neosurf)
Source	Bovine lung	Porcine lung	Bovine lipid
Phospholipid (DPCC)	25 mg/mL	76 mg/mL	27 mg/mL
Initial dose	4 cc/kg	2.5 cc/kg	5 cc/kg
Vial size (mL)	4/8	1.5/3	3/5
Storage	2–8°C	2–8°C	–10°C
Getting ready	Warm at room temperature for 10 min	Wait for 30 min	Slowly warm to room temperature

surfactant is extracted from animal sources such as bovine or porcine. Synthetic surfactant is manufactured from compounds that mimic natural surfactant properties.

Natural surfactants are preferred as they have shown to be superior to synthetic surfactant. Most of the head-to-head trials show that surfactants have similar efficacy when used in similar doses; however, there is a survival advantage when 200 mg/kg of poractant alfa is compared with 100 mg/kg of beractant or 100 mg/kg poractant alfa to treat RDS.

TIMING OF SURFACTANT THERAPY

- *Prophylactic or preventive treatment*: Surfactant is administered at the time of birth or shortly thereafter to infants who are at high risk for developing RDS from surfactant deficiency. There is no evidence to suggest that prophylactic surfactant helps in preterm babies (Box 2).
- *Rescue or therapeutic treatment*: Surfactant is administered following onset of respiratory distress meeting the treatment criterion as above (Flowchart 1).

Using CPAP immediately after birth in infants with respiratory distress with subsequent selective surfactant administration is preferred as an alternative to routine intubation with prophylactic or early surfactant administration in preterm infants.

Box 2 Concerns with prophylactic therapy.

- Interference with resuscitation
- Associated risk of invasive intervention
- Over treatment
- Added cost

EARLY ADMINISTRATION OF SURFACTANT FOLLOWED BY BRIEF VENTILATION AND EXTUBATION TO CONTINUOUS POSITIVE AIRWAY PRESSURE (INSURE STRATEGY)

This technique features early surfactant replacement therapy with prompt extubation to nasal CPAP. In the trials prior to use of routine CPAP, this technique is associated with less need for mechanical ventilation, lower incidence of BPD, and fewer air leak syndromes, when compared with later, selective surfactant replacement therapy, mechanical ventilation, and extubation from lower ventilator settings.

Technique of Surfactant Administration

Surfactant has traditionally been administered through an endotracheal tube (ETT) either

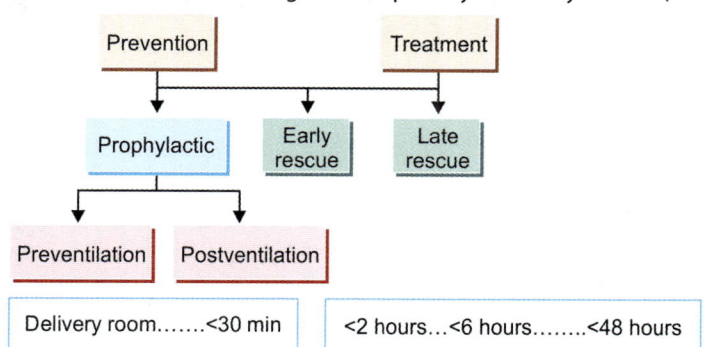

Flowchart 1: Surfactant strategies for respiratory distress syndrome (RDS).

as bolus, in smaller aliquots or by infusion through an adaptor port on the proximal end of the endotracheal tube (Box 3). Changing the chest position after installation is not recommended.

INSURE–surfactant administration after intubation and brief ventilation of less than 60 min.

LISA/ MIST-Uses a fine catheter placed in the trachea under direct or video-laryngoscopy, with the infant spontaneously breathing on CPAP/ NIV. Specialised catheters designed for this method are available. Recent evidence is suggesting that LISA is superior in terms of reducing need for MV and the combined outcome of death or BPD.

Number of Dosages

The evidence in randomized trials supports two doses is better than a single dose. The repeat dose can be given after 6–12 hours based on surfactant preparation used. Criteria for repeat dose are:
- Persistent or recurrent oxygen requirement of 30% or more
- No change in FIO_2 requirement by 6 hours
- Still intubated at 12 hours from the last dose
- a/A ratio of <0.22.

> **Box 3**
> Steps for surfactant administration.
> - Assess, support and maintain temperature, airway, breathing, circulation, and sugar
> - Ensure the infant has heart rate, SpO_2 monitor
> - Ensure strict asepsis
> - Calculate the dose based on weight. Keep the surfactant in room temperature for at least 20 minutes. Do not shake or agitate
> - Prepare a sterile field and keep syringe and the 5 Fr feeding tube ready. Cut the feeding tube to the desired length—the length of the cut endotracheal tube (ETT) plus 3 cm for the adaptor
> - Draw the surfactant dose with a big bore needle with the assistant holding the vial in an inverted position
> - Prime the catheter with surfactant (approximately 0.4 cc). The dose to be given should equal the amount in the syringe
> - Administer surfactant dose in 2–4 aliquots by disconnecting the ET, inserting the feeding tube to premeasured distance via the ET. Hand ventilate the baby allowing the baby to stabilize over next few minutes to administer the next aliquot
> - After the complete dose has been administered monitor bedside over next 30–60 minutes the clinical course (Table 2). Anticipate and prepare for complications (Table 3)
> - Do not attempt suction postsurfactant administration for at least 6 hours unless there is acute threatening event
> - Consider an arterial blood gases (ABG), 30 minutes postsurfactant administration

Table 2: Monitoring for surfactant administration.

During therapy	After therapy
• Heart rate and respirations • Chest expansion • Skin color, and vigor • Chest-wall movement • Oxygen saturation • Proper placement and position of delivery device • FiO_2 and ventilator settings • Reflux of surfactant into ETT • Position of patient (i.e. head direction)	• Heart rate and respirations • Chest expansion • Skin color, and vigor • Breath sounds • Blood pressure • Chest radiograph • Ventilator settings (PIP, PEEP, Paw) and FIO_2 • ABG

(ABG: arterial blood gases; ETT: endotracheal tube; Paw: mean airway pressure; PEEP: positive end-expiratory pressure; PIP: peak inspiratory pressure)

Table 3: Complications of surfactant administration.

Procedural	Physiologic
• Plugging of endotracheal tube • Hemoglobin desaturation • Bradycardia • Tachycardia • Pharyngeal deposition • Administration to only one lung • Suboptimal dose delivery secondary to miscalculation or error in reconstitution	• Apnea • Pulmonary hemorrhage • Mucus plugs • Increased necessity for treatment for patent ductus arteriosus (PDA) • Barotrauma

Administering more than three doses has not been shown to have added benefit.

Role of Antenatal Steroids in Surfactant Era

- Use of antenatal steroids has an additive and synergistic effect on outcomes of RDS when treated with surfactant (Flowchart 2).
- All mothers with threatened preterm labor should be administered antenatal steroids irrespective of availability of surfactant (Table 4 and Fig. 1).
- An important additional benefit of antenatal steroids is a reduction in risk of intraventricular hemorrhage, an advantage not found with surfactant replacement alone. The effects of antenatal steroids on other neonatal morbidities, such as necrotizing enterocolitis and patent ductus arteriosus, have been inconsistent. However, antenatal steroids have not significantly decreased the incidence of BPD.

Nonresponders to Surfactant Therapy

Consider wrong dose, wrong technique, wrong disease, or wrong baby in addition to following:
- Lung injury prior to birth
- Lung injury after birth and prior to treatment
- Pulmonary hypoplasia
- Cardiovascular disease

SECTION 5
Specific Therapies

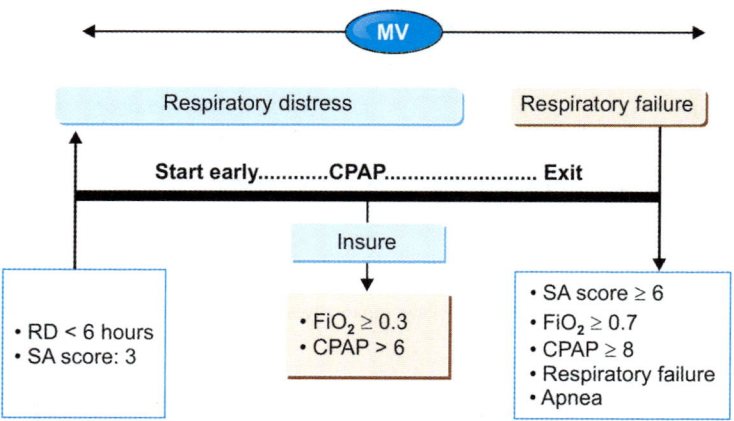

Flowchart 2: Timeline for surfactant.

(CPAP: continuous positive airway pressure; FiO$_2$: fraction of inspired oxygen; InSurE: intubate, surfactant, extubate; MV: mechanical ventilation; RD: respiratory distress; SA score: Silverman-Anderson Score)

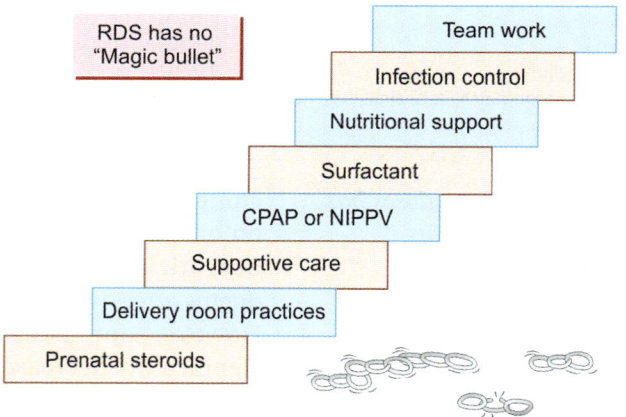

Fig. 1: "Chain of interventions" for best RDS outcome.

(CPAP: continuous positive airway pressure; NIPPV: nasal intermittent positive pressure ventilation; RDS: respiratory distress syndrome)

Table 4: Algorithm for surfactant replacement therapy.

GA < 26 weeks	*GA 29–31 weeks*	*GA ≥ 32 weeks*
Prophylaxis in delivery room (100 mg/kg) especially if no antenatal steroids or if need intubation	Early nCPAP	Observe
Extubate to nCPAP	Early rescue with 100 mg/kg if FIO$_2$ > 0.30	Rescue with 100–200 mg/kg if FiO$_2$ > 0.40

(GA: gestational age; nCPAP: nasal continuous positive airway pressure)

SUGGESTED READING

1. Polin RA, Carlo WA, Committee on Fetus and Newborn. Surfactant replacement therapy for preterm and term neonates with respiratory distress. Pediatrics. 2014;133:156-63.
2. Sardesai S, Biniwale M, Wertheimer F, et al. Evolution of surfactant therapy for respiratory distress syndrome: past, present, and future. Pediatr Res. 2017;81(1-2):240-8.
3. Sweet DG, Carnielli V, Greisen G. European consensus guidelines in management of neonatal RDS in preterm infant. Neonatology. 2013;103:353-68.

CHAPTER 62

Continuous Positive Airway Pressure

Nandkishor Kabra

INDICATIONS

- Respiratory distress syndrome (RDS)
- Postextubation from ventilation support
- Apnea of prematurity
- Transient tachypnea of newborn
- Pneumonia
- Meconium aspirations syndrome
- Pulmonary edema
- Pulmonary hemorrhage
- Laryngo/tracheo/bronchomalacia.

CONTRAINDICATIONS

- Poor respiratory efforts not improving by continuous positive airway pressure (CPAP) therapy
- Shock/hypotension/severe cardiovascular instability
- Congenital malformations of the airway such as choanal atresia, cleft palate, tracheoesophageal fistula, congenital diaphragmatic hernia.
- Progressive respiratory failure with pH < 7.2 and PCO_2 > 65 in arterial blood gases (ABGs).

COMPONENTS OF CONTINUOUS POSITIVE AIRWAY PRESSURE

- Pressure generator:
  - *Continuous flow devices*: Ventilator, conventional CPAP, bubble CPAP (bCPAP)
  - *Variable flow devices*: Infant flow driver, SiPAP.
- Gas source and circuit that provides warm humidified blended air and oxygen mixture.
- *Patient interface*: Nasal prongs, nasal masks, nasal cannulae, nasopharyngeal prongs, etc.

Initiation and Adjustments

- Preparing the device/machine and circuit
- Fixing the cap
- Securing CPAP interface (choose appropriate size as per infant's weight and size)
- Connecting the circuit to interface
- Insertion of orogastric tube
- Setting positive end-expiratory pressure (PEEP), FiO_2, and flow:
  - Start with PEEP of 5 cm and adjust upward or downward between 4 and 8 cm as needed

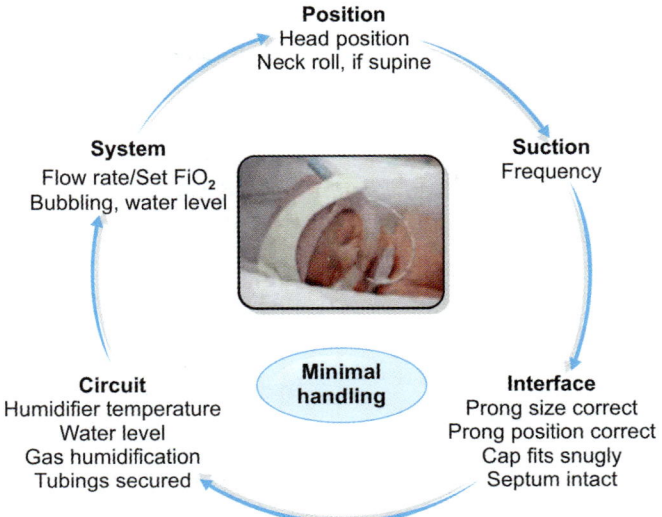

Fig. 1: Setting of continuous positive airway pressure (CPAP) in a neonate.

Flowchart 1: Algorithm for managing a newborn baby with respiratory distress syndrome (RDS).

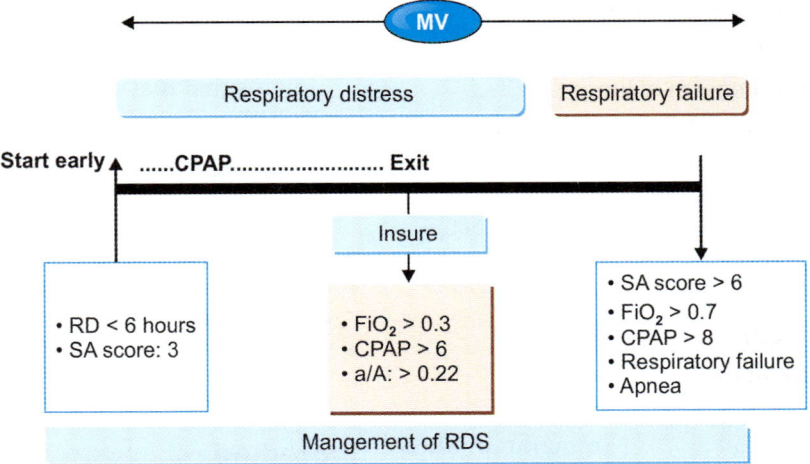

(CPAP: continuous positive airway pressure; SA score: Silverman–Anderson score; MV: mechanical ventilation).

- In bubble CPAP devices, set minimal flow to produce continuous bubbling in the bubbling chamber. Generally, started at 5 L/min and adjusted as needed.
- Start with FiO_2 of 40–50% and adjust to keep SpO_2 in target range (91–95%) (Flowchart 1).

Monitoring (Fig. 1)

- Continuous monitoring of temperature, HR, RR, SpO_2
- Monitoring chest retractions and signs of respiratory distress by SAS or Downe's score

- Sensorium
- *Perfusion*: Capillary refill time, blood pressure, peripheral pulses, and urine output
- Chest X-ray
- Periodic blood gases as per unit's policy
  - Abdominal distension by monitoring circumference.

Adequate Continuous Positive Airway Pressure

- Infant appearing comfortable
- Nil or minimal chest retractions
- Normal perfusion and blood pressure
- SpO_2 in target range (91–95%)
- Acceptable blood gases.

Complications

- Air leaks
- Shock due to decreased cardiac output due to over distension of lungs
- Decreased pulmonary blood flow with increased pulmonary vascular resistance due to inappropriately high CPAP
- Gastric over distension and CPAP belly
- Nasal trauma.

Continuous Positive Airway Pressure Failure

- CPAP pressure more than 8 cm
- $FiO_2 > 80\%$
- Recurrent apnea

  (To maintain SPO_2 more than 90%)

- Arterial blood gas showing respiratory acidosis
- Severe distress Silverman score > 6.

Potential Best Practices to Prevent Continuous Positive Airway Pressure Failure

- Early intervention if no AN steroids
- Consider T-piece resuscitator (<28 weeks)
- Prefer bCPAP over variable flow for extubation
- Early use of caffeine (<3 days in <28 weeks)
- Keep airway clear (suction 3–4 hours)
- Consider sustained lung inflation (<28 weeks)
- Dedicated team work.

INTUBATE, SURFACTANT AND EXTUBATE (INSURE) PROCEDURE

Indications

Any nonintubated infants with clinical signs of respiratory distress or other evidence of RDS like abnormal gas (respiratory acidosis), worsening FiO_2 requirement or abnormal chest X-ray can be considered for the procedure.

- Eligible infants should have good respiratory effort
- Preferably less than 6 hours old (earlier the age of INSURE, better the outcomes).

Infants that may not be good candidates for INSURE:

- Intubated at birth for apneas/poor respiratory effort, unless strong respiratory efforts established after appropriate resuscitation
- Neonates who have received extensive resuscitation
- Any associated medical issues, e.g. anemia, hydrops.

Procedure

- No premedication
- Intubation as per existing Neonatal Clinical Guidelines
- Tube size according to the gestational age and weight or a smaller sized ETT
- Check tube placement with auscultation.
- Surfactant to be administered in bolus aliquots as per standard surfactant administration procedure
- Extubate to nCPAP following re-establishment of airflow.

Before Extubation Ensure

- Heart rate and oxygen saturations are stable
- FiO_2 less than the presurfactant level
- No apneas
- Adequate airflow without clinical evidence of airway obstruction
- Nasal CPAP prongs/masks are in position to ensure smooth transfer from ETT CPAP to nasal CPAP and minimize risk of lung collapse.

Other Recommendations

- One-to-one nursing is recommended for the duration of the administration and observations
- Medical supervision is recommended. Senior registrar/consultant to supervise administration of appropriate dose of surfactant
- Ventilate using the T-piece resuscitator until stable
- Keep ventilator as a standby
- Extubate to nCPAP as soon as possible.

ASSESSMENT CHECKLIST FOR CONTINUOUS POSITIVE AIRWAY PRESSURE

Note the following:
- Nose:
    - Note the size, shape, and position in relation to the rest of the face
    - Are the nares symmetrical, stretched out?
    - Is there any blanching of skin at nares?
    - Is there a skin breakdown?
    - Septum position; is it straight or does it appear crooked?
    - Is there nasal flaring?
    - Compress the tip of the nose and note whether the nares remains symmetrical If they do not remain symmetrical, the neonate may have a dislocated septum
    - Note the color, consistency, and quantity of nasal secretions
    - Is the nasal interface component twisted because of tension on the tubing?
    - Is the nasal prong of appropriate size?
    - Is the cap appropriately placed?
- Chest:
    - Divide the chest into right and left sides and then divide each side into thirds
    - Auscultate and compare the differences between the right side and the left side
    - Note the quality of breath sounds in each area.
- CPAP system:
    - What is the actual pressure and FiO_2 reading at versus the medical orders?
    - Is there bubbling?
    - Is the humidification appropriate?
    - Is the flow rate adequate?
- Newborn:
    - What is the color, activity, posture, comfort?
    - How is the work of breathing (WOB): Rate, effort, pattern, retraction, chest movement, grunt, air entry?
    - How is the temperature setting?
    - What are the monitor readings?
    - What is the urine output?

SUGGESTED READING

1. Gupta S, Donn SM. Continuous positive airway pressure: physiology and comparison of devices. Semin Fetal Neonatal Med. 2016;21(3):204-11.
2. Jensen EA, Chaudhary A, Bhutta ZA, et al. Non-invasive respiratory support for infants in low- and middle-income countries. Semin Fetal Neonatal Med. 2016;21(3):181-8.
3. Sahni R, Schiaratura M, Polin RA. Strategies for the prevention of continuous positive airway pressure failure. Semin Fetal Neonatal Med. 2016;21(3):196-203.
4. Subramaniam P, Ho JJ, Davis PG. Prophylactic nasal continuous positive airway pressure for preventing morbidity and mortality in very preterm infants. Cochrane Database Syst Rev. 2016:(6):CD001243.

CHAPTER 63

INtubate, SURfactant, Extubate (INSURE) Procedure

Nandkishor Kabra

INDICATIONS

- Clinical signs of respiratory distress
- Increasing oxygen requirement
- Increasing continuous positive airway pressure (CPAP).

ELIGIBILITY CRITERION

- Infant has good respiratory effort
- Age preferably less than 6 hours old [earlier the age of INtubate, SURfactant, Extubate (INSURE), better the outcomes].

POOR CANDIDATES

- Need for intubation at birth.
- Neonates with prolonged resuscitation
- Comorbid conditions, e.g. hypothermia, shock, sepsis, anemia, and hydrops.

PROCEDURE

- Intubate with standard precautions and continuous monitoring
- Use appropriate size of endotracheal tube (ETT) based on gestation or weight
- Check appropriate placement of ETT
- Administer surfactant in separate aliquots with intermittent ventilation
- Extubate to nCPAP after the last dose.

BEFORE EXTUBATION ENSURE

- Stable heart rate and oxygen saturation
- Regular breathing
- Nasal CPAP prongs/masks are in position to ensure smooth transfer from ETT CPAP to nasal CPAP and minimize risk of lung collapse.

CLINICAL PEARLS

- Ensure continuous monitoring and an attendant to help, if required
- Ventilate using the T-piece resuscitator or positive pressure ventilation until stable
- Keep ventilator as backup
- Extubate to nCPAP as soon as possible.

SUGGESTED READING

1. Gupta S, Donn SM. Continuous positive airway pressure: physiology and comparison of devices. Semin Fetal Neonatal Med. 2016;21(3):204-11.
2. Jensen EA, Chaudhary A, Bhutta ZA, et al. Non-invasive respiratory support for infants in low- and middle-income countries. Semin Fetal Neonatal Med. 2016;21(3):181-8.
3. Sahni R, Schiaratura M, Polin RA. Strategies for the prevention of continuous positive airway pressure failure. Semin Fetal Neonatal Med. 2016;21(3):196-203.
4. Subramaniam P, Ho JJ, Davis PG. Prophylactic nasal continuous positive airway pressure for preventing morbidity and mortality in very preterm infants. Cochrane Database Syst Rev. 2016;(6):CD001243.

CHAPTER 64

Blood Component Therapy

Pramod Gaddam, Deepak Sharma, Tejopratap Oleti

INTRODUCTION

Blood transfusion therapy is an integral part of modern neonatal care. Sick neonates are one of the most heavily transfused groups of patients in modern medicine; nearly 85% of extremely low birth weight (ELBW) babies get transfusions during their hospital stay. As newer evidence favors restricted transfusion guidelines in comparison to liberal transfusion policy, the guidelines for blood transfusion have changed in recent times. The audit of blood transfusion should be integral part of quality care management in all nursery. The current concept is using a component rather than whole blood.

Blood components used in transfusion are:
- Whole blood
- Packed red blood cells (RBCs)
- Platelets
- Plasma
- Cryoprecipitate.

INDICATIONS FOR TRANSFUSION

Whole Blood

Indications of use:
- Exchange transfusions
- Pre- or postcardiac surgery with measured blood loss
- Priming circuit of extracorporeal membrane oxygenation (ECMO) or cardiopulmonary bypass
- Blood replacement after acute blood loss.

Now-a-days, its use has been limited to exchange transfusion therapy in neonates. The advantage of whole blood for exchange transfusion is a lower risk of posttransfusion polycythemia. Whole blood should have hematocrit between 50% and 55%.

Which Blood Group to use?

As maternal RBC might be circulating in neonatal blood in first few days of life, therefore, before blood transfusion, blood must be cross-matched with both mother and neonatal blood for initial 3 months of life (Table 1).

Table 1: Choice of blood group for whole blood transfusion.

Mother's blood group	Infant blood group	Donor blood group
O	O, A, B, or AB	O
A, B, AB	O, A, B, or AB	Baby blood group or O group
Rh negative	Rh negative or Rh positive	Rh negative

Volume of Blood to be used for Exchange Transfusion

- *Single volume*: 80–90 mL/kg
- *Indication*: Sepsis, metabolic acidosis
- *Double volume*: 160–180 mL/kg
- *Indication*: Severe hyperbilirubinemia.

PRECAUTIONS BEFORE TRANSFUSION

- Fresh donor blood should be less than 5 days old (maximum 7 days)
- Use donor blood that is irradiated within 24 hours before transfusion to prevent graft versus host disease
- Before the procedure, the blood should be warmed to body temperature using either a water bath or by wrapping the container in a warmed towel
- Avoid warming under radiant warmer
- Transfusion should be given either by syringe pump or pediatric intravenous (IV) set and infusion pump should be avoided
- Exchange transfusion should be through a standard blood giving set with a clot screen filter (170–200 μm) *(see also general principles of transfusion).*

Table 2: Transfusion guidelines.

Hematocrit	Clinical features
≤20%	• Asymptomatic neonate after 28 days of age with reticulocyte count <1%
≤25%	• Experiencing weight gain <10 g/day over at least 4 days while receiving 100 kcal/kg/day • Tachycardia, poor feeding • Receiving any supplemental oxygen
≤30%	• Requiring continuous positive airway pressure or mechanical ventilation with mean airway pressure <6 cm H_2O and FiO_2 less than 35% • Undergoing surgery within 72 hours
≤35%	• Requiring >35% oxygen with continuous positive airway pressure or mechanical ventilation with mean airway pressure of more than 6 cm H_2O
Acute blood loss	• Greater than 10% of blood volume with features of decreased oxygen delivery or greater than 20% of blood volume

PACKED RED BLOOD CELLS

Packed red blood cells (PRBCs) is used for resolution of symptomatic anemia and to improve tissue oxygenation.

When to Transfuse?

There is limited scientific evidence on thresholds at which newborn infants should be transfused (Table 2).

Transfusion triggers vary with etiology, age, and general condition of the neonate.

Severe anemia of antenatal onset: Anemia occurring before birth, characterized by Hb < 8/dL at birth and it requires prompt transfusion.

- In severe anemia associated with immunohemolysis, chronic fetomaternal, or fetofetal hemorrhage, the most appropriate treatment is "partial" exchange transfusion (PET) with PRBC for reducing the volume overload.
- In severe anemia with hypovolemic shock due to causes like placenta previa, abruption placentae, rupture of the cord, requires blood transfusion for correction of anemia.

Early neonatal anemia: For anemia developing after birth or in the first 4 week of life, in which the values of Hb are moderately decreased, transfusion treatment is necessary in the case of severe cardiopulmonary diseases, in order to maintain the packed cell volume (PCV) greater than 35–40%.

Late neonatal anemia: The below guidelines can be used.

Which Blood Group to Choose for Blood Transfusion?

Blood should be of newborn's ABO and Rh group, cross matched with both mother and neonate.

Volume and Rate of Transfusion

- Volume of PRBC

$$\frac{\text{Blood volume (mL/kg)} \times (\text{Desired} - \text{Actual hematocrit})}{\text{Hematocrit of transfused RBC}}$$

- A dose of 20 mL/kg is well tolerated and results in an overall decrease in number of transfusions compared to transfusions done at 10 mL/kg
- Hematocrit of transfused PRBC should be 60–65%.
- Rate of not more than 10 mL/kg/h in the absence of cardiac failure and in presence of cardiac failure rate is 2 mL/kg/h. Transfusion should be done always through a clot screen filter 170–200 μm.
- PRBC transfusion in preterm neonates should be restricted to minimum to prevent complications such as increased incidence of retinopathy of prematurity (ROP), cytomegalovirus (CMV) infection, and even necrotizing enterocolitis (NEC).
- Each transfusion of 9 mL/kg of body weight should increase hemoglobin level by 3 g/dL *(see also general principles of transfusion).*

Platelets

Thrombocytopenia is defined as platelet count less than 1.5 lakh/mm³. The incidence is 1–5% in newborns at birth. Severe thrombocytopenia is defined as platelet count

Table 3: Indications for platelet transfusion.

Platelet count	Symptoms
<30,000	None
30,000–50,000	• Sick or bleeding • Less than 1,000 g • <7 days old • Concurrent coagulopathy • Major IVH grade 3 or 4 • Requiring surgery, exchange transfusion
50,000–90,000	Actively bleeding

(IVH: intraventricular hemorrhage)

less than 50,000/mm³. In neonatal intensive-care units (NICUs), the incidence is as high as 22–35%.

In neonatal alloimmune thrombocytopenia (NAIT) and idiopathic thrombocytopenic purpura (ITP), aim is to maintain the platelet count above 30,000/mm³ (Table 3).

In NAIT, washed and irradiated maternal platelet is first choice, in the absence of which single donor platelets (SDP)/random donor platelets (RDP) can be used.

Indications for Platelet Transfusion in Nonimmune Thrombocytopenia

Random Donor Platelets versus Single Donor Platelets (Table 4)

- Infant and donor should be ABO identical or compatible
- Never use a *filter* during platelet transfusion
- Platelets should be stored at 22–24°C with continuous gentle agitation in platelet incubator and agitator
- "Washed platelets" can be used in patients with anaphylactic reactions to the plasma component *(see also general principles of transfusion).*

Plasma Derivatives

Plasma contains about 1 unit/mL of each of the coagulation factors as well as normal

Table 4: Random donor versus single donor platelet transfusion.

	Random donor platelets (RDP)	Single donor platelets (SDP)
Preparation	From multiple whole blood units by pooling	From single donor by plateletpheresis
Platelet density	0.5×10^{11}/unit	3×10^{11}/unit
Dosage	15 mL/kg	15 mL/kg
Predicted improvement	20,000/mm^3	60,000/mm^3
Duration of administration	Over 30 minutes	Over 30 minutes
Storage period	5 days, needs constant agitation	7 days, needs constant agitation
Advantage	Less cost	Avoids multiple donor exposure

Table 5: Storage characteristics of blood and blood products.

Product	Storage temperature	Shelf life	Transport temperature
Whole blood			
• CPD	1–6°C	21 days	1–10°C
• CPDA1/A2	1–6°C	35 days	1–10°C
PRBC (CPDA1/A2)	1–4°C	35 days	1–10°C
PRBC (SAG-M)	1–4°C	42 days	1–10°C
Platelets constant agitation	22°C	3–5 days	20–24°C
Granulocyte	4°C	<24 hours	
FFP	–20°C	1 year	1–10°C once thawed
Cryoprecipitate	–18°C	1 year	20–24°C once thawed

(CPD: citrate phosphate dextrose; CPDA: citrate-phosphate-dextrose-adenine; FFP: fresh frozen plasma; PRBC: packed blood red cell)

concentrations of other plasma proteins. Labile coagulation factors, like factors V and VIII, are not stable in plasma stored for prolonged periods at 1–6°C; therefore, plasma is usually stored frozen at –18°C or lower (Table 5).

Fresh Frozen Plasma

Fresh frozen plasma (FFP) is stored within 8 hours of collection. It contains about 87% of factor VIII at the time of collection and must contain at least 0.70 IU/mL of factor VIII.

Indications for Transfusing Fresh Frozen Plasma

1. Disseminated intravascular coagulopathy
2. Vitamin K deficiency bleeding
3. Inherited deficiencies of coagulation factors
4. Hepatic failure
5. Prophylaxis of bleeding for an invasive procedure in the presence of coagulopathy
6. Circuit priming for cardiopulmonary bypass
7. Circuit priming for ECMO
8. Exchange transfusion for hyperbilirubinemia with PRBC.

Dosing: 10–20 mL/kg is usually adequate dose. Dose of 10 mL/kg should increase clotting factors and inhibitor levels by approximately 10 IU/dL (10%).

Fresh frozen plasma (FFP) should be group AB, or compatible with recipient's ABO red cell antigens.

Cryoprecipitate

Cryoprecipitate contains about 80–100 U of factor VIII in 10–25 mL of plasma, 300 mg of fibrinogen, and varying amounts of factor XIII. It is stored at a temperature of –20°C or below.

Indications for use of Cryoprecipitate

- Congenital factor VIII deficiency
- Congenital factor XIII deficiency
- Afibrinogenemia and dysfibrinogenemia
- Von Willebrand disease.

Dose: Cryoprecipitate: 5 mL/kg.

Storage and Shelf Life of Blood and Blood Products

General Principles of Transfusion

1. Select appropriate donor:
   - Avoid blood donation from first and second degree relatives.
   - Donor should be seronegative for human immunodeficiency virus (HIV), hepatitis B, hepatitis C, malaria, and cytomegalovirus
2. Use appropriate component
3. Parent's consent should be obtained prior to transfusion explaining about all the risk associated
4. Blood should ideally be:
   - Less than 5 days old, with hematocrit of 0.5–0.6
   - Leukodepleted by using preissue (blood bank) or postissue (bedside) filters:
     ♦ Irradiated especially for preterm. Dosage 25–50 Gy. To be used within 48 hours
     ♦ Use piggyback bags to avoid multiple donor exposure (*no guidelines for usage of reconstituted blood in India*).
5. Treat patient not laboratory values in deciding upon transfusion
6. Checklist during transfusion:
   - Check donor and recipient details
   - Monitor vitals during and posttransfusion
7. Awareness of hazards of transfusion (Table 6)
   - Infectious: HIV, hepatitis B, malaria, febrile reaction
   - Noninfectious-like volume overload, metabolic-like hypoglycemia, hyperkalemia, immune-mediated hemolysis
8. How to minimize transfusion:
   - Minimize iatrogenic blood loss: Minimizing sampling, using microanalysis techniques, in-line arterial sampling
   - Delayed cord clamping at birth
   - Use of early erythropoietin in minimizing transfusion in preterm infants. Cochrane meta-analysis concludes that early administration of erythropoietin (EPO) reduces the use of RBC transfusions and the volume of RBCs transfused. These small reductions are of limited clinical importance. There was also a significant increase in the rate of ROP (stage ≥ 3).
   - *Recombinant granulocyte-macrophage colony-stimulating factor (GM-CSF):* Currently, there is insufficient evidence to support the introduction of either G-CSF or GM-CSF into neonatal practice, either as treatment of established systemic infection to reduce resulting mortality, or as prophylaxis to prevent systemic infection in high-risk neonates. The limited data suggesting that CSF treatment may reduce mortality when systemic infection is accompanied by severe neutropenia should be investigated further in adequately powered trials which recruit sufficient infants infected with organisms associated with a significant mortality risk.

Table 6: Complications of blood product transfusion.

Name of reaction	Definition	Age of onset	Prevention
Acute hemolytic transfusion reaction	These reactions are because of incompatibility of donor RBCs with antibodies in the patient's plasma. The antibodies usually responsible for it are isohemagglutinins (anti-A, anti-B). These reactions are very rarely seen in neonatal period as they do not make isohemagglutinins until they are 4 to 6 months old	Less than 24 hours	Blood compatible to both mother and neonate Watch for acute drop in PCV or urine output after transfusion. Administer fluids and diuretics for protecting kidneys. Treat hypotension with vasopressor
Allergic reaction	Due to antibodies in the patient's plasma that react with proteins in donor plasma. Rarely seen in neonatal period as they do not make isohemagglutinins until they are 4–6 months old	Less than 24 hours	Blood compatible to both mother and neonate Watch for hemodynamic parameters during transfusion Keep hydrocortisone and adrenaline available in NICU
Volume overload	All the blood components have high oncotic pressure and rapid infusion can cause excessive intravascular volume, leading to hemodynamic decompensation	Less than 24 hours	Using fixed volume of blood transfusion
Hyperkalemia	RBC leakage during storage increases the concentration of potassium in the unit. In stored blood, potassium levels tend to be high. It has been seen that after storage for around 42 days, potassium levels may reach 50 mEq/L in a RBC unit	Less than 24 hours	Use blood less than age of 5 days
Hypocalcemia	Citrate, commonly used to anticoagulate blood components, chelates calcium and thereby inhibits the coagulation cascade. This is mainly seen with massive blood transfusion (>60 mL/kg)	Less than 24 hours	Calcium supplementation if massive blood transfusion is done
Hypothermia	Refrigerated (4°C) or frozen (−18°C or below) blood components can result in hypothermia when rapidly infused	Less than 24 hours	Transfuse prewarmed blood using blood warmers
Transfusion associated acute lung injury (TRALI)	Refers to noncardiogenic pulmonary edema complicating transfusion therapy. This is often due to antibodies in donor plasma that react with the patient's histo-compatibility (HLA) antigens	Less than 24 hours	Blood compatible to both mother and neonate Monitor for symptoms and stop
Transfusion associated acute gut injury (TRAGI)	Characterized by severe neonatal gastro-intestinal reaction temporally related to a transfusion of packed blood red cells (PRBCs)	Less than 24 hours	Nil per orally during blood transfusion

Contd...

Contd...

Name of reaction	Definition	Age of onset	Prevention
Febrile nonhemolytic transfusion reaction	Usually due to cytokines released from leukocytes in the donor unit	Less than 24 hours	Leukodepleted blood transfusion. Keep hydrocortisone and adrenaline available in NICU
Infectious complication	Transmission of HIV, HBV, HCV, HTLV 1, HTLV 2, CMV, malaria		Prescreening of transfused blood
Graft versus host disease	Lymphocytes from donor blood components can mount an immune response against the patient	Less than 24 hours	Leukodepleted and irradiated blood transfusion. Dedicated allocation of single donor blood and platelets to the neonate
Iron overload	PRBC contains significant amount of iron		To check for iron overload parameters when the baby requires multiple transfusion

(CMV: cytomegalovirus; HBV: hepatitis B virus; HCV: hepatitis C virus; HIV: human immunodeficiency virus; HTLV 1: human T-lymphotropic virus 1; HTLV 2: human T-lymphotropic virus 2; NICU: newborn intensive care unit; RBC: red blood cell)

- *Granulocyte transfusion:* Granulocyte transfusion is indicated for severe bacterial and fungal sepsis with neutropenia that is unresponsive to therapy with antimicrobials. Currently, evidence is not conclusive regarding its usage.

SUGGESTED READING

1. Bell EF. Transfusion thresholds for preterm infants: how low should we go? J Pediatr. 2006;149:287-9.
2. Joint United Kingdom (UK) Blood Transfusion and Tissue Transplantation Services Professional Advisory Committee guidelines. http://www.transfusionguidelines.org.uk/transfusion-handbook/10-effective-transfusion-in-paediatric-practice/10-2-neonatal-transfusion
3. Maier RF, Obladen M, Muller-Hansen I, et al. Early treatment with erythropoietin beta ameliorates anemia and reduces transfusion requirements in infants with birth weights below 1000 g. J Pediatr. 2002;141:8.
4. Rothenberger S. Neonatal alloimmune thrombocytopenia. Ther Apher. 2002;6:32-5.
5. Tucci M. Goal-directed blood transfusion therapies. Current Concepts in Pediatric Critical Care Refresher Course available at http//sccmcms.scom.org. Accessed on April 15, 2008.

CHAPTER
65

Total Parenteral Nutrition

Tushar B Parikh

INTRODUCTION

Birth of a preterm, low birth weight (LBW) baby is considered as a "nutritional emergency." Inadequate nutrient intake for even 1 day can put extremely preterm neonate into catabolic stress and negative nitrogen balance. Published literature suggests that "extra-uterine growth retardation" is a major universal clinical problem in preterm infants. Total parenteral nutrition (TPN) refers to provision of total spectrum of nutrients through the intravenous route.

There is a considerable body of evidence to suggest that nutrition at this early age not only determines long-term physical growth but also intellectual development.

Who should give total parenteral nutrition?
All level II B and level III units should have facility for parenteral nutrition (PN). The level II B and level III units look after sick neonates and preterm neonates who cannot be fed enterally. These units should provide space for preparation and dispensing PN.

Which babies need total parenteral nutrition?
Following are broad common indications for use of TPN in neonatal intensive care unit (NICU).

- Prematurity <28 weeks gestation and/or <1,000 g should start TPN on day 1.
- Prematurity <32 weeks gestation and/or <1,500 g who are unable to achieve reasonable enteral feeds by day 3.
- Infants >32 weeks and/or >1,500 g who are unlikely to achieve at least 50% enteral feeds by day 5.
  - Necrotizing enterocolitis (NEC)
  - Surgically correctable gastrointestinal tract anomalies (exomphalus, gastroschisis, atresia of intestine, volvulus, etc.), both preoperatively and postoperatively
  - Short bowel syndrome.

BROAD OUTLINE OF TOTAL PARENTERAL NUTRITION THERAPY

Preparation of Total Parenteral Nutrition

- Parenteral nutrition can be prepared by anyone who is trained in PN preparation such as, by the neonatologist pediatrician, pediatric residents, nursing staff, or nutritionist.
- Identifying nutrient requirements and their dosage calculation is the first step in preparation of TPN.

- A strict sterile aseptic technique with surgical scrub is essential during mixing of nutrients (compounding). Use of laminar flow is desirable. Strict aseptic technique with surgical scrubbing should be continued during connecting TPN to the central venous catheter.

Administration of Total Parenteral Nutrition

- Parenteral nutrition can be delivered through peripheral or central venous lines. TPN solution with glucose concentration more than 12.5% should be infused through central line. Peripherally inserted central catheter (PICC) or umbilical venous catheter can be used.
- Position of central line should be confirmed by X-ray or point-of-care ultrasound, before starting infusion. The venous access used for PN should not be interrupted for giving antibiotics or other medications.
- Lipid solution is infused by a syringe pump and rest TPN contents, viz. dextrose, amino acids, electrolytes, etc. are mixed together in a sterile bottle or syringe and infused separately.
- The two preparations can be infused through same line/cannula by joining together with a three-way connector (Fig. 1). At the time of connecting TPN through a central line, one has to follow strict asepsis guidelines.
- A bacterial filter is used in-line with the amino acid, dextrose, and electrolyte infusion (Fig. 1).

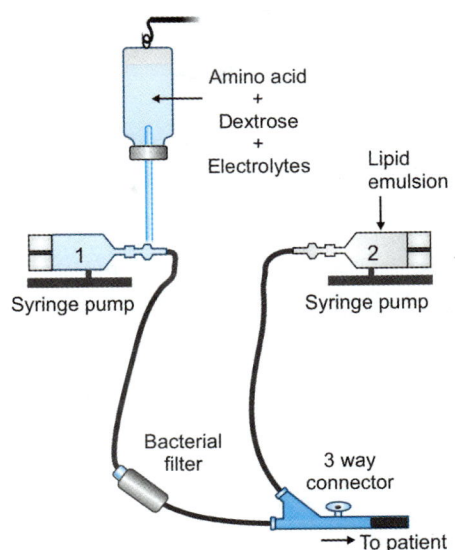

Fig. 1: Total parenteral nutrition (TPN) infusion assembly.

NUTRIENTS IN TOTAL PARENTERAL NUTRITION

Fluid and Electrolytes

Fluid intake for a baby depends upon the gestational age, weight, and day of life. One has to also take into account insensible losses due to radiant warmer, phototherapy, ambient humidity, etc. Starting volume of fluids recommended is given in Table 1.

The initial fluids should be 10% dextrose in order to maintain glucose infusion rate of 4–6 mg/kg/min. Subsequently, fluid intake is increased depending on clinical examination, weight, urine output, and serum electrolytes (Tables 2 to 4).

Table 1: Day-wise recommended fluid volume (mL/kg/day).

	Day 1	Days 2–3	Days 4–5	Days 6–7	Days >7
<1,000 g	80–100	120	140	150	150–170
1,000–1,500 g	80	100	120	140	150
>1,500 g	60	80	100	120	150

Table 2: Guidelines for starting electrolytes in fluid therapy.

Electrolytes	Day 1	Day 3 onward
Sodium (Na)	Nil	3 mEq/kg/day
Potassium (K)	Nil	2 mEq/kg/day
Chloride (Cl)	Nil	3–5 mEq/kg/day

Na:
- Normal Na$^+$: 135–145 mEq/L
- Supplementation: 2–3 mEq/kg/day (may be higher in ELBW)
- Begin supplementation on Day 3 of life generally after 6–10% weight loss of the baby.

K:
- Normal K$^+$: 3.5–5.2 mEq/L
- Supplementation: 1–2 mEq/kg/day
- Levels rise in first 24–72 h in extreme preterms, known as "nonoliguric hyperkalemia."
- Begin supplementation on Day 3 of life after ensuring good urine output (>1 mL/kg/h).

Cl:
- Normal serum Cl: 90–110 mEq/L
- Supplementation: 2–3 mEq/kg/day (same as Na).

Table 3: How to monitor fluid therapy?

Parameter	Frequency of monitoring	Normal limits	Fluid deficit	Fluid overload
Clinical signs*	12 hours		Features of dehydration	Features of over hydration
Weight	Daily	1–3% loss/day	>4%/day	Weight gain/no loss
Urine volume	12 hours	1–3 mL/kg/h	<1 mL/kg/h	>3 mL/kg/h
Urine specific gravity	12 hours	1,008–1,012	>1,020	<1,008
Serum sodium	24 hours (as per need)	135–145 mEq/L	>145	<125 mEq/L
Blood urea	24 hours	20–40 mg/dL	>50 mg/dL	

*Heart rate, blood pressure, skin turgor, mucous membranes, eyes, AF tension, edema, capillary refill time, hepatomegaly (BP changes occur late in response to decreased cardiac output).

Table 4: Goals of fluid therapy.

Parameter	Goal
Urine output	1–3 mL/kg/h
Urine specific gravity	1,010–1,020
Daily weight loss	1–3% of body weight
Clinical signs	Absence of edema/dehydration
Sodium	135–145 mEq/L
Urea	20–40 mg/dL
Serum osmolality	285 mOsm/kg

Table 5: Daily recommended energy intake for preterm infants.

Committee	Recommended intake (kcal/kg/day)
American Academy of Pediatrics	105–130
Canadian Pediatric Society	105–135
European society of Pediatric Gastroenterology and Nutrition	98–128
Life Sciences Research Office	110–135

ENERGY NEEDS

Minimal energy needs for a neonate are met by 50–60 kcal/kg/day. For growth on parenteral nutrition, energy needs for preterm and term neonates are 110–120 kcal/kg/day and 90–100 kcal/kg/day, respectively (Table 5).

Balance of Calories

A correct balance of calories is essential to avoid nutritional side effects of TPN.
- *CHO calories*: 40–50%
- *Fat calories*: 35–45%
- *Protein calories*: 15%.

Carbohydrate (Dextrose)

Dextrose is a source of energy. Each gram dextrose provides 3.4 kcal of energy. Dextrose is started on Day 1, and intake should be calculated as glucose infusion rate (Table 6).

In most of clinical scenarios, 10% dextrose is used. The GIR will increase correspondingly with daily increment in fluid rate. Glucose concentration above 12.5% will require infusion through central line.

Proteins (Amino Acids)

Each gram of protein can provide 4 kcal energy. Neonatal amino acid solution is available as 10% concentration. Neonatal amino acid solution is different than adult solution in that they contain conditionally essential amino acids (cysteine, tyrosine, glutamine, arginine, proline, glycine, and taurine). Therefore, adult amino acid preparations should not be used for neonatal PN.

For a preterm baby: Amino acid supplementation should start on first postnatal day. A minimum amino acid dose should be 1.5 g/kg/day. Higher dose needed to achieve positive nitrogen balance. Daily amino acid dose should be increased by 1 g to achieve maximum dose of 3.5–4 g/kg/day. Studies have shown that higher first week protein intake has direct correlation with better neurodevelopment scores in preterm neonates.

For a term baby: A minimum amino acid intake of 1.5 g/kg/day is recommended to avoid a negative nitrogen balance while a maximum amino acid intake should usually not exceed 3 g/kg/day.

Protein Calorie Ratio

In order to get protein accretion, 30 nonprotein calories (NPC) per gram of amino acid should be provided. If NPC intake is less, the amino acids are utilized for energy generation purpose rather than protein synthesis. Other way of expressing the protein calorie balance is nonprotein energy ratio (NER) or calorie nitrogen ratio (CNR), which can be calculated and maintained between 150 and 250.

$$NER = \frac{NPC\,(Carbohydrate + lipid\ calories)}{1.6 \times protein\,(g)}$$

LIPIDS IN TOTAL PARENTERAL NUTRITION

Lipids are calorie dense source of energy and with low osmolarity. The commercial IV lipid emulsions are aqueous suspensions containing neutral triglycerides derived from soybean, safflower oil, egg yolk to emulsify, and glycerin to adjust tonicity. 1 g of lipid gives 9 kcal energy. In preterm neonates, lipids should be started on Day 1 of life to prevent occurrence of essential fatty acid deficiency. The recommended dose of lipids on Day 1 is 1 g/kg/day. Gradually daily dose is increased to maximum 3 g/kg/day. In preterm, infant's tolerance of lipid emulsions is improved by continuous infusion over 24 hours versus an intermittent regimen with lipid-free intervals. Rate of infusion should be less than 150 mg/kg/min.

Table 6: Carbohydrate (dextrose) in total parenteral nutrition.

• Recommended GIR for preterms on day 1	4–8 mg/kg/min
• Recommended GIR for terms on day 1	3–6 mg/kg/min
How much should be increased daily?	1–2 mg/kg/min
Target blood sugar level	50–150 mg/dL
• Maximum GIR for preterms	12 mg/kg/min

(GIR: glucose infusion rate)

Lipid preparations are available as 10% and 20% but 20% lipid emulsion is preferred over 10%, because the higher phospholipid content of the 10% solution impedes plasma triglyceride clearance, resulting in higher triglyceride and plasma cholesterol concentration. Lipids are potentially vulnerable to photo-oxidation leading to peroxide formation. Hence, the lipid emulsion should be covered with sterile opaque paper or aluminum foil (Table 7).

MULTIVITAMINS IN TOTAL PARENTERAL NUTRITION

Both fat- and water-soluble vitamins are essential for positive growth in the neonate on PN. Vitamins should be started as soon as possible, preferably on Day 1 of TPN.

Vitamins should preferably be added to lipid emulsion to increase stability and reduce peroxide formation. Pediatric MVI solutions are not available in India. Since adult MVI has questionable compatibility with lipids, it is infused through dextrose–amino acid solution. PN solution containing MVI should be protected from light to prevent photo-degradation of photosensitive vitamins. Dose of adult MVI in neonatal PN is 0.5 mL/kg/day.

MINERALS (TABLE 8)

Calcium (Ca), phosphorus (P), and magnesium (Mg) are the three important minerals required in the neonatal period. Estimated requirement is equal to third-trimester fetal accretion rates of 90–140 mg/kg/day for calcium and 30–75 mg/kg/day for phosphorus. If preterm baby does not receive appropriate mineral intake it is prone to osteopenia of prematurity and rickets.

Calcium is provided as 10% calcium gluconate, added to dextrose amino acid solution. Recently, phosphorous preparation is available in India. Magnesium preparation is available as 50% solution and dose is 5–15 mg/day. If phosphorous is added one must ensure that there is no precipitation in the solution.

These minerals should be added from Day 1 and suggested doses are described in Table 8.

Iron

Iron is not routinely provided in parenteral nutrition and is not part of trace element solutions. Whether or not, there is a need for routine iron supplementation in PN remains controversial. During long-term

Table 7: Summary of dosing guidelines for initiation and maintenance of total parenteral nutrition (TPN).

Substrate	Initiation	Advancing	Goals	Comments
Dextrose	5–7 mg/kg/min (10% D)	2–3 mg/kg	10–12 mg/kg/min	• Increase as tolerated • Consider insulin if hyperglycemic
Amino acids	1.5–2 g/kg/day	1 g/kg/day	3–4 g/kg/day	Maintain calorie to nitrogen ratio at approximately 200:1
20% Lipids	1 g/kg/day	1 g/kg/day	3 g/kg/day	Only use 20%

Table 8: Recommended mineral intake.

Mineral	Term neonate	Preterm neonate
Calcium (mg/kg/day)	32	42–120
Phosphate (mg/kg/day)	14	28–64
Magnesium (mg/kg/day)	5	5

PN (>3 weeks), the child's iron status should be monitored closely and supplementation begun as soon as impending deficiency is identified. The preferred modality of iron administration is as regular daily doses. The ideal formulation (dextran, citrate, etc.) has not been adequately studied but data in adults regarding iron dextran shows it to be safe and efficacious.

Trace Elements

Trace elements are elements found in microscopic amounts in the blood but are essential for well-being. Zinc is universally recommended from day 1 of TPN, whereas the other trace minerals are generally indicated if PN is administered for ≥2 weeks. Essential trace elements include zinc, copper, selenium, chromium, manganese, molybdenum, iodide, and iron. Commercially in India, Celcel (Claris) of three varieties (3/5/7 trace elements) is available. Dose is 1 mL/100 mL or 0.2 mL/kg/day. The aim is to provide zinc 400 mcg/kg/day (preterm infants) and 300 mcg/kg/day (term infants), chromium 0.2 mcg/kg/day, and selenium 2 mcg/kg/day. Discontinue chromium, selenium, and molybdenum with patients with renal impairment. Copper and manganese are discontinued from TPN solutions with the complication of cholestasis.

CALCULATION FOR TOTAL PARENTERAL NUTRITION

Calculation of TPN is done with automated software is preferable. These software are accurate, validated, and reduce errors of compounding. Manual method is used when software is not available. Following are the steps in calculation of TPN nutrients, manually:
- Determine total fluid requirement for the day.
- Subtract amount of fluid to be used for medications (e.g. diluting and infusing antibiotics) and enteral feeds.
- Calculate amount of nutrients amino acid, lipids, and glucose to be infused over 24 hours. Lipid is infused separately with a syringe pump. Remaining nutrients are mixed in a bottle/syringe for infusion.
- For calculating amount of each PN component, use following formula:

Amount of PN Compoent

$$= \frac{\text{Amount to be given per kg} \times \text{Body weight}}{\text{Strength of Solution}}$$

For example, for a baby weighing 1.5 kg to be given 3 mEq/kg of sodium, amount of 3% NaCl to be used is:

Amount of 3% NaCl

$$= \frac{3\,\text{mEq/kg} \times 1.5\,\text{kg}}{0.5\,\text{mEq/mL}} = 9\,\text{mL}$$

- Finally, calculate concentration of glucose required to make desired glucose infusion rate. Achieve the desired concentration of glucose by using combination of 5%, 10%, 25%, or 50% dextrose.

COMPOUNDING AND SETTING-UP TOTAL PARENTERAL NUTRITION (FIG. 2)

Compounding is the process of mixing all nutrients for administration. Once the quantity of nutrients is calculated, it should be double-checked. The compounding can be done by automated machines or manually. It should be done under strict aseptic precautions, preferably under laminar flow hood. The working surface and all the nutrient vials should be kept under UV sterilizer lights for 45 min before starting compounding. During process of compounding UV light should be kept off and high-efficiency particulate air (HEPA) filter should be turned on.

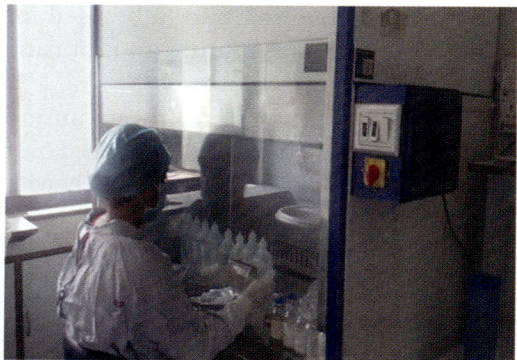

Fig. 2: Total parenteral nutrition compounding.

The TPN calculation sheet should be kept open and easily referable while preparing TPN. TPN is prepared as two parts (Table 9):

1. *Contents in the bottle* [usually a 500 mL bottle or 50 mL syringe for extremely low body weight (ELBW) baby]:
   - *Carbohydrates*: Dextrose
   - *Proteins*: Amino acids
   - *Electrolytes*: Sodium, potassium, calcium, magnesium, chloride
   - *Minerals*: Zinc, iron, manganese, copper, iodine, sulphur, selenium, molybdenum
   - Vitamins (water soluble)/adult MVI preparation.
2. *Contents in the syringe* (usually a 20 or 50 mL syringe):
   - 20% Lipids
   - *Vitamins (fat soluble)*: If available (currently not available in India).

Table 9: Availability of total parenteral nutrition solutions in India.

	Preparation	Manufacturer	Available (mL)
Dextrose	Dextrose 5%, 10%, 25%, 50%	Many manufacturers	25, 100, 500
Amino acids	Aminoven Infant 10%	Freseinus Kabi India Pvt Ltd	100
	Primene 10%	Baxter Healthcare	100
	Aminoplan 10%	Abbott Healthcare	50
Lipids	Intralipid 10% PLR	Freseinus Kabi India Pvt Ltd	100, 500
	Intralipid 20% (soya based)	Freseinus Kabi India Pvt Ltd	100, 500
	Clinoleic 20% (olive oil base)	Baxter Healthcare	500
	SMOFlipid 20% (combination of soya oil, MCTs oil, olive oil, and fish oil)	Freseinus Kabi India Pvt Ltd	100, 500
Sodium	3% NaCl (0.5 mEq/mL)	Denis Chem Lab Ltd	100
	Concentrated ringer lactate (3.3 mEq Na/mL)	T. Walker's Pharmaceuticals Pvt Ltd	20
	0.9% Normal saline	Many manufacturers	10, 25, 100, 500
Potassium	Potassium chloride (2 mEq K/mL)	Many manufacturers	10
Calcium	10% Calcium gluconate	Many manufacturers	10
	10% Calcium chloride	Neon Laboratories Ltd	10
Magnesium	Magnesium sulphate 25%, 50%	Carewin Pharmaceuticals	2
Vitamin	Multivitamin infusion (adult composition)	Martin & Brown Biosciences	10
Trace elements	Celecel 4, Celecel 5	Claris Lifesciences Ltd	1, 3, 10
Phosphorus	Potphos (potassium phosphate injection)	Neon Laboratories Ltd	15

(MCTs: medium-chain triglycerides)

MONITORING WHILE ON TOTAL PARENTERAL NUTRITION

Growth Monitoring

Combination of antenatal growth chart and postnatal growth chart such as Fenton charts can be used to monitor growth.

Reference growth for growing premature babies:
- *Weight gain*: 15–18 g/kg/day
- *Length gain*: 0.75–1 cm/week
- *Head circumference*: 0.5–1 cm/week.

Biochemical Monitoring (Table 10)

Following is the suggested monitoring schedule to help minimize PN related complications.

COMPLICATIONS RELATED TO TOTAL PARENTERAL NUTRITION

Metabolic and sepsis-related complications are most common. Catheter-related problems and calculation errors need continuous vigilance.

Complications of PN can be nutrient-related or venous access-related. Nutrient-related complications include hypoglycemia (plasma sugar <54 mg%), hyperglycemia (plasma sugar >150 mg%) (glucose related); azotemia, metabolic acidosis, hyperammonemia (protein related); hypertriglyceridemia (triglyceride >200 mg/dL) (lipid-related), cholestasis, and trace element deficiency. Most of these complications can be avoided by proper monitoring and provision of nutrients. PN-related cholestasis is usually complication of long-term PN and can be avoided by provision of minimal-enteral nutrition (MEN). Catheter-related complications include dislodgement and infection.

CONCEPT OF AGGRESSIVE NUTRITION

The concept of aggressive nutrition is based on the concept that if, a preterm newborn continues to receive uninterrupted transfer of nutrients after birth, it should achieve in utero growth rates.

Aggressive practice is understood either as practice that ranks toward the upper end of the range of established practices, or as practice that goes beyond the established and into untested territory. Aggressive nutritional approach states that "In-eligible preterm

Table 10: Biochemical monitoring during total parenteral nutrition.

Parameter	Initial period (first 3–4 days)	Established PN
Blood sugar	Twice daily + as clinically indicated	Once daily
Urine sugar	Once daily	Once daily
Blood gas	Depending on hemodynamic stability	Once weekly
Serum sodium, potassium	• Baby <30 weeks, first testing around 12–24 hours then 12–24 hours. • Baby ≥30 weeks, every 24–48 hours, can be given more frequently if clinical signs demand.	Once weekly
Serum calcium	Every 24–48 hours, can be done more frequently if clinical signs demand	Once weekly
Urea, creatinine	Every 48–72 hours	Once weekly
Serum triglyceride	Before initiating and with increment of lipid dose	Once weekly
Liver function tests	Before initiating lipids	Depending on clinical signs
Hemogram	Depending on clinical need	Once weekly

babies, PN should be started within a few hours of birth, with a starting dose of amino acids 2.5–3.0 g/kg/day and lipids of at least 1 g/kg/day, with gradual increase to 3 g/kg/day." (Ziegler, MD 2002).

Current practice of parenteral nutrition is more conservative than proposed aggressive nutrition by Ziegler, et al. However, we have to remember that today's aggressive practice may become tomorrow's standard practice.

STARTER PACKS IN TOTAL PARENTERAL NUTRITION

Starter packs are TPN solutions with standard combination of nutrients. Standardized PN offers advantages over routine individualized PN in terms of providing adequate nutrition to the majority of neonates without significant alteration in biochemical responses, with the potential for reduced cost and prescription error. It can be started even at odd hours after baby's admission to NICU. Standardized starter packs have longer shelf life than PN solutions prepared in the NICU. Presently, such starter packs are not available in India.

SUGGESTED READING

1. Adamkin DH, Radmacher PG. Current trends and future challenges in neonatal parenteral nutrition. J Neonatal Perinatal Med. 2014;7(3):157-64.
2. Bolisetty S, Osborn D, Sinn J, et al. Standardised neonatal parenteral nutrition formulations—An Australasian group consensus 2012. BMC Pediatr. 2014;14:48
3. Chaudhari S, Kadam S. Total parenteral nutrition in neonates. Indian Pediatr. 2006;43(11):953-64.
4. Embleton ND, Simmer K. Practice of parenteral nutrition in VLBW and ELBW infants. World Rev Nutr Diet. 2014;110:177-89.
5. Koletzko B, Goulet O, Hunt J, et al. Guidelines on Paediatric Parenteral Nutrition of the European Society of Paediatric Gastroenterology, Hepatology and Nutrition (ESPGHAN) and the European Society for Clinical Nutrition and Metabolism (ESPEN), Supported by the European Society of Paediatric Research (ESPR). J Pediatr Gastroenterol Nutr. 2005;41(Suppl 2):S1-87.
6. NNF Clinical Practice Guidelines. Use of parenteral nutrition in the newborn. In: NNF Clinical Practice Guidelines. NNF Publication; 2011. [online] Available from https://www.hse.ie/eng/services/publications/clinical-strategy-and-programmes/guideline-on-the-use-of-parenteral-nutrition-in-neonatal-and-paediatric-units.pdf [Last accessed May, 2019].
7. Parikh TB. Preparation and Administration of TPN. Manual of Neonatal Nursing. New Delhi: Jaypee Brothers (Publication by IAP Neonatology Chapter); 2015.
8. Stephen BE, Walden RV, Gargus RA, et al. First-week protein and energy intakes are associated with 18-month developmental outcomes in extremely LBW infants. Pediatrics. 2009;123(5):1337-43.
9. Ziegler E, Carlson S. Early nutrition of VLBW infants. J Matern Fetal Neonatal Med. 2009;22: 191-7.

CHAPTER 66

Oxygen Therapy

Rhishikesh Thakre, Srinivas Murki

INTRODUCTION

Oxygen is the first drug of choice in care of the sick newborn. Like other drugs, there are clear indications for treatment, methods of delivery, monitoring, and risk of toxicity. Oxygen therapy must be safe, simple, effective with ease in oxygen administration. Hypoxia can occur by one of the mechanisms:

- *Hypoxemia (reduced arterial oxygen content)*:
  - Decreased partial pressure of oxygen (PaO_2)
  - Decreased oxygen saturation (SaO_2)
  - Decreased hemoglobin content (anemia).
- *Reduced oxygen delivery*:
  - Decreased cardiac output
  - Left-to-right systemic shunt (e.g. septic shock).
- *Decreased tissue oxygen uptake*:
  - Left-shift of oxygen dissociation curve (e.g. abnormal hemoglobin structure).

INDICATIONS FOR OXYGEN THERAPY

- Clinical signs such as respiratory distress, central cyanosis, grunt, tachypnea, irritability and drowsiness, shock, and hypotension.
- Anticipated hypoxia (e.g. postanesthesia recovery, intubation, etc.)
- *Documented hypoxemia*: in neonates, PaO_2 < 50 mm Hg and/or SaO_2 < 88%.

SOURCE OF OXYGEN

Oxygen need to be readily available 24 × 7. Oxygen source can be a cylinder, concentrator, or central gas line depending upon resources (Table 1). For reliable and uninterrupted oxygen delivery for a small nursery, it is desirable to have central piped oxygen line.

Table 1: Comparison of oxygen cylinders and oxygen concentrators.

	Cylinders	Concentrators
Capital cost	Low	High
Running cost	High	Low
Reliability	Excellent	Good on selected models
Regular maintenance	Simple care only	Needed
Electricity	Not needed	Needed
Continuity of oxygen delivery	Liable to run out	Good, unless they break down or power fails
Supply system	Transport needed	Transport not needed

SELECTION OF AN OXYGEN DELIVERY DEVICE

Oxygen can be delivered in several ways (Tables 2 to 6). Ventilatory minute volume (MV) and the flow rate of oxygen determine inspired oxygen delivery. The greater the respiratory rate, lower is the FiO_2 for a given flow rate of supplemental oxygen. The choice of device would depend upon the gestational age, wellness of infant, oxygen requirement, and available resources.

Table 2: Head box oxygen.

Advantages	Disadvantages
No need for humidification	Limitations on mobility
No risk of airway obstruction	Difficulty in feeding and suction procedures
No gastric dilatation	High flow oxygen required
	CO_2 buildup
Gas flow of at least 4 L/min is kept to avoid rebreathing of carbon dioxide	

Table 3: Facemask oxygen.

Advantages	Disadvantages
No risk of airway obstruction	Variable FiO_2 delivery
No gastric dilatation	Difficulty in feeding and suction procedures
	High flow oxygen required
	CO_2 buildup
There is no data in newborns and infants	

Table 4: Nasal cannula.

Advantages	Disadvantages
Positive distending pressure	Risk of airway obstruction
No need for humidification	Variables affecting are cannula flow rate, ratio of nasal prongs and nasal diameters, minute ventilation, ratio of inspiration to expiration, mouth breathing, use of sedatives
No gastric dilatation	
The maximum flow permissible is 2 L/min on nasal cannula	

Table 5: Nasal catheter.

Advantages	Disadvantages
No need for humidification	Require high oxygen flow
No gastric dilatation	
Unlikely to be dislodged	
A catheter is placed equal to the distance from the side of the nostril to the inner margin of eyebrow to reach the posterior part of the nasal cavity	
Do not allow the flow of gas more than 1 L/min	

Table 6: Nasopharyngeal catheter.

Advantages	Disadvantages
No danger of hypercarbia if the oxygen is turned off or the tubing disconnects.	Risk of airway obstruction
Continuous distending pressure	Requires humidification
	Risk of dislodgement into esophagus
	Gastric dilatation
	Removing and cleaning the catheter twice a day is required

Catheter is placed via the nose to a depth equal to the distance from the side of the nose to the front of the ear. A flow of 0.5 L/min oxygen through an 8 F nasopharyngeal catheter in newborn infants with pneumonia, and 1 L/min in infants up to 12 months is practiced

Table 7: Comparison of different modes of oxygen delivery.

Criterion	Nasal prongs	Nasal catheter	Nasopharyn-geal catheter	Head box	Facemask
Oxygen (%)	30–35	35–40	45–60	>90	>90
Safety	High	High	Medium	Low	Low
Efficiency	Medium	Medium	High	Low	Low
Simplicity	High	Medium	Medium	Low	Medium
Tolerability	High	Medium	Medium	High	Low
Availability	Medium	High	High	Low	Low

PRACTICAL CONSIDERATIONS IN OXYGEN DELIVERY

All oxygen delivery systems need to be supervised and monitored (Table 7).

Role of Humidification

Nonhumidified gas is dry and irritates the linings of the nose, throat, and airways. It is recommended to humidify oxygen for administration when nasopharynx is bypassed or if the oxygen flow rate is more than 2 L/min. This is achieved by simple humidifier filled with sterile water or temperature controlled electric humidifiers.

Dose for Oxygen Delivery

In acute conditions, administration of 100% oxygen for a brief period of time is critical and may save life until more specific treatment is initiated. Thereafter, the dose should be titrated based upon pulse oximetry and arterial blood gas.

Treatment Strategies for Hypoxia

- Treatment must be aimed at the underlying cause.
- For optimal oxygen delivery, one should take into consideration the delivery device, hemoglobin status, cardiac output, and systemic perfusion (Table 8).
- Prevention, early identification, and correction of inadequate perfusion should be the goal.
- Efforts must be directed to correct low-cardiac output and/or improve ventilation, e.g. increasing cardiac output by inotropes or reducing systemic vascular resistance; increasing hemoglobin concentration by blood transfusions; matching ventilation with pulmonary perfusion by recruitment of lung by providing continuous positive

Table 8: Choosing appropriate oxygen delivery device.

Nasal prong	Low oxygen delivery (up to 30%)
Nasopharyngeal catheter	Feed the infant without interrupting oxygen delivery
Oxygen masks	Provide supplemental O_2 (0.35–0.50, depending on size and minute ventilation) for short periods of time (e.g. during procedures, for transport, in emergency situations)
Partial rebreathing masks	Variable oxygen delivery (FiO_2 0.4–0.6)
Nonrebreathing masks	Used to deliver variable FiO_2 up to 0.60 or specific concentrations (as from a blender)
Oxygen hood	High FiO_2 (>90%) delivery

Table 9: Strategies to improve oxygenation.

Noninvasive	Invasive
• Prone positioning • Relief of pain • Reduction of noise • Supplementing oxygen • Correction of anemia • Correction of shock • Continuous positive airway pressure (CPAP) • Bilevel positive airway pressure (BiPAP)	• Conventional mechanical ventilation • Surfactant • High frequency ventilation • Nitric oxide therapy • Hyperbaric oxygen • Extracorporeal membrane oxygenation (ECMO)

airway pressure (CPAP), surfactant, prone positioning, and giving nitric oxide (Table 9). Also, strategies to reduce **oxygen** consumption by relieving pain, reducing noise, and minimal handling of the infant should be addressed.

MONITORING OXYGEN THERAPY

- Clinical assessment should include ongoing evaluation of respiratory, circulatory, and neurologic status.
- Assessment of FiO_2, SpO_2 periodically, bedside which is noninvasive:
  - Pulse oximetry is simple, bedside, noninvasive tool for continuous monitoring of oxygen therapy. The target SpO_2 should be between 90% and 95%. Arterial blood gases (ABG) should be done intermittently to define the PaO_2 status. The drawbacks of pulse oximeter are inability to detect hyperoxia, poor reliability with circulatory insufficiency, and artifacts—light, movements.
  - PaO_2 remain the gold standard for detecting arterial hypoxemia. Sample can be accessed by a peripheral arterial stab, umbilical arterial line, or by capillary blood gas.
  - *Tissue oxygenation*: Serial lactate measurements and lactate pyruvate ratio.
  - *Near-infrared spectroscopy (NIRS)*: Measures regional tissue oxygenation (cerebral, renal, splanchnic) and can be used to monitor infants with respiratory distress syndrome (RDS) on mechanical ventilator, predicting circulatory disturbance.

OXYGEN TOXICITY

No FiO_2 above 21% can be regarded as safe unless the PaO_2 or SaO_2 are measured and found to be in the normal range.

Following are complications due to oxygen toxicity:
- *Retinopathy of prematurity*: Immaturity is the most important risk factor but oxy-

gen also plays a role. Other risk factors include acidosis, shock, sepsis, apnea, anemia, necrotizing enterocolitis (NEC), blood transfusion, and patent ductus arteriosus; and prolonged ventilatory support. Current evidence suggests that retinopathy of prematurity (ROP) is linked to the duration of oxygen rather than the concentration.
- *Chronic lung disease*: With $FiO_2 \geq 0.5$, generation of oxygen free radicals leading to free radical injury to the lung altering the lung function.
- *Increased PaO_2 may cause closure or constriction of the ductus arteriosus*: A risk for infants with ductus-dependent heart lesions.
- Fire hazard.
- Bacterial contamination with associated use of humidification or nebulization.

WEANING OXYGEN

Oxygen is omitted if the breathing is regular, effortless with pulse oximeter in normal range. Oxygen should be reduced in small steps (10%) at a time. A sudden, large drop in FiO_2 may aggravate hypoxia and cause sudden collapse. However, the most appropriate way of oxygen weaning is unknown.

OXYGENATION STATUS

- While assessing the oxygenation status, knowledge regarding gestational age, postnatal age, and the inspired oxygen concentration (FiO_2) is important. Even if PaO_2 and SaO_2 is normal, where the hemoglobin is inadequate the final delivery of O_2 to the tissues will be compromised. Hence, optimum hemoglobin level has to be maintained.
- Saturation targeting in infants:
  - SpO_2 target = 90–95% all neonates.
  - PaO_2 target = 50–70 mm Hg.

KEY POINTS

- Oxygen is a *drug*, i.e. a form of therapy.
- Oxygen delivery is dependent on the type of delivery device, circulatory status, adequacy of Hb, and cardiorespiratory status.
- All patients on oxygen therapy should be continuously monitored using pulse oximeter. Target SpO_2 should be 90–95%. Ongoing clinical assessment for perfusion of skin, brain, and kidneys is must.
- Arterial oxygen saturation (SpO_2) and PaO_2 are most reliable clinical markers of arterial hypoxemia. The results should be interpreted taking into consideration, the gestational age, postnatal age, shock, and anemia.

SUGGESTED READING

1. Askie LM, Henderson-Smart DJ. Gradual versus abrupt discontinuation of oxygen in preterm or low birth weight infants. Cochrane Database Syst Rev. 2000;(2):CD001075.
2. Askie LM. Early versus late discontinuation of oxygen in preterm or low birth weight infants. Cochrane Database Syst Rev. 2000;(2):CD001076.
3. Bateman NT, Leach RM. ABC of oxygen: acute oxygen therapy. Br Med J. 1998;317:798-801.
4. Dobson MB. Oxygen concentrators for the smaller hospital: a review. Trop Doct. 1992;22:56-8.
5. Frey B, Shann F. Oxygen administration in infants. Arch Dis Child Fetal Neonatal Ed. 2003;88:F84.
6. Tin W. Oxygen therapy: 50 years of uncertainty. Pediatrics. 2002;110(3):615-6.
7. Treacher DF, Leach RM. ABC of oxygen. Oxygen transport: basic principles. Br Med J. 1998;317:1302-6.
8. World Health Organization. Oxygen Therapy for Acute Respiratory Infections in Young Children in Developing Countries. Geneva: World Health Organization, 1993. WHO/ARI 93.28.
9. AARC Clinical Practice Guideline. Selection of an oxygen delivery device for neonatal and pediatric patients. Respir Care. 1996;41(7):637.

CHAPTER

Chest Physiotherapy

Tanveer Bashir, Rhishikesh Thakre

INDICATIONS

To help clear lung secretions as with:
- Consolidation
- Lung collapse or aspiration on chest X-ray
- Excessive or tenacious secretions.

CONTRAINDICATIONS

- Unstable vital parameters, hypotension, apneas, bradycardias, or variable desaturation on handling
- Recent intraventricular hemorrhage
- Thermal instability.

Pre-requisites

- Note the heart rate and SpO_2
- *Note the settings on the ventilator*: Reduce the sensitivity of trigger to avoid false triggering due to manual vibration if on A/C or synchronized intermittent-mandatory ventilation (SIMV) mode
- Auscultate the chest. Note the air entry and chest sounds
- Perform oropharyngeal suction as necessary.

Postural Drainage

- Allows gravity to mobilize secretions toward the trachea
- Based on the affected lung segments hold and position the infant (Fig. 1)
- If the secretions are thin, the therapy is more beneficial
- Gastroesophageal reflux worsening and intracranial pressure fluctuation may be prevented by avoiding head low position.

Vibration

- The infant is in postural drainage position
- Apply gentle vibration with minimal pressure
- Cupping is done with the other hand
- Intense vibration may cause rib fractures, hence are avoided.

Percussion

- Postural drainage position is given to the patient.
- Based on the anatomy of lung, the area is identified. The finger is used to tap the space directly or via a facemask or finger interface. This is followed by vibration. The secretions are thus mobilized and removed.
- The infants head needs to be supported during the procedure.
- Infants <1,200 g or <33 weeks should not undergo this procedure.

Chest Physiotherapy

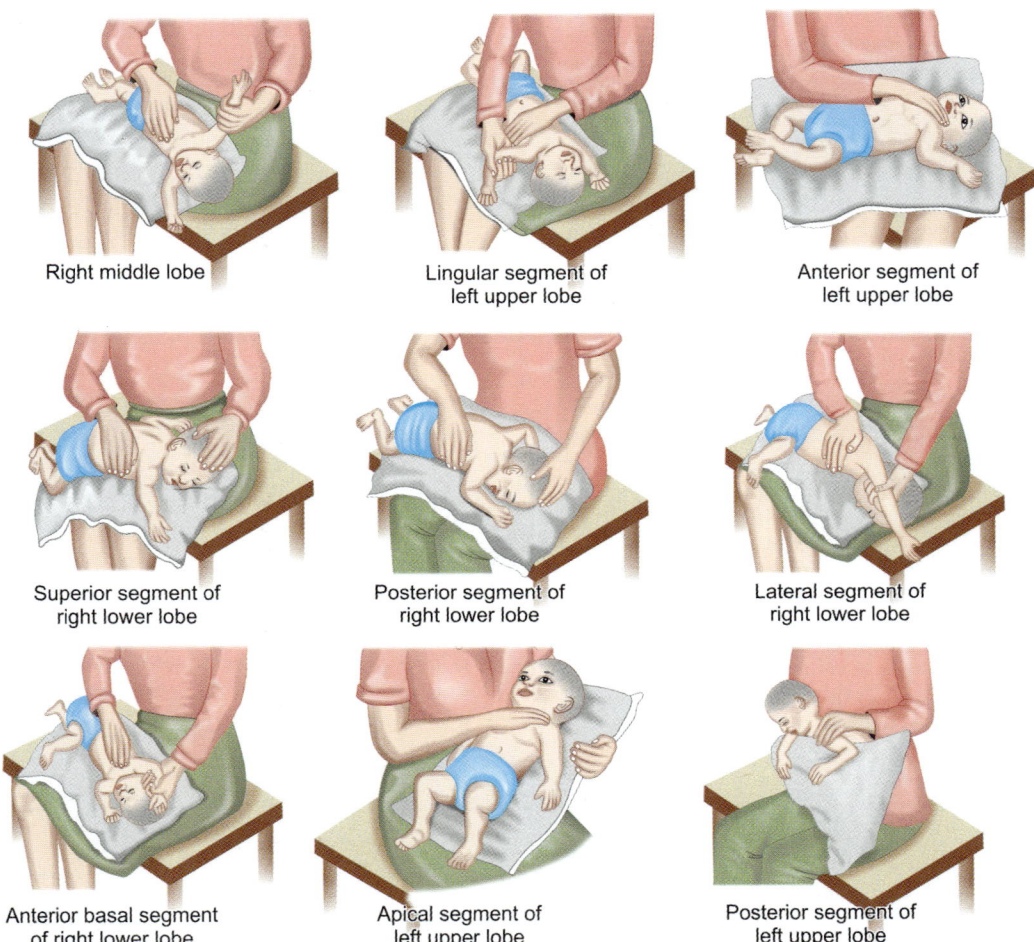

Fig. 1: Postural drainage.

SUGGESTED READING

1. Flenady VJ, Gray PH. Chest physiotherapy for preventing morbidity in babies being extubated from mechanical ventilation.Cochrane Database Syst Rev. 2002;(2):CD000283.
2. Oberwaldner B.Physiotherapy for airway clearance in paediatrics.Oberwaldner B. Eur Respir J. 2000 Jan;15(1):196-204

SECTION 6

Interpreting Tests

SECTION OUTLINE

68. Neonatal Sepsis Screen
69. C-reactive Protein
70. Blood Culture
71. Thyroid Function Test
72. Interpreting Neonatal X-rays
73. Congenital Renal Disorders

CHAPTER 68

Neonatal Sepsis Screen

Rhishikesh Thakre, Srinivas Murki

INTRODUCTION

In newborn care, the dictum appears to be "rule out sepsis" and treat with antibiotics. Following tests have been used to screen for newborn infection. There practical utility is discussed.

WHITE BLOOD CELLS COUNT

- Total count is the least useful of the blood tests.
- The count varies with gestation and postnatal age.
- With automated machines, inclusion of nucleated red blood cells (RBC) in the count causes more confusion.
- 30–40% lower values if sample obtained from central catheter compared to capillary blood.
- The complete blood count (CBC) in above cases resolves to normal within 24–36 hours.

NEUTROPHIL COUNT (BOXES 1 AND 2)

- Absolute neutrophil count (ANC) is of more value than total count.
- Standard values laid by Monroe and its extension in very low body weight (VLBW) babies are well documented and available in standard textbooks. These, however, are based on just 108 babies who were in the first 24 hours of birth.
- *Rule of thumb*: ANC < $1,500/cm^2$ is s/o infection.
- Neutropenia is more common than neutrophilia in sepsis.

PERIPHERAL BLOOD SMEAR

- The appearance of neutrophil changes in infection as immature forms enters the circulation. In severe infections, the marrow reserve may be exhausted. Hence, ratio of immature to total neutrophils should be taken (Table 1).

Box 1: Non infectious causes of neutrophilia and elevated I/T ratio.

- Maternal fever
- Difficult or prolonged labor
- Perinatal asphyxia
- Extended administration of intrapartum oxytocin
- Meconium aspiration
- Pneumothorax
- Intraventricular hemorrhage
- Hemolysis
- Seizures

> **Box 2: Non infectious causes of neutropenia.**
>
> - Maternal hypertension
> - Preeclampsia
> - Hemolysis
> - Intrauterine growth retardation (IUGR)
> - Necrotizing enterocolitis (NEC)
> - Periventricular hemorrhage
> - Seizures
> - Donor in twin to twin transfusion
> - Erythroblastosis fetalis.

Table 1: Interpreting I/T ratio.

No.	Age	Normal I/T ratio
1.	<24 h	0.16
2.	24–48 h	0.14
3.	48–60 h	0.13
4.	60 h–1 month	0.12

- *Rule of thumb*: I/T ratio > 0.2 is suggestive of infection.
- Presence of toxic granules (eosinophilic granules in cytoplasm of neutrophils), cytoplasmic vacuolations, and Dohle bodies (aggregates of rough endoplasmic reticulum which stain light blue on Giemsa stain) on the smear are suggestive of sepsis.
- Fifty percent of septic babies will have thrombocytopenia. This is, however, late in course of infection and the baby is usually septic clinically. Hence, documented thrombocytopenia is suggestive of advanced sepsis.

C-REACTIVE PROTEIN

- C-reactive protein (CRP) is an acute phase reactant. It has both diagnostic and prognostic significance. It is more informative than white blood cells (WBC) indices especially when serial measurements are done.
- C-reactive protein rises 8–10 hours following onset of neonatal infection.
- Culture proven sepsis is most unlikely if the CRP does not rise within 24–48 hours of onset of illness.
- Serial monitoring is useful in grading the severity of infection.
- The most accurate, rapid, and reliable measurement of CRP is by nephelometry. Bedside estimation can be done by latex agglutination. A positive rapid latex agglutination test on undiluted sample corresponds to a plasma CRP concentration of 0.8–1 mg/dL. Reading < 1.6 mg/dL on days 1 and 2, and <1 mg/dL, thereafter, is normal.
- Serial normal CRP has got good negative predictive value (rules out sepsis).

> *Persistently elevated CRP in spite of antibiotic therapy:*
> - Fungal infection
> - Resistant organism
> - Infective endocarditis
> - Abscess formation

> *Noninfectious causes of raised CRP*
> - Meconium aspiration syndrome
> - Perinatal asphyxia

- C-reactive protein is a good marker of bone and soft tissue infection.
- Viral infections do not have any effect on CRP.

ERYTHROCYTE SEDIMENTATION RATE

- Microerythrocyte sedimentation rate (ESR) is obtained by collecting capillary blood in a standard preheparinized micro hematocrit tube (75 mm length, internal diameter of 1.1 mm and outer diameter 1.5 mm) and reading the fall of erythrocyte column after 1 hour.
- Absolute value more than 15 mm at the end of 1 hour or more than, days of life +3 is considered to be significant.

- *False positive*: Hemolysis
- *False negative*: Disseminated intravascular coagulation (DIC).

GASTRIC ASPIRATE

- This can be viewed as sample of amniotic fluid plus or minus some swallowed secretions from the birth canal.
- Presence of >5 polymorphs/high-power field (hpf), or >75% neutrophil to epithelial cells ratio or presence of bacteria on Gram staining suggests exposure to infection in utero but not necessarily an infected fetus.
- Its utility is limited to first 6 hours of life.
- The great majority of these babies do not become septic. The value is more especially in very preterm infants.
- If antibiotics have to be started on clinical grounds, choose antibiotic based on organism isolated in the gastric aspirate.

BLOOD CULTURE

- Considered as gold standard for diagnosis of sepsis.
- Under aseptic precautions, 1 mL blood added to 5 or 10 mL liquid broth is sufficient for isolating an organism.
- A better yield is obtained if skin is cleansed for 30 seconds rather than the usual 5–10 seconds.
- Virtually all cultures that are going to be positive have grown by 48 hours whatever the culture method. Possible exceptions are Listeria monocytogenes, *H. influenzae*, and yeasts (Box 3).
- Presence of bizarre organism, mixed organism, and growth that does not appear until 72 hours of incubation should raise suspicion of contamination. Resistance to antibiotics on antibiotic sensitivity pattern favors a contaminant isolation.

Box 3: Clinically septic baby but blood culture negative.

- Culture obtained after antibiotic therapy
- Takes time to culture organism:
  - *Listeria monocytogenes*
  - *Haemophilus influenzae*
- Organism requiring special media:
  - Candida
  - Chlamydia
  - Mycoplasma
  - Viruses
- Metabolic derangement:
  - Hypoglycemia
  - Inborn errors of metabolism
- Anatomical malformation:
  - Aicardi's syndrome
- Drug effects/interactions
- Intracranial hemorrhage
- Environmental temperature fluctuation
- Polycythemia
- Technical error

- It is unwise to ignore bizarre organisms or polymicrobial growth in VLBW infant.

PRACTICAL UTILITY

- Taken into isolation, none of the above-mentioned tests are definite indicators of sepsis. A number of noninfectious conditions cause abnormality and are mistaken for sepsis and given antibiotics. Hence, a combination of tests is usually recommended (Table 2).

A practical sepsis screen would be:
- Leukopenia < $5,000/cm^2$.
- Neutropenia as per Monroe's curve.
- I/T ratio > 0.2.
- Micro-ESR > 15 mm.

If more than two tests are positive, infant should be treated with presumptive diagnosis of neonatal sepsis. If none or one test is positive repeat tests after 12 hours, if clinical suspicion persists.

Table 2: Neonatal sepsis screen.

No.	Authors	Screen	Sensitivity (%)	Specificity (%)
1.	Philip, 1980	TLC, CRP, I/T, ESR, haptoglobin	93	88
2.	Gerdes, 1987	TLC, CRP, I/T, ESR	100	83
3.	Misra, 1989	TLC, I/T, ESR, thrombocytopenia	58–60	78–96
4.	Sarkar, 1996	TLC, ANC, ESR, CRP	56	94
(Any two or more positive)				

(ANC: absolute neutrophil count; CRP: C-reactive protein; ESR: erythrocyte sedimentation rate; TLC: total leukocyte count)

- Subjective bias and interobserver variability in lab tests should be minimized by supervision and quality control.
- Following tests have no value in early onset sepsis screen unless specifically indicated:
    - Urine examination
    - CSF examination
    - Stool examination.
- The at-risk approach is the most prevalent method to evaluate an infant for sepsis. Presence of risk factors, sepsis screen positivity, clinical features, and culture positivity should guide the management. Commence with antibiotics in probable sepsis cases, but discontinue as soon as there is no supportive evidence of infection.
- I/T ratio is the earliest parameter to be abnormal, followed by elevation of band cell count and later on by neutrophilia in neonatal sepsis. Neutrophilia and thrombocytopenia are late markers of sepsis.
- Eosinopenia is marker of severity of sepsis. Eosinophilia is more common in preterms than in terms. Lymphocyte count at birth is somewhat higher than in adults (2,000–7,000/cm^2) and after a transient decline between days 2 and 6, the lymphocyte count stabilizes between 2,500 and 9,000/cm^2. Depressed lymphocyte counts are associated with maternal hypertension and neonatal sepsis. Lymphopenia (<1,500 cells/cm^2) is marker of underlying immune deficiency syndrome.
- An increase in monocytes is seen during recovery phase from sepsis.
- Babies of mothers with severe preeclampsia are more than usually vulnerable to late onset sepsis.

SUGGESTED READING

1. Escobar GJ. The Neonatal "sepsis work up": personal reflections on the development of an evidence based approach toward newborn infections in a managed care organization. Pediatrics. 1999;103(1 Suppl E):360-73.
2. Lee GR. Hematologic status of the neonate and young infant. In: Wintrobe's Clinical Hematology, 10th edition. Baltimore, MD: Lippincott Williams & Wilkins; 1999.
3. Manroe BL, Rosenfeld CR, Weinberg AG, et al. The neonatal blood count in health and disease. 1. Reference values for neutrophil cells. J Pediatr. 1979;95:89-98.
4. Marsh JC, Bogga DR, Cartwright G, et al. Neutrophil kinetics in acute infection. J Clin Invest. 1967;46:1843.
5. Mouzihno A, Rosenfeld CR, Sanchez PJ, et al. Revised reference ranges for circulating neutrophils in very low birth weight neonates. Pediatrics. 1994;94:76-82.
6. Mouzinho A, Rosenfeld CR, Sanchez PJ, et al. Effect on maternal hypertension on neonatal neutropenia and risk of nosocomial infection. Pediatrics. 1992;90:430-5.

CHAPTER 69

C-reactive Protein

Rhishikesh Thakre

INTRODUCTION

C-reactive protein (CRP), an acute phase protein, synthesized in the liver and a clinical marker of inflammation. It has a short half-life of 19 hours.

TECHNICAL ISSUES

Serum CRP concentrations can be measured by:
- *Latex agglutination assay*: Traditional method for measuring CRP is a *qualitative test*
- *Immunoassays*: These methods are considered gold standard for measuring CRP [e.g. laser nephelometry, radioimmunoassay (RIA), and enzyme immunoassays]
- Ultrasensitive or high-sensitive (hs) CRP assay.

FACTORS AFFECTING RESULTS

- Serum which is turbid, hemolyzed, or lipemic may cause incorrect results and should not be used.
- The kits should be stored at 2–8°C for best results.
- Refrigeration of the sample may cause a false-positive result.

CLINICAL IMPLICATIONS

- *Indication*: CRP is indicated in patients where sepsis is doubtful, and when negative cultures raise doubts about need for antibiotics [e.g. intrapartum maternal antibiotics, culture negative sepsis, cerebrospinal fluid (CSF) which is blood tinged, gastric residues, etc.].
- An *elevated* CRP level (greater than 10 mg/L) is abnormal. Two values of CRP 24–48 hours apart are of great value in diagnosis and treatment.
- In *early onset sepsis*, a single CRP 24 hours of onset of illness has a 93% sensitivity for "probable" sepsis. Two measures 24 hours apart are more reliable. In *late onset sepsis*, a single CRP has a sensitivity of 85%, with likelihood ratio of 0.19 (sepsis five times less likely given normal result), and two separate measures have a likelihood ratio 0.07 (sepsis 14 times less likely).
- C-reactive protein is a more sensitive and reliable than erythrocyte sedimentation rate (ESR) and the leukocyte count.
- *C-reactive protein trend*: CRP measured 24 hours after the onset of signs and symptoms of infection yields the maximum information. Serial evaluation 12–24 hours apart is more reliable.

- *Utility*: Helps to differentiate bacterial (significant elevation) from viral infection (minimal elevation).
- C-reactive protein is useful for distinguishing infants with septic arthritis and for determining whether arthrocentesis is to be performed. CRP rises rapidly and decreases to normal ranges within a week of treatment. A secondary rise may serve as a warning sign of recurrence of bone or joint infections.
- A positive test is poorly predictive of sepsis as the positive predictive value is poor. *False-positives* arise from noninfectious condition such as intraventricular hemorrhage, meconium aspiration, respiratory distress syndrome, fetal hypoxia, intraventricular hemorrhage, necrotizing enterocolitis (NEC), pneumothorax, surgery, and immunization.
- In the absence of clinical or bacteriological factors, an *isolated slight rise* in CRP is not a sufficient reason for starting antibiotics, as the rise may be a false-positive result unrelated to infection. However, the child should be monitored.
- CRP values ≤ 10 mg/L 24 hours apart, suggest that the infant is unlikely to be infected. Negative predictive value of serial serum CRP is 100% in deciding duration of antibiotics therapy in neonatal septicemia up to 7 days.

CLINICAL LIMITATIONS

- C-reactive protein evaluation on initial presentation or at birth is of no utility. CRP start rising by 24 hours of onset of infection in serum. About 60% of subsequently proven sepsis episodes will have a normal initial CRP as the sensitivity of the test is 40% only.
- C-reactive protein does not differentiate between survivors or nonsurvivors.
- C-reactive protein plasma levels remain elevated for days after the elimination of the infection.
- C-reactive protein may rise in noninfective inflammatory conditions thus mimicking bacterial infection.
- Isolated CRP value cannot be taken to discontinue antibiotics.

CLINICAL PEARLS

- Ask for CRP in doubtful sepsis after 12–24 hours after birth/onset of infection.
- Semiquantitative techniques should give way to quantitative estimation.
- The CRP level in isolation does not diagnose sepsis. Its utility lies in using as part of a sepsis screen.
- C-reactive protein in isolation should not be used to decide initiation or stopping of antibiotics.
- If the infant is symptomatic, draw a blood culture and initiate antibiotics. There is no point doing a CRP. However, when history and clinical examination is doubtful in making a decision to initiate or not to initiate treatment, one should do a CRP and better, repeat 24 hours later for decision making. Two CRP values 24 hours apart if negative, reasonably rules out bacterial infection.

SUGGESTED READING

1. Cheisa C, Panero A, Osborn JF, et al. Diagnosis of neonatal sepsis: a clinical and laboratory challenge. Clin Chem. 2004;50:279-87.
2. Malik A, Hui CP, Pennie RA, et al. Beyond the complete blood cell count and C-reactive protein: a systematic review. Arch Pediatr Adolesc Med. 2003;157:511-6.
3. Ng PC. Diagnostic markers of infection in neonates. Arch Dis Child Fetal Neonatal Ed. 2004;89(3):F229-35.

CHAPTER 70

Blood Culture

Rhishikesh Thakre, Srinivas Murki

INTRODUCTION

Blood cultures help to identify the specific type of organism responsible for blood stream infection. Combined with antibiotic sensitivity tests, it provides information about therapeutic interventions.

INDICATIONS

- Prior to initiation of antibiotics
- Clinical suspicion of sepsis.

TECHNIQUE OF BLOOD CULTURE

- Immobilize the extremity.
- Drawing blood culture is a two-person job.
- Use alcohol swabs to cleanse the skin. Apply for three times or until the area appears clean and allow to air dry.
- Use 10% povidone-iodine, or 2% tincture of iodine in 70% alcohol. Apply thrice over the site of venipuncture moving from center to outside. After third swab, allow to air dry.
- Swab the culture caps with alcohol. Ensure all supplies are in place.
- Apply alcohol to cleanse the iodine at the site of puncture.
- Prick the vein with needle ensuring that the bevel is up. Attach syringe to port and obtain blood sample. Empty the syringe to blood culture bottle.

PRACTICE POINTERS

- *Timing of specimen*: The best time to draw blood cultures is just before administering antibiotics. There is no rationale of timing it with fever.
- *The number of samples*: At least one sample is collected. Multiple samples 30 min apart may help recover organism as bacteremia is intermittent. Do not collect blood sample from the indwelling catheters for the cultures.
- *Volume of blood samples*: Approximately 1 mL sample yields maximum chance of isolation of organism in neonates.
- *Growth characteristics of the medium*: Aerobic cultures are routinely collected, unless specified. Use anaerobic cultures if suspected peritonitis, fasciitis, or immune-compromised state.
- *Method used for detection of growth in cultures*: Antibiotic removal devices are useful if patient is already on antibiotics. Resins are added to media to adsorb antibiotics and help improve microbial detection.

- *False positive culture report*: Following features suggest positive blood culture, viz.:
  - Coagulase-negative staphylococci (*S. epidermidis*) and *S. viridans* in a single bottle
  - *Corynebacterium, Propionibacterium acne*, and *Bacillus* spp. are usually contaminants
  - Multiple organisms (isolated) suggest contamination
  - Delayed isolation of growth
  - The patient has recovered or the symptoms do not suggest sepsis
  - A primary site of infection [e.g. cerebrospinal fluid (CSF) or urine] identifies a different pathogenic organism.

RATIONALE FOR A BLOOD CULTURE ON TREATMENT OR ONCE TREATMENT IS ALREADY INITIATED

Ideally one would do a blood culture before initiating antibiotics. In clinical practice, this may not be always possible. Hence, the blood culture on therapy would be needed for:
- To document presence of infection
- To decide the duration of therapy
- To decide change of antibiotics depending on the organism sensitivity
- To prognosticate
- To be medically, ethically, and legally be right.

If the culture reports are available after starting therapy and they do not correlate with the present management, do we need to change the drugs?

When the therapeutic response to initial therapy is excellent it can be continued because of lack of correlation between in vivo and in vitro antibacterial sensitivity pattern.

How does one alter antibiotic once culture sensitivity is reported?
- Select a single sensitive antibiotic. Only with *Pseudomonas* isolation, two sensitive antibiotics are justified.
- Change treatment to a narrow spectrum or low-cost antibiotic reported to be sensitive even if the patient is improving or the empiric antibiotics are sensitive.
- If there is deterioration on sensitive antibiotics, one should change the antibiotics to another sensitive one with a narrow spectrum and low-cost.
- With clinical improvement on resistant antibiotics, possibility of in vivo sensitivity should be considered and case re-evaluated. One must discontinue antibiotics with in vitro resistance even if there is improvement if the organisms isolated are *Pseudomonas, Klebsiella* and methicillin-resistant *Staphylococcus aureus* (MRSA); or the infection is affecting the central nervous system (CNS) or is deep-seated.
- If all antibiotics are reported nonsensitive, one should choose moderately sensitive antibiotic.

CAUSES OF PERSISTENCE OF POSITIVE BLOOD CULTURE

Reasons for persistent positive blood cultures include:
- Inadequate antibiotic concentration or duration
- Resistance to drug
- Colonization of indwelling line, catheter, or tube
- Focal infection (e.g. necrosis, abscess, pus)
- Osteomyelitis
- Infective endocarditis.

Table 1: Recommended interpretation of blood culture results for hospital-acquired infections.[a]

Blood culture source/result 1-mL culture from vein and each catheter if no central catheters, use 2 cultures from veins		Interpretation (Based on results at Bacterial—48 h; Fungal—72 h)	
ID	Vein	Each catheter	
NA	Negative	Negative	No infection
Coagulase negative staphylococcus	Positive	Positive	True infection
	Positive	Negative	Contaminant
	Negative	Positive	Line colonization
	Either site positive	No central catheter	Requires clinical decision
Gram-negative rods or other pathogenic species	Positive	Positive	True infection
	Any site (venopuncture or line) positive		Treat for infection

(NA: not applicable)
[a]These recommendations should be interpreted and adjusted on the basis of the clinical setting and individualized to each patient.

Why are cultures sterile in a suspected newborn with infection?

Low inoculums of blood sample, prior antibiotic exposure, intrapartum antibiotics, noninfective conditions.

Interpreting Blood Culture for Hospital-acquired Infection (Table 1)

How to interpret susceptibility/resistance data?

- Susceptibility testing does not predict in vivo efficacy as it is an in vitro phenomenon.
- Susceptibility testing is affected by type of organism tested, media used, incubation criterion, and technique of isolating bacterial growth.
- At times, the resistance may be agent specific but may be reported as class specific, e.g. resistance to ciprofloxacin may be reported as quinolone resistant.
- Studies show that area under the curve (AUC)/minimum inhibitory concentration (MIC) ratios have not been found to be superior to the traditional kill ratios comparing antibiotic serum/tissue levels to MIC as a predictor of antibiotic efficacy. Antibiotics with a relatively low AUC/MIC (e.g. ≤45) ratios do not predict therapeutic failure or resistance.
- A commensal organism is likely to be resistant to all antibiotics.

SUGGESTED READING

1. Gerdes JS. Diagnosis and management of bacterial infections in the neonate. Pediatr Clin North Am. 2004;51(4):939-59.
2. Isaacman DJ, Karasic RB, Reynolds EA, et al. Effect of number of blood cultures and volume of blood on detection of bacteremia in children. J Pediatr. 1996;128:190-5.
3. Roberts GC, Goodman NL, Land GA, et al. In: Lennette EH, Balows A, Hausler WJ, Shadomy HJ (Eds). Manual of Clinical Microbiology, 4th edition. Washington, DC: AMS; 1985. pp. 500-13.

CHAPTER 71

Thyroid Function Test

Rhishikesh Thakre

INTRODUCTION

Congenital hypothyroidism (CH) is one of the most common metabolic disorders and a preventable cause of intellectual delay. Majority of infants are asymptomatic and clinical evaluation is unreliable to detect CH early. Making a diagnosis beyond 8 weeks of age leads to irreversible brain dysfunction causing intellectual delay and coarse physical features.

HOW RELIABLE ARE CLINICAL FEATURES FOR DIAGNOSIS OF CONGENITAL HYPOTHYROIDISM?

Majority of infants are asymptomatic: Presence of coarse/puffy face, macroglossia, jaundice (>14 days), sleepiness, not waking for feeds, and dry skin should raise suspicion of CH.

When to screen?
- All newborns between D3 and D5
- Cord blood of all newborns (if follow-up is doubtful).

How to screen?
- By capillary heel prick using filter paper (D3–D5)
- Vein puncture and serum study
- Cord blood sample (if follow-up not assured) (Table 1)

Which test should be used for screening?
Screening is done by doing a thyroid stimulating hormone (TSH) or T4 (Table 2).

Practical Tips on Screening
- Screening is done respective of milk feeds, gestational age, or transfusion.

Table 1: Cord blood screening.

Advantages	Disadvantages
Painless	Not for home deliveries
Large quantity	Not for all inborn error of metabolism (IEM)
Not affected by surge	Not for sick newborns
No drop outs	
Report ready by discharge	

Table 2: Screening strategy.

	T4 first	TSH first
Primary CH	Good	Good
Central CH	Some	No
Mild CH	No	Yes
Delayed TSH rise	Yes	No
Thyroid transport, metabolism, or	No	No

(CH: congenital hypothyroidism; TSH: thyroid-stimulating hormone)

Table 3: Thyroid-stimulating hormone (TSH) cutoffs for blood sample for screening congenital hypothyroidism.

Cord Blood	>40 (mIU/L)	If values higher, do Serum study for TSH and T4
<2 weeks	>20 (mIU/L)	
>2 weeks	>10 (mIU/L)	

- Cord blood carries risk of high false positives hence different TSH cut-offs are required.
- A positive screening does not indicate initiation of treatment. Confirmatory tests are required for starting treatment.

What are TSH cutoffs for blood sample for screening CH?

Thyroid stimulating hormone cutoffs for blood sample for screening CH has been shown in Table 3.

Interpreting Screening Test (Table 4)

- Screen invalid
- Screen negative
- *Screen positive means*:
  - Further testing is required to confirm
  - Does not mean that the infant is affected.

How to interpret confirmatory tests? (Table 5)

Confirmatory tests include TSH and T4 or free T4 after 72 hours of screening.

What are criterions for starting treatment after confirmatory tests are done?

Criterion for starting treatment for CH are shown in Table 6.

Principles of Treatment for Congenital Hypothyroidism

- Start oral treatment with thyroxine, i.e. T4 10–15 µg/kg/day.
- Crush tablet in breast milk. Use syringe for administration.

Table 4: Thyroid-stimulating hormone (TSH) level interpretation.

TSH (mIU/L)	Result	Action
<20	Normal	–
20–40	Borderline	Repeat after 7–10 days
>40	Positive	Do venous TSH, fT4/T4 after 72 hours

Table 5: Interpreting thyroid tests.

Thyroid stimulating hormone (TSH)	fT4	T4	Action
High	N	N	Repeat TSH after 2 weeks
High	Low	Low	Start treatment
N	N	N	Normal
Low FT4 (<1.1ng/dL) or low T4 (<8 g/dL) irrespective of TSH			Start treatment

Table 6: Criterion for starting treatment for CH.

T4	Free T4	TSH (mIU/L)
Low T4* (<100 nmol/L or <8 µg/dL)	Low FT4 * (12 pmol/L or <1.1 ng/dL)	Any value#
Mild low T4 (<128 nmol/L or <10 µg/dL)	Low FT4 (<15 pmol/L or <1.17 ng/dL	TSH >20 (<2 weeks) or TSH >10 (>2 weeks)
Normal	Normal	TSH >10 (>3 weeks)*

*Revaluation at 3 years;
#Central congenital hypothyroidism.
(TSH: thyroid-stimulating hormone)

- Administer as single dose half an hour before feed.
- No concomitant administration of iron, calcium, or soya preparation.
- Emphasize the need for compliance.
- *Follow up*:
  - *2 weeks of starting treatment* (T4 or fT4).
  - *1 month later* (TSH and T4 or fT4)

Table 7: Compliance check.

Thyroid replacement	Clinical features
Low (under Rx)	Lethargy, constipation, weight gain
High (over Rx)	Diarrhea, palpitations, increased appetite, weight loss

Table 8: Interpreting thyroid US and scan.

USG	Nuclear scan	Diagnosis
Absent	No uptake	Agenesis
Absent	Ectopic uptake	Ectopic
Small	Absent/reduced	Hypoplasia
Normal	Increased uptake	Endemic iodine deficiency
	Reduced uptake	Perinatal iodine exposure
	No uptake	Thyroid-stimulating hormone (TSH) receptor blocking antibody or iodine trapping defect
Enlarged	Increased uptake	Endemic iodine deficiency
	Reduced uptake	Maternal antithyroid drugs

- *3 months and 6 months age* (TSH and T4 or fT4)
- *Every 3 months from 6 months to 36 months* (TSH and T4 or fT4)
- Annually thereafter (TSH)
- When compliance is in doubt.
- Sampling for blood is done 4 hours postdrug intake or 2 weeks after dose change.
- T4 will normalize in most infants by 1 week. TSH will normalize within 1 month.
- Clinical clues to under or overtreatment are given in Table 7.

What clinical work-up should be done in newly diagnosed congenital hypothyroidism?

At all visits, anthropometry should be documented on growth charts. Parental concerns should be sought. A clinical evaluation is carried out for congenital malformation, goiter, Downs syndrome, and midline defects (e.g. cleft lip/palate, micropenis). Hearing evaluation, 2D echo testing *must be done*. Thyroid function tests (TFT) of mother should be carried out.

What is the utility of nuclear scan and ultrasound study in congenital hypothyroidism?

Refer Table 8.

What are special circumstances for interpreting thyroid tests in newborn?

- *Preterm/low birth weight (LBW)/very low birth weight (VLBW)/Twins*: For preterms, < 32 weeks, repeat thyroid screening test at 28 or at discharge (Flowchart 1).
- *Sick Newborns*: Screening tests should be done at discharge or 7 days age. If transfused, collect sample pretransfusion sample, repeat testing at 28 days.

How does maternal thyroid status affect newborn thyroid testing?

- *Maternal autoimmune thyroiditis*: It has no effect on newborn or thyroid screening/tests.
- *Maternal hypothyroidism*: Increase maternal T4 dose by 25–30% on missed cycle. Aim to keep maternal TSH < 2.5 mU/L (1st) and < 3 mU/L later. Adverse newborn neuro outcomes are known even if no hypothyroidism is detected in newborn.
- *Graves' disease*: Do a thyroid receptor blocking antibody test (TRAb) in the 3rd trimester and/or cord blood. Perform fT4, fT3, and TSH on cord blood, D5, and D14.

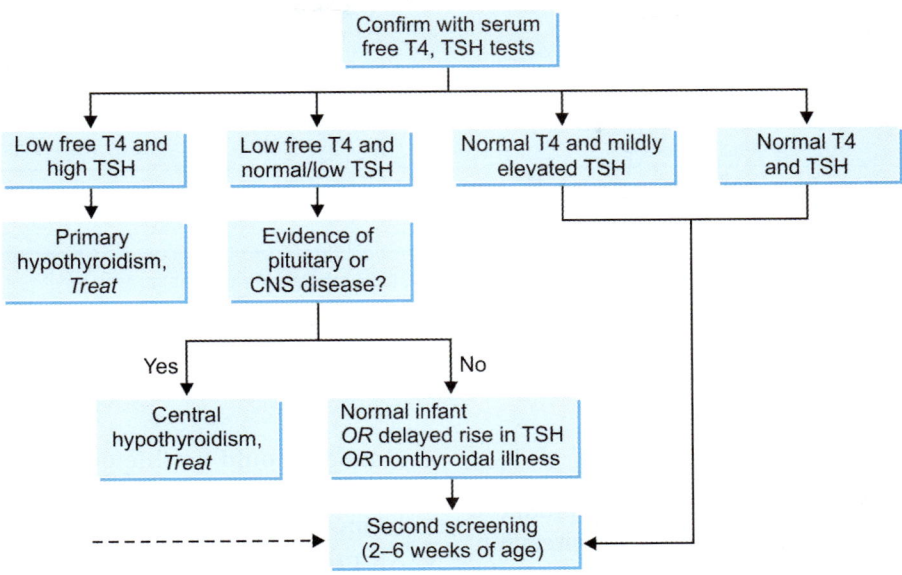

Flowchart 1: Evaluation of thyroid function tests (TFT) in preterm.

(CNS: Central nervous system; TSH: thyroid-stimulating hormone)

SUGGESTED READING

1. Agrawal P, Philip R, Saran S, et al. Congenital hypothyroidism. Indian J Endocrinol Metab. 2015;19(2):221-7.
2. Sudhanshu S, Riaz I, Sharma R, et al. Newborn screening guidelines for congenital hypothyroidism in India: recommendations of the Indian Society for Pediatric and Adolescent Endocrinology (ISPAE)–Part II: imaging, treatment and follow-up. Indian J Pediatr. 2018;85(6):448-53.

CHAPTER 72

Interpreting Neonatal X-rays

Rhishikesh Thakre, Tanveer Bashir, Srinivas Murki

INTRODUCTION

A radiograph is display of "shadows" produced by an X-ray beam. For correct interpretation, we must ensure the X-ray is technically appropriate and perform a systematic evaluation.

What decides interpretation of images on X-ray?

The object density plays a major role in image formation. There are four basic densities in human body: air, fat, water, and metal or bone (in order of increasing density). Air or gas do not absorb X-ray beam and hence appear as black or dark gray image (radiolucent) on the radiograph. Water blocks a greater proportion of X-ray beam, appearing as a light gray image. Dense objects (metal or bone) absorb a greater percentage of the rays and hence appear "white" or radiopaque.

RADIATION PROTECTION MEASURES

- All attendants should stay at a distance more than 6 feet from the patient, X-ray tube, and beam.
- A lead apron and gloves should be worn by attendant holding the patient or if within a distance of 6 feet from the beam.
- Gonads should be shielded and should be more than 5 cm away from the primary beam.
- All pregnant women should stay away during use of X-ray machine.

What simple precautions should be taken while taking X-rays?

- Do not place the baby directly in contact with the cassette. Cover the cassette with a soft cloth.
- Ensure thermal support to the newborn, as appropriate.
- Maintain hand hygiene while handling the neonate.
- Keep the infant position straight, head in midline.
- Allowing the infant to become quiet before shooting the X-ray.
- Raising the head of the bed slightly (approximately 5–10°) helps prevent lordosis from taking place.
- Restrict exposure to the area of interest only. Do not take an infantogram for lung disease.
- Have the X-ray dose as per the infant's age.
- Note the MAS/KV, duration of exposure and the energy used. This will help in consistently getting good quality films.

Chapter 72
Interpreting Neonatal X-rays

Table 1: Common landmarks on X-ray.

Type	Position
Endotracheal tube	Just above the carina (T2–3)
Umbilical arterial catheter tip	High (T6–9), low (L3–5)
Umbilical venous catheter tip	Just above the diaphragm
Nasogastric tube tip	In the stomach
Intercostal drain	Intrathoracic

STEPS FOR INTERPRETATION

- *View*: The frontal view identifies whether the abnormality is on right or left side. The lateral view is used to define whether the problem is anterior or posterior.
- *Chin position*: If the infants chin is down at the time of exposure the endotracheal tube (ET) will be higher up in trachea. If the chin is elevated, then tube will be pushed further down the trachea.
- *Check for rotation*: The spine should make a "T" with the clavicles. The lung fields should be symmetrical. Rotation can be evaluated by comparing the length of the ribs bilaterally and looking for the domes of the diaphragm.
- Adequacy of exposure is suggested by visualization of intervertebral spaces through the cardiac silhouette
- *Note the landmarks (Table 1)*: The carina is usually placed at T4 level. The last rib comes to join the T12 vertebrae
- *Age of the infant*: Secondary ossification of the proximal humerus is seen at term maturity. Typically, the presence of air may be observed in the stomach right at birth, small bowel with 3 hours of life, and in the rectum, 6–8 hours after birth.
- *Respiratory phase*: Following features help in defining the respiratory phase of film.
  - During the expiratory phase, the ribs angle down in a caudal direction or angle-off sharply to the posterior.

Box 1: Hyperinflation features.
- Lung expansion >6 ribs anteriorly and >8 ribs posteriorly
- Flattening of diaphragm
- Increased lung lucency
- Ribs more horizontal

  - Adequate inspiration is considered if the diaphragm is at or below the eighth rib.
  - Diaphragms appearing rounded or bulging into the lung fields suggest under-inflation.
  - If the stomach bubble appears to be bulging into the lower left lung border, it suggests an expiratory film.
  - If the X-ray film shows increasing haziness in a stable infant, one must consider the possibility of an underinflated or expiratory film.
  - Note for features of hyperinflation (Box 1)
- *Lung appearance (Tables 2 and 3)*: Normal lungs give an appearance of being dark or lucent as the alveoli and airways are air filled; diseased lungs appear as shades of gray across the lung fields. The lung pathology is depicted as gray or hazy areas if there are infiltrates (lung parenchyma filled with blood, pus, or fluid) or atelectactic areas (collapsed alveoli).
- *Beyond lungs*: Note the soft tissues, mediastinal structures, hilar area, diaphragms, and bony structures.

Table 2: Classical findings in respiratory disorders.

Condition	Features	X-ray
Respiratory distress syndrome	• Decreased lung volume • Air bronchogram • Reticulogranular pattern • Increased lung opacification	
Transient tachypnea of the newborn (TTNB)	• Prominent perihilar markings • Normal to increased lung volume • Fluid in the fissures • Occasional cardiomegaly and pleural effusions	
Meconium aspiration syndrome (MAS)	• *Diffuse, patchy/nodular infiltrates*: Focal or general, asymmetric or symmetric • Hyperinflated lung fields • Air leaks • Pleural effusion • Cardiomegaly	
Pneumonia	Patchy alveolar and interstitial infiltration	

Table 3: Common radiologic signs.

Radiological signs	Etiology
Low lung volume	RDS, pulmonary hypoplasia
High lung volume	MAS, TTN, cystic lung disease, hyperventilation
Air bronchograms	RDS, pneumonia
Diffuse parenchymal infiltrates	TTN, MAS, pneumonia
Lobar consolidation	Pneumonia, CLE, CCAM
Pleural effusion	Pneumonia, pulmonary lymphangiectasia
Reticular granular pattern	RDS, pneumonia
Hyperinflation	TTN, MAS, pulmonary lymphangiectasia
Fluid accumulations in interlobar spaces	TTN, pulmonary lymphangiectasia
"Cystic" mass	CCAM, CDH, pulmonary sequestration
Pneumothorax/pneumomediastinum	Spontaneous, MAS, RDS, pneumonia

(CCAM: congenital cystic adenomatoid malformation; CDH: congenital diaphragmatic hernia; CLE: congenital lobar emphysema; MAS: meconium aspiration syndrome; RDS: respiratory distress syndrome; TTN: transient tachypnea of the newborn)

INDICATIONS FOR LATERAL VIEW

- To determine the accurate position of a lesion seen on frontal view
- To assess for cardiac enlargement
- To define the tracheal width in suspected vascular rings
- To assess lymphadenopathy at the pulmonary hilum.

COMMON ERRORS IN X-RAY DUE TO TECHNICAL PROBLEM

- A differential density in the hemithoraces is often due to rotation and may be confused with unilateral disease such as infection or effusion.
- The most common cause of diffusely dense lungs is under-aeration/expiratory film.
- Skin folds may mimic a pneumothorax but are seen to extend beyond the boundaries of the chest.
- An excessively high kVp may diminish the pulmonary vasculature.
- Unilateral hyperlucency may be seen with patient rotation and mimic a pathological finding.
- Expiratory film mimics cardiomegaly or increased lung density.

CLINICAL PEARLS

- Interpretation of X-rays should take into consideration the clinical status of the patient.
- A single disease can present with varying X-ray findings and a same X-ray finding may be seen in several clinical conditions. Clinical correlation clinches the diagnosis (Table 4).
- One or more pathologies may coexist. One must do a thorough interpretation even if one pathology has been identified.

Table 4: Radiologic differential diagnosis.

Diffuse pulmonary disease	
Term	Preterm
Increased lung volume	*Decreased lung volume*
MAS Pneumonia TTN	RDS Pneumonia
Cardiac, pulmonary edema, pulmonary hemorrhage	
Focal asymmetric disease	
Opaque hemithorax	Cystic, lucent hemithorax
Pleural fluid (chylothorax, hemothorax)	Extra-alveolar air (pneumothorax, pulmonary interstitial emphysema)
Congenital diaphragmatic hernia (airless) Pulmonary sequestration Bronchogenic cyst	Congenital diaphragmatic hernia (containing air)
Congenital cystic adenomatoid malformation type III	Congenital cystic adenomatoid malformation types I and II
Fluid-filled congenital lesions in early neonatal period (CPAM I and II, CLE)	Congenital lobar emphysema (CLE)
Lung consolidation	Other obstructive hyperinflation (mucous plug, vascular anomaly)
Mass lesions (teratoma)	Compensatory hyperinflation (contralateral agenesis or hypoplasia, contralateral lung collapse) lung collapse

(CPAM: congenital pulmonary airway malformation; MAS: meconium aspiration syndrome; RDS: respiratory distress syndrome; TTNB: transient tachypnea of the newborn)

SECTION 6
Interpreting Tests

Table 5: Steps in interpreting X-ray.

- *Know the patient*:
  - Gestation/day of life/clinical status/indication/marking/previous films
  - Ensure right- or left-sided label
  - Note the date and time and if multiple X-rays, the sequence
- *Assess quality of film*:
  - Exposure
  - Alignment
  - *Breathing phase*: Inspiration/expiration

Interpret:
- Identify trachea and carina
- Assess mediastinum
- Assess hilum
- *Assess heart*: Size, shape, position
- *Assess diaphragm*: Pleura-gastric bubble
- *Assess soft tissues*: Chest/neck/extremities
- *Assess bony framework*: Ribs/clavicles/vertebrae
- *Assess lung fields*:
  - *Compare and contrast lung fields*: Symmetrical, focal, or diffuse
  - Consider areas of density and lucency.
- Look for lines/tubes/catheters, etc.
- Have a differential diagnosis
- Co-relate clinically

Box 2 Respiratory distress with normal lungs.

- Choanal atresia
- Tracheal obstruction (e.g. vascular ring)
- Neuromuscular disorder
- Persistent pulmonary hypertension (PPHN)
- Metabolic disorder
- Abdominal distention causing splinting of diaphragm
- Skeletal dysplasia

- Babies with tetralogy of Fallot (TOF) are likely to demonstrate excessive bowel gas. With esophageal atresia, there is no gas in abdomen.
- Total anomalous pulmonary venous connection (TAPVC) should be suspected, if a small heart is seen with increased interstitial markings of pulmonary edema.
- Bell-shaped thorax, thin ribs, scoliosis, and eventration of diaphragm should lead to suspicion of neuromuscular disease.
- Respiratory distress at times may be nonrespiratory in origin (Box 2).
- A systematic approach leads to appropriate diagnosis and avoids missing of any features (Table 5).
- Consider less common causes of respiratory distress when X-ray chest is normal or the findings are atypical.

SUGGESTED READING

1. Lobo L. The neonatal chest. Eur J Radiol. 2006;60:152-8.
2. Morris SJ. Radiology of chest in neonates. Curr Pediatr. 2003;13:460-8.
3. Trotter C, Carey BE. Radiology basics: overview and concepts. Neonatal Netw. 2000;19(2):35-47.

CHAPTER 73

Congenital Renal Disorders

Rhishikesh Thakre, Tanveer Bashir

ANTENATAL HYDRONEPHROSIS

- Antenatal hydronephrosis is considered significant if anteroposterior diameter (APD) is greater than 4 mm in second trimester and greater than 7 mm in third trimester. The classification of fetal hydronephrosis is done based on: (1) APD; or (2) Society for Fetal Urology (SFU) grade.
- Repeat USG at 2–3 days. If normal, repeat at 4–6 weeks. Do not start antibiotics prophylactically. No role for micturating cystourethrogram (MCU) if both USG normal (Flowchart 1).
- If postnatal hydronephrosis (>10 mm APD or SFU grade 3 or 4) present, do a MCU and if normal, do a diuretic renography. Prophylactic antibiotics are indicated till MCU in all neonates with significant hydronephrosis (Flowchart 1 and Box 1). Parents should be informed about signs and symptoms of urinary tract infection (UTI) and advised not to initiate antibiotic in case of fever without doing a urine examination.
- The severity of APD dilatation predicts major renal anomaly, especially ureteropelvic junction (UPJ) obstruction. APD does not predict vesicoureteric reflux (VUR).
- Multiple conditions like multicystic dysplastic kidney (MCDK), UPJ obstruction, or autosomal recessive polycystic kidney disease (ARPKD) have a palpable lump on clinical assessment.

VESICOURETERIC REFLUX

- Majority of grade I–III VUR undergo spontaneous resolution.
- Consult urologist for infants with VUR of grade III or higher.
- Infants with VUR should receive prophylactic antibiotics during first year of life.

MULTICYSTIC DYSPLASTIC KIDNEY

- Multicystic dysplastic kidney shows classical USG findings of cysts of various sizes, absence of renal parenchyma, and proximal ureters atresia.
- Dimercaptosuccinic acid (DMSA) scan is not required if ultrasound features are diagnostic of MCDK.
- Multicystic dysplastic kidney has a high rate of renal anomalies in the opposite kidney.
- Infants with unilateral MCDK and a normal contralateral kidney on postnatal ultrasounds do not need routine voiding

Flowchart 1: Evaluation and management plan of antenatal hydronephrosis.

```
                    Postnatal ultrasound
          Initial scan in first week, repeat at 4–6 weeks
    ┌──────────────────────┼──────────────────────────┐
    ▼                      ▼                          ▼
• No hydronephrosis   • Mild hydronephrosis      • Moderate, severe hydronephrosis
• SFU grade 0           (without ureteric dilation) • SFU grade 3–4
• APD < 7 mm          • SFU grade 1–2            • APD > 10 mm
                      • APD 7–10 mm              • Mild hydronephrosis with ureteric dilatation
    │                                                 │
    ▼                                                 ▼
No intervention*                          Micturating cystourethrography
                      ┌───────────────────┼───────────────────┐
                      ▼                   ▼                   ▼
              No vesicoureteric    Vesicoureteric       Lower urinary tract
                   reflux              reflux               obstruction
                      │                   │                   │
                      ▼                   ▼                   ▼
                  Diuretic             Antibiotic          Refer for
                 renography           prophylaxis           surgery
              ┌───────┴────────┐
              ▼                ▼
             No            Obstructed
          obstructed         pattern
              │                │
              ▼                ▼
    Ultrasound q 3–6 months   • Surgery if differential function low
       until resolution         or further declines on follow-up
                              • Monitor by ultrasound until resolution*
```

*Parents of infants with hydronephrosis should be counseled regarding the risk of urinary tract infections.
(SFU: Society for Fetal Urology; APD: anteroposterior diameter)

Box 1: Clinical parameters to indicate surgical intervention.

- Reduced differential function, less than 40%
- Deterioration of differential function greater than 5%
- Bilateral hydronephrosis with worsening dilatation
- Unilateral gross hydronephrosis, greater than 50 mm
- Severe hydronephrosis in solitary kidney
- Febrile breakthrough infection or symptoms.

cystourethrogram (VCUG) screening. Such infants are followed up clinically.
- An MCU is indicated if there are abnormalities in opposite kidney (e.g. hydronephrosis, small size, lack of corticomedullary differentiation, and dilated ureter).

SOLITARY KIDNEY

- If the infant has no other renal anomaly further imaging studies are not indicated.
- If postnatal ultrasound shows abnormality, VCUG and diuretic renography are indicated.
- Close monitoring of all such infants is required for risk of developing hypertension and/or proteinuria.

URETEROPELVIC JUNCTION OBSTRUCTION

- Ultrasound shows dilated renal pelvis with no other anomaly.

- Diuretic renography is essential for confirmation of diagnosis and for differential renal function.
- If there is decreased differential function, urologist evaluation should be called.
- If the obstruction is unilateral with a well-functioning kidney (differential function >40%), no active intervention is recommended.

POSTERIOR URETHRAL VALVES

- Presence of a distended, thick-walled bladder, posterior urethral dilatation, hydroureter, and bilateral hydronephrosis is classical of posterior urethral valves (PUV) diagnosis on ultrasound.
- With prenatally suspected bladder outlet obstruction, ultrasound and MCU study is indicated within first 2 days of life.
- Work-up includes urine examination and culture, serum electrolytes, creatinine, and blood urea nitrogen.

PRUNE BELLY SYNDROME

- All such infants should be evaluated promptly to a pediatric urologist.
- Clinical spectrum includes gastrointestinal anomalies (malrotation, volvulus, gastroschisis, omphalocele, Hirschsprung's, imperforate anus), pulmonary anomaly (hypoplasia secondary to oligohydramnios), cardiac defects (atrial septal defect, ventricular septal defect, tetralogy of Fallot), and orthopedic conditions (developmental dislocation of the hip, scoliosis, pectus excavatum, talipes equinovarus, and torticollis).

URETEROVESICAL OBSTRUCTION

Pediatric urologist referral is made at the earliest.

URETEROCELES

- The condition is characterized by cystic dilatation of the intravesical ureter.
- Early surgical evaluation is must with MCU study and at times, nuclear renography.

SUGGESTED READING

1. Aulbert W, Kemper MJ. Severe antenatally diagnosed renal disorders: background, prognosis and practical approach. Pediatr Nephrol. 2016;31(4):563-74.
2. Cohen JN, Ringer SA. Congenital kidney abnormalities: diagnosis, management, and palliative care. NeoReviews. 2010;11:e226-35.
3. Poudel A, Afshan S, Dixit M. Congenital anomalies of the kidney and urinary tract. NeoReviews. 2016;17:e18.

SECTION 7

Miscellaneous Topics

SECTION OUTLINE

74. Parent Counseling
75. Disinfection and Sterilization
76. Handwashing
77. Pain Management
78. Coping with Death
79. Birth Injury
80. Best Practices in Neonatal Intensive Care Unit
81. Checklists
82. Use of Neonatal Intensive Care Unit Charts, Algorithms, Calculators: Mobile Apps and Website Links

CHAPTER 74

Parent Counseling

Ranjan Kumar Pejaver

INTRODUCTION

Counseling is termed as a guiding relationship that helps the counseled individual (counselee) to become self-sufficient, self-dependent, and self-directed and to adjust themselves efficiently to the demands of a better and meaningful life. The process of counseling is one wherein the counselor provides accurate and up-to-date information to the counselee regarding the situation, and helps the counselee to take an informed decision which will allow him to lead a better and more meaningful life. Counseling is an art as well as science and is of utmost importance in the medical field.

QUALITIES OF A GOOD COUNSELOR

To be effective as a counselor, it is essential to possess following qualities:
- Authentic, sincere, and honest.
- Listen attentively and express thoughts and ideas clearly.
- Maintain confidentiality.
- Inform choices that are life oriented.
- Have a sincere interest in the welfare of others.
- Maintain healthy boundaries with the counselee.

Though the principles of counseling are the same across the board, some of specialties like neonatology have unique situations where parents and relatives are need to be counseled about the baby's condition. *Counseling should be nondirective and nonjudgmental at all times.*

WHEN DO WE NEED TO COUNSEL DURING PERINATAL PERIOD?

Preconception

There is a history of recurrent pregnancy loss, stillbirths, or neonatal deaths. Parents are worried about the next pregnancy and would want to know the chances of recurrence and ways to prevent the same happening.

Previous child of the parents or any members of the immediate family of either of the spouses is suffering from inherited disorder, congenital abnormalities, developmental delay, and dysmorphic features.

Health of the Parents

Parents are of advanced ages and may be suffering from conditions like severe diabetes, hypertension, and systemic diseases. Would want to know how this may affect the pregnancy, child's birth, and child's health in the short- and-long term?

Abnormal Antenatal Ultrasound Scan

It has revealed some congenital abnormalities or findings like growth restriction, oligo or polyhydramnios. Parents need information and guidance regarding the seriousness of it and its affect on child birth and subsequent health.

At Delivery

Baby is receiving extensive resuscitation and does not seem to be responding. They may need counseling regarding continuation/ stopping resuscitation measures.

Immediately after Delivery

Baby needed extensive resuscitation, has survived. Parents need to know the repercussions. Baby is extremely low-birth weight (LBW)/ premature, or in case of congenital abnormalities, information regarding the management and prognosis.

Neonatal Period

Preterm infant has had an eventful stay in the intensive care unit (ICU). Intact survival is unlikely. Regarding possible sequelae, further continuation of care or withdrawal of care.

Predischarge Counseling

Parents of neonatal intensive care unit (NICU) graduates have to be counseled regarding danger signs to watch out, follow-up plans, and other instructions like feeding, medications, immunizations, etc. or, in case of postoperative state. Parents need information regarding home care and any follow-up procedures—timing, cost, and prognosis.

Bereavement Counseling

If a baby has demised or stillbirth has occurred.

GENERAL PRINCIPLES OF PARENT COUNSELING

The counseling should be conducted in a quiet and comfortable room.

It should be conducted by a senior member of the team in a language the parents understand. If necessary, a reliable interpreter may be used. Provide information in simple, nontechnical language. The depth of the information should commensurate with the educational level and understanding ability of the listeners.

It should be done in strict privacy, preferably with both parents being present, and may be some elders or influential family members, with the permission of the parents.

It is good to involve nurses, and other specialists who may be sharing in the care.

Be careful not to hurt the local, traditional, family, cultural, and religious sentiments of the parents. Be patient, be ready to repeat the advice, answer queries, and give time to the parents to understand, think and then convey the decisions.

If there is any written material relevant to the discussion, it is helpful and may be given to the parents.

It is a good practice to summarize the discussion, decisions arrived at, write it down, and take the signatures of the parents after they have read it. Signatures of the counselor and witness are also important. Many centers have started video recording the counseling sessions informing the parents about the same.

SOME TECHNICAL ASPECTS OF PERINATAL COUNSELING

- *Diagnosis* wherever applicable should be known as far as possible, it should be conveyed to the parents. If a visit to higher center would be helpful, then sufficient information about that should be supplied.
- *Statistical data support* should be known and quoted where necessary, e.g. survival of very LBW infants, premature infants, etc.
- *Resuscitation procedure*: Discontinuation is justified if there are no signs of life (no heart beat and no spontaneous respirations) after 10 minutes of full resuscitation. Parents should be informed, if possible about the progress and status of the baby at various steps. In major congenital abnormalities incompatible with life, discussion with parents is essential before taking decision to discontinue resuscitation. A concurrence of another colleague is ideal.

WITHDRAWAL OF CARE

Parental requests do come in for withdrawal of care in babies receiving intensive care, having multiple organ systems involved, with remote possibility for ultimate survival, or likelihood of severe neurological sequel is almost certain. Investigation results confirming the same should be discussed with parents, documented, and filed. Due deliberation, proper documentation, and authorized personnel's and parents' concurrence in black and white should be obtained. Legal sanction for any of the above does not exist at present time.

Discharge against medical care (DAMA) is one of the most complicated issues in the practice of neonatal medicine. This could be due to financial constraints or other family/social reasons. As far as possible, the parents must be counseled and convinced of the reasonable chances if present of survival of the newborn and the need for the patience to provide time for the recovery process to occur. Alternatively, other medical centers or government set-ups (affordable to the parents) can be suggested and safe transfer of the baby should be arranged. Any withdrawal request or related communication document from the parents in fact should be in their own language and handwriting. The replies from the establishment should also be in the same manner. Reliable witness signatures are important.

Please note that "discharge at request" has no meaning in the realms of the language of medical care and no standing in the court of law.

Pregnancy loss, stillbirth, death of a neonate are devastating to the family. There is a feeling of loss, guilt, shame, inadequacy, and anger in the parents. Compassionate counseling is required stressing on the point that neither of the parent is responsible for it. It is essential that a diagnosis be arrived at in view of future pregnancies even it may not help in the current one.

In cases of neonatal deaths, a meeting should be arranged with the parents a few days after the event when the parents may be more receptive. Future reproductive options, perinatal preventive strategies like folic acid consumption, investigations, antenatal management as "high risk" pregnancy, planning of delivery, and neonatal care could be discussed. Visits by a social worker to the abode of the unfortunate couple at least during the first few months after the tragedy to counsel will be very beneficial.

Parent counseling is an integral part of healthcare management in perinatal Medicine. It should be included in the medical curriculum and further training should be acquired by at least one person in a team or establishment providing perinatal care.

SUGGESTED READING

1. Freer Y, Lyon A, Stenson B, et al. BabyLink—improving communication among clinicians and with parents with babies in intensive care. Br J Healthcare Comput Inform Manag. 2005;22(2):34-6.
2. Kaempf JW, Tomlinson MW, Campbell B, et al. Counseling pregnant women who may deliver extremely premature infants: medical care guidelines, family choices, and neonatal outcomes. Pediatrics. 2009;123(6):1509-15.
3. Lam V, Kain N, Joynt C, et al. A descriptive report of end-of-life care practices occurring in two neonatal intensive care units. Palliat Med. 2016;30(10):971-8.
4. Leslie L, Harris LL, Douma C. End-of-life care in the NICU: a family-centered approach. Neo Reviews. 2010;11:e194-9.
5. Munson D. Withdrawal of mechanical ventilation in pediatric and neonatal intensive care units. Pediatr Clin North Am. 2007;54:773-85.
6. Stokes TA, Watson KL, Boss RD. Teaching antenatal counseling skills to neonatal providers. Semin Perinatol. 2014;38(1):47-51.
7. Yee W, Ross S. Communicating with parents of high-risk infants in neonatal intensive care. Paediatr Child Health. 2006;11(5):291-4.

CHAPTER 75

Disinfection and Sterilization

Srinivas Murki, Rhishikesh Thakre

BASIC CONCEPTS

Cleaning: Physical removal.

Sterilization: Destruction of all forms of microbial life.

Disinfection: Intermediate measures between physical cleaning and sterilization are carried out with pasteurization or chemical germicides or ultraviolet radiation.

What is the deciding factor for decontamination?

The *rationale* for cleaning, disinfecting, or sterilizing patient-care equipment can be understood more readily if medical devices, equipment, and surgical materials are divided into three general categories (critical items, semi-critical items, and noncritical items) based on the potential risk of infection involved in their use.

All items that will touch normally sterile tissues can be sterilized (*critical items*). Items that touch mucous membranes but do not breach the continuity (*semi-critical*), e.g. bronchoscope, endotracheal tube, and respiratory tubes, require a disinfection process. For many *noncritical* items, such as blood pressure cuffs or crutches, cleaning can consist only of: (1) washing with a detergent or a disinfectant-detergent, (2) rinsing, and (3) thorough drying. In general, items that touch only intact skin need to be cleaned.

Cleaning is always essential prior to disinfection or sterilization.

DISINFECTION

Decontamination

It involves cleaning, disinfection, and sterilization (Table 1).

The formula for making a dilute chlorine solution from any concentrated hypochlorite solution is:
- Check concentration (% concentrate) of the chlorine product you are using.
- Determine total parts (TPs) water needed using the formula below:

    Total parts water = (% concentrate)
    $-$ 1% dilute

- Mix one part concentrated bleach with the TPs water required.

For example, make a dilute solution (0.5%) from 5% concentrated solution.

Step 1: Calculate TP water: (5.0%)/0.5% $-$ 1
    $= 10 - 1 = 9$

Step 2: Take one part concentrated solution and add to nine parts water.

SECTION 7
Miscellaneous Topics

Table 1: Levels of disinfection.

High-level disinfection	Intermediate-level disinfection	Low-level disinfection	Use sterile
2% glutaraldehyde, 6% hydrogen peroxide (H_2O_2), and 1:64 bleach water	Ethanol, phenol, iodophors, and 1:64 bleach water	Phenol, iodophors, and 1:500 bleach water	
Semi-critical items	Blood spills	All reusable equipment	Syringes, needles, and catheters
Scopes, anesthesia equipment	Microbial spills	Environmental surfaces	All implantable devices
Nebulizer cups	Thermometers	Stethoscopes, ear specula	All intravascular devices
Nasal specula, breast pump accessories		BP cuffs, bed pans, and urinals	Biopsy equipment, neurologic test needles

The formula for making a dilute solution from a powder of any percent available chlorine is:

Formula for making chlorine solution from dry powders:
- Check concentration (% concentrate) of the powder you are using.
- Determine grams bleach needed using the formula below:

Grams/liter = (% dilute) × 1000% concentrate
- Mix measured amount of bleach powder with 1 L of water.

For example, make a dilute chlorine-releasing solution (0.5%) from a concentrated powder (35%).

Step 1: Calculate g/L × 1000
= (0.5%) × 100 = 14.2 g/L 35%

Step 2: Add 14.2 g (approximately 14 g) to 1 L of water.

Cleaning Methods of Housekeeping Surfaces (Table 2)

Cleaning should start with the least soiled area and move to the most soiled area and from high to low surfaces. The preferred order of housekeeping practices is discussed in Table 3.

Wet Mopping
- It is the most common and preferred method to clean floors.

Double-bucket Technique
Two different buckets are used, one containing a cleaning solution and the other containing rinse water. The mop is always rinsed and wrung out before it is dipped into the cleaning solution. The double-bucket technique extends the life of the cleaning solution (fewer changes are required), saving both labor and material costs.

Dusting
Most commonly used for cleaning walls, ceilings, doors, windows, furniture, and other environmental surfaces.

Cleaning Strategies for Spills of Blood and Body Substances

- Clean spills with a 0.5% chlorine solution
- Clean spills of blood, body fluids, and other potentially infectious fluids immediately.

For Small Spills
While wearing utility or examination gloves, remove visible material using a cloth soaked in a 0.5% chlorine solution, then wipe clean with a disinfectant cleaning solution.

For Large Spills
While wearing gloves, flood the area with a 0.5% chlorine solution, mop up the solution

Table 2: Time schedule for cleaning and disinfection.

Once a day—morning	• Sterilizer • Swab container, injection, and medicine tray • Cheatle forceps • Steel drums • Baby linen, blanket, and blanket cover • Cotton gauze
Once a day—night	• Warmer or incubator • Bed making • Infusion pump/syringe pump • Stethoscope, measuring tape, cotton, syringe, gauze, and thermometer • Weighing scale • Ambu bag • Laryngoscope • Oxygen hood, oxygen tube, and suction tube • Change water in oxygen and suction bottle
Once a day—evening	• Total parenteral nutrition (TPN) or drug preparation area • Unused medical equipment, incubator, and warmer • Crash trolley, files, and nursing stations
Once or twice—weekly	• Ambu bag to be sterilized • Refrigerator • Procedure trays (exchange, LP, ICD, and central line kit)
After every use	• Stethoscope, thermometer, laryngoscope, and feeding utensils

(LP: lumbar puncture; ICD: intercostal drain)

Table 3: The preferred order of housekeeping practices.

Order of cleaning	Responsibility	Cleaning method	Frequency
1	Suction jars, oxygen humidifiers, and suction tubing	Removed and washed with soap and water. Sent for sterilization with ethylene oxide (ETO) or in 2% cidex for 8 hours	2 times/week
2	Surface cleaning (horizontal surfaces, window sills, top of doors, door knobs, light switches, lights, furniture in nursing station, and racks)	(0.5% chlorine + detergent cleaning solution). Only wet dusting with cleaning cloth	Daily and whenever visibly soiled
3	Procedure and examination rooms	Wipe horizontal surfaces with 0.5% chlorine + detergent cleaning solution	After each procedure and whenever visibly soiled
4	Walls, windows, ceilings, window curtains, window blinds, and doors	(0.5% chlorine + detergent cleaning solution)	Spot cleaning only when soiled
5	Main scrub area and sinks	Scrub with a separate brush and 0.5% chlorine + detergent cleaning solution. Rinse with water	Daily
6	Soiled linen	Collect soiled linen in closed, leak proof containers	Daily (or more often as needed)
7	Waste	Collect waste from all areas	At least daily (or more frequently as needed). Avoid overflowing

Contd...

Contd...

Order of cleaning	Responsibility	Cleaning method	Frequency
8	Floor mopping	0.5% chlorine cleaning + detergent solution, only wet mopping	Once per shift (3 times/day) and when soiling or spill occurs
9	Slippers	Detergent solution	Every night
10	Waste disposal bins	0.5% chlorine + detergent solution and scrub to remove soil and organic material	Clean contaminated waste containers daily and noncontaminated containers when visibly soiled and at least once a week
11	Toilets	Scrub with a separate brush and harpic	3 times/day (at the end of every shift)

and then clean as usual with detergent and water.

Sterile or Unsterile Gloves

Sterile gloves is indicated when certain invasive procedures are performed or when open wounds are touched. Nonsterile gloves can be worn when hands are likely to become contaminated with potentially infective material, such as blood, body fluids, or secretions, and when objects soiled with excretions/secretions are handled.

Medical gloves made of vinyl, nitrile, neoprene, or polyethylene serve as adequate barriers, particularly when latex allergies are a concern.

Microbiologic Sampling

Routine microbiologic sampling of the air and environmental surfaces should not be done. The only routine or periodic microbiologic sampling that is recommended is of the water and dialysis fluids. Microbiologic sampling is indicated during investigation of infection problems if environmental reservoirs are implicated epidemiologically in disease transmission.

STERILIZATION

- *Steam*: Whenever sterilization is indicated, a steam sterilizer should be used unless the object to be sterilized will be damaged by heat, pressure, or moisture. Unsuitable, however, for processing plastics with low melting points, powders, or anhydrous oils. Microbiological monitoring of steam sterilizers is recommended at least once a week with commercial preparations of spores of *Bacillus stearothermophilus* (a microorganism having spores that are particularly resistant to moist heat, thus assuring a wide margin of safety).
- Flash sterilization [270°F (132°C) for 3 minutes in a gravity displacement steam sterilizer].
- Ethylene oxide gas sterilization.

SUGGESTED READING

1. Centers for Disease Control and Prevention (CDC). (2013). Preventing Healthcare-associated Infections. [online] Available from https://www.cdc.gov/hai/prevent/prevention.html. [Last accessed May, 2019].

2. Dieckhaus KD, Cooper BW. Infection control concepts in critical care. Crit Care Clin. 1998;14(1):55-70.
3. Garner JS, Favero MS. CDC guidelines for the prevention and control of nosocomial infections. Guideline for handwashing and hospital environmental control, 1985. Supersedes guideline for hospital environmental control published in 1981. Am J Infect Control. 1986;14(3):110-29.
4. Laboratory Centre for Disease Control, Bureau of Infectious Diseases, Health Canada. Hand washing, cleaning, disinfection and sterilization in health care. Can Commun Dis Rep. 1998;24 Suppl 8:1-55.
5. Larson E. Current handwashing issues. Infect Control. 1984;5(1):15-7.
6. World Health Organization (WHO).(2002). Prevention of hospital-acquired infections: A practical guide. [online] Available from https://www.who.int/csr/ resources/ publications/whocdscsreph200212.pdf. [Last accessed May, 2019].

CHAPTER 76

Handwashing

Srinivas Murki, Rhishikesh Thakre

INTRODUCTION

Handwashing is single, simple, effective, evidence-based intervention to help reduce hospital-acquired infections. Handwashing is a part of normal duty of care.

INDICATIONS (WORLD HEALTH ORGANIZATON, FIVE MOMENTS OF HAND HYGIENE)

1. Before touching a patient
2. Before clean/aseptic procedure
3. After body fluid exposure/risk
4. After touching a patient
5. After touching patient surroundings.

PURPOSE OF HANDWASHING

- Remove all dirt and debris
- Reduce cross contamination
- Interrupt fecal oral route of infection
- Reduce risk of hands acting as vectors
- Break link in chain of infections.

STEPS OF HANDWASHING (TABLE 1)

- Remove jewelry, watch, etc. of hands. Roll-up the sleeves above the elbow.
- Place hands under running water. The following steps should take at least 45–60 sec.
- Lather with soap using friction both the hands. Vigorously wash hands (Fig. 1).
- Wash the arms with form circular motions.

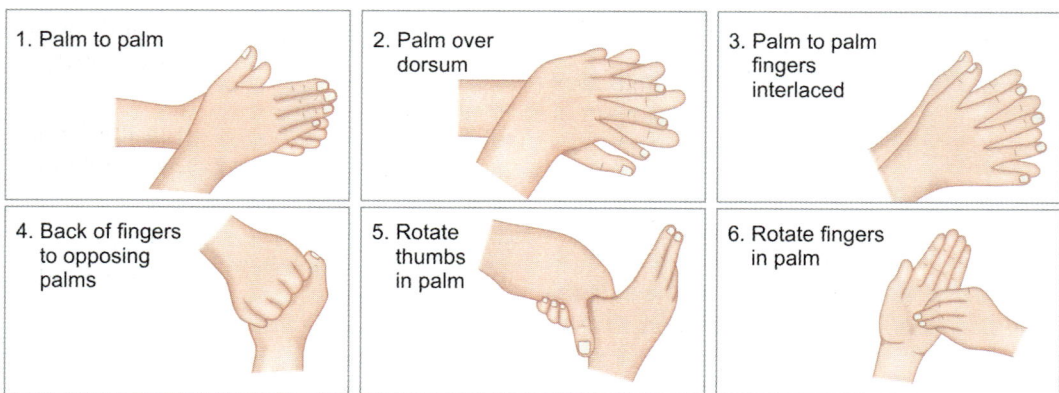

Fig. 1: Handwashing steps.

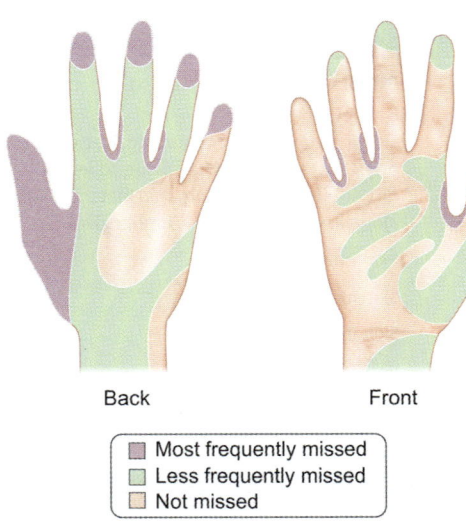

Fig. 2: Missed portions during handwashing.

Table 1: Tips on Handwashing.	
Do's	*Don'ts*
• Keep basins, dryers, soap at convenient sites • Educate and demonstrate hand wash • Keep vigilance • Use sink for hand wash only and not for any other purpose	• Do not use nail polish or artificial nails • Do not use washed hands for turning off the water source • Do not substitute hand washing by wearing gloves

- Rinse each arm thoroughly by allowing the water to run off the elbows.
- Frequently missed areas are nails, nail bed, under surface of nails, thumbs, web spaces, back of fingers, and hands (Fig. 2).
- Turn-off the water soap by foot or elbow.
- Dry hands thoroughly using a dry cloth or autoclaved towel.

TYPES OF HAND HYGIENE

- *Mechanical*: Use of soap and water.
- *Chemical*: Use of antimicrobials.

MICROORGANISMS ON SKIN

- *Resident*: Always present in deep layers of skin and can be cultured repeatedly, e.g. coagulase–negative Staphylococci, *Acinetobacter*, *Corynebacterium* (diphtheroids or coryneforms).
- *Transient*: Recent contamination and are the common sources of nosocomial infections, e.g. Gram-negative coliforms and *Staphylococcus aureus*.

PRE-REQUISITES OF HANDWASHING AGENTS

Handwashing agents must have immediate and persistent antimicrobial effects.

Immediate antimicrobial effectiveness is determined by type and amount of antimicrobial agent used, time spent in handwashing, the pressure and friction exerted, and water temperature.

The persistent antimicrobial effect (the ability of the hand wash to keep the microorganisms at a low level after washing) is dependent upon the product used.

CHOICE OF HANDWASHING AGENTS: SOAP VERSUS ANTIMICROBIAL (TABLE 2)

For most of the times, handwashing with plain soap is sufficient. Antimicrobial handwashing products should be used preferably in following conditions:

- *During suspected or proven epidemics*: Intensive care unit (ICU), neonatal intensive care unit (NICU)
- In immunocompromised patients
- In barrier nursing leaving an isolation room.

Table 2: Comparision of handwashing agents.

Agent	Immediate effect	Residual effect	Remarks
Plain soap	Yes	No	Skin irritation, time consuming. Need to be dried. Not effective if hands are soiled with dirt or blood or other organic material. Not alone for surgical scrub. Cumbersome.
Ipodophor iodine	Yes	Yes	Skin irritation
Chlorhexidine gluconate (4%)	Yes	Yes	Skin irritation if >4%
>50% alcohol	Yes	No	Skin irritation
Sodium hypochlorite	Yes	No	Very irritating to hand
Hexachlorophene	Yes	No	Only against gram-positive

PRECAUTIONS IN SOAP USE

- Any soap can be used such as liquid, bar, granule, or soap-impregnated tissue form.
- If liquid soap is used, it must be placed in disposable jars. If reusable jars are used prior to refilling complete, thorough cleaning of the jar is mandatory. The jar should be emptied and replaced. If reused, it should be thoroughly cleansed. Fresh liquid should not be added to a partially full dispenser.
- If bar soap is used, it should be ensured that is dry and not dispersed in water.

CHOICE OF ANTIMICROBIAL SOLUTION

The choice is based on efficacy, safety, cost, and acceptability.

The most commonly used antimicrobial hand wash in emergency care are alcohol based (70%) (Table 3). Following precautions must be followed for its effective use:

- The hands must not be visibly soiled with blood or organic material.
- The hand surface must be completely covered with antiseptic.
- Hands must be allowed to dry.
- Not less than 0.5 mL should be used.

Table 3: Alcohol-based handwash.

Advantages	Disadvantages
• Rapid reduction in microbial counts • Easy to use • Time saving • Better compliance • Eliminates use of water and drying • Does not need sink, dryers	• May cause skin irritation • Sensitive to dilution with water • Costly

HAND DRYING

Air hand dryers are avoided in critical patient care areas. Drying by single use autoclaved towel is beneficial. Autoclaved paper napkins are also beneficial. Drying of hands by wiping to the personal wears or common towel is not advisable.

METHODS TO IMPROVE HANDWASHING

- Senior staff should serve as role models
- Policing each other
- Educating the need for handwashing
- Demonstrating the technique
- Convenient placement of infrastructure like sinks, dryers, etc.
- Cognitive aides in the form of pictures of handwashing technique.

KEY POINTS

- Handwashing remains the single most important practice in the control of nosocomial infections. Handwashing with a suitable detergent agent should be done for at least 40–60 sec initially and 20–30 sec in between two babies.
- Handwashing is necessary after touching body surface or body fluid.
- Gloving does not replace handwashing; handwashing is essential after removing gloves.
- The efficacy of a hand wash depends on the technique and time spent on hand wash.

SUGGESTED READING

1. Canada Health and Welfare Canada. Infection control guidelines. Hand Washing, Cleaning, Disinfection and Sterilization in Health Care. Can Commun Dis Rep. 1998;24(Suppl 8):i-xi, 1-55, i-xi, 1-57. ISSN 1188-4169.
2. Garner JS, Favero MS. CDC Guideline for hand washing and hospital environmental control; 1985.
3. Larson E. Current hand washing issues. Infect Control. 1984;5:15-7.
4. Supersedes guideline for hospital environmental control. MMWR. 1988;37(24).

CHAPTER 77

Pain Management

Somashekhar Nimbalkar

INTRODUCTION

Pain inducing procedures are invariable in the intensive care setting. In the first 14 days of stay, almost 10–16 painful procedures can be done on each infant with almost 90% being needle pricks in the first week. It is imperative for the treating clinician to assess it every time, reduce the number of such procedures and offer available therapies to reduce or avoid pain. The failure to treat pain leads to various short-term complications and long-term sequelae, such as altered pain processing, attention-deficit disorder, impaired executive functions, and impaired visual perceptual ability or visual-motor integration (Table 1).

Factors that need to be considered during pain assessment are:
- Gestational age
- Postnatal age
- Health status of the newborn
- Duration and type of pain
- Environmental stimuli
- Interval between last painful procedure
- Response to previous pain reliving efforts
- State of alertness.

Pain Assessment

The commonly used pain assessment scales evaluate multidimensional parameters, such

Table 1: Procedural pain.

Mild painful procedures	Moderate painful procedures	Severe pain	Chronic pain
• Physical examination • Heel prick • Venipunctures • Arterial puncture • Feeding tube insertion • SC/IM injection • Handling for X-ray • Umbilical catheterization • Adhesive tape removal	• Lumbar punctures • ICD insertion • ET suction • Elective intubation • ROP testing • Ventricular tap • PICC lines • Bladder catheterization	Surgical correction	• NEC • Ventilation • Meningitis • Osteomyelitis

(IM: intramuscular; NEC: necrotizing enterocolitis; PICC: peripherally inserted central catheter; ROP: retinopathy of prematurity; SC: subcutaneous)

Table 2: Neonatal infant pain scale (NIPS).

Variable	0 point	1 point	2 points
Facial expression	Relaxed muscles	Grimace	
Cry*	No cry	Whimper	Vigorous
Breathing patterns	Relaxed	Change in breathing	
Arms	Relaxed/restrained	Flexed/extended	
Legs	Relaxed/restrained	Flexed/extended	
State of arousal	Sleeping/awake	Fussy	

*Silent cry may be scored if intubated neonates present mouth and facial movement.
- The tool can be used in newborns up to 1 month of age.
- NIPS is a nonintrusive assessment that does not require the use of any equipment.
- Can be used assess the sleeping bundled newborn undisturbed.
- Scores greater than 3 indicate the presence of pain.

Table 3: Neonatal Facial coding system (NFCS).

Facial movement	0 point	1 point
Brow lowering	Absent	Present
Eyes squeezed shut	Absent	Present
Deepening of the nasolabial furrow	Absent	Present
Open lips	Absent	Present
Vertical horizontal mouth stretch	Absent	Present
Horizontal mouth stretch	Absent	Present
Taut tongue	Absent	Present
Lip pursing	Absent	Present
Chin quiver	Absent	Present

Pain is considered present when a cluster of at least three facial movements is present.

Box 1

CRIES.

- **C**: Crying—no cry, cry but consolable, or inconsolable
- **R**: Requires increased oxygen administration for saturation >95%—no requirement from baseline, <30% from baseline or >30% from baseline
- **I**: Increased vital signs—heart rate and blood pressure both unchanged or less than baseline, heart rate or blood pressure increased by <20%, or heart rate or blood pressure increased by >20%
- **E**: Expression—no grimace, grimace present, grimace, and nonaudible grunt present
- **S**: Sleeplessness—continuously asleep, awakens at frequent intervals, or awake constantly.

Developed to assess postoperative newborn pain in newborns greater than or equal to 32 weeks' gestation.

as physiologic and behavioral parameters (Tables 2 to 4, Box 1). The tools most commonly used in the neonatal intensive care unit (NICU) for acute pain assessment include the Premature Infant Pain Profile (PIPP), Neonatal Pain Agitation and Sedation Scale (N-PASS), Neonatal Infant Pain Scale (NIPS), and the crying, requires oxygen saturation, increased vital signs, expression, sleeplessness (CRIES) scale. None of these evaluate chronic or persistent pain. All evaluate acute pain and some postoperative pain too. Hence, while using any scale, it is necessary to understand what kind of pain evaluation it can be used for. It is preferable to have in the NICU scale which everyone understands and is suitable for the kind of population it serves. Since the scales may be used often, it will be beneficial to print them out and use them with in the case sheet of patients. A comparison of commonly used scales is given in Table 2 to 5 and Box 1.

SECTION 7
Miscellaneous Topics

Table 4: Premature Infant Pain Profile (PIPP).

- Score the corrected gestational age before beginning the assessment
- Assess baseline heart rate and oxygen saturation
- For procedural pain, assess before the event
- If pain is already present, review the chart for earlier baseline
- Score the behavioral state by observing the infant for 15 sec immediately before the event
- Observe the infant for 30 sec immediately after the event.

Action	Variable	0 point	1 point	2 points	3 points
	GA (weeks)	≥36	32–35	28–31	<28
Observe 15 sec Record baseline HR/SaO$_2$	Behavioral state	Active/awake Eyes open Facial movements	Quiet/awake Eyes open No facial movements	Active/asleep Eyes closed Facial movements	Quiet/asleep Eyes closed No facial movements
Observe 30 sec	Minimum HR change	0–4 beats/min	5–14 beats/min	15–24 beats/min	≥25 beats/min
	Minimum SaO$_2$	0–2.4%	2.5–4.9%	5–7.4%	≥7.5%
	Brow bulge	None	Minimum	Moderate	Maximum
	Eye squeeze	None	Minimum	Moderate	Maximum
	Nasolabial furrow	None	Minimum	Moderate	Maximum

Scores of less than 7 indicate absence or minimum pain, and scores of more than 12 indicate moderate or intense pain.
None: 0–9% of time; Minimum: 10–30% of time; Moderate: 40–69% of time; Maximum: 70% of time inter-rater reliability >0.93

(GA: gestational age)

Table 5: Pain assessment tools.

Acute pain	Prolonged pain	Postoperative pain
PIPP	EDIN	PIPP
NIPS	N-PASS	CRIES
N-PASS		
NFCS		

(CRIES: crying, requires oxygen saturation, increased vital signs, expression, sleeplessness; NFCS: Neonatal Facial Coding System; NIPS: Neonatal Infant Pain Scale; N-PASS: Neonatal Pain Agitation and Sedation Scale; PIPP: Premature Infant Pain Profile)

Pain Management

Evidence-based nonpharmacologic strategies and pharmacologic agents are available for most procedures.

NONPHARMACOLOGIC STRATEGIES

Nonpharmacological pain intervention is a prophylactic and complementary approach to reduce pain. Most nonpharmacological measures have an effect in reducing pain and/or stress in procedures causing mild-to-moderate pain. Hence, they can be co-opted during procedures that cause pain (Table 6).

Swaddling, Containment, and Facilitated Tucking

Swaddling involves wrapping the infant in a sheet or blanket with the limbs flexed; the head, shoulders, and hips neutral, without rotation; and the hands accessible for exploration.

Table 6: Recommended nonpharmacologic methods of pain relief in newborns.

Intervention	Procedures
Modification of environmental stimuli	• Shade infant's eyes • Cover isolette/crib with blankets • Close doors gently • Avoid loud noises/voices • Set telephone ring at lowest volume possible • Decrease amount of noise • Cluster nursing-care activities • Allow periods of undisturbed rest • Gentle manipulation of tubes and lines • Careful removal of tape from skin
Positioning	• Swaddling • Nesting using blanket rolls to tuck around sides/back/feet and head to promote boundaries • Hugging • Holding—kangaroo care (skin-to-skin contact) • Proper body alignment
Touch	• Stroking, rocking, caressing, cuddling and massaging • Simple massage or rubbing of painful areas can relieve pain and spasm and mobilize contracted muscles
Pacifier/sucrose	Give sucrose via pacifier 2 min before painful procedures
Distraction	• Use materials that have auditory and visual stimulation such as music, colored objects, and mobiles • Rhythmic rocking

Containment involves restricting the infant's motions by holding or using an arm to place the neonate's arms and legs near the trunk to maintain a flexed in utero posture, with limbs placed in body midline. Facilitated tucking is when containment is provided by a care provider in which they use their hands to hold the infant in a side-lying, flexed, fetal-type position. Containment also can be given by rolled blankets and neonatal boundaries.

Non-nutritive Sucking

Non-nutritive sucking is efficacious in reducing pain-related distress reactivity in preterm neonates and improving immediate pain-related regulation in preterm and term neonates up to 1 month of age. It can be done by placement of a pacifier in the infant's mouth to stimulate a sucking response or by getting the neonate to suck on a breast that has been emptied.

Rocking/Holding

Rocking is a gentle back-and-forth motion that stimulates a vestibular response while holding is holding of a clothed infant by either a parent or care provider. Both have beneficial effects especially if skin contact is present.

Breastfeeding or Breast Milk

Breastfeeding or breast milk alleviates procedural pain in neonates undergoing a single painful procedure. There are practical difficulties in preterm babies who have impaired sucking ability, are critically ill, etc.

Kangaroo Care

Kangaroo care is an effective modality for pain management of common needle procedures and can be effective even after 15 min of skin-to-skin contact.

Sucrose

Sucrose administered on the infant's tongue with a pacifier, syringe, or cup is effective in reducing pain during common needle procedures. The usual single dose is 0.5–2.0 mL of 12–24% strength (weight/volume); however, lower doses are typically used in preterm infants (as little as 0.05 mL of 24%) and larger doses in older infants (as much as 10 mL of 25%). The onset of action is quick (within seconds); the peak effect occurs at 2 min; the duration of action is up to 10 min. At the point of writing, sucrose is not available in India. Glucose has similar effects but has fewer studies conducted on its use.

Music Therapy

Music may be beneficial for relieving procedural pain in both full-term and preterm infants. However, the optimal type or decibel level of the music or potential differences among various gestational age groups are not well-known.

Sensorial Saturation

Sensorial saturation is defined as a multisensory stimulation consisting of delicate tactile, gustative, auditory, and visual stimuli whereby, during the procedure, the infant's attention is attracted by massaging the face, speaking to the infant gently, and instilling a sweet solution on the infant's tongue. It combines many of the nonpharmacologic modalities and may end up with more stimulation than necessary.

PHARMACOLOGIC AGENTS

Many analgesics and sedatives are available. Yet the possibility of short- and long-term side effects and few studies in neonates may hamper their use. However, there are many drugs that have found good use in neonates (Table 7).

Table 7: Pharmacologic agents.

Type of pain	Useful agent
Mild pain	Oral sucrose
Moderate pain	Oral or rectal paracetamol
Severe pain	Opioids like fentanyl or morphine
Local pain relief	Local infiltration of lignocaine/topical analgesic creams

Lidocaine Topical Agents

Lidocaine inhibits axonal transmission by blocking sodium ion channels. Lidocaine infiltration is used for penile blocks for circumcision and has been shown to decrease the pain response to immunizations as long as 4 months after circumcision.

Topical anesthetics, such as eutectic mixture of lidocaine/prilocaine 5% cream (eutectic mixture of local anesthesia (EMLA)) and tetracaine 4% gel, are effective for certain types of procedural pain, such as venous cannulation, lumbar puncture, or venipuncture. However, they are not very useful in heel pricks. Recommended doses of EMLA are 0.5–2 g, under an occlusive dressing between 1 hour and 2 hours before the procedure, which achieves effect for a depth of penetration of approximately 2–3 mm.

Opioids

Opioids provide the most effective therapy for moderate-to-severe pain as they produce both analgesia and sedation, have a wide therapeutic window, and also attenuate the physiologic stress responses of neonates.

Morphine

Morphine is a drug that has been investigated and continues to be investigated in term and preterm neonates in various circumstances that have pain as an important component. The routine use of morphine infusions is not recommended for ventilated preterm neonates but may be beneficial for term neonates following birth asphyxia (there may be an increase in the duration of ventilation). Morphine is safe and effective for postoperative pain in term neonates and older infants but the status in preterms is not well-defined. Also, the preparation of morphine infusions involves the manual dilution of small volumes, leading to significant inaccuracies in the concentrations delivered to neonates.

Fentanyl

Fentanyl provides rapid analgesia with minimal hemodynamic effects in term and preterm newborns. Fentanyl should be used when a rapidly acting opioid is required for analgesia in a controlled setting, where any associated side effects (bradycardia, hypotension, laryngospasm, and chest wall rigidity) can be addressed rapidly and adequately. Other indications include postoperative pain (following cardiac surgery) or for patients with pulmonary hypertension (primary or secondary). The routine use of fentanyl infusions in ventilated preterm infants is not recommended except for neonates undergoing tracheal intubation, central line placement, or surgery.

Remifentanil, Alfentanil, Sufentanil

Detailed safety and efficacy is not known though they have been used in neonates. Remifentanil has twice its analgesic potency of fentanyl with an ultrashort duration of action (3–15 min). Alfentanil is more potent than morphine but has about one-third the potency of fentanyl and a short duration of action (20–30 min).

Benzodiazepines

Benzodiazepines provide sedation and muscle relaxation but they have no analgesic effects.

Midazolam

It is the most commonly used drug during mechanical ventilation or procedural pain in spite of little evidence and known side-effects. A starting dose of 100 µg/kg with a maintenance dosage of 50–100 µg/kg/h can be used in neonates to provide sedation. Oral midazolam is also effective, with 50% bioavailability compared with the intravenous (IV) preparation.

Lorazepam

Lorazepam is a longer-acting drug than midazolam, with duration of action 6–12 hours, so it does not have to be given as an infusion.

Ketamine

Ketamine is a dissociative anesthetic that provides analgesia, amnesia, and sedation.

For pain caused by endotracheal suctioning in ventilated neonates a dose of 2 mg/kg can be used. However, few studies exist and its use should be restricted to invasive procedures only (Table 8).

Chloral Hydrate

Chloral hydrate should be used for sedation without analgesia and with caution in preterm and young-term neonates.

Paracetamol

Intravenous (IV) paracetamol decreases the amount of opioids needed after surgery and is particularly useful for routine postsurgical care with opioid-sparing effects. It is safe and effective when used appropriately. Paracetamol rarely causes hepatic or renal toxicity in newborns, neither does it induce hypothermia. In preterm and term infants, the clearance is slower than older children, so

SECTION 7
Miscellaneous Topics

Table 8: Strategies for the prevention and management of procedural pain.

Procedures	Nonpharmacologic management	Pharmacologic management
Adhesive removal	Sweet analgesia/NNS or breastfeeding. Other NP techniques (swaddling or FT), parental presence	Inappropriate
Heel lancing	Sweet analgesia/NNS or breastfeeding. Other NP technique (swaddling or FT). Parental presence. Use of a mechanical rather than manual lancet. Squeezing the heal is the most painful part	Ineffective
Venepuncture/arterial puncture/LP	Sweet analgesia/NNS or breastfeeding. Other NP technique. Parental presence	Topical anesthetic (EMLA). Sucrose. Subcutaneous infiltration of lidocaine for LP
Percutaneous venous/arterial catheter insertion	Sweet analgesia/NNS or breastfeeding. Other NP techniques (swaddling or FT)	Topical anesthetic (EMLA). Subcutaneous infiltration of lidocaine. Opioid bolus if baby is ventilated
Subcutaneous/Intramuscular injection	Avoid if possible, use nonpharmacologic measures and topical local anesthetics if procedure cannot be avoided	EMLA cream
Oro/nasogastric tube insertion	Sweet analgesia/NNS or breastfeeding. Other NP technique. Parental presence	Ineffective
Nasal/ET suction	Sweet analgesia/NNS. Other NP technique (FT). Parental presence	Opioid bolus for ET seems ineffective
Tracheal intubation	NP techniques before sedation/analgesia	Give fentanyl (1 μg/kg) or morphine (10–30 μg/kg), with midazolam (50–100 μg/kg), ketamine (1 mg/kg), use muscle relaxant only if experienced clinician, consider atropine
Chest drain insertion	NP techniques before sedation/analgesia	EMLA creama. Subcutaneous infiltration of lidocaine. Combination of strong opioid with propofol or ketamine
Circumcision	Nonpharmacologic measures	Topical local anesthetic, lidocaine infiltration, IV/PO paracetamol before and after procedure
Suprapubic bladder aspiration	Nonpharmacologic measures	Topical local anesthetic, lidocaine infiltration, consider IV fentanyl (0.5–1.0 μg/kg)
Umbilical catheterization	Nonpharmacologic measures	IV paracetamol (10 mg/kg), avoid sutures to the skin
Tracheal extubation	Use solvent swab for tape, consider nonpharmacologic measures	
Dressing change	Nonpharmacologic measures	Topical local anesthetic, consider deep sedation if extensive
Wound treatment	Nonpharmacologic measures	Topical local anesthetics, consider low-dose opioids, or deep sedation based on extent of injury
ECMO cannulation	None	Propofol 2–4 mg/kg, ketamine 1–2 mg/kg, fentanyl 1–3 μg/kg, muscle relaxant as needed

(EMLA: eutectic mixture of local anesthesia; NNS: non-nutritive sucking; ECMO: extracorporeal membrane oxygenation)

oral/rectal dosing is required less frequently. Single oral doses of 10–15 mg/kg may be given every 6–8 hours, and 20–25 mg/kg can be given rectally at the same time intervals. The recommended total daily doses based on postmenstrual age are 20–30 mg/kg/d (24–30 weeks GA); 35–50 mg/kg/d (31–36 weeks GA); 50–60 mg/kg/d (37–42 weeks GA), and 60–75 mg/kg/d (1–3 months' postnatal).

Nonsteroidal Anti-inflammatory Drugs

Little is known about the use of nonsteroidal anti-inflammatory drugs (NSAIDs) for analgesia in neonates. They are expected to be useful but their side effect profile leads to restricted use.

The various management strategies can be used in tandem for managing common neonatal pain causing procedures as outlined in Table 8.

REDUCTION OF PAINFUL PROCEDURES (TABLE 9 AND FIG. 1)

One of the best ways to manage pain is to prevent its occurrence. Policies that limit handling and invasive procedures, while clustered care is done need to be promoted. A few approaches that can be considered are as follows:
- Decrease bedside disruptions by timing routine interventions (daily physical examinations) with other procedures (diaper change or suctioning).

Table 9: Protocol for pain assessment/scoring.

When to assess pain?
- On admission
- When pain is suspected
- Before and 10–30 min after additional pain medication
- A high pain score suggests high probability of pain and/or distress
- Reduce pain or stress, e.g. by giving sucrose 2 min beforehand

How frequently to assess pain?
Acute procedures:
- Scoring basically not required
- Focus on performing the procedure optimally

Severe painful events:
- Newborns with (suspected) NEC with distended abdomen, every shift
- Newborns after vacuum extraction every shift during first 24 hours
- Newborns with fractures: every shift till further notice (decision during rounds)
- Newborns with extended hematoma (e.g. after breech extraction) every shift
- Intestinal surgery related to necrotizing enterocolitis (NEC), cardiac surgery (thoracotomy), every shift till further notice (decision during rounds)
- Wound dressing—on demand and every shift till further notice (decision during rounds).

Which pain tool for assessment?
- *Acute pain*: PIPP (Premature Infant Pain Profile)
- *Prolonged pain*: N-PASS (Neonatal Pain Agitation and Sedation Scale)

Source: Adapted from Seminars in Fetal and Neonatal Medicine. 2006;11:237-45.

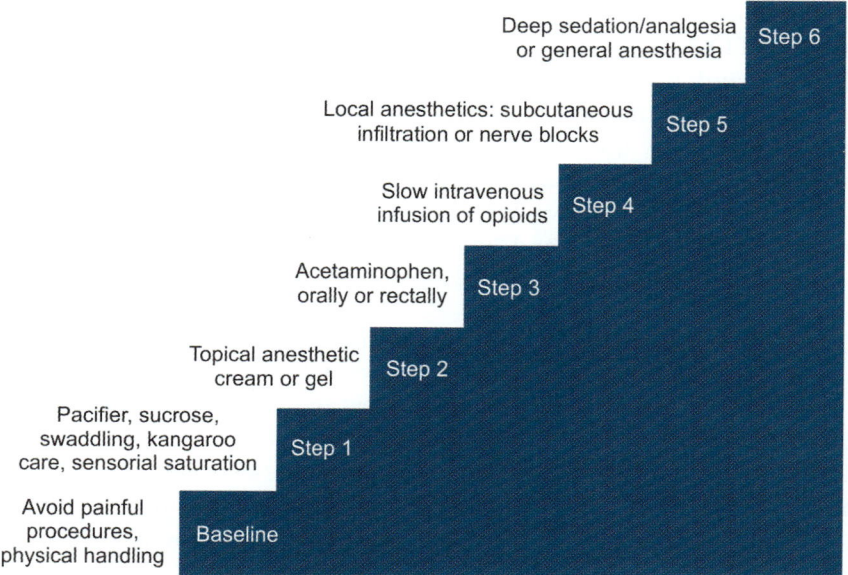

Fig. 1: Pain management steps.

- Anticipate laboratory testing to minimize blood sampling frequency.
- Use point-of-care devices that can perform several analyses (pH, PaO_2, $PaCO_2$, electrolytes, calcium, bilirubin, lactate) from a single small blood sample.
- Place peripheral arterial or central venous catheters in patients who need more than 3–4 heel sticks per day.
- If clinically appropriate, use noninvasive monitoring, such as transcutaneous PaO_2, $PaCO_2$, oxygen saturations, glucose or bilirubin levels, or near infrared spectroscopy, to avoid the need for blood sampling.

SUGGESTED READING

1. Cong X, McGrath JM, Cusson RM, et al. Pain assessment and measurement in neonates: an updated review. Adv Neonatal Care. 2013;13(6):379-95.
2. Hall RW, Anand KJ. Pain management in newborns. Clin Perinatol. 2014;41(4):895-924.
3. Johnston C, Campbell-Yeo M, Fernandes A, et al. Skin-to-skin care for procedural pain in neonates. Cochrane Database Syst Rev. 2014;1:CD008435.
4. Maxwell LG, Malavolta CP, Fraga MV. Assessment of pain in the neonate. Clin Perinatol. 2013;40(3):457-69.
5. Walter-Nicolet E, Annequin D, Biran V, et al. Pain management in newborns: from prevention to treatment. Paediatr Drugs. 2010;12(6):353-65.

CHAPTER 78

Coping with Death

Rhishikesh Thakre

IMPLICATIONS FOR PRACTICE

- Bereaved parents never forget the understanding, respect, and genuine warmth they receive from caregivers, which can become as lasting and important as any other memories of their lost pregnancy or their baby's brief life.
- End-of-life care supports a peaceful, dignified death for the infant and the provision of loving support to the family.
- Caring for a dying baby is a team approach involving the doctor, parents, social worker, and nurse.
- Parents who are psychologically prepared for the baby's death may cope better when it really happens.
- Give chance to let parents ventilate their feelings. Active listening is the key.
- Handle parents with empathy, genuineness, and compassion. Be nonjudgmental (Table 1).

BEFORE DEATH

- Pay attention to parents of critically-ill babies most "at risk" of sudden deterioration or likely to develop cardiopulmonary failure.
- Establish a good rapport with the parents at the very beginning.
- Explain the situation to them concisely.
- Keep the parents informed periodically about the progress.
- Make the best effort to let parents have more chance to visit, see, touch, and participate in the baby care.
- Always give them consistent answers.
- Help parents to plan what they want to do for the baby when he/she is still alive.
- Let the parents fulfill their parent role.
- Try to create memorable moments for the family.

Table 1: Communication pointers.

What to say and do	What NOT to say or do
Use simple and straight forward language	Do not say:
• "I wish things would have ended differently"	• "It is best this way"
• "I feel sad" or "I am sad for you"	• "It could be worse"
• "Do you have any questions?"	• "You can have more children"
• "We can talk again later"	• "It's good your baby died before you got to know him or her well"
• Answer questions honestly	• Do not use medical jargon
	• Do not argue with parents

- Always communicate using name of the baby.
- When giving bad news, both parents or one parent with another support person should be present.

DURING THE LAST MOMENTS

- Be prepared to face the intense emotions of the parents.
- Ask the doctor to talk to the parents as soon as they are available.
- Provide privacy—preferable a quiet room.
- Let the parents hold and accompany their baby in his/her last journey.
- Inform other family members.
- Mute the alarms/pagers/mobiles while communicating with undivided attention.
- Accompany the parents, if they need.
- Encourage the parents to say their last words to their baby.
- Ask parents for anything they wish to do for the baby.
- Ask doctor to certify death when it is appropriate.
- Do not take the parents anger personally.
- Reassure parents that their baby was not alone, not afraid, and not in pain at the time of death.
- Reassure parents that nothing more could be done.

AFTER DEATH

- After certifying death, remove all tubings and cover all wounds or intravenous (IV) access sites.
- After tidying and dressing the baby, provide a quiet place and allow adequate time for the family members to stay, to grieve, and to settle.
- Keeping the baby a nice and peaceful appearance is one of the most important things that can help to soothe the parent's pain.
- Do not hurry the parents. Assure parents that it is normal to feel uncomfortable at this time.
- Briefly explain the aftermath to the parents (e.g. the procedure of death registration, funeral arrangement, relevant documents, postmortem, etc.)
- Clarify anything that the parents do not understand or are not clear about.
- Discuss about the need for postmortem, as applicable.
- Handover details of the patient summary and advice for follow-up appointment with the doctor for counseling.

SUGGESTED READING

1. Dietz D. Debriefing to help perinatal nurses cope with a maternal loss. MCN Am J Matern Child Nurs. 2009;34(4):243-8.
2. Dyer KA. Identifying, understanding, and working with grieving parents in the NICU. Part I: identifying and understanding loss and the grief response. Neonatal Netw. 2005;24(3):35-46.
3. Dyer KA. Identifying, understanding, and working with grieving parents in the NICU. Part II: strategies. Neonatal Netw. 2005;24(4):27-40.
4. Frischer L. The death of a baby in the infant special care unit. Pediatr Clin North Am. 1998;45(3):691-9.
5. Gold KJ, Dalton VK, Schwenk TL. Hospital care for parents after perinatal death. Obstet Gynecol. 2007;109(5):1156-66.
6. Janvier A, Barrington K, Farlow B. Communication with parents concerning withholding or withdrawing of life-sustaining interventions in neonatology. Semin Perinatol. 2014;38(1):38-46.
7. Kersting A, Wagner B. Complicated grief after perinatal loss. Dialogues Clin Neurosci. 2012;14(2):187-94.

CHAPTER 79

Birth Injury

Rhishikesh Thakre

CAPUT SUCCEDANEUM

- Characterized by serosanguinous fluid collection above the periosteum
- Is present at birth. It extends across suture lines.
- Does not require active intervention.

CEPHALHEMATOMA

- Characterized by appearance of a firm, nodular swelling, after birth during first few days. The swelling is limited by the suture with no associated discoloration or signs of inflammation
- May contribute to anemia or hyperbilirubinemia due to trapped intravascular blood
- Presence of neurologic symptoms or skull fracture may warrant a computed tomography (CT) scan
- No aspiration is to be done routinely.

SUBGALEAL HEMORRHAGE

- Characterized by swelling typically noticed in first few hours of birth. It crosses the suture line to progress in first few days
- Risk of aggravation of jaundice, anemia, and shock need to be anticipated and promptly managed
- Studies indicate mortality ranges from 14% to 22%.

SKULL FRACTURES

- Consider a surgical evaluation if the newborn has any of the following features: (i) bone fragments in cerebrum on imaging; (ii) localizing signs on central nervous system (CNS) examination; (iii) features suggestive of raised intracranial pressure; (iv) cerebrospinal fluid (CSF) accumulation below the galea and; (v) nonresponsiveness to closed manipulation.
- Nonsurgical management is indicated if there is depressions less than 2 cm in width and if the depression is over a major venous sinus but without neurologic symptoms.

EPIDURAL HEMORRHAGE

- Epidural hemorrhage occurs from injury to the middle meningeal artery. Cephalohematoma or skull fracture are common associations.

- Surgical drainage is required in most of these infants.

SUBDURAL HEMORRHAGE

- Subdural hemorrhage frequently occurs postbirth trauma. Apnea and dusky episodes are most common manifestations.
- A coagulation profile should be done in all such infants.
- Cerebral infarction is most commonly seen in such infants.
- Majority of infants do not need active intervention. Surgery is indicated if there are signs of brainstem compression or shift of midline.

SUBARACHNOID HEMORRHAGE

- Should be suspected if a well-baby in first few days of life has a unexplained seizure
- Cranial ultrasonography is not a good modality for diagnosis as it may miss such cases. CT brain is choice of investigation
- With massive subarachnoid hemorrhage there is a risk of developing posthemorrhagic hydrocephalus. Monitoring head size and ventricule size is, therefore, recommended.

ERB'S PALSY

- Erb's palsy, involves injury to the C5, C6, and C7, and accounts for majority of cases of brachial plexus injury.
- The infant is characterized by absent biceps reflex, asymmetric Moro reflex, and intact grasp reflex.
- At times, there may be associated injury to phrenic nerve.

KLUMPKE'S PALSY

- It is a form of brachial plexus injury affecting C8-T1 segments. The biceps reflex is present and the Moro reflex is asymmetric. The grasp reflex is lost.
- Presence of ptosis, miosis, and anhidrosis suggests ipsilateral Horner's syndrome. With associated phrenic nerve injury, there may be respiratory distress.
- Complete plexus involvement and Klumpke's palsy have a guarded outcome. Prognosis is defined by antigravity movement of biceps and shoulder abduction, which if present by 3 months of age, has good outcomes.
- The arm is immobilized during the first few days to reduce pain and discomfort. Physiotherapy with passive range-of-motion exercises at the shoulder, elbow, and wrist are mainstay of treatment and started after the first week. Parents are counseled about need to perform range-of-motion exercises frequently.
- Surgical exploration may be required if there is no improvement by 6 months of age. Electrodiagnostic and imaging studies (CT myelography or magnetic resonance imaging (MRI)) are indicated prior to surgery.

FACIAL NERVE PALSY

- *Infant has characteristic facies*: Inability to close the eye on affected side, asymmetric nasolabial fold, and absence of wrinkling of the forehead on crying. The mouth is deviated to opposite side.
- Presence of bilateral facial palsy should arise suspicion of genetic abnormality. Following are common associations reported with bilateral facial palsy, viz: Mobiou's syndrome, Goldenhar's syndrome, Poland's syndrome, DiGeorge syndrome, Trisomy 13, and Trisomy 18.
- Recovery from traumatic palsy is expected by 2 weeks. Efforts are made to avoid

corneal injury by use of artificial tears. Electrodiagnostic studies are indicated when the pathology does not recover. Nerve surgery may be an option for nonresponsive cases after 1 year of age.
- *Congenital hypoplasia of the depressor anguli oris muscle* is a common mimicking condition. It is characterized by an asymmetric facies on crying with the mouth pulled downward and laterally. There is no involvement of the eyes, forehead, and nasolabial fold.

PHRENIC NERVE INJURY

- The infant has features suggestive of brachial plexus injury. In addition respiratory insufficiency, with diminished air entry on the affected side is present. Symptoms appear at any time during infancy. X-ray of chest is diagnostic and it shows elevation of the affected side of diaphragm, and shift of mediastinum to the opposite side.
- Initial treatment is conservative with ongoing stabilization. Surgery is indicated if respiratory distress persists.

LARYNGEAL NERVE PALSY

- Infant manifests with stridor, respiratory distress, hoarse cry, dysphagia, and aspiration. There may be history of assisted delivery.
- Direct laryngoscopy confirms the diagnosis.
- Recovery is known with no intervention.

SPINAL CORD INJURY

- The infant has paucity of spontaneous movement, deep tendon reflexes not elicitable with apnea or shallow breathing. There is absent response below the level of the lesion to pain.
- Apnea is characteristically present if the lesion is above C4. Respiratory distress is seen if the lesion is between C4 and T4. Ultrasonography is the investigation of choice.
- Plain radiographs are misleading for diagnosis.
- Therapy is supportive. Overall the prognosis is guarded.

NASAL SEPTAL DISLOCATION

- The infant shows evidence of deviation of the nose to one side. Nostrils are unequal with loss of contour on the affected side. A simple bed side test is to apply firm pressure which leads to prominence of the septum with collapse of the nares.
- Rhinoscopy clinches the diagnosis. Manual reduction is performed at earliest by ear, nose, and throat (ENT) surgeon.

CONGENITAL MUSCULAR TORTICOLLIS

- The infant presents between 1 week and 4 weeks with inability to move head to one side. There may be a palpable mass which is firm, nontender, immobile, and located in the mid-way of the sternocleidomastoid muscle. There is no overlying discoloration or inflammation.
- Ultrasonography is investigation of choice.
- Early treatment is recommended. Active and passive stretching is carried out frequently. The severity of the limitation of passive neck range of motion determines the outcome.
- Indications for surgery are no improvement by 6 months of manual stretching; persistent head tilt with a more than 15° loss in passive rotation, and posture of lateral tilting of the head.

CLAVICULAR FRACTURES

- The infant is asymptomatic in majority of cases. No intervention is required in asymptomatic infants and when the fracture is incomplete.
- Complete fractures need immobilization of the arm for 7–10 days.
- Recovery is the rule with no complications.

FRACTURE LONG BONES

- There is history of difficult labor.
- Callus formation is noted by 7–10 days which makes X-ray unreliable. Early diagnosis is made on ultrasound study.
- Immobilization and splinting is treatment of choice if the bones are not displaced.
- Displaced bones need closed reduction and cast application. A spica cast or use of a Pavlik harness is indicated if there is femoral fracture.

SUGGESTED READING

1. Abid A. Brachial plexus birth palsy: management during the first year of life. Orthop Traumatol Surg Res. 2016;102(Suppl 1):S125-32.
2. Akangire G, Carter B. Birth injuries in neonates. Pediatr Rev. 2016;37(11):451-62.

Best Practices in Neonatal Intensive Care Unit

Srinivas Murki, Rhishikesh Thakre

INTERVENTIONS TO PREVENT PRETERM BRAIN INJURY

Prenatal

- Prevention of prematurity:
  - Identification of high risk pregnancy
  - Progesterone prophylaxis in high risk pregnancies
  - Screening and treatment of asymptomatic bacteriuria
  - Tocolysis [till antenatal steroids (ANS) coverage]
  - Screening for cervical length
  - Cerclage for cervical incompetence
- Antenatal steroids
- Antibiotics for preterm prelabor rupture of membranes (PPROM)
- In utero transport to tertiary care perinatal center
- Magnesium sulphate prior to delivery (in <32–34 weeks gestation) for neuroprotection
- Appropriate mode of delivery.

Optimize Peripartum Management

- Temperature maintenance by:
  - Delivery room temperature ≥25°C
  - Plastic wraps
  - Phase change material
  - Radiant warmer
  - Transport incubator
  - Kangaroo mother care (KMC)
- Resuscitation:
  - Trained personnel for preterm delivery
  - Starting positive pressure ventilation (PPV) with 21–30% FiO_2
  - Optimum use of fractional oxygen concentration to reach target saturation
- Delay cord clamping
- Delivery room continuous positive airway pressure (CPAP)
- Early rescue surfactant.

Management of Preterm Baby

- Cerebral perfusion:
  - Optimize therapy for systemic hypoperfusion
  - Use postnatal indomethacin judiciously
  - Implement measures to minimize pain and stress responses (fluctuations in cerebral perfusion)
  - Judicious use of fluids (avoiding fast blouses)
  - Maintaining normal metabolic milieu (glucose, calcium)

- Optimize respiratory management:
  - Noninvasive ventilation (CPAP, NIV)
  - Synchronized patient triggered ventilation
  - Volume targeted ventilation
  - Permissive hypercapnia
  - Avoid hypocapnia and hyperoxia
  - Avoid routine suctioning
  - Avoid neuromuscular paralysis
  - Sedation only when indicated
  - Use postnatal dexamethasone judiciously
  - Limit sodium bicarbonate use
  - *Caffeine therapy for all preterm infants <32 weeks gestation at birth.*
- Optimum nutritional policy:
  - Protocolized feeding policy
  - Aggressive parenteral nutrition [first drip total parenteral nutrition (TPN)]
  - Early colostrum feeding
  - Minimal enteral nutrition
  - Exclusive mothers' own milk
  - Use of human milk fortifiers
  - Early breastfeeding
  - Avoiding antihistaminic/proton pump inhibitor (PPI) use in neonates
- Developmental supportive care:
  - Protected sleep
  - Involving family in patient care
  - Kangaroo mother care
  - Prevention and treatment of pain

Screening and Diagnosis of Preterm Brain Injury

- Clinical examination:
  - Head circumference
- Popliteal angle
- Neurosonographic screening for intraventricular hemorrhage (IVH), periventricular leukomalacia (PVL) and ventriculomegaly on day 1–3, day 7, day 14 of life and postmenstrual age (PMA) 36–40 weeks
- Tone assessment (Amiel-Tison)

INFECTION CONTROL PRACTICES

- Increased compliance with hand hygiene standards
- Improved accuracy of the diagnosis of bacteremia
- Reduced line and line connection (hub) bacterial contamination
- Maximal barrier precautions for central line placement and *central line-associated blood stream infection (CLABSI) bundle* approach
- Decreased number of skin punctures
- Decreased duration of intravenous (IV) infusion
- *Optimize ventilation and ventilator-associated pneumonia (VAP) bundle*
- Breast milk for feeding newborns
- Optimum nutrition policy
- Optimum use of antibiotics (antibiotic stewardship)
- Probiotics.

RESPIRATORY DISTRESS SYNDROME MANAGEMENT

- Antenatal steroids for mothers between 24 weeks and 34 weeks gestation
- Early and aggressive use of CPAP
- Short binasal prongs are more effective than nasopharyngeal or single prong CPAP
- Early rescue surfactant therapy
- Early surfactant replacement therapy with extubation to CPAP is better than later, selective surfactant replacement and continued mechanical ventilation with extubation
- Early surfactant therapy for "at risk" for respiratory distress syndrome (RDS) (<28 weeks, with no antenatal steroids) is more beneficial than treating established RDS with surfactant
- Natural surfactants are superior to synthetic surfactants

- Nasal CPAP is effective in preventing failure of extubation in preterm infants following a period of endotracheal intubation and intermittent positive-pressure ventilation (IPPV)
- Patient triggered ventilation and volume targeted ventilation
- Caffeine therapy before extubation in preterm infants less than 32 weeks.

NEONATAL JAUNDICE MANAGEMENT

- Promote and support successful breastfeeding
- Recognize that visual estimation of the degree of jaundice and those under phototherapy can lead to errors
- Interpret all bilirubin levels according to the infant's age in hours
- Recognize that infants at less than 38 weeks' gestation are at higher risk of developing hyperbilirubinemia and require closer surveillance and monitoring
- Perform a systematic assessment on all infants before discharge for the risk of severe hyperbilirubinemia and follow-up using Bhutani nomogram.

POSTASPHYXIA MANAGEMENT

- Avoid hyperthermia
- Ensure adequate oxygenation and ventilation (avoid hypoxia/hyperoxia and hypocapnia/hypercapnia)
- Ensure adequate perfusion (avoid hypo/hypertension)
- Ensure normoglycemia (avoid hypo/hyperglycemia)
- Diagnosis and treatment of seizures [clinical and/or electroencephalogram (EEG)]
- Therapeutic hypothermia if indicated and available.

INEFFECTIVE INTERVENTIONS IN NEONATAL INTENSIVE CARE UNIT

- Evidence does not support the use of phenytoin or phenobarbitone as first-line anticonvulsant with respect to benefits and harm.
- Postnatal corticosteroid treatment (early, intermediate, or late) is of no benefit in the treatment or prevention of chronic lung disease (CLD) in the preterm infant and lead to long-term neurodevelopmental impairment.
- Acetazolamide and furosemide therapy is neither effective nor safe in treating posthemorrhagic ventricular dilatation.
- There are no current data to support routine diuretic administration in preterm infants with RDS. Elective administration of furosemide or any diuretic to any patient with RDS should be carefully weighed against the risk of precipitating hypovolemia.
- There is no role of routine intravenous fluids for treatment of jaundiced newborns.
- Routine endotracheal intubation at birth in vigorous term meconium-stained babies has not been shown to be superior to routine resuscitation including oropharyngeal suction.
- There is not enough evidence to support the administration of furosemide to premature infants treated with indomethacin for symptomatic patent ductus arteriosus.
- Furosemide is not recommended as treatment for transient tachypnea of the newborn.
- Use of gowns is not effective in limiting death, infection, or bacterial colonization in infants admitted to newborn nurseries.

- Intravenous immunoglobulin (IVIG) administration for preventing sepsis is not associated with any decrease in mortality from any cause or from infections. Routine administration of IVIG preparations investigated to date to prevent mortality in infants with suspected or subsequently proved neonatal infection has been found to be of no benefit.
- Use of intraventricular antibiotics in addition to intravenous antibiotics for neonatal meningitis is not beneficial and associated with increased complications.
- Routine use of pancuronium or any other neuromuscular blocking agent in ventilated newborn infants is of no benefit.
- Postnatal administration of phenobarbitone cannot be recommended as prophylaxis to prevent IVH in preterm.
- Routine use of doxapram to assist endotracheal extubation in preterm infants is of not much benefit.
- Vitamin E supplementation in preterm infants increases the risk of sepsis hence routine supplementation to all preterm is not beneficial.
- Routine prophylaxis with vancomycin should not be undertaken for the prevention of late-onset sepsis.
- Routine antifungal prophylaxis in extremely low birth weight (ELBW) infants recommended only in those centers with high incidence (>10%) of fungal infection.

SUGGESTED READING

1. American Academy of Pediatrics Committee on Fetus and Newborn https://neonatal.cochrane.org/our-work/guidelines/american-academy-pediatrics-committee-fetus-and-newborn. Accessed 1 June, 2019.
2. Cochrane Neonatal, https://neonatal.cochrane.org/node/8 Accessed 1 June, 2019.

CHAPTER 81

Checklists

N Chandra Kumar

PREDISCHARGE CHECKLIST FOR VLBW INFANT

Name: Date of birth: Birth weight:	Sex: Gestation: Discharge weight:			Hospital ID: CGA:
		Yes	No	NA
Anthropometry				
Weight:	Percentile:			
Length:	Percentile:			
Head circumference:	Percentile:			
Anthropometry plotted on postnatal growth chart				
Predischarge examination				
Head and scalp: • Fontanels normal • Sutures normal • Flattening/plagiocephaly				
Eyes: • Normal • Red reflex • Eye discharge				
Nose: • Normal • Deviation • Choanae checked				
Ear: • Pinna normal • Meatus patent • Preauricular tag/sinus				
Mouth: • Normal • Cleft lip • Cleft palate • Natal teeth • Palatal groove				

Contd…

Contd...

	Yes	No	NA
Neck: • Normal appearance • Any swelling			
Chest and respiratory: • Clavicles normal • Tachypnea • Retractions • Breast nodule normal			
Cardiovascular: • Heart sounds (S1 and S2 normal) • Murmur, if any • Femoral pulses felt both sides			
Abdomen and trunk: • Umbilicus normal • No organomegaly • Hips stable			
Genitalia: • Normal appearance • Testes descended			
Anus: • Position normal			
Limbs: • Digits X 20 • Tone normal • Limbs normal • Talipes			
Skin: • Color pink • Birthmarks • Others			
Cry: • Normal • High-pitched			
Reflexes: • Moro • Sucking • Rooting			
Postnatal investigations			
Blood group of the baby done			
Newborn screening done			
Hearing screening done			
Pulse oximetry for congenital heart disease done			
Ultrasound cranium performed			
Retinopathy of prematurity (ROP) screening performed			
Postnatal routines			
Injection vitamin K given at birth			
Bacillus-Calmette Guérin (BCG), oral poliovirus vaccine (OPV), hepatitis B, diphtheria, pertussis, tetanus (DPT) vaccines given			

Contd...

Contd…

	Yes	No	NA
Nutrition			
Mode of feeding explained: • Breastfeeding • Spoon feeding/paladai feeding			
Type of feed: • Expressed breast milk (EBM) • EBM with fortification • Preterm formula			
Mother confident of feeding			
Mother aware of formula preparation			
Mother aware of fortification of EBM			
Feeding supervised			
Thermal care			
Mother aware of how to assess for cold stress			
Mother shown how to dress and swaddle (cap, socks, mitten)			
Kangaroo mother care (KMC) demonstrated and supervised			
Discharge advice			
Hygienic practices reinforced			
Do's and *Don'ts* explained			
Supplements and other medications explained: • Multivitamins • Iron • Vitamin D • Calcium supplement • Others			
Danger signs explained: • Cardiopulmonary resuscitation (CPR) demonstrated • Next vaccination due date informed			
Date for follow-up visit informed			
Next ROP examination due on ………………………………………			
USG cranium on follow-up			
Magnetic resonance imaging (MRI) on follow-up			
Any special consultation required			
Discharge summary handed over			
Investigation reports handed over			

Doctor:	Name:	Signature:
Nurse:	Name:	Signature:

PREDISCHARGE CHECKLIST FOR NORMAL NEWBORN

Name: Date of birth: Discharge weight:		Sex: Gestation: Weight loss (%):			Hospital ID: Birth weight:
			Yes	No	NA
Anthropometry					
Weight checked					
Length checked					
Head circumference checked					
Predischarge examination					
Head and scalp: • Cephalohematoma • Forceps marks • Abrasions • Fontanels normal • Sutures normal					
Eyes: • Normal • Red reflex • Eye discharge					
Nose: • Normal • Deviation • Choanae checked					
Ear: • Pinna normal • Meatus patent • Preauricular tag/sinus					
Mouth: • Normal • Cleft lip • Cleft palate • Natal teeth					
Neck: • Normal appearance • Any swelling					
Chest and respiratory: • Clavicles normal • Tachypnea • Retractions • Breast nodule normal					
Cardiovascular: • Heart sounds (S1 and S2 normal) • Murmur, if any • Femoral pulses felt both sides					
Abdomen and trunk: • Umbilical cord healthy • Umbilical cord separated and healing • Umbilical discharge • Hips stable					

Contd...

Contd…

	Yes	No	NA
Genitalia: • Normal appearance • Testes descended			
Anus: • Position • Patency			
Limbs: • Digits X 20 • Tone normal • Limbs normal • Talipes			
Skin: • Color pink • Jaundice • Birthmarks • Others			
Cry: • Normal • High-pitched			
Reflexes: • Moro • Sucking • Rooting			
Postnatal investigations			
Blood group of the baby done			
Predischarge bilirubin and risk stratification			
Newborn screening done			
Hearing screening done			
Pulse oximetry for congenital heart disease done			
Postnatal care			
Injectable vitamin K given at birth			
BCG, OPV, hepatitis B vaccines given			
Breastfeeding			
Positioning and attachment proper			
Mother confident of breastfeeding			
Top-up feeds required			
Method of preparation explained			
Mode of feeding demonstrated and supervised			
Discharge advice			
Hygienic practices reinforced			
Dry cord care adviced			
Do's and *Don'ts* explained			
Exclusive breastfeeding for 6 months			
Supplements and other medications explained			

Contd…

Contd...

	Yes	No	NA
Danger signs explained			
Next vaccination due date informed			
Date for follow-up visit informed			
Any special consultation required			
Discharge summary handed over			
Investigation reports handed over			
Emergency contact numbers			
Doctor:	Name:		Signature:
Nurse:	Name:		Signature:

SURGICAL CHECKLIST FOR NEWBORN

Name:		Age:		Hospital ID:	
Gestation:		Birth weight:		Current weight:	
Indication for surgery:					
Planned surgery:					
Preoperative		Yes		No	NA
Anesthetic clearance obtained					
Informed consent taken					
High-risk consent taken					
Case sheet prepared (shifting notes)					
Procedure risk explained—by pediatrician/neonatologist					
Procedure risk explained—by pediatric surgeon/anesthetist					
Baseline investigations sent					
Preoperative medications given					
Other routine medications, if required					
Any special preparation of the baby, if required					
Vital signs recorded					
Nil per oral-last feed—hours prior to surgery					
Blood requirement: Type and cross-match volume required					
Preoperative investigation results attached					
Operation theater (OT) informed to be kept warm for the baby					
Transport incubator kept warm and ready					

Contd...

Contd...

Preoperative	Yes	No	NA
Adequate number of infusion pumps kept ready			
Pulse oximeter kept ready			
Battery back-up of infusion pump and pulse oximeter checked			
Transport ventilator and circuit checked			
Oxygen cylinder checked			
Resuscitation equipment and kit checked			
Before induction of anesthesia			
Patient identity has been confirmed?			
Is the site marked?			
Is the anesthesia machine and medication check complete?			
Is the pulse oximeter on the patient functioning?			
Difficult airway or aspiration risk?			
Risk of blood loss?			
Adequate venous access (at least two)			
Before skin incision			
Antibiotic prophylaxis given?			
Are there any concerns for the surgeon?			
Are there any concerns for the anesthetist?			
Equipment check by the nursing team?			
Essential imaging displayed?			
After completion of the surgery			
Completion of instrument, sponge and needle counts			
Specimen labeling			
Any concerns in the recovery of the patient?			
Any postsurgery concerns for the surgeon?			
Postoperative orders written?			
Postoperative vitals recorded?			
Neonatal intensive care unit (NICU) informed about the preparation for receiving the baby			
Ventilator ? kept ready?			

Designation	Name	Signature	Date and Time
Neonatologist			
Surgeon			
Anesthetist			
Nurse			

SECTION 7
Miscellaneous Topics

CHECKLIST FOR PREPARATION OF FORMULA FEED

Preparation of formula feed	Yes	No
Hands washed before cleaning and sterilizing feeding utensils		
Dedicated sink used for cleaning feeding utensils		
Cleaning: Feeding and preparation utensils (e.g. palada, cups, spoons, bottles) washed in hot soapy water. Dedicated soap and sponge/brush used for cleaning		
After washing, utensils rinsed thoroughly in safe water.		
Sterilizing: Washed utensils completely submerged in large pan filled with water, pan covered with a lid, brought to a rolling boil and kept covered until utensils needed		
Surface cleaned and disinfected before feed preparation		
Hands washed before utensils removed with a sterilized forceps		
Sterilized cheatle/forcep used to remove utensil has a date <24 hours old		
Kettle filled with at least 1 liter fresh safe drinking water (water boiled previously not re-used).		
Safe drinking water boiled until a rolling boil (bottled water preferably not used, if used its also boiled)		
Water used within 30 minutes of boiling (so that it remains at a temperature of at least 70°C)		
Appropriate amount of boiled water poured into sterilized feeding vessel (30 mL for every scoop). Water poured before formula added (if a batch made in a larger container, the container used was cleaned and sterilized and maximum 1 liter prepared at one time)		
Mixed thoroughly with a cleaned and sterilized spoon		
Formula cooled by holding the bottom half of the utensil/bottle under cold/tap water without contaminating contents		
Labeling: Type of formula, infant's name or ID, time and date of preparation, and preparer's name.		
Temperature of formula feed tested on inside of wrist before giving to baby		
Left over feed thrown away		

CENTRAL LINE-ASSOCIATED BLOODSTREAM INFECTION (CLABSI) BUNDLE CHECKLIST

Name: Date of birth: Birth weight:		Sex: Hospital ID: Gestation: CGA: Catheter days:		
Is the central venous catheter indicated (ask yourself daily): YES/NO				
	Yes	No	NA	
During insertion				
Central line insertion kit ready				
Vein identified and measurements done before the procedure				
Upper limb veins preferred				
Hand hygiene ensured				
Clinician/nurse wears cap, mask, sterile gown, and gloves				
Skin disinfected as per local protocol				

Contd...

Contd…

	Yes	No	NA
Number of pricks minimized			
Hemostasis ensured before dressing			
Transparent dressing used			
Catheter tip positioned properly and checked			
Access ports covered with sterile pads			
Access ports placed away from diaper area			
Maintenance and handling of catheter			
Hand hygiene before accessing the catheter			
Sterile gloves used before access			
Catheter entry site checked for inflammation/swelling			
Replace dressings that are wet, soiled, or dislodged			
Perform dressing changes under aseptic technique using clean or sterile gloves			
Scrub the hub with antiseptic as per local policy			
Flushing done under aseptic precaution			
Central catheter used only for infusions			

EXCHANGE TRANSFUSION CHECKLIST

Name: Date and time of birth: Birth weight: Doctor in charge: Mother's blood group:	Hospital ID: Gestation: Nurse on duty: Baby's blood group:	Date: Postnatal age (hours): DCT:
Pre-exchange TSB		
Cause of hyperbilirubinemia		
Blood product details		
Packed red blood cells (RBCs) suspended in plasma/whole blood		Donor bag number
Blood group and Rh		Time since collection (days)
Total volume of blood		
Cross checked by		(Name and signature)
Baby's vitals before procedure		
Temperature	Heart rate	Respiratory rate
Blood pressure	Capillary refill time (CRT) (sec)	SpO_2
Bilirubin encephalopathy: Yes/No		
Other findings if any		
Exchange transfusion details		
Total volume to be exchanged		
Volume per aliquot (mL)	Total no. of aliquots	
Access: Umbilical/peripheral		

	Yes	No
Equipment list		
For asepsis/universal precautions		
Sterile gloves (two pairs)		
Cap/mask/gown (two pairs)		
Spirit/betadine/chlorhexidine 2%		
Drapes (2)		
For cannulation and procedure		
Surgical blade (1)		
Umbilical catheter: 3.5 Fr, 5 Fr, 6 Fr		
Two 3-way stop cock (2)		
Syringes: 2 mL (2), 5 mL (2), 10 mL (2)		
Blood transfusion set (1)		
Intravenous (IV) set (2)		
Peripheral IV cannula (1)		
Saline bottle for disposal of exchanged blood		
Gauze pieces (6)		
Umbilical cord tie (1)		
Tegaderm/Durapore		
Procedure checklist		
Preprocedure		
Umbilical catheter flushed		
Two 3-way stopcock assembled in tandem and flushed		
Blood bag warmed		
Blood bag connected with blood transfusion set		
Container for exchanged blood ready with IV set connected to three way		
Umbilical vein catheter (UVC) catheter in place and back flow ensured		
Pre-exchange blood sample drawn for investigations, if required		
Umbilical vein cannulation		
Umbilical vein identified		
Appropriate size umbilical catheter inserted until free flow of blood		
Exchange transfusion procedure		
Aliquot volume rechecked once before start		
Back flow checked again		
Cycle started with pull-out from the baby		

Contd...

Contd…

	Yes	No
Push-in from the blood bag to baby		
Blood bag mixed intermittently		
Blood glucose checked during the procedure		
Vitals monitored at regular intervals		
Sample sent for packed cell volume (PCV), TSB from the last cycle		
Medications repeated after exchange		
Intravenous immunoglobulin (IVIG) administration ensured if indicated		
Restart phototherapy if stopped during procedure		

Cycle no.	Time	Volume in	Volume out	Heart rate	SpO$_2$	CRT	Blood pressure (BP)	Remarks

SECTION 7
Miscellaneous Topics

VENTILATOR-ASSOCIATED PNEUMONIA (VAP) BUNDLE CHECKLIST

Name: Date of birth: Birth weight:	Sex: Gestation: Mechanical ventilation days:			Hospital ID: CGA:
		Yes	No	NA
Hand hygiene				
Hand washing with soap and water (all six steps for minimum 60 sec)				
Baby or baby's environment not touched without glove				
Hand wash/hand rub after removing the gloves				
Positioning of the baby				
Thirty degree elevation of the head				
Lateral decubitus position duration (in hours)				
Change of position every 2 hourly				
Endotracheal tube (ET) care				
Asepsis during intubation and reintubation				
Oral intubation performed				
ET suctioning done only when indicated				
Respiratory equipment care				
Ventilator circuit changed every week				
Ventilator tubing to be positioned parallel to the baby				
Bedside resuscitation equipment disinfected daily				
Humidification				
Humidifier temperature at 37°C				
Distilled water used in humidifier				
Auto fill method used to refill humidification chamber				
No condensation in the inspiratory limb				
Water trap in the expiratory limb emptied at regular intervals				
Oral hygiene				
Oral suctioning performed if pooling of secretions				
Disposable suction catheters used				
Enteral nutrition				
Trophic feeding as early as possible				
Mother's milk used				
Mechanical ventilation				
Noninvasive ventilation preferred if possible				
Unplanned extubation avoided				
No emergency reintubation				
Drugs to be avoided				
Ranitidine or proton pump inhibitors used				
Sedatives used				
Muscle relaxants used				

CHAPTER 82

Use of Neonatal Intensive Care Unit Charts, Algorithms, Calculators: Mobile Apps and Website Links

Baswaraj Tandur

INTRODUCTION

In most business sectors, including healthcare, it is widely claimed that the use of smartphones or tablets either alone or in combination with existing desktop resources, has the potential to achieve significant increases in the efficiency of work practices.

There are many good websites that one can use as resources—some of them are free, and some of them are not.

This chapter is about mobile applications and internet resources that are useful in neonatal intensive care units (NICU) and for neonatologists. Because of the scarcity of specific neonatal applications, even general application that may serve very useful for those who care for the neonates are also included here.

As you review the following resources, pay attention to which apps work with your device. Web-based apps will work with almost any device with a browser and an active web connection. Downloaded apps may work even without a web-connection, but may not be available on your device. Throughout the following lists, priority has been given to tools that are free or have only a trivial cost to users. If you are willing to pay more for access, many more valuable tools are available through your device's marketplace.

CHARTS

Growth charts help pediatricians and health professionals to calculate growth centiles for babies, infants, and children. Growth centile calculations are often prone to error with paper charts, and these tools aims to make this process quicker and more reliable. Plenty of apps on growth monitoring are available in the mobile stores but most of them are not authenticated. One needs to be careful before using them or suggesting to parents.

Web-Based Growth Charts

- *Baby Infant Growth Chart Calculator*: This chrome app uses World Health Organization (WHO) tables and data for weight for age calculations. The calculator is valid for babies, infants, toddlers, and preschoolers with an age range of birth to 5 years. This is a mobile ready and can be used with ease on any smartphone browsers.
  URL: http://www.infantchart.com/
- *MedCalc—Interactive Growth Charts*: After entering the baby's detail, it provides option to select various growth charts and also the option of selecting newborn baby, premature baby, or Down's syndrome. It is very quick and easy to use. The data is based on CDC growth charts.
  URL: http://www.medcalc.com/growth/

Mobile Apps

STAT Growth Charts™ WHO: Calculate childhood height, weight, body mass index (BMI), head circumference, and weight for height percentiles based on the new WHO Child Growth Standards. Available on iOS for free.

m-NEONATE: All growth parameters, percentage changes in weight, head circumference (HC), length are captured and plotted on various charts for comparison. It provides quick understanding of baby's growth as against standard values for given GA. Available for free on android. Good app but is unrated yet.

Growth Charts UK-WHO: Calculate growth centiles for babies, infants, and children based on UK-WHO growth data provided by the Royal College of Pediatrics and Child Health (RCPCH). Available for free on Android and iOS.

Two Apps are available based on the 2013 Fenton Growth Charts. Both of them are available only on iOS.
- *Preterm growth chart*: Designed to help parents and medical professionals track the growth of preterm infants. Tracking preterm infants with gestational age at birth from 20 weeks to 37 weeks. Tracking measurements up to 67 weeks. Family version allows tracking of two children (through in-app purchase). Professional version allows tracking an unlimited number of children (through in-app purchase).
- *Neonatal growth chart 2013*: It is intended for preterm infants born at <37 weeks gestational age and tracks them through 50 weeks gestational age corrected. It allows the user to enter the corrected weeks gestational age, weight, length, HC and then calculates the percentages and Z-scores of those values.

IAP Growth Charts: It is based on revised IAP growth chart 2015. It can plot the entered data efficiently on the reference graphs and analyzes the data to give a diagnostic interpretation instantly. Available for both Android and iOS devices.

Ped(z)—Pediatric Calculator: Available free for android phones. Preterm growth plotting based on Fenton or Voigt data is available. Calculates the percentages and Z-Scores but does not display it against graph. Neonatology: Birth percentiles.

ALGORITHMS

There are hundreds of clinical prediction algorithms available, via medal.org and the iOS app. Medal-Advanced medical decisions, is one of the leading resource for medical algorithms, calculators, and decision making tools. Free to use but you need to register. Under pediatrics/neonatal perinatal and neurodevelopmental disabilities various neonatal-related algorithms can be found.
https://www.medicalalgorithms.com
http://www.medal.org/browse?tab=specialty&id=19&level=1

DISEASE DIAGNOSIS TOOLS

There are many web-based, diagnosis checklist systems designed to assist clinicians that may have diagnostic doubt or want reassurance on a particular diagnosis. These tools provides a practical and dynamic diagnosis checklist within the normal workflow. These tools matches symptoms with diseases. Some of the most popular one are mentioned below.
- *SAGIL symptom checker*: It is a medical diagnosis symptom checker available online. It is free, easy to use, and the most used by physicians.
  URL: http://esagil.org/
- *ISABEL*: Very popular but requires annual subscription to use. Give 1 week full access on trial registration.
  URL: http://www.isabelhealthcare.com/home/default

- *Diagnosaurus*: One can search by symptom, by disease or by organ system. Access: Pediatrics full site access requires annual subscription which is very expensive. There is an alternative option of "timed access" for 24 hours or 48 hours is also available.
   URL: http://accesspediatrics.mhmedical.com/index.aspx
- *Uptodate*: It is one of the most reputed and widely used point of care evidence-based medical resource. It includes a collection of medical and patient information, access to Lexicomp drug monographs and drug-to-drug and drug-to-herb interactions information, and a number of medical calculators. It requires a subscription for access which is US$ 399 per year as of 2015. Student subscription is almost 70% cheaper. It is available both via the Internet and offline on personal computers or mobile devices.
- Other cheaper alternatives to Uptodate:
   - Essential evidence
   - Dynamed
   - Medscape: Free!

Websites for Computer-aided Syndrome Diagnosis

Making a diagnosis for a dysmorphic patient requires a high degree of experience and expertise since many dysmorphic diseases are very rare. A dysmorphology database can be useful for the clinician in the task of diagnosing multiple malformation syndromes in children. Generally, these web sources support doctors who wish to diagnose their patients with dysmorphic diseases quickly, effectively, and successfully.
- *Simulconsult*: On entering patient findings into the software, you get an initial differential diagnosis and suggestions about other useful findings, including tests. Provide link to Online Mendelian Inheritance in Man (OMIM). Free for individual medical professionals.
   URL: http://simulconsult.com/
- *Orphanet*: Freely available. It contains a new facility for searching by clinical sign.
   URL: http://www.orpha.net/consor/cgi-bin/index.php
- *The Phenomizer*: Freely available but not expert-curated.
   URL: http://compbio.charite.de/phenomizer/
- *POSSUMweb*: Although requires purchase very useful for diagnosis of dysmorphic child.
- *London Dysmorphology Database (LDDB)*: This is a software for using on a standalone computer. Expensive but very useful.
- *OMIM*: It is a database that catalogues all the known diseases with a genetic component, and—when possible—links them to the relevant genes in the human genome and provides references for further research and tools for genomic analysis of a catalogued gene. Free to use.
   URL: www.omim.org

MOBILE APPS

Most of the above-mentioned web sources can also be accessed through their app versions on smartphones or tablets.
- *AIIMS-WHO CC STPs*: For management of sick newborn at small hospitals with limited resources (newborn stabilization units and first referral units). Available for free for android phones. For iOS phones, it is available as "sicknewborn."
- *AIIMS-WHO CC ENBC*: Essential Newborn Nursing for Small Hospitals with limited resources. The participatory learning tool. Core contents are based on current evidence, based practices advocated by WHO and experts' opinion. Available for

free for android phones. For iOS phones, it is available as "newborncare"
- *LactMed@NIH*: LactMed is a peer-reviewed database containing information about drugs and chemicals for breastfeeding mothers and the clinicians who provide care for them. LactMed describes potential adverse effects of drugs and chemicals on infants of breastfeeding mothers and details the levels of the drugs and chemicals in breast milk and infant blood.
- *CCHD Wheel*: The cyanotic congenital heart disease (CCHD) wheel provides a practical guide approach and algorithm arranged in wheel format easy to read, screening and subsequent management of CCHD. Based on current guidelines, this wheel takes you through steps that are needed to make tentative diagnosis of CCHD, which should then be confirmed by pediatric cardiologist and manage accordingly. Paid: Available only on iOS.
- *TnECHO*: This application focuses on neonatologist-performed targeted neonatal echocardiography (TnECHO). This application is aimed at familiarizing neonatologists with basic echocardiography views and aiding self-directed learning, but does not represent complete training. It is available only on iOS and is free.

Decibel X: This noise meter app helps in measuring sound level in NICU. It is highly reliable, pre-calibrated and supports dBA, dBC. This is extremely useful tool to know how quiet is your NICU. Available for android and iOS and is free.

CALCULATORS

App stores are flooded with hundreds of calculators. Some of the useful ones are presented here.

Web-based

Many of these are also mobile ready sites which can be used conveniently on any mobile web browsers.
- *BiliTool*: It is designed to help clinicians assess the risks toward the development of hyperbilirubinemia or "jaundice" in newborns over 35 weeks gestational age. Required values include the age of the child in hours (between 12 and 146 hours) and the total bilirubin. Results are based on the hour-specific nomogram for risk stratification published in "Management of Hyperbilirubinemia in the Newborn Infant 35 or More Weeks of Gestation" (2004) by the AAP journal.
  URL: http://bilitool.org/
- *NICU tools*: Provides range of useful calculators free of charge in the care of newborn infant.
  - $AaDO_2$
  - Altitude physiology
  - Baby check
  - Body surface area
  - Diaphragmatic hernia
  - Survival probability
  - Endotracheal tubes and umbilical catheters
  - Extreme preterm birth outcomes
  - Gestational age
  - Glucose delivery
  - Low flow O_2 FiO_2
  - Nitric oxide delivery
  - Partial exchange transfusion
  - Percutaneous central lines
     URL: www.nicutools.org
- *Peditools*: Provide medical calculators and links to references useful for the practicing pediatrician. Following are the useful neonatologists.
  - Growth calculator for preterm infants
  - Hyperbilirubinemia management assistance

CHAPTER 82
Use of Neonatal Intensive Care Unit Charts, Algorithms, Calculators: Mobile Apps and Website Links

- Olsen 2010 growth calculator for preterm infants
- "NEW" Olsen 2015 BMI curves for preterm infants
- Gestational age calculator for newborn infant
- Parenteral nutrition calculations
- WHO growth standard for 0–24 months.
  URL: http://peditools.org/
- *Neonatology on the web*: Under the section on "computers in neonatology" various web-based calculators/links are available free of cost.
  - Extreme prematurity outcome calculator (NICHD)
  - Bilirubin management guide at www.bilitool.com (Stanford)
  - Medical calculators from Cornell University
  - NICU tools from Wellington Hospital, New Zealand
  - Quick drip calculator for neonates from Cedars-Sinai Medical Center
  - Quick IV calculator for neonates from Cedars-Sinai Medical Center
  - Clinical calculators by Charles Hu
  - Neonatal infusion calculators by Denis Azzopardi
  - Clinical calculators at Perinatology.com
  - Calculators at GlobalRPh.com
  - Stats calculator at center for evidence-based medicine
  - PICU tools from Michael Verive
  - Medical calculators from Supermagnus Software
    URL: http://www.paediatrics.co.uk/nicu/
- *TPN calculators*: Calculating TPN for premature and sick babies is a very tedious process and chances of errors are very high. With the use of these tools, one can save a lot of time and at the same time avoid complications.

- *Kimaya NICU*: It is easy to use single page application which also incorporates enteral feeding while calculating TPN. Multiple patients/hospitals can be registered. It is backed by KEM Hospital, Pune. On registration, you get 6 months free usage.
  URL: http://kimayanicu.com/
- *Neonatal fluids, electrolytes, and nutrition*: This one is from medcalc.com. This is free to use. Many other neonatology-related calculators can be found here. Useful ones are NICU quick drip, NICU quick IV calc, dosing calc, immunization, etc.
- *Early onset sepsis calculator*: Using this tool, the risk of early-onset sepsis can be calculated in an infant born >34 weeks gestation. The interactive calculator produces the probability of early onset sepsis per 1,000 babies by entering values for the specified maternal risk factors along with the infant's clinical presentation.
  URL: http://www.dor.kaiser.org/external/DORExternal/research/InfectionProbability Calculator.aspx

Mobile Applications (Table 1) Resources for e-learning

ONTOP: The ONTOP-IN (Online Neonatal Training Orientation Program: in India), an online web-based teaching learning program was conceptualized by senior faculty members of the Division of Neonatology, AIIMS, New Delhi. At present, it offers three certified courses.
1. Sick newborn care course: 3 months
2. Newborn nursing course: 10 weeks
3. CPAP course: 8 weeks
   URL: http://www.ontop-in.org/login/index.php

NOTE VPS—Neonatal Online Training and Education: It offers a new international online Masters (M) level educational program in neonatal medicine. The aim of the program is to provide high-quality postgraduate neonatal

SECTION 7
Miscellaneous Topics

Table 1: Mobile applications.

Product/Apps	Description	Devices	Cost
NeoMate	The app offers drug, infusion, and fluid calculations, concise checklists for common clinical problems, and quick reference information to guide acute neonatal intensive care. NeoMate is based upon established guidelines used by the London Neonatal Transfer Service (NTS)	iOS Android	Free
NICU calculator	Perform calculations that are commonly performed in the NICU.	Android	Free
NICU fluids	NICU fluids is an all-in-one calculator for IV fluids, GIR, electrolytes, and FENa	iOS	Free
INOMAX NICU PRO	Oxygenation index calculator AaDO$_2$ calculator Pregnancy/gestational age calculator Fractional excretion of sodium (FENa) calculator SNAP-II and SNAPPE-II	iOS	Free
Bili QuikCalc	It is the fastest, clearest bilirubin calculator for viewing bilirubin risk zone interpretations, plotting bilirubin on the risk, phototherapy, and exchange transfusion nomograms based on AAP guidelines	iOS Android	Paid
NICU nutrition calculator	Extremely easy, quick and error-free TPN calculator	iOS Android	Paid
Drug Center—Pediatric oncall	Drug index and interaction checker. Provides dosages for neonates, can be used offline once installed and logged in using the pediatric oncall account	iOS Android	Annual subscription

(GIR: glucose infusion rate; IV: intravenous; NICU: neonatal intensive care unit)

education within a unique global Neonatal Virtual Learning Environment (VLE).
URL: http://www.neonataltraining.eu/

NICU University: All the latest news related to neonatology can be found here. Also one can access many online courses.
URL: http://www.nicuniversity.org/

Pedialink: The AAP online learning center: Various neonatology-related online courses can be found here from time to time. This is by American Academy of Pediatrics.
URL: http://pedialink.aap.org/visitor/home

EdX Courses: EdX is a massive open online course (MOOC) provider and online learning platform. It hosts online university-level courses in a wide range of disciplines to a worldwide audience, some at no charge. Many courses related to medical field can be found here. On successful completion, certificate will be issued.

URL: https://www.edx.org/Stanford University—Stanford Medicine

This also works on open-Edx platform and many health-related free online courses can be found here. Both timed and self-paced courses are available.
URL: http://online.stanford.edu/courses

MedEd ON THE GO: It is a mobile-friendly platform that delivers comprehensive education in short video episodes (<10 minutes), designed to fit busy schedule of physicians. It offers a host of educational opportunities, including:

- Weekly online publications delivered by leading experts
- Free certified CE/CME programs
- Quiz challenges to test your knowledge and review in-depth explanations for incorrect answers

Downloadable assets for many videos (PDF, PPT)

Hot topics in Neonatology, Neoflip classrooms, etc., are very popular.

Apps to get journal articles: Keeping up with the medical literature is increasingly difficult. Following are some of the good apps to access the medical literature. Select the field of interest and journals you wish to follow. Alerts allow you to see new articles on topics of interest. Viewing abstracts is simple, and these can easily be shared via email or major social networks. Automatically checks for availability of free full text article and can be directly downloaded in pdf format.

- QxMD Read
- Docnews (formerly Docwise)
- Docphin

As apps stores are flooded with plenty of health-related apps, one has to be careful in selecting them. It is best to read the review over internet. Best place to find the review of most of the health-related apps is www.imedicalapps.com

Index

Page numbers followed by *b* refer to box, *f* refer to figure, *fc* refer to flowchart, and *t* refer to table

A

Abdomen 188
Abdominal distension 4, 94, 158, 159*fc*, 159*t*, 160*t*
Abdominal mass 160*t*
　causes of 158, 160*f*
Abruptio placentae 346
Absolute neutrophil count 34, 35, 383, 386
Acceptable, feasible, affordable, sustainable, and safe criteria 307*t*
Acid suppressants 326
Acidosis 43, 346
　correction of 72
　metabolic 9, 32, 49, 208
Acrocyanosis 8
Activated partial thromboplastin time 97, 99, 101
Acute kidney injury, rule out 204
Acyclovir 317
　role of 316
Acyl carnitine profile 129
Addisonian crisis 145
Adenosine 64, 156
Adhesive tape 156
Adrenal deficiency, congenital 142*t*
Adrenal insufficiency 81
Adrenocorticotropic hormone 141, 142, 145
Aerophagia 158
Afibrinogenemia 361
Aggressive nutrition, concept of 371
Air
　leak syndromes 152
　tanks 155
　transport 153

Airway 5, 150
　assessment of 5*fc*
　congenital malformations of 352
　malformation, congenital pulmonary 399
　oral 156
Albumin, serum 85
Allogenic transplant 331
Alpha 1 antitrypsin deficiency 200
Amenorrhea, primary 139
American Academy of Pediatrics 49, 113, 223
Amiel tison 275
Amikacin 340, 343, 343*t*
Amino acid 45, 367
　metabolism, disorders of 127
　profile, quantitative 129
Aminoglycosides 340
Aminophylline 166*t*
Ammonia
　levels 127
　serum 130
Amniotic fluid, meconium stained 15
Amphotericin 340, 341, 345
Ampicillin 156, 340, 341, 343, 344*t*
Anaerobic organisms 340
Analgesia 169
Analgesics 324
Androgen
　insensitivity syndrome 143, 145
　　clinical classification of 147*f*
　synthesis, abnormal 147
Androstenedione 143
Anemia 107, 108*fc*, 109, 109*t*, 113
　etiology of 113
　evaluation of 110
　forms of 110

hemolytic 107, 109
hemorrhagic 109
hypoplastic 110, 113
investigations 111*t*
late neonatal 359
physiologic 108
severe 358
Anesthesia, before induction of 445
Angiotensin-converting enzyme 73, 178, 204
Anogenital ratio 140
Anorectal malformations 210
Antenatal hydronephrosis 401
    causes of 217*t*
    management plan of 402*fc*
Antenatal steroids 94, 291, 292, 435
    role of 349
Antenatal ultrasound scan, abnormal 408
Anthropometry 442
Antibiotic 19, 63, 237, 325, 341
    choice of 38*t*
    duration of 39, 39*fc*
    prescription protocol 343
    prophylaxis 219
    resistant organisms 339
    stewardship program 342
    therapy 384
Anticoagulants 325
Anticonvulsants 325
    medication 47
Antidepressants 325
Antiemetics 326
Antiepileptic drug 45, 47
    alternative 48*t*
Antifetal platelet membranes antibody 104
Antifungal 325
    agents 173*t*
    prophylaxis 173
Antihistaminics 326
Antimicrobial solution, choice of 418
Antimüllerian hormone 138, 142, 146
Antiphospholipid syndrome 320
Antiplatelet antibodies 99
Antiretroviral prophylaxis 305
Antiretroviral therapy 304-306
Antiseptic solution 156
Anti-tuberculous therapy 100

Anus 188
Aorta, coarctation of 58
Aortic arch 58
Aortic stenosis 58, 59
Apgar score 33, 43, 334*t*
Apnea 8, 32, 42, 89, 94, 163, 165, 165*t*, 263
    causes of 163
    common causes of 163*t*
    management 164*fc*
    mimic 163
    nonepileptic 42
    prematurity 165, 165*t*, 352
Apneic episode, acute 163
Apneic infant, stabilization of 164
Apt test 99
Arachidonic acid 258
Arrhythmias 64
    cardiac 149
Arterial blood gas 17, 26, 45, 90, 104, 349, 352, 376
    sampling 124
Arterial oxygen
    content, reduced 373
    saturation 377
Arteriovenous malformations, pulmonary 65
Artery, pulmonary 62
Arthritis, septic 32
Asepsis 237
Aspergillosis 174
Asphyxia 49, 179*b*
    perinatal 72
Atonic neck reflex 121
Atresia, pulmonary 58
Atrial flutter 64
Atrial septal defect 59, 60
Atropine 156
Attention deficit hyperactivity disorder 273
Auditory brainstem response 262
Auditory steady state response 271
Auscultation 60
Autism, red flag signs for 277*t*
Autoantibody, maternal 104
Autoimmune diseases 320
Autosomal dominant 129, 169
Autosomal recessive 129, 169
    polycystic kidney disease 401

B

Baby infant growth chart calculator 451
Bacillus Calmette-Guérin 262
    vaccination 312
Bacillus stearothermophilus 414
Bacteria, gram-positive 38
Bacterial colonization 339
Balloon
    atrial septostomy 65
    valvuloplasty 65
Benzodiazepines 326
Betamethasone 291
Bifid scrotum 137*f*
Biliary atresia, extrahepatic 212
Bilirubin
    encephalopathy 49, 117
    transcutaneous 56
Bilitool 454
Biochemical 194
    monitoring 371
Birth injury 431
Birth weight 6, 55, 149, 182, 295
    extremely low 33, 74, 109, 234, 281, 340, 357, 408, 438
    very low 29, 32, 227, 383, 394
Bleeding
    disorders 97, 100*t*, 296
        evaluation of 97
        neonatal 97
    in early pregnancy 178
    newborn 97, 100*t*
        clinical examination 98*t*
        history 98*t*
    prevention of 100
    umbilical 225
Blindness, permanent 263
Blood
    ammonia 45
    and blood products 360*t*, 361
    component therapy 357
    culture 17, 385, 389
        sensitivity 34
        technique of 389
    exchange transfusion 53
    flow, pulmonary 62
    glucose screening 78*t*
    group, choice of 54, 357*t*
    loss 25
    presence of 282*f*
    pressure 15, 28, 65, 71, 366
        role of 23
    product transfusion, complications of 362*t*
    sample
        collection of 127
        site of 88
        volume of 389
    smear, peripheral 383
    sugar 17, 45
        estimation 117
        monitoring of 119
        random 46
    transfusion 112*t*, 263, 357*t*, 359
        therapy 357
    viscosity 89
    volume of 358
Body fluid
    compartment, composition of 69*t*
    compositions 67*f*
Body mass index 452
Body weight 70, 310
Bowel
    loops, visible 94
    motility, immature 161
    obstruction, medical management of 161
Bradycardia 8, 32, 75, 94
Brain injury 72
Brainstem evoked response audiometry 270, 271
Breast
    discharge 223
    engorgement 224*f*, 232
    milk 94, 229, 255
        expressed 256, 257
        fortification 252, 256
        storage and handling 293
        transporting 293

Breastfeeding 312, 328*t*
   and medications 324, 327
   and vaccination 295
   cues 230
   early 436
   exclusive 182
   football positioning for 230*f*
   initiation and maintenance 229
Breathing 150
   assessment of 5, 5*fc*
   spontaneous 333
   work of 65
Bronchomalacia 352
Brucellosis 320
Bulb syringe 155

C

Caffeine 166*t*
   citrate 165
Calcium 45, 65, 69, 256, 435
   concentration 84
   gluconate 156
Callus formation 434
Calories, balance of 367
Candida
   albicans 171, 224
   dermatitis 220*f*
   glabrata 171
   krusei 171
   lusitaniae 171
   parapsilosis 171
   stellatoidea 171
Capillary refill time 5, 15, 22, 366
Caput succedaneum 431
Carbohydrate 367, 367*t*
   metabolism, disorders of 127
Carbon dioxide, end tidal 156
Cardiac catheterization 65
Cardiac failure 63
   congestive 60, 65
Cardiac function 125
Cardiac index 29
Cardiomyopathy 58
Cardiorespiratory support 263

Cardiovascular disease 349
Cardiovascular drugs 326
Cardiovascular examination 58
Cardiovascular system 16, 187
Cardioversion 64
Cataract 267
Catecholamine, use of 27
Catheter
   handling of 447
   maintenance of 447
Cefotaxime 344*t*, 345
Centers for Disease Control and Prevention
   growth charts 254
Central line associated bloodstream infection
   bundle 342
   approach 436
   checklist 446
Central nervous system 17, 42, 117, 124*t*, 390, 395, 431
   depression 9
   infection 43
   malformations 117
Central venous oxygen saturation 29
Central venous pressure 29
Cephalhematoma 431
Cephalosporins 340
Cerebral
   artery infarction 43
   palsy 117, 123, 124
      diagnosis of 276
   perfusion 435
Cerebrospinal fluid 34, 46, 117, 124, 312, 319, 387, 431
   analysis 35
Cerebrovascular accidents 89
Cesarean section 305
Chest 355
   indrawing 58, 187
   physiotherapy 378
   X-ray 17, 36, 60
Chickenpox 315, 316, 316*t*
   infection, timing of 315
   maternal 315
   severe 315

Chloramphenicol 172
Cholestasis 52
    medical management of 215*t*
    neonatal 213*t*, 214*fc*, 215*t*
Chorioamnionitis, maternal 33
Choroid plexus hemorrhage 43
Ciprofloxacin 340
Circulation 150
    assessment of 5, 5*fc*
Circulatory blood volume 25
Citrate phosphate dextrose 360
    adenine 360
Clavicles 188
Clavicular fractures 434
Clitoral size 140
Clitoral width 140
Clotrimazole 224
Cloxacillin 340, 341
Coagulation screening tests 104
Colic 221, 238
    etiology of 238
    infantile 238, 240
    management of 239
Colistin 340
Colorimetric method 78
Colostrum feeding, early 436
Commercial endotracheal tube holders 156
Complete androgen insensitivity syndrome 138
Complete blood count 34, 37, 95, 97, 101, 102, 124, 383
Computed tomography 45, 126, 160
Computer-aided syndrome diagnosis, websites for 453
Congenital heart defect, suspected 57
Conjunctivitis 32
Consanguinity, history of 139
Consciousness, assessment of 6*fc*
Constant positive airway pressure 112
    system 355
Continuous flow devices 352
Continuous positive airway pressure 19, 22, 36, 95, 152, 158, 164, 166, 234, 341, 250, 347, 350, 352, 353, 355, 356, 435

adequate 354
components of 352
failure 354
setting of 353*f*
Convulsions, benign neonatal 44
Coombs' test, direct 50, 51, 223
Cord
    blood 112
        banking, types of 331
        screening 392*t*
    care 181
    clamping 181, 235
        delayed 112, 332
Corticosteroids, antenatal 291
Corynebacterium 390
Co-trimoxazole prophylaxis 308*t*
    therapy 306, 308
Coxsackievirus 43
Cradle cap 225
Cranial ultrasound 106, 280
C-reactive protein 26, 34, 35, 37, 39, 95, 124, 384, 386-388
Creatinine phosphokinase 124
Crying infant 239*fc*
Cryoprecipitate 357, 361
    use of 361
Cryptorchidism 137*f*, 301
Cyanosis 57, 58, 61*t*, 89, 187
Cystic adenomatoid malformation, congenital 18, 22, 398
Cystic fibrosis, rule out 161
Cystoscopy 142
Cytology 36
Cytomegalovirus 32, 43, 111, 164, 212-215, 361, 363
    infection 14, 359

D

Danger signs 182, 187, 228*b*, 238
Day-wise recommended fluid volume 365*t*
D-dimer test 99
Death
    after 334, 430
    before 429
    declaration 335

Decongestants 326
Decontamination 411
Deep tendon reflex 124, 126
Dehydration 209
Dehydroepiandrosterone 142
Delivery, mode of 168
Deoxycorticosterone 142, 144
Deoxyribonucleic acid 194
Depressor anguli oris muscle, congenital hypoplasia of 433
Development observation chart 275*t*
Developmental supportive care 287
Dexamethasone 291, 291*t*
Dextrose 70, 150, 367, 367*t*
    solution 156
Diabetes 346
    insipidus 43
Diaper
    dermatitis 220, 220*f*
    rash 220
Diaphragmatic hernia, congenital 14, 398
Diarrhea 94, 225
Diethylenetriaminepentaacetic acid 206, 219
DiGeorge syndrome 432
Digoxin 63
Dihydrotestosterone 142-145
Dimercaptosuccinic acid 206, 401
Discordant genitalia 139
Disinfection 411
Disseminated intravascular coagulation 50, 99, 100, 103, 108
Docosahexaenoic acid 258
Dohle bodies 384
Donor
    blood group 54*t*
    human milk 256
Double volume exchange transfusion 39, 100
Double-bucket technique 412
Double-catheter pull push technique 54
Downe's score 13, 20*t*, 353
Doxapram 165
Dubin-Johnson syndrome 212
Ductus arteriosus 58
    constriction of 377

Ductus dependent lesions 58
Duodenal atresia 159, 210
Dysautonomia, familial 121
Dyselectrolytemia 105
Dysfibrinogenemia 361
Dysplasia, bronchopulmonary 14, 72, 165

E

Echovirus 43
Ectopic testis 301
Edema 366
    pulmonary 58, 352
Electrocardiogram 61, 236, 333
Electrocardiography 62, 124, 125
Electroencephalogram 124, 437
Electroencephalography 41, 42, 45-47
Electrolyte 455
    imbalance 32, 68
    maintenance of 169
    serum 71
    supplementation 69
Electromyography 124-126
Emesis 94
Empiric antibiotic therapy, selection of 339
Encephalitis 117
Encephalopathy 116, 133
    severity of 117
Endocarditis 320
    infective 390
Endotracheal intubation 155
Endotracheal tube 155, 347, 349, 356
    care 450
Enzyme
    deficiency 142
    replacement therapy 136
Eosinophilic granules 384
Epidermolysis bullosa 168, 169, 169*t*
    management of 169
Epilepsy 47
Epinephrine 156
Epstein-Barr virus 320
Erb's palsy 432
Erythrocyte sedimentation rate 384, 386

Erythropoietin 108, 112, 361
Escherichia coli 33, 43
Esophageal atresia 152
Ethylenediaminetetraacetate 104, 105
Evoked otoacoustic emission test 270
Exchange transfusion 53, 55, 103, 263, 339
    checklist 447
External genitalia, virilization of 141*f*
External masculization score 139*t*
Extracellular fluid 67, 71
Extracellular water 71
Extracorporeal membrane oxygenation 22, 28, 29, 103, 357
Eye
    care 181
    complications 267
    discharge 227
    manifestations 128*t*
    preparation 264

F

Facemask oxygen 374*t*
Facial
    dysmorphism 212
    nerve palsy 432
False positive culture report 390
Fat
    calories 367
    soluble 202
    subcutaneous 221*f*
Fatty acid
    oxidation
        defect 80
        disorders of 124, 127
    very long chain 126
Feed intolerance 94, 253
    clinical symptoms of 94
Feeding 125, 169, 198, 251
    method 248
    oral 251
    skills, maturation of 248
Feet 189
Female external genitalia 141

Fentanyl 156
Fenton fetal-infant chart 192
Ferritin, serum 214
Fetal infant growth charts 191
Fever
    with rash 178
    without rash 178
Fibrillation, ventricular 64, 75
Fibrosis, cystic 200
Floppy infant 120, 121*t*
    etiology of 123*t*
    phenotype 123*t*
Fluconazole 173, 340, 341, 345, 345*t*
Flucytosine 172
Fluid 67, 69, 207, 455
    administration, rate of 69
    and electrolyte 237, 365
        management 67
        status, monitoring of 70
        therapy 67
    deficit therapy, replacement of 71
    intravenous 19, 55
    maintenance of 169
    replacement 92
    restriction 72
    solution 76
    supplement 55
    therapy 366*t*
        goals of 366*t*
Fluorescence *in situ* hybridization 124, 126*f*
Fluorescent treponemal antibody absorption 319, 320
Follicle-stimulating hormone 140, 302, 303
Foramen of Monro 283*f*
Fracture long bones 434
Free fatty acid 80
Fresh frozen plasma 100, 360
    transfusion 99, 360
Functional intestinal obstruction 161
Fungal infection 171, 171*b*, 174
    systemic 171
Fungal sepsis 33, 36
Fungus 340

G

Galactosemia 81
Galeazzi's sign 189*f*
Gamma-glutamyl transferase 213
Gamma-glutamyl transpeptidase 213
Gas chromatography mass spectrophotometry 45
Gasping respiration 32
Gastric
   aspirate 385
   decompression 65
   residual 94, 95
      volume 253
Gastroesophageal reflux 14, 95, 163
   disease 14
      management of 125
Gastrointestinal tract 158
   anomalies 364
Gastroschisis 364
Gene therapy 136
Gene Xpert 312
Genitalia 141*t*, 188
Gentamicin 156, 172, 340
Gestation 165*t*
Gestational age 43, 53, 149, 182, 209, 209*t*, 248, 295, 333, 350
   large for 15, 16, 77, 85, 182
   small for 15, 16, 77, 80, 182, 319
Glaucoma 267
Gliding testis 301
Glomerular filtration rate 204
Glucose 36, 435
   6-phosphate dehydrogenase 51, 108, 111
      deficiency 50, 53
   concentration 78
   infusion 82
      rate 22, 68, 70*t*, 79, 80, 82, 237, 367, 456
      tapering of 81
   oxidase 78
   sampling 78*t*
   screening 78
   status 68
Glycerine 45

Glycogen storage
   disease 81, 124
   disorder 80
Goldenhar's syndrome 432
Gonads 139
   dysgenetic 147
   palpable 138*f*
Graft versus host disease 330
Gram-negative organisms 340
Gram-positive organisms 340
Granulocyte
   colony-stimulating factor 39
   transfusion 363
Granuloma, umbilical 226, 226*f*
Graves' disease 394
Great artery 57
   transposition of 59, 62, 63, 65
Gross Motor Function Classification System 274, 275
Growth
   and nutrition follow-up 276
   characteristics of medium 389
   charts 451, 452
      longitudinal postnatal 192
      neonatal 452
      web-based 451
   monitoring 191, 371
   red flag signs for 277*t*

H

Hand
   drying 418
   hygiene 450
      five moments of 416
      types of 417
Handwashing 416
   agents 418*t*
      choice of 417
      pre-requisites of 417
   purpose of 416
   steps of 416, 416
   tips on 417*t*
Head box oxygen 374*t*

Head circumference 193
Health and disease, developmental origins of 254
Hearing
　assessment 270*t*
　follow-up 277*fc*
　impairment 269*b*
　　severity of 270*b*
　loss 270
　　signs of 269
　　symptoms of 269
　red flag signs for 275*t*
　screening 269
　　importance of 269
　　neonatal 271*fc*
　tests 270
Heart
　block, congenital 64
　defect
　　congenital 57*f*
　　critical congenital 58, 59
　　cyanotic 58, 62*t*
　disease 59*t*
　　congenital 14, 16, 17, 17*b*, 22, 57, 59, 60, 65*fc*, 88, 149, 178
　failure, congestive 210
　rate 15, 28, 64, 65, 86, 112, 366
　　characteristics, monitoring of 33
Heat loss, source of 11
Heel prick, site of 196*f*
Hemangioma 222
　capillary 222*f*
　cavernous 222*f*
　strawberry 222
Hematocrit 22, 45, 91
Hematopoietic progenitor cells 330
Hemodialysis 208
Hemofiltration 208
Hemoglobin 17
Hemolysis, signs of 50
Hemolytic diseases 53
Hemorrhage
　epidural 431
　fetal 263
　germinal matrix 280
　intracerebral 104
　intracranial 43, 117
　intraventricular 121, 124, 163, 262, 263, 280, 282*f*, 359, 388, 436
　periventricular 43
　pulmonary 352
　subarachnoid 43, 432
　subdural 43, 432
　subgaleal 431
Hepatic oxygen sensors 108
Hepatitis 320
　B 361
　　immunoglobulin 310
　　immunoprophylaxis scheme 296*t*
　　surface antigen 309, 310
　　vaccination 295
　　virus 309, 363
　C 361
　　virus 363
　fulminant 315
Hepatobiliary iminodiacetic acid 213, 214
Hermaphrodite 137
Herpes simplex 46
　virus 32, 111, 212-215
High efficiency particulate air 174
Hips 189
　developmental dysplasia of 272
Hirschsprung's disease 161, 210
Hormone, luteinizing 140, 142, 143, 302, 303
Hospital-acquired infection 391
Housekeeping surfaces, cleaning methods of 412
Human breast milk, role of 255
Human chorionic gonadotropin 143-146
　stimulation test 142
Human immunodeficiency virus 304, 306, 307*t*, 361, 363
　care of 308
　transmission 304*t*, 305
Human milk 293
　fortifier 95, 253, 256
　　use of 436
　optimizing use of 250*t*, 255*t*

Human platelet antigens 106
Human T-lymphotropic virus 363
Humidification 10, 450
　role of 375
Hydration 71*t*
Hydronephrosis 216*t*, 219
　classification of 216
　congenital 216
　fetal 216
Hydrops fetalis 346
Hydroxyprogesterone 144
Hydroxysteroid dehydrogenase 142-146
Hyperammonemia 129, 130*fc*
　management of 135
Hyperandrogenism, gestational 146
Hyperbilirubinemia
　conjugated 212
　direct 32, 212
　management of 454
　severe 149
　treatment of 119
Hypercapnia, permissive 436
Hyperechogenic lesions 283*f*
Hyperekplexia 41
Hyperglycemia 32
Hyperglycinemia, nonketotic 45
Hyperinsulinemia 81
Hyperinsulinism 81
Hyperkalemia 72, 75, 207
Hypernatremia 43, 71, 74
　correction of 75
Hyperoxia 436
　test 61, 61*t*
Hyperphosphatemia 85
Hyperplasia, congenital adrenal 88, 139, 146
Hypertension
　persistent pulmonary 16, 20, 22, 28, 29, 103
　pregnancy induced 346
Hyperthermia 187
Hypertrophy, left ventricular 62
Hypocalcemia 43, 62, 84, 86*t*
　asymptomatic 86
　clinical suspicion of 84
　early onset 43

etiology of 85*t*
late-onset 43
neonatal 84*b*
specific treatment of 86
symptomatic 86
Hypocapnia 436
Hypoglycemia 9, 32, 43, 62, 77, 77*t*, 79*fc*, 82, 89, 90, 116, 117, 129, 130
　asymptomatic 80
　clinical detection of 78
　control 82
　etiology of 80*t*
　hyperinsulinemic 82*t*
　management of 79, 80*t*
　neonatal 77
　persistent 80*fc*, 81, 81*t*, 131*fc*
　prolonged 81
　recurrent 80*fc*
　symptomatic 80
Hypoglycemic episode 81
Hypokalemia 75
　management of 75*t*
Hypomagnesemia 43
Hyponatremia 43, 71, 73*fc*, 74, 74*fc*, 193, 208
Hypoperfusion, systemic 435
Hypopituitarism 81
Hypoplasia, pulmonary 349
Hypoplastic left heart syndrome 58, 63
Hypospadiasis 137*f*, 139
Hypotension 24, 25*t*, 105
Hypothermia 7, 32, 187
　clinical manifestations of 8
　consequences of 9
　management of 9
　prevention of 11*t*
　severity of 7*t*
　therapeutic 118
　treatment strategies for 9*t*
Hypothyroidism 209
　congenital 392, 393, 393*t*, 394
　maternal 394
Hypotonia 8, 32, 120, 126*fc*
Hypoxemia 373

Hypoxia 9, 58, 346
　fetal 388
　intrauterine 88
　perinatal 121
　treatment strategies for 375
Hypoxic ischemic encephalopathy 116, 121, 122, 124, 126
　prevention of 119
　treatment of 118
Hypsarrhythmia 45

I

Iatrogenic blood loss, reduction of 112
Ibuprofen 100
Icterus 49
Idiopathic thrombocytopenic purpura 105
Immune
　disorders 331
　thrombocytopenic purpura 98, 100
Immunization 388
Immunoglobulins 39
Immunosuppressant 327
Imperforated anus 159
Implantable cardioverter-defibrillator 22
Incomplete screening test 198
Incubators 9
Indian Academy of Pediatrics growth charts 452
Indomethacin 100
Infant feeding, principles of 306
Infant Health and Development Program 276
Infantile neuroaxonal degeneration 121
Infection 346
　control 19
　　practices 436
　focal 390
　intrauterine 44
　perinatal 44
　suspected 32
　suspicion of 6
Infertility 139
Infusion
　device 156
　intravenous 156

Inguinal hernia 161
Inguinal region 137f
Inspired oxygen, fraction of 350
Intensity 53
Intensive care unit 33, 408
Intersex 137
Intestinal obstruction 158
　acquired 161
Intestine, atresia of 364
Intracellular fluid 67
Intrauterine growth 119
　restriction 7, 46, 49, 80, 88, 103, 178, 185, 213
Intravenous immunoglobulin 28, 55, 100, 438
　role of 55
Intraventricular antibiotics, use of 438
Intussusceptions 161
Invasive candidiasis 345
Iron 256, 368
　supplementation 113
Ischemia, hypoxic 42
Isoniazid prophylaxis 312
Isovaleric academia 134

J

Jaundice 49, 52fc, 56f, 223, 223f, 232
　assessing severity of 49
　direct 212
　etiology of 49, 50fc
　evaluation of 51, 51t
　management of 54, 55t, 56b
　onset of 50
　physiological 4
　prolonged 52
　rapid progression of 50
　severe 4, 339
Jejunoileal atresia 210
Jitteriness 4, 41, 89
Jugular venous pressure 71

K

Kangaroo care 243
Kangaroo discharge 243

Kangaroo feeding policy 243
Kangaroo mother care 243, 244, 246, 247, 250, 435
 advantages of 243
 benefits of 244*t*
 chart 245
 components of 243
 discontinuation of 246
 don'ts of 246
 duration of 245, 245*t*
 implementation 247
 initiation of 247*fc*
 monitoring in 246, 246*t*
 position 244, 245*f*
 ward 247
Kangaroo position 243
Kasai's portoenterostomy 214
Kidney
 congenital anomalies of 216
 injury, acute 206
 solitary 402
Kimaya 455
Klebsiella 33, 390
Klumpke's palsy 432
Knees, asymmetry of 189*f*
Koebner phenomenon 168

L

Labia majora 139, 140
Labial fusion, posterior 137
Lactate 129, 130
Lactic acidosis 129
 congenital 135
Large intestine, disorders of 210
Laryngeal mask airway 155
Laryngeal nerve palsy 433
Laryngomalacia 352
Laryngoscope spare
 batteries 155
 bulbs 155
Laser nephelometry 387
Latest Newborn Resuscitation Program 112
Latex agglutination assay 387

Left ventricular outflow tract 60
Legal issues 154
Length 193
Lethargy 89
Leukemia 331
Leukocyte filtration 111
Levene staging 118*t*
Levofloxacin 341
Lidocaine 48
Light, types of 53
Light-emitting diode 312
 fluorescence microscopy 312
Limb, upper 16, 17, 57, 65, 188
Linear fractional transformation 124
Lipid storage disease 121
Liquid-based mycobacteria growth indicator tube 312
Liver 173, 315
 disease, chronic 320
Lobar emphysema, congenital 18, 22, 398
London dysmorphology database 453
Low birth weight 4, 6, 7, 33, 243, 244, 250, 250*t*, 251, 252*fc*, 295, 364, 394
 baby 248, 250, 295
 feeding 248
 nutritional management of 248
Low molecular weight heparin 100
Lower chest retraction 20
Lower limb 16, 17, 57
 pulses 65
Lower motor neuron
 disease, suspected 124
 lesion 122, 126
Lumbar puncture 40, 413
Lung
 appearance 397
 disease, chronic 22, 263, 377, 437
 injury 349
 normal 400*b*
 pathology 17*t*
Lymphogranuloma venereum 320
Lymphoma 331
Lysosomal disorder 121, 127

M

Magnesium 45
Magnetic resonance imaging 43, 51, 82, 126, 262, 432
　brain 45
　chest, role of 18
　role of 135
Major congenital anomalies 4, 149
Malaria 320, 361
Malassezia furfur 173, 225
Malrotation 210
Maple syrup urine disease 45, 198
Mastitis 233
Mean airway pressure 29, 112, 349
Mean arterial pressure 28
Mean blood pressure 22
Mean corpuscular volume 107, 108, 111
Measles 320
Mechanical obstruction, congenital 158
Mechanical ventilation 22, 33, 350, 353
Meconium 209
　aspiration 388
　　syndrome 14, 16-18, 339, 352, 398, 399
　first passage of 209
　ileus 161, 210
　plug syndrome 161, 210
Medium-chain
　triacylglycerols 256, 258
　triglycerides 370
Membrane
　premature rupture of 37, 40, 44, 346
　prolonged rupture of 33
Menaquinone 202
Meningitis 32, 38, 40, 117
　signs of 35
　symptoms of 35
Meningomyelocele 152
Meperidine 324
Mercaptoacetyltriglycine 206
Meropenem 340, 341, 344
　dosing interval for 344t
Mesenteric thrombosis 161
Metabolic crisis 121

Metabolic disorders 43, 81
Metabolic inherited disorders 198, 199t
Metabolic screening, types of 196, 196t
Metabolism
　inborn errors of 14, 43, 80, 116, 117, 124, 127, 128t, 149, 163
　suspected inborn errors of 127
Methicillin-resistant *Staphylococcus aureus* 390
Methylmalonic academia 134
Methylxanthines 165
Metronidazole 340
Microcentrifuge 90
Microerythrocyte sedimentation rate 384
Microhemagglutination tests 320
Micturating cystourethrogram 160, 206, 218, 401
Midazolam 156
Minerals 368
Minimal enteral nutrition 250t, 371, 436
Minimum inhibitory concentration 340, 391
Mitochondrial disorder 121, 129
Mitochondrial metabolism, disorders of 127
Mitral atresia 57
Mixed gonadal dysgenesis 147
M-neonate 452
Mobile applications 452, 453, 456t
　resources for e-learning 455
Mobiou's syndrome 432
Molecular genetic study 125
Monitoring oxygen therapy 376
Monovalent hepatitis B vaccine 310
Moro reflex 432
Morphine sulfate 156
Mortality rate, infant 195
Mother-to-child transmission 304, 309
　prevention of 304, 309, 309t
Motor system 122t
Motor unit disease 121
Mucopolysaccharidosis 123
Mucous membranes 366
Müllerian duct syndrome, persistent 146
Müllerian inhibiting substance 145, 302
Multicystic dysplastic kidney 401

Multiorgan dysfunction 116, 149
Multiple births 346
Multiple carboxylase deficiency 134
Multiple pregnancy 178
Multivitamins 256, 368
Mumps 320
Murmur 58
　pathological 61*t*
Muscle biopsy 125
Muscular torticollis, congenital 433
Myopia 263

N

Nail involvement, importance of 170
Nares dilatation 20
Nasal
　cannula 155, 374*t*
　catheter 374*t*
　continuous positive airway pressure 350
　intermittent positive pressure ventilation 164, 166, 350
　septal dislocation 433
Nasopharyngeal catheter 375*t*
Natal tooth 223, 224*f*
National Institute for Health and Care Excellence 223
　Guidelines 52
National Institute of Child Health and Human Development 192
Near-infrared spectroscopy 376
Necrotizing enterocolitis 8, 72, 94, 95, 100, 103, 158, 163, 291, 359, 364, 377, 388
Neonatal anemia 107
　approach of 109
　causes of 109
　early 358
　management of 110
Neonatal convulsions
　causes of 47*t*
　incidence of 47*t*
　outcome of 47*t*
Neonatal encephalopathy 116, 118
　causes of 116
　early detection of 118
　treatment of 118

Neonatal intensive care unit 6, 94, 107, 182, 193, 234, 250, 260, 269, 272, 274, 342, 359, 364, 408, 435, 437, 451, 456
　antibiotic policy in 339
　charts, use of 451
　environment 289
　tools 454
Neonatal jaundice management 437
Neonatal online training and education 455
Neonatal reflexes, absent 32
Neonatal resuscitation 155, 156
　equipment checklist 179*t*
Neonatal seizures 41, 42, 47, 48*t*
　drug therapy of 48
　management of 46*fc*, 48
Neonatal sepsis 32, 34*t*, 38*t*, 263
　antibiotic choice in 340*t*
　classification of 33
　early onset 179*b*
　screen 383, 386*t*
Neonatal transport 149
　equipment 154
Neonatal virtual learning environment 456
Nerve
　biopsy 125
　conduction
　　study 125
　　velocity 125
Neurofibromatosis 44
Neurologic dysfunction score, bilirubin-induced 49, 49*t*
Neutropenia, non-infectious causes of 384*b*
Neutrophilia, non-infectious causes of 383*b*
Neutrophils
　count 383
　immature 35
Nevirapine 305
　prophylaxis 305*t*
Newborn intensive care unit 264, 287
Newborn screening 58, 136, 194
Nikolsky's sign 168
Nipple
　flat 230
　inverted 230
　sore 232

Nitric oxide, inhaled 22
Noise 153
Nonductal-dependent cyanotic lesions 58
Noninvasive positive pressure ventilation 22
Nonsteroidal anti-inflammatory drugs 324
Nontreponemal antibody tests 318, 319
Nuclear scan 394
Nutrition 19, 208, 237, 441, 455
    maintenance of 169
    parenteral 364
Nutritional supplementation 255, 257

O

Occupational therapy 125
Odor 128*t*
Oligoanuria 204, 206
    diagnosis of 204
Oligohydramnios 346
Oliguria 72
    presence of 72
Ophthalmology 170
Optimum nutritional policy 436
Oral antidiabetic agents 326
Oral polio vaccine 262
Oral thrush 32, 224, 224*f*
Organic academia 135
Organic acidemia 132*fc*
Organic acids 45
    metabolism, disorders of 127
    urine for 129
Ornithine transcarbamylase deficiency 134
Orphanet 453
Oscillometric method 24
Osteomyelitis 32, 390
Otoacoustic emission 262, 271
Oxygen 19, 373, 374
    administration 235
    analyzer 155
    blender 155
    concentrators 373*t*
    cylinders 373*t*
    delivery 375
      device 374, 376*t*
      different modes of 375*t*
      dose for 375
      reduced 373
    hood 155
    masks, neonatal 155
    source of 373
    tanks 155
    therapy 373
      prolonged 263
    toxicity 376
    tubing and adapters 155
Oxygenation 376*t*
    index 13
    status 377

P

P450-oxidoreductase 138
Packed cell volume 22, 50, 51, 262
Packed red blood cell 112, 357, 358, 360
Pallidum particle agglutination 320
Pallor 50
    severe 4
Pancytopenia 102
Paralytic ileus 161
Parenteral glucose therapy 79
Parkins score 182
Partial androgen insensitivity syndrome 138
Partial exchange transfusion 91
    technique of 92
Partial thromboplastin 97, 99-101
    time 105, 201
Patent ductus arteriosus 22, 28, 29, 60, 72, 100, 163, 291
    management of 95
Peak inspiratory pressure 235, 349
Pedialink 456
Peditools 454
Pelvic ureteric junction 218, 219
Penicillin 340
Penile
    length 139
    width 139
Perinatal intensive care 272
Peripheral smear 104
    examination 99

Peritoneal dialysis 208
Peritrigonal blush 285
Periventricular hemorrhagic infarction, presence of 283f
Periventricular leukomalacia 262, 284, 285f
   classification of 284
Peroxisomal disorders 127
Phallic length nomogram 140f
Phenobarbital 156
Phenomizer 453
Phenylketonuria 198
Phimosis 224
Phosphorus 256
Phototherapy 49, 55
   administration of 52
Phrenic nerve injury 433
Physiotherapy 125
Phytonadione 202
Piperacillin 340, 341, 344
Placental transfusion 88
Plasma 357
   derivatives 359
   loss 25
Plastic wraps 435
Platelet 357, 359
   count 359
   transfusion 99, 105, 105t, 106, 359, 359t
Pneumatosis intestinalis 94
Pneumonia 32, 38, 315, 342, 352
Pneumoperitoneum 158
Pneumothorax 388
Poland's syndrome 432
Polyarteritis nodosa 320
Polycythemia 88-90, 91fc
   assessing severity of 88
   neonatal 88
   signs of 90t
   symptoms of 89, 90t
Polymerase chain reaction 117, 214, 312, 320
Poor postnatal weight gain 263
Positive blood culture, causes of persistence of 390

Positive end-expiratory pressure 235, 349, 352
Positive ferric chloride reaction 129
Positive pressure ventilation 116, 235, 180, 435
   intermittent 437
Postasphyxia management 437
Postural drainage 378, 379f
Potassium 69, 75
Prader grading 141, 141f
Prebiotics 95
Pregnancy loss 409
Prenatal steroids 292
Pressure gages 155
Pressure manometer 156
Preterm
   birth 255, 364
   brain injury
      diagnosis of 436
      prevent 435
      screening of 436
   golden hour care for 234
   growth chart 191, 452
Probiotics 95
Procalcitonin 35
Progressive familial intrahepatic cholestasis 213
Prophylactic therapy 347b
Propionibacterium acne 390
Propionic academia 134
Prostaglandin 63, 65, 165
Protein 36, 367
   calorie 367
Prothrombin time 105, 201
Prune Belly syndrome 403
Pseudohermaphrodite 137
Pseudomonas 390
Public umbilical cord blood banking 331fc
Pulmonary function test 125
Pulse oximeter 16, 16t, 45, 234, 236
Pyelography, intravenous 160
Pyloric stenosis 158
Pyridoxine dependency 43
Pyruvate 45, 129, 130, 131fc

R

Radiant warmer 435
Radiation protection measures 396
Radioimmunoassay 387
Raised intracranial pressure 431
Random donor 360t
   platelets 359
Rapid plasma reagin 318, 319
Rashes 4
Rashtriya Bal Surakhsa Karyakram 264
Real time polymerase chain reaction 312
Recombinant granulocyte-macrophage colony-stimulating factor 361
Red blood cell 99, 107, 111, 112, 363, 383
Red flag sign 121
Reflexes 189
   absent 9
Refractory thrombocytopenia, causes of 103
Regurgitation 228
Renal disorders, congenital 401
Renal failure 72
Renal function 173
Renal replacement 208
Renal scars 218
Renal ultrasound 205
Renal vascular thrombosis, bilateral 206
Renal vein thrombosis 103
Renography, diuretic 218
Respiratory arrest 13
Respiratory disorders 398t
Respiratory distress 13, 14, 16, 17, 18b, 21fc, 32, 57, 89, 149, 152, 350, 400b
   cardiac cause of 16t
   history 14t
   management of 18
   quantify 20
   risk factors 14t
   severe 58, 121
   syndrome 14, 16-18, 20, 22, 50, 72, 103, 263, 291, 348fc, 350, 352, 353fc, 376, 388, 398, 399
      management of 346, 436
Respiratory equipment care 450
Respiratory failure 13
   hypoxic 149
Respiratory phase 397
Respiratory rate 15, 20, 65, 71, 112
Respiratory support 125, 237
Respiratory system 16, 187
Restlessness 4
Resuscitation 178, 179b, 333, 334
   cardiopulmonary 154
   procedure 409
Reticulocyte count 50
Retinal detachment 263
Retinopathy of prematurity 113, 262-264, 265f, 267, 359, 376, 377
   care 267fc
   classification of 265t
   examination 264, 267t
   screening 263, 266fc
      technique of 264f
Retractile testis 301
Rotor-wing aircraft 152
Rubella 32, 43, 111
Rule of three 221, 238
Rule of thumb 384

S

Sabouraud dextrose agar 172
SAGIL symptom checker 452
Sclerema 32
Sclerosis, tuberous 44
Screening test 195t
   systemic candidiasis 172b
Scrotal fusion, complete 141
Scrotum 139, 302
Seborrheic dermatitis 225, 225f
Seizure 32, 46, 89, 121, 149, 187
   clinical types of 42t
   clonic 41
   disorder, chronic 47
   drug-associated 43
   epileptic 41
   evaluation of 42
   mimics 41

monitoring 125
nonepileptic 41
persistent 132
refractory 135
treatment 125
Sensorium 71
Sepsis 36, 49, 117, 210
   calculator, early onset 455
   culture
      negative 38
      positive 38, 342
   early onset 33, 37-39, 340, 387
   late-onset 32-34, 39, 340, 387
   management of 95
   prevention of 119
   rule out 383
   screen positive 342
   signs of 40
   symptoms of 40
   screen 17, 40, 149
Septicemia 32, 38
Serum creatinine phosphokinase 124
Serum glutamic
   oxaloacetic transaminase 213
   pyruvic transaminase 213
Severe hypoxic ischemic injury 149
Sexual development
   46 XX disorder of 146, 146*fc*
   46 XY disorder of 145*fc*, 146
   disorders of 137, 138*t*, 139, 143*t*, 144, 146
   sex chromosome disorder of 147
Sexual differentiation, disorders of 144*fc*
Sexually transmitted diseases 322
Shock 23, 24, 25*t*, 30, 57, 346
   cardiogenic 25
   clinical manifestations of 25*t*
   compensated 23
   diagnostic of 71
   distributive 25
   hypovolemic 25
   irreversible 23
   neonatal 23, 24*t*, 30, 30*t*
   obstructive 25
   phases of 23, 23*t*

   thermal 9
   types of 24, 24*t*
   uncompensated 23
Silverman Anderson score 13, 20*t*, 21, 350, 353
Simethicone 240
Simple replacement transfusion 110
Single catheter pull push technique 53
Single donor platelet 359
   transfusion 360*t*
Skin 189
   care 169, 227, 236
   disorders, blistering 168
   incision 445
   infection, suspecting 169
   mottling 8
   to-skin contact 243
      early 182
   turgor 366
Skull fractures 431
Sleep myoclonus
   benign 41
   neonatal 228
Small intestine, disorders of 210
Small left colon syndrome 210
Society for Fetal Urology 401, 402
Sodium 69, 72, 73
   bicarbonate 156
   serum 45
   valproate therapy 127
Special care neonatal unit 6
Spectrum beta-lactamase, extended 38, 340
Spinal cord injury 433
Spinal muscular atrophy 121-124
Spine 188
Staphylococcus aureus 33, 38, 417
Stem cell 330
   banking 330
   hematopoietic 330
Stenosis, pulmonary 59
Sterile
   equipment 181
   linen 181
   water 156

Sterilization 411, 414
Steroids 30
    role of 292
Stillbirth 409
    declaration form 334
Stools not passed in first 48 hours 209
Stork bites 222*f*
Strabismus 263, 267
Stress behaviour, signs of 288
Stroke 117
Sturge-Weber anomaly 44
Superior vena cava 26, 29
Supportive care 9, 18, 36, 105
Surfactant replacement therapy 346, 350*t*
    benefits of 346*b*
Surgery 388
Surgical therapy 82
Symptomatic neonatal hypocalcemia, management of 87*fc*
Syndrome of inappropriate antidiuretic hormone 73, 74
Syphilis 156, 320, 322, 323
    congenital 318, 322
    early 322
        congenital 318
    late congenital 319
    maternal 322
        therapy for 323*t*
    serologic tests for 319
Syringe infusion pumps 151
Systemic lupus erythematosus 178, 320

T

T pallidum particle agglutination 320
Tachycardia 32, 64, 75
    paroxysmal supraventricular 64
    supraventricular 75
    ventricular 64, 75
Tachypnea 13, 58
    transient 14, 18, 352, 398, 399
Tandem mass
    spectrometry 136, 214
    spectrophotometry 45

Tazobactam 341, 344
Teicoplanin 340
Temperature
    airway breathing circulation dextrose 65
    assessment of 4, 4*fc*
    instability 32, 94
    monitoring 7
    normal 8
Tensilon test 125
Term growth charts 192
Testicular activity, abnormal 146
Testosterone 142, 143
Tetralogy of Fallot 58, 59, 62, 400
Thawing breast milk 293
Theophylline 165
Thermal
    care 18, 234, 441
        strategies 10
    issues 153
    management 10*fc*
Thermometer, types of 8
Thermoneutral environment 7
Thiomersal issue 296
Thrombocytopenia 102, 102*t*, 103*t*
    alloimmune 104
    autoimmune 104, 104*t*
    neonatal 102, 103*fc*
        alloimmune 106, 359
    nonimmune 359
Thyroid
    function test 392
        evaluation of 395*fc*
    replacement 394
    status, maternal 394
    stimulating hormone 210, 213, 262, 392, 393, 393*t*, 395
    testing 393*t*, 394
Thyroiditis, maternal autoimmune 394
Tigecycline 340
Tissue oxygen delivery 27*fc*
Total anomalous pulmonary venous connection 14, 58, 59, 62, 63, 400

Total body
  water 70
    composition 68*t*
  weight 67
Total leukocyte count 34, 45, 386
Total parenteral nutrition 171, 197, 237, 364, 365, 367, 368, 368*t*, 371, 371*t*, 373
  administration of 365
  calculation for 369
  compounding 370*f*
  preparation of 364
  solutions 370*t*
  therapy, broad outline of 364
Total serum bilirubin 52, 56
  levels 55*t*
Toxicology screen 125
Toxoplasmosis other rubella cytomegalovirus and herpes infections 32, 122, 123
Tracheoesophageal fistula 14, 16, 22
Tracheomalacia 352
Transfusion 197
  general principles of 361
  guidelines 110, 358*t*
Transmission, risk of 304, 315
Transport
  incubators 151, 435
  indications of 149
  modes of 152*t*
  preparation 150
  team
    responsibilities 153
    types of 151
Trauma, avoidance of 169
Tremors 89
Treponema pallidum 319
  particle agglutination 319
Treponemal tests 320
Tricuspid atresia 57
Trisomy 13 432
Trisomy 18 432
Truncus arteriosus 58
Tube feeds 251
Tuberculosis 311, 320
Tubular necrosis, acute 205
Twin-to-twin transfusion 88

U

Ultrasonography 124, 160, 217, 284
Umbilical artery catheter 206
Umbilical cord blood 330
  advantages of 330
  banking 330
Umbilical discharge 225, 226*f*
Umbilical hernia 226, 226*f*
Umbilical vein 54*f*
  catheter 65
Undescended testis 302*fc*
Upper chest retraction 20
Upper motor neuron lesion 122, 126
Urea cycle defects 131
Ureteroceles 403
Ureteropelvic junction obstruction 401, 402
Ureterovesical obstruction 403
Urethral opening 140, 302
Urethral valves, posterior 403
Urethrogram, retrograde 142
Urinary sodium excretion 205, 205*t*
Urinary tract
  congenital anomalies of 216
  infection 32, 38, 178, 218, 219
  obstruction 216
Urine
  analysis 205
  culture 34, 36, 218
  not passed in first 48 hours 204
  output 71, 72, 236
  specific gravity 71
Urogenital sinus, opening of 141

V

Vaccination 296
Vaccine administration 295
Vaginal bleeding 4, 227, 227*f*
Vaginal discharge 227*f*
Vaginoscopy 142
Vancomycin 340, 341, 344, 344*t*
Vanillylmandelic acid 160
Varicella zoster immune globulin 317
Vasoconstriction, pulmonary 9

Venereal Disease Research Laboratory 318, 319
  Test 45
Ventilation
  high frequency 22
  intermittent mandatory 166
  noninvasive 436
  system 174
Ventilator-associated pneumonia 436, 450
  compliance of 342
Ventilatory minute volume 374
Ventricular septal defect 58, 59
Vesicoureteral reflux 216, 219, 401
Vibration 153, 378
Viral infections 212
Virilization 140
Vision, red flag signs for 275*t*
Vitamin 370
  A 215, 256, 258
  B12 109, 113
  D 85, 256
  E 109
    supplementation 438
  K 200, 201
    absence 201
    administration of 9, 181
    deficiency bleeding 201, 360
    forms 202, 203*t*
    levels 202
    oral 202
    prophylactic 200
    risk of 202
    storage of 203
    supplementation 202, 202*t*
    therapeutic 200
  K1 202
  K2 202, 203
  K3 202
Voiding cystourethrogram 217
Volpe's classification 281
Volvulus 210, 364
von Willebrand disease 361

W

Warm chain 10, 11*b*
Weaning oxygen 377
Weight 193
  gain 72
    poor 9
Wet mopping 412
White blood cells 384
  count 383
Wolff-Parkinson-White syndrome 64

X

Xiphoid retraction 20

Z

Zidovudine 305, 306*t*
Zoster immune globulin 315, 316